OXFORD MEDICAL PUBLICATIONS

Sexual Deviation

Third Edition

Sexual Deviation

Third Edition

Edited by

Ismond Rosen

Honorary Consultant Psychiatrist
Parkside Clinic, London

Oxford   New York   Tokyo
Oxford University Press
1996

Oxford University Press, Walton Street, Oxford OX2 6DP

Oxford   New York

Athens   Auckland   Bangkok   Bombay
Calcutta   Cape Town   Dar es Salaam   Delhi
Florence   Hong Kong   Istanbul   Karachi
Kuala Lumpur   Madras   Madrid   Melbourne
Mexico City   Nairobi   Paris   Singapore
Taipei   Tokyo   Toronto

and associated companies in
Berlin   Ibadan

Oxford is a trade mark of Oxford University Press

Published in the United States
by Oxford University Press Inc., New York

First edition published 1964 (as 'The Pathology and Treatment of Sexual Deviation')
Second edition published 1979

© Oxford University Press, 1964, 1979, 1996

A catalogue record for this book is available from the British Library

Library of Congress Cataloging-in-Publication Data
Sexual deviation / edited by Ismond Rosen. -- 3rd ed.
p. cm.
Includes bibliographical references and index.
ISBN 0-19-262516-0 (hbk.)
1. Sexual deviation.   I. Rosen, Ismond.
RC556.S477   1996
616.85'83--dc20   95-49028
CIP

Typeset by Hewer Text Composition Services, Edinburgh
Printed in Great Britain on acid-free paper by
Biddles Ltd, Guildford

Preface

The special character of this series has established it as the leading reference work on sexual deviation. The three editions should be regarded as a whole, as new subject matter is introduced with each publication, and some chapters, often of classical content, are omitted. Most chapters in this third edition are new contributions. Appearing for the first time are sections on child sexual abuse and its effects in adulthood, as well as sexual boundary violations by professionals. The importance of gender identity for subsequent sexual development is given due space. Those subjects requiring an historical approach, incorporating previous material, are updated.

Chapters are not uniform in length as in a textbook. Authors are encouraged to deal comprehensively with their subjects and in depth. The international contributors are all highly expert in the theory as well as the practice of their subject, be it clinical, experimental, or legal. Many have made important contributions to knowledge in their field. They describe original work and review the cutting edge of research in a personal style.

Expertise in one area of a spectrum of rapidly accumulating data does not confer knowledge of other aspects. In this regard we are all somewhat ignorant of much of what is presented here. Hence the emphasis is on clear exposition, the explanation of basic concepts and technical terms, and the avoidance of jargon.

While this refers to the biological, genetic, developmental, unconscious, psychological, social, and legal aspects, the aims of the book are primarily clinical. Many of the various approaches described here apply simultaneously. This must be accepted in order to appreciate what is happening within a particular person with sexual deviation, their interaction with a partner or victim, and their need for care.

The prevailing attitudes to sexuality in Western society are now more liberal. Sexual behaviour hitherto regarded as intolerably abnormal, is now viewed as passable, provided it does not offend publicly or harm others. The effect of this alteration in public opinion has been to bring patients to the attention of caring authorities because their sexual deviation has manifested itself as an offence. Non-offenders, however, still seek help on their own account. But experience with large numbers of sexual deviants is now the province of the forensic psychiatrist or specialist in this field.

The opening psychiatric chapter is by two forensic psychiatrists, Dr Bee Brockman and Professor Robert Bluglass from Birmingham, UK. They deal with the latest psychiatric nomenclature and the need for an integrated approach to sexual deviation. This combines, where necessary, cognitive, psychotherapeutic, social and drug therapies. Professor Gene Abel and Dr Candice Bergen from Atlanta, Georgia, succinctly describe the behavioural therapies which have developed in the last fifteen years. These are becoming widely applied in the treatment of the sexual offender.

When sexual offenders require treatment in a Special Hospital such as Broadmoor, skilled forensic psychotherapy is available along the lines described and updated by Dr Murray Cox. His use of Shakespearian metaphor in the psychotherapy of resistant and often dangerous sexual criminal patients has led to a new and growing area of experience between the theatre and psychotherapy.

Dr Mervin Glasser of the Portman Clinic examines the relationship between sex and aggression from a psycho-analytic point of view, with the emphasis on treatment.

Several other chapters deal with their clinical material psycho-analytically. Dr Ismond Rosen's chapter on integrating the psycho-analytic theory of perversion with modern practice deals with the concept historically. It then examines the controversial area of homosexuality as a perversion, and makes new observations on the development of sado-masochism and its relation to self-esteem. The section on perversion as a regulator of self-esteem is updated by Rosen to include new ideas on the formation of the ego ideal.

Specific clinical syndromes are studied in separate chapters. Exhibitionism and voyeurism are updated by Rosen and include a new section on obscene telephone calls. The chapter on fetishism by Phyllis Greenacre is reprinted as a classic of its kind for the benefit of new readers.

The gender disorders occupy three chapters. Stoller's chapter is reprinted as a basic text covering the field. I judged this to be convenient not only for new readers but as a background for the other two chapters in this section. They contain many references to advances on and disagreements with some of Stoller's ideas. Professor Vamík Volkan and Dr William Greer, Jnr, from Charlottesville, Virginia provide new insights into the psychopathology and treatment of adult transsexuals and discuss the controversy over surgical sex change. Professor Loretta Loeb of Portland, Oregon, outlines her successful use of transference interpretations with children suffering from gender identity disorders.

Transference and in particular, the use of counter-transference in the analysis of female homosexual patients is a feature of the chapter by Dr Joyce McDougall from Paris. In the second edition she dealt extensively with the psychopathology in female homosexuality. Building on this background, she examines Freud's views on female psychology historically. She then points out the many similarities and analogies, rather than divergence, in the psychosexual development of both boys and girls. Using clinical cases she describes in detail the exchanges between patient and analyst, where the need for understanding the analyst's unconscious response to the patient's material allows of progress in the treatment. Finally she discusses the acceptance of homosexual aspects within the self as positive for creativity.

Professor Charles Socarides has rewritten his section on male homosexuality. As the doyen of US psychoanalysts in this field, his ideas, based on wide experience in the treatment of male homosexuals, command great respect. They are nevertheless controversial in part, making for a very lively presentation. Dr Adam Limentani has updated his views on homosexuality. He is a former President of the International Psychoanalytic Association, who died during the compilation of this edition, and will, like other deceased contributors before him, be sadly missed.

As friends depart, new friends and fresh subjects are welcome in the shape of Professor Issy Kolvin and Dr Judith Trowell from the Tavistock Clinic, London. They deal with the most prodigious growth area in the psychological knowledge of our time, that of child sexual abuse.

Dr Ismond Rosen's chapter on the adult sequelae of childhood sexual abuse examines the sociology, psychopathology, and treatment. Because such persons are liable to further sexual abuse by others, including professional carers, the implication for such sexual boundary violations during therapy is discussed in detail. Special attention is given to the treatment needs and hazards of such patients in psychotherapy. The importance of transference and countertransference in therapy is described.

Professor Michael Freeman of University College London has rewritten the legal chapter to incorporate the many changes in English and US law, and other relevant law dealing with sexual offenders. His approach has been to examine the principles underlying the legal requirements and their changes.

Professor Richard Michael and Professor Doris Zumpe from Emory University, Atlanta, are among the foremost experimental researchers in neuroendocrinology. They have provided a new chapter to include our latest understanding of the biological basis of sexual behaviour, including first published reports of their most recent work. Richard Michael shares with me the distinction of having contributed to all three editions.

I would like to thank all the present and former contributors for their prodigious efforts. Thanks are also due to Oxford University Press and their helpful staff.

Looking back over the 31 years of publication of the three editions, I am amazed not by the passage of time, but by the vitality of the work that has grown from strength to strength. May it continue.

London   I.R.

March 1995

Contents

Contributors

Gene G. Abel, M.D.
Director, Behavioral Medicine Institute of Atlanta
Clinical Professor of Psychiatry, Emory University School of Medicine.

Robert S. Bluglass, C.B.E., M.D., F.R.C.PSYCH., M.R.C.P., D.P.M.
Professor of Forensic Psychiatry, University of Birmingham,
Clinical Director, Reaside Clinic, Birmingham, U.K.

Bee Brockman, M.B., CH.B., D.C.H., M.R.C.PSYCH.
Consultant Forensic Psychiatrist, Reaside Clinic, Birmingham;
Senior Clinical Lecturer, Dept of Psychiatry, University of Birmingham

Murray Cox, M.A., F.R.C.PSYCH., D.P.M., M.Inst. G.A. (Hon).
Consultant Psychotherapist, Broadmoor Hospital;
Hon. Research Fellow, The Shakespeare Institute, University of Birmingham.

Michael Freeman, LL.M.
Professor of English Law, University College London;
Barrister, Gray's Inn, London.

Mervin Glasser, B.A., F.R.C.PSYCH., D.P.M.
Hon. Consultant Psychiatrist, Portman Clinic, London;
Training Analyst, British Psycho-Analytical Society.
Director, London Clinic of Psycho-Analysis.

Phyllis Greenacre, M.D.
Member of Faculty of the New York Psychoanalytic Institute;
Clinical Professor of Psychiatry (Emeritus), Cornell Medical College, New York.

William F. Greer, Jnr., Ph.D.
Asst. Professor, Dept. of Psychology, Hampton University, Hampton, Virginia;
Asst. Professor, Community Faculty, Medical College of Hampton Roads, Norfolk,
VA

Israel Kolvin, B.A., M.D., F.R.C.PSYCH., Dip. Psych., M.F.P.H.M.
Bowlby Emeritus Professor of Child and Family Mental Health, The Royal Free Hospital
and The Tavistock Clinic, London.

Adam Limentani, M.D., F.R.C.PSYCH., D.P.M.

Hon. Consultant Psychotherapist, Portman Clinic, London;
Former President, International Psychoanalytic Association;
Hon. Member & Former President, British Psycho-Analytical Society.

Loretta Loeb, M.D.

Member, American Psychoanalytic Association;
Clinical Professor of Psychiatry, Oregon Health Sciences University.

Joyce McDougall, D.Ed.

Membre titulaire Societe Psychanalytique de Paris;
Full Member, International Psychoanalytic Association;
Hon. Member, Association for Psychoanalytic Medicine, New York;
Member, New York Freudian Society.

Richard P. Michael, M.D., D.Sc., Ph.D., D.P.M., F.R.C.PSYCH.

Professor of Psychiatry and Behavioural Sciences;
Professor of Anatomy and Cell Biology;
Director, Biological Psychiatry Research Laborotories;
Emory University School of Medicine, Atlanta, Georgia.

Candice A. Osborn, M.A.

Behavioral Medicine Institute of Atlanta, Georgia.

Ismond Rosen, M.D., F.R.C.PSYCH., D.P.M.

Hon. Consultant Psychiatrist, Parkside Clinic, London;
Member, British Psycho-Analytical Society.

Charles W. Socarides, M.D.

Clinical Professor of Psychiatry, Albert Einstein College of Medicine/Montefiore
Medical Centre, New York; Member, American Psychoanalytic Association; Fellow,
American College of Psychoanalysis. President, National Association for Research and
Therapy of Homosexuality.

Robert J. Stoller, M.D.

Professor of Psychiatry, University of California at Los Angeles School of Medicine;
Member, Los Angeles Psychoanalytic Society and Institute.

Judith Trowell, M.B.B.S., D.C.H., D.P.M., F.R.C.PSYCH.

Consultant Child and Adolescent Psychiatrist, The Tavistock Clinic;
Hon. Senior Lecturer and Consultant, Royal Free Hospital;
Hon. Senior Lecturer, Children's Dept., Institute of Psychiatry, London.

Vamík D. Volkan, M.D.

Professor of Psychiatry; Director, Centre for the Study of Mind and Human Interaction,
University of Virginia School of Medicine, Charlottesville;
Training Analyst, Washington Psychoanalytic Institute, Washington D.C.

Doris Zumpe, Ph.D.

Professor of Psychiatry, Emory University School of Medicine, Atlanta.

1
A general psychiatric approach to sexual deviation

Bee Brockman and Robert Bluglass

INTRODUCTION

Developments in the understanding of normal human sexual behaviour in the 1960s and 1970s coincided with a more tolerant social attitude and healthier climate in which to encourage the scientific study of the sociological, physiological and endocrinological aspects of sexuality. Wakeling (1979), for example, reviewed the development of sexual dysfunction clinics, describing how change in social attitudes enabled patients with sexual deviancy to come forward and seek help. However, the more recent past has shown a change to less tolerant societal views with frequent dramatic media coverage of sex-offenders and associated clamour for harsher sentencing. Current UK criminal statistics do not demonstrate a rise in sexual offences overall, but they still account for 1 per cent of all indictable crimes, and the percentage clear-up rates have remained stable at 75 per cent for the past decade. Chiswick (1983) draws attention to the disproportionate public concern and associated high investment of psychiatric interest and enquiry. Becker (1992), acknowledging society's fear and concern about sentencing practices and the release of sexual offenders highlights the need for adequate understanding and treatment of sexual deviancy. Sexual recidivism is well known to be a significant problem with rates ranging widely to over 50 per cent (Furby et al. 1989). There are significant difficulties in the evaluation of recidivism studies, the area requiring further research. What is not in dispute is the need to develop adequate definitions, classifications, and typologies of sexual deviancy and offending. Apart from legal definitions, attempts have been made to classify offenders by their psychopathology, type of offence, motivation, victim, and situational factors, or typology of denial (Grubin and Gunn 1990). Models or theories, reviewed by Quinsey (1977), Howells and Hollin (1991), Langevin et al. (1988), Araji and Finkelhor (1986), Marshall and Barbaree (1990), Lanyon (1991), and Becker (1992) highlight the inadequacy of any single factor model.

Early psychodynamic theories (Freud 1953) concentrated on the diversion of sexual desire away from normal arousal stimuli, coining the term 'perversion'. Developmental abnormalities were explained in the form of oedipal conflicts, anxiety, repression, and regression. Recent global theories of paraphilias develop this theme (Money et al. 1975; Money 1986, 1990). Social psychiatry and behavioural learning theory (Abel et al. 1987), Lanyon (1991), Langevin et al. (1988) Woolf (1985), Levine and Troiden (1988), Laws and Marshall (1990) has developed to explain the acquisition and maintenance of sexual deviancy. Biological models seeking the origin of deviancy in physical abnormalities have been described by Flor-Henry (1987), Bradford (1985), Berlin (1983), Rada *et al.* (1983). No single causative biological factor has been found to account for deviancy, which is more often due to multi-factorial aetiology. Araji and Finkelhor (1986) reviewed the empirical evidence for child sexual abuse and summarized the various theories.

To date, no satisfactory classification of sexual deviancy exists. Traditional attempts divide the problems loosely into disorders of orientation and gender dysfunction. These descriptive accounts have parallels in lepidoptery but do little to help our understanding of the aetiology of the problem. For example, cross-dressing is usually categorized as deviant arousal but clinicians are aware that it may be no more than a vehicle for effective tension reduction in an immature, insecure, isolated man. It would be just as simplistic to make an assumption that all rapes are sexually motivated. Again, clinicians are aware that sexual behaviour may be a vehicle for expressing aggression.

THE PARAPHILIAS

Sexual deviation is a term which is particularly applicable to a subclass of sexual disorder termed 'paraphilia'. The distinguishing feature of the paraphilias is that they are associated with arousal in response to sexual objects or stimuli that are not associated with normal behavioural patterns and may interfere with the capacity to establish sexual relationships. DSMIIIR (American Psychiatric Association 1987) describes the essential feature of the paraphilias as recurrent, intense, sexual urges, and sexually arousing fantasies generally involving one of the following: (1) non-human objects; (2) the suffering or humiliation of one's self or one's partner (not merely simulated); or (3) children or other non-consenting persons. 'Paraphilia' is considered a preferable term to 'sexual deviation' in modern classifications in that it emphasizes the essential nature of this group of behaviours; arousal in response to an inappropriate stimulus.

Some behaviours discussed here may occur as a harmless variation or stimulus in sexual activity between consenting partners, rather than as a preference or as a necessary source of arousal. Examples which, of course, exploited by commerce, are clothing, particularly items such as shoes or underwear, odours (perfumes), and soft pornography (and its influence on advertising). Sexually sadistic or masochistic behaviour may play a harmless or injurious part as a variation of sexual activity, depending on the level of consent between the partners. General psychiatrists and other therapists who specialize in sexual dysfunction will see some of the commoner paraphilias frequently. Others only present as a consequence of an offence or complaint and are more likely to be revealed to specialist forensic teams. However, the extent of the market in sex aids and paraphilic pornography in a variety of media suggests a higher prevalence of paraphilic activity in the general community than can be recognized simply from clinical presentation and criminal statistics.

DSMIIIR specifically describes eight paraphilias as among those more commonly seen, but makes reference to several other examples. Money (1986) lists more than 30 categories, including some which have rarely been described. Paraphilic preference, fantasy, or imagery will frequently influence choice of occupation, partner, interests, and hobbies. Often paraphilic activity is experienced in isolation and may be carefully concealed from others for many years. Exposure not infrequently results in denial of the behaviour or the assertion that it causes neither the individual or others any harm. Alternatively, it results in guilt and severe depression and a breakdown in relationships with partners, family, and friends. Partners and spouses have often been kept in ignorance of the behaviour until it is revealed and may find difficulty in coping with it subsequently. Individuals who experience a paraphilia may suffer from more than one variety or may progress from one to another. They may exist as an isolated and discrete anomaly in an otherwise apparently stable personality structure but, not uncommonly, people with paraphilias have personality disorders, psychoactive substance dependence, neurosis, or affective disorders.

Exhibitionism

This is the most common of the paraphilias and the behaviour which is most frequently seen by clinicians. Older studies of cohorts of remanded or convicted sex-offenders in England (e.g., East 1924; Taylor 1947) found that about a third were exhibitionists and similar proportions were reported elsewhere (Mohr *et al.* 1964; Arieff and Rotman 1942). The essential nature of exhibitionism is recurrent intense sexual urges, and sexually arousing fantasies to expose the genitals to a stranger. There is no intention to have sexual contact with the stranger, but there is sometimes a desire to shock or the fantasy that the (female) observer will be impressed and sexually aroused by the exposure. However, the exhibitionist will often admit that he would be terrified, or unable to proceed to contact, if such a response was achieved. The offenders are almost exclusively male, although exhibitionism in females does occur rarely (see below) in psychosis or mental handicap. Most cases come to attention via the courts and are charged under Section 4 of the Vagrancy Act 1824 which refers to the offence of indecent exposure and, by implication, it is an offence which only applies to males. Rooth (1971) summarized previous literature on exhibitionism and constructed a single classification: Type I, the inhibited flaccid exposer and, Type II, the sociopathic, erect exposer who may have a history of other asocial conduct. There are thus a wide variety of determinants and patterns to this syndrome and several psychological and psychodynamic explanations, but no single theory which satisfies all cases.

The dangerousness of male genital exhibitionists has been underestimated in the past, but more recent work indicates that exhibitionism is an indicator of future contact sexual offences in some individuals and the literature reporting follow-up studies is reviewed by Sugarman *et al.* 1994. Bluglass (1980) reported a follow-up study of up to eight years of 100 exhibitionists during which time 7 per cent were convicted of contact sexual offences, including rape. This group were characterized by psychiatric problems in childhood, juvenile court appearances, low intelligence, unstable work records, unsatisfactory sexual relationships, unco-operativeness in treatment, and a diagnosis of personality disorder. All had prior convictions for sexual offences including indecent exposure. These 100 cases, together with a further 110 referred subsequently, were all reviewed again for up to 25 years (Sugarman *et al.* 1994)—26 per cent had a conviction for a contact sexual offence including rape, buggery, attempted buggery and 60 offences were recorded against children. Two-thirds of the contact sexual offences occurred some time after the first known arrest for indecent exposure. An analysis of variables taken from the histories of the subjects confirmed the predictive markers identified in the earlier study and assists in identifying risk factors at an early stage in those who present with exhibitionist behaviour, indicating those who may most benefit from treatment or supervision to prevent more serious behaviour occurring.

Hirschfeld (1936) linked 'verbal exhibitionism' as a variant of genital exhibitionism and also added a category of 'psychological exhibitionism' whose exaggerated urge for frankness causes them to reveal to the world weaknesses which others endeavour to conceal. Classic examples cited are the confessions of Rousseau and the memoirs of Frank Harris. Contemporary examples are easily found. In criminal cases, a defence of urinating in public is sometimes successful and needs to be excluded clinically, as the English offence requires proof of an intention 'to insult' the observer. In Scotland the offence is, interestingly, included within the category of 'lewd and libidinous practices'.

Until recently, magistrates courts would request a psychiatric report on a person charged with indecent exposure, certainly on a second appearance, but during the last decade this practice appears to have decreased and it is not known whether this is because of a change in policy or because of rising costs. Although generally thought of as a problem seen from adolescence to middle age it is periodically seen *de novo* in the elderly when it often represents the disinhibition resulting from a dementing process. An organic origin should always be considered in the older age group.

Fetishism

The word fetish and its use in other cultural contexts denotes magic, idol, or an object of reverence. Sexual fetishism implies an erotic idolatry and like some other paraphilic behaviours is an exaggeration or perversion of tendencies or behaviour that is commonplace in normal sexual interaction. The essential feature of fetishism is the use of non-living objects to stimulate recurrent sexual urges and sexually arousing fantasies. The fetish may be the only or preferred stimulus for sexual arousal and relief and its absence may result in impotence. In some cases the wearing or use of the fetishistic object by a partner may be essential to achieve potency.

Fetishistic objects commonly include a variety of female underwear; rubber, plastic or leather garments, and specific articles such as shoes or boots. Parts of the body may act as fetish objects such as hair (which may be collected) or odours or faeces may act as alternatives. Pitcher (1990) provides a helpful review of this paraphilia with five case descriptions providing different examples of presentation drawn from individual cases reported in the literature. Forensic psychiatrists are commonly referred individuals who have stolen female underwear such as bras or pants from clothes lines or bathrooms to use to stimulate sexual excitement during masturbation, sometimes linked with fantasies relating to their known or believed owner. Fetishism is revealed by way of a charge of theft or, in other cases, during forensic evaluation of other sociopathic or violent behaviour. Frustration or inhibition arising from failure to own or touch the fetishism object can occasionally release violent or uncontrolled anger. A boot fetishist who had been convicted for indecent assault was released from 15 years of secure psychiatric care and almost immediately murdered a young woman wearing calf-length boots. It had been generally agreed that his original problems were now in the past.

DSMIIIR lists the diagnostic criteria for fetishism as:

1. Over a period of at least six months, recurrent intense sexual urges and sexually arising fantasies involving the use of non-living objects by themselves.
2. The person has acted on these urges, or is markedly distressed by them.
3. The fetishes are not only articles of female clothing used in cross-dressing (transvestic fetishism) or devices designed for the purpose of tactile genital stimulation (e.g. a vibrator).

The disorder is more common among males than females and its prevalence is unknown, but it can often be traced from adolescence, and usually persists. Treatment of the specific condition (rather than primary disorders such as neurosis, organic pathology, or psychopathy) is generally considered disappointing, although a variety of approaches are often tried, including aversive conditioning, cognitive therapy, and psychotherapy, which may allow a greater understanding of the origins of the behaviour in an individual case.

Frotteurism

This is another example of an ultimately deviant behaviour which is an exaggeration of activity which is not pathological within the context of normative sexual interplay. The essential feature (DSMIIIR) is recurrent, intense, sexual urges, and sexually arousing fantasies of at least six months' duration, involving touching and rubbing against a non-consensual person. Characteristically, frotteurism occurs in crowded places, such as underground trains, and a particular victim is selected, usually of the opposite sex. The person rubs his genital area against the person's thighs or may touch with his hands. The offender achieves sexual arousal from this behaviour repeatedly and as the main source of sexual excitement, although commonly other paraphilias are also found in a particular individual. Some authors distinguish 'toucherism' from 'frotteurism' but it is a fine distinction. Usually the disorder is reported between the ages of 15 to 25 years but we have noted it equally commonly among older, shy, inhibited individuals. Fantasies of such behaviour, without action, are also often reported and are used to encourage sexual arousal.

Voyeurism

It is difficult to define clearly the dividing line between innocent enjoyment in nudity, the disrobed human figure, the enjoyment of observing sexual activity and behaviour which is similar but deviant in other circumstances. The paraphilia of voyeurism sometimes referred to as scopophilia (Hirschfeld 1936) or scoptophilia (the love of seeing) is distinguished by the passivity and ignorance of the observed. The essential feature (DSMIIIR) is recurrent, intense, sexual urges, and sexually arousing fantasies, of at least six months duration, involving the act of observing unsuspecting people, usually, but not always, strangers in a state of undress or in the course of sexual activity. The individual has often acted on these urges or is distressed by them. Presentation to doctors not uncommonly occurs because the person is so plagued by guilt and an inability to cease the behaviour. Sometimes the behaviour is revealed as a result of a criminal offence or creating a nuisance or because an obsessive preoccupation with an observed individual leads to a contact offence, occasionally a serious or violent one. In such cases, as in exhibitionism, voyeurism is linked to other paraphilias and the prognosis should be guarded. The fantasies of power and control link erotic pleasure with aggression. Preferences for witnessing defecation or spying on small children, for example, are also warning signals of a more serious underlying tendency.

The exploitation of the common desire to indulge in voyeurism provided for by live shows, prostitutes, and pornography indicate the extent of voyeuristic tendencies generally.

Paedophilia

There has been a wide recognition in recent years that child sexual abuse is much more widespread than had been previously recognized. Hirschfeld's *Sexual anomalies and perversions*, an undated *festschrift* by his students published early this century, barely mentions this disorder (see Hirschfeld 1936). Paedophiles now cause considerable concern, although the incidence and prevalence of paedophilia are only roughly known and are implied from the known figures for childhood sexual abuse as reported by adults and from criminal statistics. Baker and Duncan (1985), for example, estimated that over 4.5 million adults in Great Britain were sexually abused as children (from a large sample interviewed in a MORI survey). Glasser (1990) reports that 13 per cent of 784 sexually deviant patients referred to the Portman Clinic, London, for assessment in 1976–8 were paedophiles. Figures in various studies vary considerably, however, and are often subject to differing criteria so that self-reports must be critically scrutinized. The essential feature of this disorder (DSMIIIR) is recurrent, intense, sexual urges, and sexually arousing fantasies, of at least six months duration, involving sexual activity with a prepubescent child. The age of the child is generally 13 years or younger and the age of the person is arbitrarily set at 16 years or older, and at least five years older than the child.

Paedophiles frequently report a variety of instability in child/parent relationships as children, with evidence of inhibition, prudity, and restraint in the course of their own psychosexual development and, not infrequently, of experience of sexual abuse in childhood themselves. Paedophiles vary in their predispositions. Many are attracted exclusively to children (boys or girls) of a specific age range. Some are attracted only to children; (exclusive type) and others also to adults (non-exclusive type). Glasser (1990) categorizes paedophilia as primary or secondary. The primary paedophile is an individual who has a consistent interest in children (invariant type) or his persistent preference is masked by an apparent adult interaction which is superficial and is abandoned as a result of stress or failure in a relationship (pseudo-neurotic type). Paedophilic fantasies may be necessary for successful adult sexual performance.

Paedophiles vary on the level of contact they may seek with young children from touching, masturbating (or mutually masturbating), undressing, to more explicit contact such as fellatio, cunnilingus, penetration with objects or fingers, together with varying degrees of force and threat towards the child. The victim may be a stranger, a member of the paedophile's family, or from within his social circle and a variety of threats, subterfuges or seduction may be used to achieve his objectives. Some individuals are genuinely kind and affectionate but a dominant characteristic is egocentricity, using the child object to achieve personal sexual gratification but with the fantasy that the child finds pleasure in his attentions. The child cannot give consent to such activities and is inevitably exploited and frequently is physically and psychologically damaged. Facile justifications are sometimes put forward in defence of such behaviour, that it has a historical background in other cultures or that it occurs as an expression of affection or love for children. Such explanations can be summarily dismissed. Persistent paedophilic behaviour must be distinguished from isolated acts occurring as a result of loneliness, stress, marital discord, or isolation when the child is a transient adult substitute, albeit an inappropriate one.

Sexual masochism

The essential feature of this disorder is the urge to gain sexual gratification from the experience of being cruelly treated or humiliated. Storr (1990) observes that the number of people who engage in sadomasochistic behaviour cannot be small, but is greatly exceeded by those who merely experience sadomasochistic fantasies. At a trivial level, there are commonly elements of sadomasochistic behaviour in ordinary sexual interplay. DSMIIIR gives the diagnostic criteria of this disorder as recurrent, intense, sexual urges, and sexually arousing fantasies, of at least six months' duration, involving the act (real not simulated) of being humiliated, beaten, bound, or otherwise made to suffer. The urges are distressing or have been acted on.

The range of activity is extensive and may be found through a partner including forms of restraint, beating, cutting, pinning, bonding, or being defiled by being defecated or urinated on. Others behave on their own through self-mutilation, arranging elaborate apparatus to inflict pain (for instance electrically), or engage in bondage. Some engage in group activity, perhaps seeking to be treated as a victim or a child, and may find these services provided by prostitutes. Some require to be forced to cross-dress to obtain sexual relief.

A subgroup deliberately induces cerebral hypoxia to gain sexual excitement (described as sexual asphyxia by Brittain (1968) or hypoxyphilia (DSMIIIR). The individual will indulge in complex practices involving ligatures or nooses to induce oxygen deprivation, sometimes while cross-dressing. This induces sexual stimulation and sexual fantasies but can be dangerous. Hucker (1990a) has provided an extensive review of the literature on this condition and from this suggests that there are a possible 150 to 200 deaths per year in the United Kingdom as a consequence of this activity. Few cases come to psychiatric attention.

Sexual sadism

There is no distinct dividing line between sexual sadism and sexual masochism and the two predispositions are often interchangeable and exist in the same individual, sometimes in association with other paraphilias. The intense urge to obtain control or dominance over a victim, through a range of behaviours, characterizes this paraphilia. The recurrent, intense urge to give psychological or physical suffering to another provides sexual excitement. The behaviour may exist in fantasy or be acted on with, for example, torture, stabbing, whipping, mutilation, cutting, or otherwise hurting the victim, who may or may not be consenting and willing (and masochistic) although terrified. The suffering of the victim is sexually arousing.

Sadomasochistic practices come to light when the partner is an unwilling victim, when the physical or psychological damage requires medical attention or when a crime is revealed. The seriousness and severity of the behaviours often increases with time although, as with other paraphilias, can be concealed without the knowledge of others. Sometimes the end result is a victim's death.

Some other paraphilias

Sexual arousal may be obtained from a wide range of other bizarre and unusual behaviours, which in some cases is the only stimulus or principal fantasy allowing sexual relief. Some prostitutes will provide one or other of these activities for paying customers; others will otherwise find willing partners, where a partner is necessary.

Other paraphilias include:

1. *Necrophilia*. Fantasies involving sexual activity with corpses, which may be acted upon and can be associated with homicide or with obtaining access to a corpse (Hucker 1990*b* reviews the literature).
2. *Zoophilia*. A deviant preference for animals usually a particular category of animal (see Bluglass 1990).
3. *Coprophilia and urophilia* Involving the fantasy or real experience of sexual arousal from being sprayed with excreta or ingesting it. *Klismaphilia* refers similarly to enemas.
4. *Telephone scatalogia* or obscene telephone calls also enter the category of the paraphilias (see Cordess 1990).

UNDERSTANDING SEXUAL DEVIANCY

One approach to understanding the aetiology of the paraphilias, is based on the analysis of groups who commit the same offence and, not surprisingly, researchers find that, on the whole, they are heterogeneous. The offending behaviour is the final outcome of a sequence of external and internal factors, due to a variety of causative factors. Since the acknowledgement of women, adolescents, and children as possible perpetrators of sexual offences, in addition to men, researchers have attempted, without success, to define differences between the varied perpetrator groups. This search to find a 'uniqueness' about a certain group of offenders is most evident in the papers about female offenders which strive to demonstrate differences between male and female when they may not exist.

Previous theories of sexual offending, whether psychodynamic, behavioural, or biological, can be integrated with the more recently acknowledged important cognitive model. Lanyon (1991) discussed integration of the three traditional theoretical approaches with the cognitive model. It is possible to produce a formulation of offending behaviour based on sound psychodynamic theory, using additional techniques of functional analysis from behaviour theory, give consideration to the possibility of organic factors, and obtain an understanding of how the patient construes themselves and others. This integrated approach to assessment, formulation, and treatment has been used by cognitive analytical therapists in the United Kingdom for the past 15 years. The technique has been successfully used to treat patients suffering from such wide-ranging disorders as brittle diabetes, depression, anxiety, self-harming, eating disorders as well as the paraphilias, and borderline personality disorder (Ryle 1990).

INTEGRATED MODEL OF SEXUAL OFFENDING

Most sexual offenders or people with paraphilias are not mentally ill or handicapped, and many do not fulfil formal psychiatric diagnostic criteria, although a significant percentage demonstrate personality disorder and alcohol and/or substance abuse problems (Prins 1990; Gibbens and Robertson 1983; Chiswick 1983). Some fulfil ICD 10 or DSMIVR criteria for deviancy and hypersexuality. Lanyon (1991), referring to Abel *et al.* (1987) discussed the dimension of deviant sexual preference with 'fixated' paraphilias at one end of a continuum with situational 'regressed' neurotic offenders at the other. Docter (1988) and Burgess (1984) describe an episodic versus continuous or lifestyle format of sexual offending.

It is known that most adults are capable of demonstrating arousal to deviant stimuli in the laboratory. However, there is limited explanation for the variation in sexual deviance expressed in the population, and why some act on the deviant urge and others do not. It is likely that a balance exists between desire/motivation to deviation (the forward propulsion) and the internal and external inhibitors (the brakes). If we consider the antecedent predisposition or internal factors, the most important factor is that of the individual's cognitions. His or her attitude towards him- or herself and others; repeated faulty attribution and misinterpretation in relationships, and thought or visual fantasy form the foundation stones of deviancy. The individual's childhood experience is emphasized by psychodynamic and behavioural theorists and widely researched in children and adults who were sexually abused themselves prior to offending. Degrees of mood disturbance, ranging from irritability to neurotic anxiety and depression, colour the patient's thoughts and behaviours. Individuals with a predisposition for affective disorder or schizophrenia may be disinhibited or act in response to command hallucinations and delusions during a psychotic episode. Patients with personality disorders associated with problems of self-esteem, tension, frustration and anger management, poor tolerance to delayed gratification, lack of empathy with others, and faulty cognitions are particularly vulnerable.

Organic risk is carried in factors such as the chromosome abnormality of Klinefelter's syndrome, temporal lobe epilepsy, and tumours or brain injury, which may result in disinhibition, hypersexuality or deviant arousal. Endocrine abnormalities may rarely be an important internal factor. Patients suffering from mental handicap can be vulnerable because of impaired social learning, poor interpersonal skills, frustration

Table 1.1 Integrated model of sexual offending

Antecedent predispositions: Internal factors	Triggers or releasers: External factors
All have ability to respond to deviant cues	
Degrees of potential deviance	
Cognitions Attitudes Faulty attribution and interpretation Fantasy	Visually triggered memory 'Child like abused self' 'Woman like abusive mother' Person to fit fantasy image
Childhood experience	
Mood Irritability	Loss event Perceived rejection Interpersonal difficulties
Neurosis Anxiety Depression	Loss event Perceived rejection Interpersonal difficulties

Mental illness
Affective disorders
Schizophrenia
	Psychotic episode
	   Disinhibition
	   Command act
	(Internal factor stimulated
	by external factors)

Personality disorder Low self-esteem Tension Frustration Poor tolerance delayed gratification Faulty cognitions Lack of empathy Victim as object Propensity for violence	Interpersonal difficulties Alcohol/substance abuse Visually triggered memory
Chromosome abnormalities	
Temporal lobe epilepsy Deviant arousal	Emotional conflict, or Fetish object triggers a fit
Tumour/brain injury Disinhibition Hypersexuality Deviant arousal	
Mental handicap Impaired social learning Poor interpersonal skills Frustration of normal sex drive Associated PD mental impairment	No appropriate sexual outlet Misinterpret friendliness Opportunistic
Endocrine Hormonal imbalance	

of normal sexual drive, or mental impairment associated with seriously irresponsible and aggressive behaviour to others.

The likelihood of offending behaviour occurring, and whether it is subsequently repeated, depends on the proportional contribution and interplay between the patient's internal predisposition which contributes to the strength of deviant arousal, the presence or absence of hypersexuality, the propensity or motivation to carry out a deviant act, inhibiting internal and external factors, and the triggers or releasers. The latter are usually external factors such as important events in relationships, environmental opportunities, and victim characteristics. Faulty cognitions may be triggered by a direct visual stimulus such as seeing a person who fits a prior fantasy image or indirectly by visually triggered memories such as seeing a child who reminds the offender of his 'abused self' or a woman like 'his abusive mother'. Internal factors such as mood and the presence of neurosis may be triggered by loss events such as loss of employment or bereavement, perceived or real rejection in a close relationship, or other interpersonal difficulties. Psychotic episodes of mental illness may be released by social stimuli or substance abuse in addition to inherent biological releasing factors. In personality disordered patients, interpersonal difficulties, alcohol and substance abuse may act as releasing factors in addition to seemingly minimal provocation from others. Temporal lobe epilepsy can be triggered by emotional conflict or sight of a fetish object. Vulnerable mentally handicapped patients entering puberty with poor social skills may misinterpret the friendliness of others as an invitation to sexual behaviour.

Lanyon (1991), developing his hypothesis, noted that those with marked internal factors are more likely to offend with minimal external triggers and to repeat the behaviour, whereas those with less powerful internal factors are likely to require strong or multiple external releasing factors, and to show episodic or one-off behaviours.

In our opinion, the integrated model has utility, and is applicable to all types of offences and offenders. More importantly, it allows planning of appropriate intervention. Assessment of the possibility of modifying the antecedent internal factors and manipulating external factors, allows clinicians to consider the risk of both frequency and cost of any future offending, and to decide on the appropriate treatment. The model allows the therapist to engage the patient in accepting responsibility for his or her own behaviour at an early stage, to empower him or her, by way of self-knowledge and recognition, of the ability to change, so that he or she may be able to predict for him or herself the circumstances which may lead to a high risk of re-offending. Physical intervention in the form of adjunctive pharmacotherapy can be assimilated into the integrated model and treatment approach with the patient's informed consent and co-operation. The integrated model not only explains how different antecedent factors can cause one type of offending behaviour, but also how the behaviour is maintained by reverberating circuits of faulty cognitions and mood states, leading to inevitable repetition. The model can be used to explain repetition within the individual, intra-familial, and inter-generational cycles of abuse. (See Table 1.1)

Case study

The following case example, first presented by one of us (BB) at a meeting of cognitive analytical therapists in London (1988), illustrates how a patient presenting with a variety of antecedent problems and repeated intermittent sexual aggression can be explained using the integrated model.

Mr AB is a 20-year-old, single, unemployed, Caucasian man. He was born with multiple congenital abnormalities and was not expected to survive an emergency operation after birth. He spent most of his infancy in hospital, had multiple operations, and did not develop a close relationship with his parents who did not expect him to survive. Although of normal intellect, he was educated in a school for the physically and mentally handicapped because of profound physical difficulties. He was unhappy, did not develop a sense of belonging, and remained friendless. He obtained qualifications allowing him to attend college, graduating at 18 as a chef. His subsequent employment was disrupted by repeated offending.

From the age of 18 with the onset of episodes of depressed mood, he abused solvents and drank alcohol to excess for symptomatic relief. Two members of his family suffered from bipolar affective disorder.

He entered puberty at the age of 12 and was of heterosexual orientation. The congenital abnormalities (one kidney, anal and oesophageal atresia) resulted in multiple operations. After closure of a colostomy he suffered from intermittent faecal incontinence, pain, and bleeding which were not amenable to further surgery. Because of his physical symptoms he was extremely shy and unable to make close relationships. He was most attracted by younger women or those whom he perceived not to pose a threat to him with his sense of sexual inadequacy. He was of normal sexual drive but felt sexually frustrated due to his lack of appropriate outlet. He rarely masturbated because of intense pain prior to ejaculation, combined with retarded ejaculation and intermittent impotence when depressed and anxious.

Aged 17, he was first assessed by a psychiatrist after self-disclosure of his first episode of indecent assault on a 7-year-old girl. At that time he was diagnosed to be of deviant sexual orientation due to his preference of girls between the age of 8 and 13. He attended for outpatient treatment which included individual behaviour therapy, a social skills group, group therapy, and liaison with the family. He did not engage in therapy, and it is of note that his sister was a member of staff in the hospital. He was assessed again a year later by a forensic psychiatrist and psychologist and diagnosed again to be of deviant orientation, preferring girls of approximately 14 when aged 18 himself. Outpatient therapy was planned but did not occur due to lack of staff. He was admitted briefly a year later after an episode of serious self-harm. His second admission to psychiatric hospital occurred a year later when he was noted to be depressed with suicidal intent, to be abusing alcohol and solvents, and he received inpatient individual and group therapy for six weeks. His third informal admission to hospital occurred some months later after a grave overdose. His admission followed an episode of depression with pronounced suicidal ideas and an attempt to kill himself via inhalation of cooking gas. Each of the admissions was preceded by a period of extreme tension, anxiety, and depressed mood, following thoughts of his previous offending behaviour. Each suicide attempt was seen to be the only solution to his problems as he was fearful of hurting others.

The internal factors, predisposing him to repeated self-harm or sexual offending, were based on three main components, physical, cognitions, and mood. He had a familial predisposition to suffer from episodes of depression. Subsequent to the

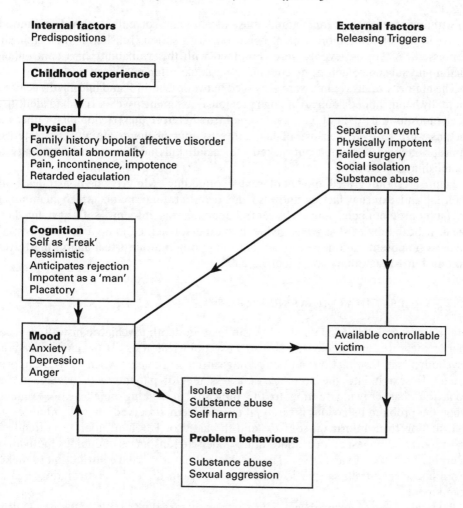

Fig. 1.1 Integrated model of sexual offending, Mr A B.

congenital abnormalities he suffered pain, incontinence, ejaculatory dysfunction, and impotence. These factors, combined with his childhood experience, led to the psychological components of long-standing low self-esteem, poor social relationships, and persistent faulty cognitions. He viewed himself as a freak, was pessimistic about his future, was unusually vulnerable to set-backs, and had a tendency to misinterpret occurrences as deliberate rejection by others. He viewed himself as a failure as a 'man'. The physical and psychological predispositions led to repeated episodes of abnormal mood with significant anxiety, depression, anger, and frustration of his normal sexual drive.

Prior to each of the six indecent assaults he experienced a significant personal loss such as separation through bereavement or change of location of another person close to him, together with failed surgical treatment of his pain and incontinence, or an episode of physical impotence. Although his usual faulty coping strategy was to withdraw from social contact and abuse alcohol and solvents to elevate his mood, he could demonstrate more violent behaviour with serious self-harm when clinically depressed. When loss events were combined with the availability of a controllable victim and substance abuse, he committed a sexual offence.

The majority of his victims were girls aged between 7 and 14, and one an offence on a mentally handicapped adult. Although previously assessing psychiatrists had identified deviant arousal, he did not have evidence of true heterosexual paedophilia, rather the victims were selected because of his ability to control them. He was interested in appropriately aged women but lacked the social skills and confidence necessary to establish a relationship.

Figure 1.1 (integrated model of sexual offending, Mr AB) demonstrates both internal and external factors and also the reverberating circuits which maintained his faulty problem behaviours. His central dilemma was 'it seems as if I have lived my life as if I can only exist as *either* giving in to others; when I end up feeling depressed, anxious, impotent, and hopeless; *or* controlling others when I feel angry, masterful, potent, but I hurt others and I feel a freak'.

PSYCHIATRIC ASSESSMENT OF SEXUAL DEVIANCY

Multi-professional assessment should include an in-depth psychiatric history, psychometric measures including standardized psychological tests, behavioural analysis, psychodynamic formulation, and physiological measurements when they are appropriate. Research into the accuracy of assessment of patients with deviant sexual behaviour has drawn attention to the difficulty in making objective assessments when the problem behaviour is rarely, if ever, directly observed; there is often scanty information from informant sources; and the assessor is reliant upon the offender's self-report and honest co-operation, often under circumstances of dubious motivation (Perkins 1982; Lee-Evans 1986). The psychiatrist has a specific contribution to make, given his eclectic training, particularly in cases where there is a contributing organic component.

Physical causes of sexual deviancy are extremely rare but the role of the psychiatrist as part of a multi-professional assessment remains critical. Physical treatments can provide dramatic and enduring improvement in some cases. Whatever procedures the assessor uses, the following questions need to be answered:

1. Is the patient suffering from mental illness, whether functional or organic, or other mental disorder?
2. If so, is the illness or disorder related to the offending behaviour?
3. Can the nature of the sexual deviancy, likely aetiology, treatability, and risk of future offending be described?
4. Does the formulation of the deviation or offending behaviour allow the assessor to make treatment recommendations and risk predictions?

The assessor must consider whether the patient suffers from an abnormality of sexual drive and/or deviant arousal, and provide an offence formulation.

Regardless of the type of assessment technique used, the most important instrument in taking a psychosexual history is the interviewer himself. For interviewing and

- Sexual knowledge and sources

- Sexual attitudes to self and others

- Age onset   Interest
                                Masturbation
                                Dating
                                Sexual Intercourse

- Frequency   Masturbation
                                Sexual Intercourse
                                Other sexual behaviours

- Relationships   Age self/partner
                                Gender(s)
                                Duration
                                Quality/problems/abuse

- Fantasy   Content/use

- Orientation

- Drive

- Experience

Fig. 1.2 Taking a psychosexual history.

information-gathering to be successful, it is essential that the interviewer is capable of putting the patient at ease, and is a good facilitator. Facilitation is aided by the interviewer having at his finger-tips a wide vocabulary to describe sexual matters and sufficient sensitivity to pitch the conversation at the right level. An interrogative style is likely to be unproductive. It is important to ask open questions and not make assumptions about orientation or experience that might alienate the patient.

The gathering of information about sexual dysfunction, deviation, and any associated offending must be part of a comprehensive psychiatric history. This allows the interviewer to understand deviant behaviour in the context of developmental, social, psychological, and organic factors. It is usually appropriate to elicit the detailed psychosexual history when taking the patient's chronological life history. In this way, questions about puberty, the development of sexual interest, close relationships, and later sexual activity can be discussed as part of a natural progression in gaining an understanding of the individual and his previous life's experience. This is less threatening or intimidating than a direct confrontational approach. The interviewer needs to determine the patient's current sexual knowledge and understanding, the methods by which he gained that information, and his sexual attitudes in general. Details of puberty, the age of onset of interest in sexual relationships, the orientation of that interest over time, the onset and frequency of masturbation in association with masturbatory fantasies, and the onset of dating and sexual intercourse (when appropriate) should all be established.

It is important, when discussing sexual experience and chronological relationships, to determine the ages of both the patient and the partner on each occasion, the partner's gender, the duration of the relationship, and the type of sexual relationship in each case. Sensitive questioning about relationships and sexual experience can often elicit a spontaneous account of sexual abuse experienced by the patient with the avoidance of direct questioning.

In the interview, the clinician is looking for indicators of sexual or social dysfunction, in addition to building up a comprehensive picture that will allow formulation of the patient's current sexual orientation or arousal, and the level of his or her sexual drive. (See Fig. 1.2.)

AVOIDING PITFALLS IN TAKING A PSYCHOSEXUAL HISTORY

It is important to remember to distinguish between sexual behaviour associated with normal arousal, and seemingly normal sexual behaviour actually stimulated by deviant arousal. In order to make this distinction, it is essential to explore the patient's thoughts and visual imagery, use of material for stimulation, and under what conditions arousal can be achieved, in addition to the description of the sexual behaviour carried out. For example, a man may report that he has no problem in having sexual intercourse with his wife, and cannot understand why he has committed a sexual offence against a child. On enquiry, it is evident that he is only able to achieve an erection and have intercourse with his wife whilst using visual images or thoughts of children in his head.

Patients may spontaneously report that they are perfectly able to be aroused and have normal sexual intercourse with their partners, and will only tell you about cross-dressing, bondage, or other fetish if you enquire about it specifically. It is also important to remember that aggression may be the primary ingredient necessary for the individual to obtain arousal, or that a sexual offence may be a vehicle for aggression rather than sexual expression. In the assessment of the predominant orientation or arousal of the patient, it can be useful to employ an arousal check-list for both sexual intercourse and masturbation. (See Fig. 1.3.)

Primary Arousal/orientation	Sexual intercourse	Masturbation
Mood		
Thoughts		
Visual images		
Material used/ collected		
Conditions for arousal		

Fig. 1.3 Arousal checklist.

Gathering data in a structured manner can, for example, reveal when masturbation is used for tension reduction, rather than its use for pleasure or to obtain relief from sexual frustration. Similarly, details of conditions necessary for arousal during

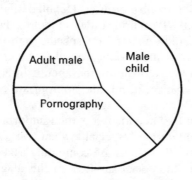

Fig. 1.4 Deviant arousal.

seemingly normal heterosexual intercourse may elicit details such as the patient requires darkness so that he cannot see his adult female partner, a preference that she does not speak so that she does not remind him of her presence, and a preference for shaving of his partner's pubic hair, all indicating a preference for prepubertal girls. This detail enables the clinician to probe appropriately for deviant thought and imagery of children. Under these circumstances, the adult woman is but a vehicle for sexual expression in a man with a primary paedophilic arousal pattern. When patients report various types of arousal it is helpful to them to create a pie chart, 'cut up a cake' to show the proportional contributions of each arousal stimulus. (See Fig. 1.4.)

In order to evaluate the the patient's sexual drive, the interviewer needs to know the frequency of masturbation and sexual intercourse. Comprehensive history-taking may be augmented by the use of attitude questionnaires, self-rating scales, and diary-keeping by the patient. (Perkins 1986; Lanyon 1991). The clinician may also find it necessary to carry out physical investigations in addition to the detailed history-taking, in order to clarify whether there is an underlying chromosomal, hormonal, or other organic cause contributing to the abnormal behaviour. Penile plethysmography may be necessary (Lanyon 1991) in order to clarify sexual interest patterns, and provide the basis for discussion with the patient during subsequent treatment sessions.

For the assessment of offending behaviour, it is important to gain a detailed description not only from the patient himself, but also from other informant sources such as depositions, spouse, relatives, and co-assessing professionals. Data can then be collated and allow formulation that takes into consideration the external and internal antecedent factors, the behaviour itself, and consequences of the behaviour that may act as offending reinforcers. Future risk assessment is beset with difficulties and limited.

In assessing the risk of future offending, the assessor is looking for a progression or escalation in the type or frequency of offending, an assessment of the patient's attitude to his offence and victim in addition to external factors such as social stresses or substance abuse. When considering the antecedents to the offence behaviour, particular attention should be directed to the content of fantasy, whether it has been progressively acted out or incorporated into offences over time and/or used in repeated masturbatory/intercourse arousal. Detailed analysis commonly reveals a procedural sequence (Ryle 1989) or 'firing order' of feelings leading to cognitions, then behaviours, which are repeatedly enacted and specific to the individual. Identification of the faulty neurotic behaviour and deviant arousal enables the assessor to understand the offence, identify target areas for future therapeutic intervention, elicit a baseline against which to measure change, decide the appropriate therapeutic environment, and make risk predictions.

Having gathered data on the individual it is then important to consider them with reference to the available literature, especially when considering types of treatment intervention and future risk. Physicians are commonly asked to advise the civil and criminal courts, probation, and social services on the diagnosis and treatability of sexual offenders. When making recommendations to the courts the clinician must consider the appropriate placement for treatment with regard to public safety as well as the appropriate therapeutic environment for the patient. Recommendations must be realistic. The clinician should only intervene when appropriate, and not make treatment proposals *unless* there are achievable treatment goals. Given the uncertainty about long-term efficacy, treatment should be recommended thoughtfully and risk assessment carried out cautiously. Many sexual offenders are treated in the group setting without specific medical intervention. Some require adjunctive medication for hypersexuality or deviant arousal. Mentally ill offenders usually require inpatient treatment of the primary pathology before psychosexual assessment can be carried out. The majority of serious offenders receive custodial sentences and those receiving a sentence of four years or more in the United Kingdom are now automatically referred for assessment within a prison sex-offender treatment programme, some going on into treatment. It is generally acknowledged that many first-time offenders do not repeat the behaviour, but for recidivists imprisonment does nothing to reduce future risk.

RELATIONSHIP BETWEEN SEXUAL OFFENDING AND MENTAL DISORDER

Most sexual offenders and people with paraphilias are neither mentally ill nor mentally handicapped, many do not fulfil formal psychiatric diagnostic criteria, although a significant percentage demonstrate personality disorders and alcohol or substance abuse problems (Gibbens and Robertson 1983; Chiswick 1983; Prins 1990).

Care must be exercised in making comparisons between US and UK literature due to the different meaning of terms used. Many sex-offenders are detained under mentally disordered offender statutes in US mental health facilities. Monahan *et al.* (1983) highlight the problem of patients being labelled as mentally disordered simply because of their behaviour; akin to the UK controversy over the diagnosis of personality disorder.

United States law allows detention in hospital of patients diagnosed as sexually deviant. However, patients with this sole diagnosis are specifically excluded from detention under the Mental Health Act 1983 in the United Kingdom. Few of the United States detained mentally disordered sex-offenders (MDSOs) (11 of 260 in Sturgeon and Taylor's 1980 study) were diagnosed as suffering from affective or functional psychosis, affective disorder or mental handicap. Similarly, caution must be exercised in drawing general epidemiological conclusions from studies of sexual offenders referred for outpatient psychiatric assessment or detained in hospitals because of inherent selection bias.

Detailed discussion of personality disorder is beyond the remit of this chapter. The association between antisocial personality disorder and violent crime is well documented, a similar link has been found in rapists. Alcohol and drug abuse are common secondary diagnoses in personality disordered and paedophilic offenders (Henn *et al.* 1976).

RELATIONSHIP BETWEEN SEXUAL OFFENDING AND MENTAL ILLNESS

The association between mental illness and sexual offending has been documented historically including reference to schizophrenia, affective disorder, and neuroses.

Schizophrenia and sexual offending

Clinicians are aware of the general disinhibiting effect of schizophrenia. Nurses are often so habituated to inappropriate sexual remarks, gestures, and managing disinhibited sexual behaviour in the patient, that they may 'accept' the sexual problems as part of acute illness and not report them. Although the majority of such behaviours cease when psychosis remits, it cannot always be assumed that it exists purely as a function of illness.

Schizophrenia is not only associated with disinhibited non-contact offences such as indecent exposure, but occasionally also serious contact offences including indecent assault and rape. In general there is a paucity of literature on the mentally ill sex offender. Tidmarsh (1990) reviewed the evidence for disturbance in sexuality and sexual deviancy in schizophrenics. Bleuler (1911) described an association with gender identity disturbance. Klaf and Davis (1960) in their survey of 150 paranoid schizophrenics found that 27 per cent had experienced delusions or hallucinations of a sexual nature. Planansky and Johnstone (1962) described 15 per cent of their cohort as confused about their sexual identity, 51 per cent concerned about homosexuality, and 74 per cent about heterosexual problems when acutely ill. Gittleson and Levine (1966) identified genital hallucinations and delusions of sex change in approximately 30 per cent of their cohort. Craissati and Hodes (1992) analysed data from 10 schizophrenic patients admitted for treatment following sexual offences and found evidence of antecedent deterioration in the mental state with irritability, withdrawal, deterioration in self-care, unprovoked outbursts, and sexual disinhibition prior to the offence. It appeared that the predominant motivation for offending was impulsivity and inability to resist a sexual urge. There was no evidence that their behaviour was secondary to command hallucinations or delusional drive. As in mentally well sex-offenders, some patients reported deviant offence-related fantasy prior to the index offence. The authors noted the difficulty in obtaining full psychosexual histories, both at the time of original assessment and in the follow-up research interview. Their paper suggests that mental illness was not the primary source of the sexual pathology, but acted as a disinhibiting agent.

Jones *et al.* (1992) report sexual assaults in four patients suffering from schizophrenia following the orders of command hallucinations. Murrey *et al.* (1992) compared IQ, offence, and victim data in 106 male patients detained in maximum secure hospital for treatment.

Clinicians treating schizophrenics need to consider the possibility that:

(1) the patient may be unable to conceal/control sexual deviancy when unwell;
(2) acute illness may 'disinhibit' the patient; or
(3) the patient may be acting on a delusional drive or in response to command hallucinations.

Full psychosexual evaluation needs to be completed prior to considering discharge in patients suffering from schizophrenia who demonstrate abnormal sexual behaviour. Rogers *et al.* (1990) summarize the problem of accurate history-taking and patients withholding information about command hallucinations, highlighting the risk of offending associated with passivity phenomena.

Affective disorder and sexual offending

Little work is published on the relationship between affective disorder and sexual offending. Higgins (1990) observed that the entire literature contains such a relatively small total number of patients who committed a wide range of offences (including non-sex offences) and stated that drawing definitive conclusions is clearly unwise. Wulach (1983), Gibbens and Robertson (1983), and Bearcroft and Donovan (1965) observed that most offences committed by patients suffering from hypomania were not serious. Clinicians are aware of the symptoms of social and sexual disinhibition in hypomania which are associated with the unusual offence of indecent exposure in women in some cases O'Connor (1987). Snaith and Bennett (1990) in their discussion of exhibitionism, refer to female exhibitionists 'who uncover breasts or buttocks in a seductive manner', but do not elaborate the relationship with mental illness. They observe that men who commit indecent exposure at irregular intervals without evidence of persistent deviancy should be assessed for the presence of depressive illness. Wulach (1983) series of 100 patients suffering from manic illness included two rapes. Unfortunately, neither of the two recent studies of mentally ill sex-offenders (Craissati and Hodes 1992; Murrey *et al.* 1992) give details of the form of mental illness in their subjects. It is generally accepted that treatment of the primary complaint rapidly produces control of sexual disinhibition and deviancy, but is worthwhile for clinicians to consider in depth psychosexual assessment if the problem is repeated and/or preceded by deviant sexual fantasy and planning prior to the offence, thus suggesting an additional problem of sexual deviancy.

Mentally handicapped offenders

The relationship between mental handicap and sexual offending is sparsely reported in the literature; Day (1990) noted limitations in both the quantity and nature of the data. In his descriptive paper of 26 male patients admitted to a medium-secure unit (Day 1988) he analysed the sexual history of 20 handicapped patients in depth. Day (1990) in his review of the literature, noted the preponderance of male mentally handicapped sexual offenders and observed that they share many of the social characteristics typical of non-mentally handicapped offenders. He compared the patterns of offending in the general population with the studies of the mentally handicapped offender and noted that sexual offences were over-represented in the mentally handicapped patients, a finding consistent with that of Walker and McCabe (1973). Their study of patients suffering from a variety of diagnoses, including mental handicap, who were admitted on hospital orders in a 12-month period between 1963 and 1964, demonstrated that a third of the mentally handicapped men were convicted of sexual offences in contrast to 5 per cent of all males convicted of any indictable offence in the same time period. Reid (1990) in his discussion of the relationship between low IQ and sexual offending refers to the Walker and McCabe study, observing that a third of the mentally handicapped group accounted for 59 per cent of the sexual offences in the whole sample. Craft (1984) described a subgroup of mentally handicapped offenders who had antecedent difficulties with personality disorder, promiscuous sexual behaviour, and often bisexual arousal.

Mentally handicapped patients committing more serious sexual offences tended to have significant past histories of family disturbance, evidence of conduct and personality disorder, and to commit a range of other non-sexual crimes. Reid (1990), referring to the work of Gibbens and Robertson (1983) and Murrey *et al.* (1992), observed that mentally handicapped offenders tended to commit their first offence and be detained at a younger age than mentally ill patients committing similar offences.

Clarke (1989) doubts the methodology of early studies reporting an excess of mentally handicapped sex offenders. 'More recent studies with sounder methodology have demonstrated that the prevalence of mental retardation among male offenders differs little from the prevalence of mental retardation among the general population' (MacEachron 1979; Craft 1984, 1985). Day (1990) noted that the mentally handi-capped exhibitionists did not appear to require a response from their victim, rather they appeared to be driven by frustration of normal sexual drive and to be using exposure as an inappropriate form of sexual invitation.

In the indecent assault group, the patients appear to be impulsive, the offence of a minor nature, and associated with the patient's misinterpretation of 'friendliness' in others. Mentally handicapped offenders tend to attribute sexual intent and meaning to others non-sexual warmth. Cooper *et al.* (1993), reporting the case of a moder-ately mentally handicapped man possibly suffering from Asperger's syndrome, who presented with auto-erotic fetishistic transvestism, frotteurism, and minor indecent assaults on adult women, explained the patient's behaviour as being due to factors such as social gaucheness, failure to learn appropriate courtship techniques, and a lack of appropriate outlet for his normal sexual drive. Raboch *et al.* (1987) reported two cases of sexually motivated homicide, where one patient suffered from Klinefelter's syndrome. Berlin (1983), reviewing the evidence for biological factors in 34 men who had committed sexual offences, reported three as suffering from Klinefelter's syndrome and homosexual paedophilia. This rare syndrome which can cause mental handicap and typically causes hypogonadism with low serum testosterone is of interest as it may indicate a biological aetiology of offending. Murrey *et al.* (1992), report their comparative study of 106 (mentally ill, psychopathic, and mentally handicapped) patients detained in Rampton maximum-secure hospital, who had committed sexual offences. Increasing violence was association with higher IQ. Although the number of sexual offences in total in the mentally handicapped group were significantly larger than in the mentally ill group, they were generally of less severity.

Day (1990), Reid (1990), and Murrey *et al.* (1992) all note that victims tend to be significantly younger than those of non-mentally handicapped sexual offenders. Most patients did not have evidence of paedophilia, their choice of victim reflecting the patient's immaturity, naivety, and gullibility, rather than deviant arousal. Day (1988, 1990) and Cooper *et al.* (1993) note the problem of general re-offending, Gibbens and Robertson (1983) in the 15-year follow-up of patients discharged from hospital orders noted the increased tendency to re-offend in general, with an increased incidence of sexual offending in the mentally handicapped group. Day postulates that mentally handicapped offenders are less capable of predicting the consequences of their actions, more impulsive and gullible, and have little appreciation of the effects of their actions on others. He notes the mentally handicapped offenders' associated problems of physical and mental health difficulties which contribute to poor social learning and impaired development of appropriate social skills.

Female mentally handicapped sexual offenders are even more difficult to evaluate, given the sparse literature. Walker and McCabe (1973) identified 86 female offenders (a fifth of the mentally handicapped group) of whom 9 per cent had committed sexual offences. The majority were described as young women with antecedent histories of severe family disturbance, conduct disorder, and disturbed behaviour including repeated self-harm. Hospital orders were made following offences of soliciting, prostitution, incest, or for their own care and protection: 24 per cent were prosecuted for vagrancy which including 'sexual misconduct'. Reid (1990) observed that these women were on the whole both victims and offenders. The problem of promiscuity in female mentally handicapped offenders was related to their learned behaviour whereby sex was used as a currency, or to seek emotional closeness via brief sexualized relationships.

Sexual offending in mentally handicapped women is rare and does not often put others at serious risk. However, it is important to remember the risk to self because of deviant behaviour. In addition to the risk of exploitation, infection, and pregnancy through promiscuity, women can cause serious harm to themselves by repeated penetration with a variety of unsuitable objects during excessive masturbation. In addition to routine education, counselling, and behavioural interventions, pharmacological treatment with antilibidinal agents, such as cyproterone acetate, can be essential.

Other paraphilias are rarely reported in the mentally handicapped. Berlin (1983) described transsexualism in a patient with Klinefelter's syndrome, Cooper *et al.* (1993) auto-erotic fetishistic transvestism in a moderately mentally handicapped man. Bowler and Callacott (1993) describe four handicapped men with transvestic fetishism, one transvestism.

There are no specific treatment guidelines for the mentally handicapped sexual offender, their treatment programme and site of treatment being determined by individual need and degree of security. Day (1988), Hoare and O'Brien (1991) describe treatment in medium-secure units. Programmes to treat underlying factors of under-socialization, poor impulse control, lack of social and occupational skills, education deficits, and low self-esteem usually involve personal and social skills training, education, behaviour modification programmes, counselling and, when indicated, antilibidinal medication. Day observed a re-conviction rate of 55 per cent similar to that of other follow-up studies (Wildenskov 1962; Walker and McCabe 1973; Gibbens and Robertson 1983; Craft 1984), highlighting specific vulnerability to re-offend in the immediate post-discharge period. Hoare and O'Brien (1991) noted the decline in admissions for all mentally handicapped offenders in the United Kingdom following the Mental Health Act 1983, with admission limited to the more serious male offenders. The trend in reduction could be secondary to the legislative change requiring treatability for those diagnosed as mentally impaired, but they also noted the introduction of the Police and Criminal Evidence Act (1984) and the trend for mentally handicapped offenders cases being discontinued by the police and prosecution service.

Organic factors and sexual offences

Little progress has been made in recent years in establishing organic determinants of sexual offending in the majority of cases. Although rare, links have been made between sexually deviant behaviour and chromosome, brain, and hormone abnormalities.

Chromosome abnormalities are reviewed by Berlin (1983) who noted an association between men suffering from Klinefelter's syndrome (47,XXY and XXY mosaics) and offending. Most men were hypogonadal non-offenders but some demonstrated sexual offending with associated paedophilia, transsexualism, and rarely sexual murder (Rabock *et al.* 1987).

A variety of *brain abnormalities* have been diagnosed in patients presenting with sexual deviancy ranging from tumours, epilepsy (especially temporal lobe epilepsy), degenerative disorders (such as the dementias, multiple sclerosis, and Huntington's chorea), damage secondary to alcohol abuse, surgery or head injury, and infectious deterioration as in Creutzfeldt–Jakob disease. Lishman (1987) noted the association between frontal lobe tumour, frontal lobe syndromes, disinhibition, and exhibitionism. Langevin *et al.* (1988) report sexual sadism in a man with frontal temporal glioma and associated alcohol abuse.

The association between sexual disorder and *temporal lobe epilepsy*, especially early onset temporal lobe epilepsy, has been described in papers since 1939 (Klüver and Bucy 1939; Mitchell *et al.* 1954; Epstein 1961; Hunter *et al.* 1963; Kolarsky *et al.* 1967; Blumer 1970), there are reports of links with masochism and sado-masochism (Kolarsky *et al.*1967; Taylor 1947) and hypersexuality in the post-ictal state (Blumer 1970). Most of the case reports refer to an association with exhibitionism, disinhibition, and fetishism (Mitchell *et al.* 1954; Epstein 1961; Kolarsky *et al.* 1967; Hunter *et al.* 1963; Davies and Morgenstern 1960). Although not all patients reported responded to treatment, in some sexual deviancy was controlled by treatment with carbamazepine or psychosurgery.

Head injury has been identified as linked with sexual behaviour leading to exhibitionism, hypersexuality, deviant arousal including sexual sadism (Money 1990; Langevin *et al.* 1988). Hypersexuality has developed following unsuccessful brain surgery for temporal lobe epilepsy. Non-contact and contact offences following frontal lobe injury and frontal lobe syndrome have also been described.

Sexual deviancy associated with *degenerative disease*, including the dementias, Alzheimer's disease, Pick's disease alcoholic dementia, and frontal lobe dementia are described in the work of Burns *et al.* (1990) and Haddad and Bembo (1993). Although sexual deviancy is uncommon generally, in Alzheimer's disease it was identified in 7 per cent of the patients studied by Kumar *et al.* (1988) and Burns *et al.* (1990). Deviancy was defined as verbal disinhibition, indecent exposure, public masturbation, and minor sexual assaults, occurring equally in male and female patients. Pick's disease and alcoholic dementia specifically effect the frontal lobes and are associated with disinhibited sexual offending. The development of sexual delusions leading to erotomania and morbid jealousy are known to occur with Alzheimer's disease and alcoholic dementias.

Hypersexuality, disinhibition, and fetishism were described in the case report of patients suffering from multiple sclerosis with lesions in the frontal and temporal lobes (Huws *et al.* 1991). Although patients suffering from multiple sclerosis more often suffer from hyposexuality, erotomania has also been described. Dewhurst *et al.* (1970) described the development of erotomania and hypersexual drive in Huntington's chorea, Mullen and Maack (1985) noted the association between erotomania and Creutzfeldt–Jakob disease.

Research into a *hormonal basis* for sexual offending has failed to demonstrate any firm causation, Berlin (1983). Raboch *et al.* (1987), Langevin *et al.* (1988), and Hucker and Bain (1990) review the evidence in depth. No conclusive link with raised testosterone levels has been identified apart from a small group of violent rapists. No explanation has been found for the reason why men with low testosterone commit sexual offences. Low testosterone levels are found in patients with abnormal chromosomes (47,XXY), post-castration, and primary pituitary failure.

Other physical factors

Prescribed drugs have been implicated in causing sexual disinhibition and excessive masturbation with L-dopa prescribed for Parkinson's disease, and benzodiazepines (Goodwin 1971; Di Mascio 1973). One of us has assessed two cases, one of indecent exposure and one of an indecent assault in previously well-adjusted men without evidence of deviant behaviour prior to injection with testosterone for pituitary hypogonadism.

Offenders

In the past twenty years researchers and practitioners have become increasingly aware that the problem of sexual deviancy and the capacity for sexual offending is more ubiquitous than previously thought. The problem being demonstrated, not only by adult men, but also by women and young adolescents as well. Male offender epidemiology and profiles are discussed in depth in the literature (Araji and Finkelhor 1986). Data on the relatively under-researched female and adolescent offenders is described here.

Female abusers

Historically, women have been known to have had sexual contact with young children. Banning (1989) refers to the culturally acceptable behaviour in ancient civilizations and 19th-century France when children have been 'introduced' to sexual activity by adults. Wilkins (1990) refers to the mother/son soothing behaviour, 'for centuries mothers have been known to soothe boy babies to sleep by stroking and sucking their penises' and yet the thought of women as sexual abusers was considered unlikely until relatively recently. Jennings (1993) in her review of female sexual abuse literature, notes the observation of Katahara 'Japanese mothers typically initiate the sexual acts with their sons'. Earlier opinion was that women who sexually abuse tend to suffer from mental illness or handicap, most being psychotic, and the incidence rare. Mathis (1972) wrote: 'reports of female paedophilia were so rare as to be of little significance . . . in our society women are viewed as sexually harmless to children.' This view was upheld by the feminist movement (Banning 1989), hence their tenet 'no penis, no harm'. Female abusers were perceived solely as frightened co-abusers, too afraid to go against their male partner's wishes.

The problems of sexual stereotyping in the scientific investigation of female sexual abusers has been discussed in depth by Okami (1982). Welldon (1988) examines the issues of stereotyping and sexual deviancy in women, discussing the reluctance of society and indeed professionals to address the problem. Welldon (1993), referring to the BBC2 television documentary Open Space, 'Unspeakable Acts' highlighted the plight of women victims and offenders who have difficulty obtaining help because of their fear of professionals' disbelief.

Discrepancies in attitude towards female offenders are demonstrated within the criminal justice system as well as the psychiatric services. Wilkins (1990) refers to leniency and inconsistency in sentencing in comparison with sentences given to men convicted of similar offences.

The 1980s saw a growth of research, citing evidence of women as perpetrators (Banning 1989; Sheldrick 1991) with the development of public awareness in the late 1980s. Evidence to demonstrate the problem of female sexual offending against children can be found in the analytical literature, criminal statistics, offender case reports, victim studies, and general population surveys. Examination of the criminal statistics gives evidence of women prosecuted of sexual crimes ranging from pornography, soliciting, and exhibitionism through incest, indecent assault, and child abduction. In 1989, seven women were convicted of rape and 15 of other sexual offences in the United Kingdom. Many of the early case reports are contained in the analytical literature Welldon (1988) and refer to inter-generational incestuous relationships. Research into the incidence of child sexual abuse demonstrates increasing evidence for the role of women. Groth (1979) in his study of 348 adult male offenders identified that 31 per cent were the victims of child sexual abuse themselves, 41 per cent of this group abused by women. Petrovich and Templer (1984), examining 89 rapists, demonstrated that 59 per cent had experienced childhood sexual abuse by a woman before the age of 15. The abuse was described as often repeated and involving sexual intercourse. Finkelhor and Russell (1984), examining histories of abused boys and girls, demonstrated that 25 per cent of their sample of abused boys and 13 per cent of their abused girls had been assaulted by women. Becker and Kaplan (1988), examining boys charged with sexual offences, found that 27 out of 139 reported childhood sexual abuse, 40 per cent of this group by women. Although there was initial scepticism about reports of their own childhood sexual abuse by adult male perpetrators, the significance of childhood abuse, whether by male or female, as one of the multi-factorial components in the development of later sexual offending, is now acknowledged (Travin *et al.* 1990; Cooper 1990; Sheldrick 1991; Higgs *et al.* 1992). It is estimated that women currently comprise 5 per cent of the child sexual abusers in the United Kingdom.

Information from victims rather than victim/perpetrators is available in recent literature. In 1990, a telephone help-line 'Childline' was set up, and out of the 8600 callers, 9 per cent reported a woman as the abuser between 1 April 1990 and 31 March 1991. The mother was identified in 34 per cent, other female relative or acquaintance 22 per cent, sister 11 per cent, aunt 11 per cent, step-mother 11 per cent, and both parents together 11 per cent (Harrison 1993). Kidscape, a registered charity held the first British conference on female sexual abusers in 1992. Analysis of the telephone calls received from adults to their confidential help-line identified 32 men in an 18-month period who reported abuse by single female abuser in 23 cases, dual female abusers in one case, and duel female/male abusers in eight cases. In this group, the mother was identified as the abuser in 26 per cent. Of the 95 women who contacted in the same time period, 68 reported a single female abuser, six having dual female abusers and 21 dual male/female abusers. In this group of women the mother was identified in 68 occasions (Elliott 1993).

It is acknowledged that all samples from victim and perpetrator studies may be the subject of selection bias and not reflect true incidence in the general population. In the United States, Fritz *et al.* (1981), in a survey of male undergraduate psychology students obtained an incidence of 4.8 per cent reporting sexual abuse, of whom 60 per cent reported the abuser was female. Sexual abuse was defined as 'physical contact of an overtly sexual nature'. Also in the United States, Johnson and Shrier (1987), carried out a two-year survey of more than 1000 adolescent males attending a medical clinic, placing sexual questions in their general questionnaire given to all attendees. During the two years of the survey, 11 of the 25 patients identified as victims of sexual abuse, reported having been assaulted by females, 14 by males. Female abusers were usually acquaintances, 'often a neighbour, baby-sitter or other trusted older adult or young adult'. A quarter of the abused men reported sexual dysfunction at the time of assessment, all experienced the assault as highly traumatic. In their opinion it is likely that other abused subjects did not disclose, and that the incidence is higher. In Fromuth and Burkhart's (1989) study of US male college students, they identified a prevalence of between 13 and 15 per cent, with women identified as the abuser in approximately 75 per cent. Interpretation is limited by their definition of abuse including non-contact abuse and single abuse encounters.

Travin *et al.* (1990) summarized the epidemiological studies, and concluded that the apparently disparate reports of the incidence of female perpetrators illustrate the under-reporting typical of sexual abuse in general, and perhaps to a greater degree specifically when the abuser is female. They reviewed the types of offences committed by women. Knopp and Lackey (1987) demonstrated that 71 per cent of 911 offences of sexual abuse by females involve physical contact with the victim. Wolfers (1993) in her review of 10 women co-accused of abuse describes sexual, physical and emotional abuse of a serious nature. The myth that women can do no harm is still perpetuated by some, despite ample evidence that some *women are sexual aggressors*. Knopp and Lackey (1987) noted that there were slightly more male child/adolescent victims than female victims—61 per cent of the offences were incestuous.

The question of mother/son incest is considered by Banning (1989) and Travin *et al.* (1990). Estimates range from an identified incidence 2 per cent by Mrazek (1987) in the UK population, to more recent US studies by Finkelhor (1986), of 24 per cent in the offender population. The earlier view (Mathis 1972) that most incest female offenders were handicapped or mentally ill was examined by Margolin (1986), McCarty (1986), Faller (1987), and Krugman (1986); reviewed by Banning (1989). O'Connor (1987) studied 81 convicted female prisoners. This selected sample of imprisoned female sex-offenders demonstrates an association with mental illness, handicap, personality disorder, and substance abuse.

There is little evidence to support illness and handicap as causative factors in the majority of female offenders. Increasing evidence identifies social factors such as impoverished childhood associated with emotional, physical, and sexual abuse, multiple caretakers, traumatic parental separation, and alcoholic parents as developmental characteristics of female abusers (McCarty 1986). The women's need for an adult relationship regardless of cost overrides their ability to provide for the needs of their children. These women were often isolated, had married young, and in the case of co-offenders to have features of sexual indiscretion and multiple marriages. Accomplice (facilitating) offenders victims were more often their daughters (75 per cent) with an average age of the victim being 13. Co-offenders, male and female victims, were abused equally, their average age being slightly younger, between 7 and 9. Alcohol and substance abuse, including administration to children and violence is noted in multi-offender networks (Wolfers 1993).

In contrast, the independent offender, although having a troubled childhood and suffering significant sexual abuse, often by a brother (67 per cent) also married young but the majority lived independently as an adult without repeated marriages. Drug abuse was more prevalent in this group as was the estimation of emotional distress at the time of onset of abuse. In these cases, the victim was the daughter in 60 per cent with a mean victim age of 6 for girls and 10 for boys. The women in this group demonstrated a common theme of perceiving the child, especially daughter, as an extension of themselves.

Other typologies have been described by Faller (1987), Matthews *et al.* (1989), and Marvasti (1986). Researchers, such as Finkelhor and Russell (1984), attempt to explain the low incidence of child sexual abuse by women, given the accepted evidence that more female children are abused than boys and therefore could theoretically produce more female offenders. Factors identified as predictors of risk in males likely to go on to be an abuser themselves (Friedrich *et al.* 1989) are a high frequency of sexual abuse, close relationship between the perpetrator and victim, and severe forms of sexual abuse (e.g.), penetration, threats, and physical abuse). This view was supported by the work of Hindman (1989) who emphasized that violence formed the major risk factor for becoming a later offender. Browne and Finkelhor (1986), adding other predicting factors of serious sequelae of childhood sexual abuse, include the question as to whether the child was believed or not when they disclosed and the amount of support given at the time of disclosure. There is no reason why these risk factors should be limited to male children but it would seem that many more abused boys than girls go on to perpetrate sexual offences themselves. The effects of socialization and biological factors are reviewed by Finkelhor and Russell (1984), Sheldrick (1991), and Jennings (1993). A general trend of women tending to internalize the abuse, is the development of social and psychosexual dysfunction, phobias, eating disorders, somatization disorder, non-epileptic seizures, self-harm, substance abuse, and depression. In addition to neurotic disorders they may become sexually promiscuous, exhibit grave repeated self-harm, and in some cases fulfil the diagnostic criteria for borderline personality disorder. In contrast, male victims are purported to externalize the abuse, some acting-out in later offending behaviour. Although previous opinion was that sexual behaviour with an older woman was non-harmful, men now report sexual dysfunction, sexual orientation, and neurotic difficulties secondary to childhood abuse by females.

Rape perpetrated by women is still little researched, the nine cases reported in the criminal statistics 1989, referring to women who were accomplice offenders. O'Connor (1987) examined Home Office criminal statistics between 1975 and 1984 in England and Wales, identifying 462 female offences in comparison to the 48 234 sexual offenders (0.95 per cent) committed by men. He collected data on 81 women convicted of sexual offences in Holloway Prison over a 21-month period. In the 23 cases prosecuted for unlawful sexual intercourse, 21 of the women were accomplices to men, four were the mother, one a step-mother. In a comparable US study 1985, Musk and Gallagher (1985) reported that the majority of the 202 women prosecuted were charged as independent offenders. Travin *et al.* (1990) note that female arrests for rape have only been included in the uniform crime reports of the US Department of Justice since 1975.

Sadistic sexual fantasy described by patients suffering from borderline personality disorder with gender orientation difficulties is well known to clinicians dealing with the forensic patient population (Cooper *et al.* 1990; Sarrel and Masters 1982). Although extremely rare, murders of children as part of a sexual assault are committed by women. Myers' (1967) study of 93 children killed in Detroit over a 25-year survey identified three killed in a sexual assault. The majority of these murders were intra-familial, mothers implicated in 42 per cent of the cases. Psychosis was noted in 38 cases, especially marked in the accused mothers. Whether mental illness was implicated in the sexual killing is unclear. Kaplun and Reich (1976), analysing 112 child victims killed in New York City between 1968 and 1969, found that 2 per cent were killed as part of a sexual assault. Although the authors identified the mother as the most frequent assailant it is not clear from the data whether the mother was implicated in these sexual killings.

Male adolescent sex-offenders

Research into the age of onset of offending from interviews with adult offenders demonstrates that many begin in adolescence but are undetected (Longo and Groth 1983; Abel *et al.* 1987). In 1992, 14 persons were sentenced for sexual offences under Section 53 of the Children and Young Persons Act 1933 out of a total of 93 recorded offences. Recent research acknowledges the importance and adverse effects of sibling and cousin incest, child/child, and adolescent/child sexual abuse (Watkins and Bentovim 1992; Bentovim 1993). The authors note the change in attitude with recent acknowledgement of adverse effects on the victim, the associated finding that many of the abusing children and adolescents have themselves already been abused and the link with inter-generational abuse.

Davis and Leitenberg (1987) in their literature review report that approximately 20 per cent of all American rapes and 30–50 per cent of all cases of child sexual abuse can be attributed to adolescent offenders. Kempton and Forehand (1992) compared 15 adolescent sexual offenders with other non-sexual offenders, finding less evidence of conduct disorder and emotional difficulties than in the non-sexual offender group. Okami (1992) notes the change in social trend from the sexually permissive 1960s and 1970s to the moral crusade of the 1980s and 1990s. He warns that emotional over-reactive 'activism within this crusade' against child perpetrators of sexual abuse may have the effect of stimulating long entrenched cultural tendencies to respond to childhood sexuality with exaggerated, near hysteric alarm, thus contributing to the occurrence of another common form of child sexual trauma: adult over-reaction to discovery of voluntary peer sexual interaction.

Further research is required to identify the antecedent factors in adolescent offenders and specifically explain why non-abused patients of normal orientation and drive commit sexual assaults.

Female adolescent sex-offenders

Banning (1989), in her paper reviewing the evidence on female sexual offenders, highlights the poverty of data on female adolescent offenders. Davis and Leitenberg (1987) in their lengthy review of the literature on sexual offences committed by adolescents noted that they were not able to identify a comparative study of male and female adolescent offenders. They observed the limitations of the National Crime Survey as it does not include victims under the age of 12. Fehrenbach *et al.* (1986, 1988) described a group of 28 girls aged between 10 and 18 seen over a period of seven years who had been charged with sexual offences. They noted that baby-sitting often preceded the offence, that the girls offended alone, and had few prior criminal convictions, although all in the study had committed significant offences.

Female offenders have described a progression from genital fondling to oral sexual contact, digital masturbation, and finally, repeated sexual intercourse in some cases. Fehrenbach et al noted the victim's mean age to be 5.2 years. Fifty per cent of the offenders had previously been sexually abused, 20 per cent physically. Cavanagh Johnson (1989) describe 13 girls aged between 4 and 13 who used force and coercion in their sexual offences. Their victim's mean age was 4 years 4 months with an average number of victims per girl of 3.5 (range 1–15). Boys were abused twice as often as girls and 10 of the cases were intra-familial. All 13 girls had been sexually abused themselves, four physically abused and in a third of the cases this was by a family member.

Further work is necessary to understand sexual offending in young women. To date, there is no adequate explanation why young women who do not appear to have been sexually or physically abused themselves offend against young children. Available evidence on the incidence of child sexual abuse in general suggests that more female than male children are abused and yet proportionally fewer female child sexual abuse victims than men progress to become offending adults.

TREATMENT

The mainstay of treatment for the majority of sexual offenders is psychological intervention which is discussed in Chapters 11, 13, and 16. Psychiatrists increasingly tend to act in an assessment and advisory capacity, but often do not themselves provide psychological interventions. Physicians are specifically concerned with advice on the use of physical treatments. This section will therefore concentrate on an historical review of physical treatments used in the past and current practice.

Physical treatments

In the research of treatment efficacy reviewed by Marshall *et al.* (1991), there is good evidence that successful outcome is associated with psychological, cognitive, and behavioural interventions, in conjunction with adjuvant chemical therapy. The psychiatrist and general practitioner have a specific contribution to make in the assessment and treatment of offenders requiring pharmacological intervention. Historically, there have been two main forms of physical treatments for sex offenders, surgical and pharmacological.

The two main surgical interventions used have been psychosurgery and bilateral orchidectomy, 'castration'. Psychosurgery using sterotaxic tractotomy and limbic leucotomy, is reviewed by Bradford (1985). The technique was primarily used in Germany with evidence of success in the treatment of paedophilia, hypersexuality, and exhibitionism. Evidence is limited due to the small number of subjects in studies reported (Roeder 1966; Roeder *et al.* (1972). Consideration of the non-reversible invasive procedures, the issues of non-coerced informed consent, and the physical, intellectual, and emotional side-effects of the operations means that they are unlikely to be widely used given the available alternative pharmacological intervention.

Bilateral orchidectomy—castration—was used as a therapeutic intervention in Europe and America from the 19th century. Bradford reviewed the use and efficacy of orchidectomy in the 20th century. The treatment was mainly used for offenders convicted of rape but also paedophilia, other paraphilias, and exhibitionism. He notes the significant negative physical consequences for the offender with weight disturbance, gynaecomastia, and hot flushes, osteoporosis and bone pain in the older age group, and psychological sequelae such as depressive syndromes. Gunn (1993) reviewing the outcome of castration noted that 2–3 per cent of the rapist cohort reported by Stürup (1968) in Denmark committed suicide. The efficacy of the non-reversible surgery in reducing sexual recidivism reviewed by Bradford gives a range of re-offending between 1.3 and 10.8 per cent in the cohorts studied. Other studies (e.g., Heim and Hursch 1979), demonstrate that a proportion (18 per cent) continue to be potent despite castration.

Although studies demonstrate a significant reduction of the risk of recidivism from the pre-castration risk, ranging from 58 to 84 per cent, to post-castration rates of 1.2 to 2.3 per cent, the studies do not assist clinicians in being able to identify those offenders who are most likely to benefit from orchidectomy. It is known that 5 per cent of the body's testosterone is produced by the adrenal glands, which may explain the continued potency and associated sexual offending in some patients. The ethical dilemmas of therapeutic castration and medicolegal considerations are significant deterrents to the use of the technique, especially when reversible pharmacological alternatives exist. Therapeutic castration has not been used in Western European medicine since the 1970s. The issue was recently debated (Alexander 1993) by psychiatrists and a lawyer when a patient with a long history of paedophilia repeatedly requested therapeutic castration, having refused pharmacological intervention. The Mental Health Act Commission was consulted over the issue of consent and recommended that a decision be made on the basis of a consensus expert decision, having decided that the patient was capable of giving informed consent. The view of the Mental Health Act Commission is only relevant in cases where the patient suffers from a mental disorder in addition to sexual deviancy. Overall, expert opinion did not favour orchidectomy but recommended psychological intervention and adjunctive pharmacological therapy.

In the past twenty years the most important physical treatment method used has been pharmacological. The types of medication used to suppress sexual behaviour include the major tranquillizers, oestrogens, progestogens, luteinizing hormone-releasing analogue, antiandrogens, and serotonin re-uptake inhibitors. Clarke (1989) and Bradford (1990) review the use, efficacy, side-effects, and treatment outcome of the antiandrogen and hormonal treatments of sex offenders. The antipsychotic buterophenone, benperidol (Anquil), was first used in the 1960s in Belgium to control deviant and antisocial sexual behaviour because of the observed antilibidinal actions in patients with psychosis and associated inappropriate sexual behaviour (Sterkmans and Geerts 1966). The mode of action is uncertain, there is no demonstrable effect on testosterone or luteinizing hormone concentrations. It was used for both male and female patients, but largely fell out of favour due to the limited efficacy, side-effects, and alternative treatments.

Oestrogens were prescribed because of their action to suppress testosterone production, however the severity of side-effects including significant cardiovascular events and gynaecomastia associated with irreversibility of some of the effects led to its use declining. Progestogen, medroxyprogesterone acetate (MPA, Depo-Provera) is licensed and commonly used in North America and Australasia to treat a variety of paraphilias. Its mode of action is to accelerate testosterone metabolism, and inhibit pituitary secretion of luteinizing hormone, it needs to be given by weekly injection. Efficacy has been demonstrated in numerous studies since the first clinical report (Money 1986). Overall, studies demonstrate moderate efficacy (Kelly and Cavanaugh 1982). However, Kiersch (1990) failed to demonstrate unequivocal efficacy in a study of eight subjects in a double-blind trial of MPA and saline with each patient providing their own control. In addition to the problem of commonly reported side-effects, studies demonstrate that improvement is lost on cessation of treatment.

Although not licensed for the treatment of sexual deviancy, the luteinizing hormone-releasing analogue, goserelin acetate (Zoladex), has been used to reduce sexual drive in paedophilia. The use led to consideration as to whether consent to treatment from the Mental Health Act Commission was necessary under Section 57 of the Mental Health Act 1983. The matter was subject to judicial review reported by Dyer (1988). The High Court ruled that Section 57 was not appropriate as the treatment was not a hormone and not administered by surgical implantation. It was clarified that medication may only be given in such cases where it is prescribed for treatment of mental disorder and not when the diagnosis is solely sexual deviancy, which is excluded from the provisions of the 1983 Mental Health Act. Setting aside the controversy, goserelin acetate has not been subject to clinical trial in the treatment of sexual deviancy and is not the treatment of choice because of side-effects.

The antilibidinal synthetic antiandrogen, cyproterone acetate (CPA, Androcur), is recommended because of the antiandrogenic antigonadotrophic, and progestogational effects. Treatment is given by oral daily dose or weekly depot (the latter on a named patient basis in the United Kingdom). Bradford (1990) reviews the clinical studies of treatment with CPA since 1971. There is evidence of its application in a wide range of presenting sexual difficulties from the least serious exhibitionist to its use in the treatment of patients who have committed grave sexual crimes. Efficacy has been demonstrated with hypersexuality and deviant arousal (Jeffcoate *et al.* 1980; U. Laschet and L. Laschet 1975; Marshall *et al.* 1991; Neumann and Kalmus 1991). Scepticism has been expressed by Kockott (1983) and Torpy and Tomison (1986), but overall opinion supports its efficacy when appropriately prescribed. Bradford and Pawlak (1987) reported success in a case when all other treatment interventions had failed. Studies demonstrate a 75–80 per cent response rate, thereby demonstrating greater efficacy for CPA in contrast to other pharmacological agents (Neumann and Kalmus 1991). Studies of recidivism not only report significant reduction of risk whilst on medication but also lack of recurrent sexual deviancy on cessation of treatment in some cases. In addition to lowered sexual interest, drive and physical arousal, some patients report loss of deviant thought. Unfortunately, few clinicians acknowledge this important effect, believing wrongly that the medication produces chemical castration alone without modification of deviant thought. Cyproterone acetate is associated with side-effects but to a lesser degree than those reported in subjects treated with MPA.

Whether clinicians use MPA or CPA is largely dictated by their location, training, and product licensing. Overall, there is good evidence of the benefit of antiandrogenic treatment as adjunctive therapy. As in all treatment interventions, treatments should be selected for a specific task and not just prescribed because of sexual offending *per se*. Overall, patients who are not distressed by the effects of their offences on others are not suitable, the hypothesis being that antilibidinal agents are contraindicated for patients who make external causation or attributions about both positive and negative events.

When appropriately prescribed, antiandrogens reduce sexual drive, grant the patient greater capacity for self-control, relief from intrusive fantasy, and hence decrease their general anxiety level and increase their confidence and self-esteem. Compliance can be increased by engaging the patient in daily monitoring of their deviant thoughts and actions pre-treatment, and continued via monitoring during prescribing. As in other therapeutic interventions, self-monitoring can assist the patient to make the links between mood, cognitions, and actions, and enable them to learn how to use interventions including self-medication to avoid repetition of problem behaviours. By titrating the dose it is possible to enable the patient to engage in normal sexual behaviour whilst controlling unacceptable offending.

Adjunctive therapy can avoid the necessity for quarantine by imprisonment and allow time for psychological intervention. Unfortunately, despite good evidence of efficacy, the use of adjunctive therapy is still under-utilized by both treating psychologist and psychiatrist.

Numerous authors (Clarke 1989; Bradford 1985, 1990; Ferracuti 1977) have raised the ethical medicolegal issues of informed non-coerced consent, including the difficult area of treatment of patients in secure hospital and prison. Gangé (1981) suggests practical guidelines to ensure informed consent in the treatment of pre-trial cases by explaining the nature of the treatment to the patient and (when applicable) their lawyer and emphasizing that the treatment could be refused at any time. However, he unfortunately refused to treat imprisoned sex-offenders. Progress has been made over the years with opinion changing from the position that it would be incorrect to prescribe in the prison setting (Money *et al.* 1975; Ferracuti 1977; Gagné 1981) to a more considered point of view that there are conditions when it is appropriate to offer treatment or respond to prisoners' requests for treatment whilst detained or at the pre-parole stage (Halleck, 1981; Berlin 1983; Bradford 1990). Bowden (1991), drew attention to the inherent prejudice towards sexual offenders which contaminates clinicians' objectivity on occasions. Bowden raised the uncomfortable question of whether lack of medical treatment for offenders was linked to subconscious punitive attitudes. Clinicians who work regularly with offenders will be aware of numerous spontaneous accounts of patients/prisoners who report having requested medication from general practitioners, prison health care doctors, and psychiatrists in the past, only to be greeted with a response 'there is nothing for people like you'. Similarly, patients report their medication being stopped when received into prison. No clinician would consider stopping a patient's treatment, say thyroxine, on the grounds that he had a mild thyroid disorder and would be able to cope in prison without replacement therapy, but prison clinicians do stop antilibidinal agents on reception as they think they are no longer necessary. Patients have been observed to make serious suicide attempts because of the recurrence of intrusive deviant sexual imagery and thoughts on cessation of treatment. Treatment, albeit moderately expensive, should be continued in appropriate cases during detention to avoid distress, despair, and potential death. Although there is no obligation in law to obtain written consent, practitioners may feel less uneasy if they complete a simple contractual consent form. This can help to remind prescribers to explain fully the required effects and possible side-effects of the medication as well as document informed consent.

Pharmacological treatment of female deviant sexuality

Rothschild (1970) described 10 female patients in a group of 27 patients treated with cyproterone acetate (CPA). Saba *et al.* (1975) included four women in their cohort of 24 treated with CPA, Jost (1975) six women in a total of 16 patients. Mellor *et al.* (1988) reported a case of female hypersexuality treated with CPA; they referred to the work of Levine (1982) and Appelt and Strauss (1984). Medication was used for a variety of presenting complaints including hypersexuality, 'nymphomania', schizophrenia with associated sexual delusions, erotic aggressiveness, and exhibitionism not responsive to treatment with antipsychotic medication, patients with learning disability with associated hypersexuality, and depression and psychopathy associated with sexual deviancy. Treatment in most cases was in the form of a combination of CPA, 50 mg per day on days 5–15 of the menstrual cycle and ethinyloestradiol, 50 microgram per day on days 5–25. Although none of the three early papers break down results specifically into male and female cases, the overall comment was of treatment response in the women. Prolonged treatment is not recommended for women of reproductive age

Antidepressants

Kafka (1991*a*) summarizes the evidence for the role of antidepressants in the treatment of paraphilias, noting they have responded to imipramine, lithium, electroconvulsive therapy, and Busperidone. He describes clinical improvement in a patient diagnosed as suffering from voyeurism, paraphilic coercive disorder, and major depression when fluoxetine hydrochloride was prescribed as an adjunct to supportive psychotherapy. In addition to the expected improvement in the symptoms of depression and anxiety, the patient reported cessation of daily masturbation, loss of deviant fantasy, and the development of normal heterosexual fantasy. Deviant thoughts returned when medication was ceased. In the further case reports, Kafka (1991*b*), describes improvement in sexual deviancy and depression treated with fluoxetine, imipramine or lithium.

Eysenck and Rachman (1965) discussed the similarity of obsessional compulsive disorders and the compulsive quality of the paraphilias. They noted the similarity in the build-up of tension preceding compulsive acts and masturbation and the subsequent tension reduction.

The effect of antidepressant, fluoxetine, causing reduction in masturbation was observed by Perilstein *et al.* (1991) in two patients presenting with chronic depression and compulsive daily masturbation. Subsequent prescription and response to fluoxetine in three patients with paedophilia, exhibitionism, and voyeurism/frotteurism was reported. The patients had previously received a variety of other pharmacological agents and psychotherapy without success. Stein *et al.* (1992) reviewed the outcome in 13 patients presenting with paraphilias, sexual obsessions, and other sexual addictions treated with serotonin re-uptake blockers (clomipramine, fluoxetine, and fluoxamine). Nine of the patients studied had coexisting diagnoses of obsessional compulsive disorder, three of major depression. They observed a difference in the response to treatment with sexual obsessions and compulsions demonstrating better outcome in comparison with paraphilias and non-paraphilic sexual addiction. They discussed whether the treatment response was due to the side-effects of medication, but came to the same conclusion as Kafka that the response to treatment was different from medication side-effects. Their findings indicated that there may be a differential treatment response for sexual symptoms with a compulsive quality from those symptoms with a primarily impulsive component similar to other pleasurable or gratifying symptoms. Although the reason for the improvement following the serotonin re-uptake inhibitor is unclear, it merits further research.

The review of pharmacological interventions highlights the necessity for accurate case formulation, and drug treatment with antilibidinal agents or antidepressants where appropriate. The clinical observations should fuel future research which may unravel some of the enigmatic causes of sexually deviant behaviour.

Summary

Although much research and treatment of sexual offenders in the past 10 years has been carried out by psychologists, the psychiatrist continues to play an essential role in assessment and treatment because of their eclectic training and specific skills. Their continued involvement in research, specifically in areas of the relationship between mental disorder and offending and physical treatment should lead to better scientific understanding and more effective treatment interventions.

REFERENCES

Abel, G. G., et al. (1987). Self reported sex crimes of non-incarcerated paraphiliacs *J. Interper. Viol.* **2**, 3–25.

Alexander, M. (1993). Should a sexual offender be allowed castration? Ethical considerations in using orchidectomy for social control. *Brit. Med. J.* **307**, 790–3.

American Psychiatric Association (1987). *Diagnostic and Statistical Manual of Mental Disorders*, (3rd edn, revised. APA, Washington D.C.

Appelt, H. and Strauss, B. (1984). Effects of anti-androgen treatment on the sexuality of women with hyperandrogenism. *Psychother. Psychosom.* **42**, 177–81.

Araji, S. and Finkelhor, D. (1986). Abusers: A review of the research. In *Source book on child sexual abuse*, (ed. D. Finkelhor). Sage, London.

Arieff, A. J. and Rotman, D. B. (1942). Psychiatric inventory of one hundred cases of indecent exposure. *Arch. Neurol. Psychiat.* **47**, 495–8.

Banning, A. (1989). Mother–son incest: confronting a prejudice. *Child Abuse Negl.* **13**, 563–70.

Bearcroft, J. S. and Donovan, M. D. (1965). Psychiatric referrals from courts and prisons. *Brit. Med. J.* **ii**, 1519–23.

Becker, J. V. (1992). Sexual deviance. *Curr. Opin. Psychiat.* **5**, 788–91.

Becker, J. V. and Kaplan, M. (1988). The assessment of adolescent sexual offenders advances. *Behav. Assess. Child. Fam.* **4**, 97–118

Becker, J. V., Kaplan, M. S., Tenke, C. E., and Tartaglini, A. (1991). Incidence of depressive symptomatology in juvenile sex offenders with a history of abuse. *Child Abuse Negl.* **15**, 531–6.

Bentovim, A. (1993). Why do adults sexually abuse children? *Brit. Med J.* **307**, 144–5.

Berlin, F. (1983). Sex offenders: a biomedical perspective and status report on biomedical treatment. In *The sexual aggressor: Current perspectives on treatment*, (ed. J. G. Greer and I. R. Stuart). Van Nostrand Reinhold, New York.

Bleuler, E. (1911). *Dementia praecox: or the group of schizophrenias*. International University Press, New York.

Bluglass, R. (1980). Indecent exposure in the West Midlands. In *Sex offenders in the criminal justice system*, (ed. D. West). Cambridge University Press.

Bluglass, R. (1990). Bestiality. In *Principles and practice of forensic psychiatry*, (ed. R. Bluglass and P. Bowden). Churchill Livingstone, Edinburgh.

Blumer, D. (1970). Hypersexual episodes in temporal lobe epilepsy. *Am. J. Psychiat.* **126**, 1099–1106.

Bowden, P. (1991). Treatment: use, abuse and consent. *Criminal Behaviour and Mental Health*, **1**, 130–41.

Bradford, J. M. W. (1985). Organic treatments for the male sexual offender. *Behav. Sci. Law*, **3**(4), 355–75.

Bradford, J. M. W. (1990). The anti-androgen and hormonal treatment in sex offenders. In *Handbook of sexual assault*, (ed. W. Marshall, D. R. Laws, and H. E. Barbaree). Plenum, New York.

Bradford, J. M. W. and Pawlak, A. (1987). Sadistic homosexual paedophilia: treatment with cyproterone acetate: a single case study. *Can. J. Psychiat.* **32**, 22–30.

Brittain, R. P. (1968). Sexual asphyxia. In *Gradwohl's legal medicine* (2nd (edn), ed. F. E. Camps). Williams and Wilkins, Philadelphia.

Browne, A. and Finkelhor, D. (1986). Impact of child sexual abuse: a review of the research. *Psychol. Bull.* **99**(1), 66–77.

Burgess, A. W. (1984). *Child pornography and sex rings*. Heath, Lexington, MA.

Burns, A., Jacoby, R., and Levy, R. (1990). Psychiatric phenomena in Alzheimer's disease. IV: Disorders of behaviour. *Brit. J. Psychiat.* **157**, 86–94.

Cavanagh Johnson, T. (1989). Female child perpetrators; children who molest other children. *Child Abuse Negl.* **13**, 571–85.

Chiswick, D (1983). Sex crimes *Brit. J. Psychiat.* **143**, 236–42. Clarke, D. J. (1989). Anti-libidinal drugs and mental retardation: a review. *Med. Sci. Law*, **29**(2), 136–46.

Cooper, A. J. (1990). A female sex offender with multiple paraphilias, a psychologic, physiologic endocrine case study. *Can. J. Psychiat.* **35**, 334–7.

Cooper, S. A., Mohamed, W. N., and Collacott, R. A. (1993). Possible Asperger's Syndrome in a mentally handicapped transvestite offender. *J. Intell. Disabil. Res.* **37**, 189–94.

Cordess, C. (1990). Nuisance and obscene telephone calls. In *Principles and practice of forensic psychiatry*, (ed. R. Bluglass and P. Bowden). Churchill Livingstone, Edinburgh.

Craft, A., Craft, M., and Spencer, M. (1984). Sexual offences: intent and characteristics. In *Mentally abnormal offenders*, (ed. M. Craft and A. Craft), pp. 60–87. Baillière Tindall, London.

Craft, M. (1984). Low intelligence, mental handicap and criminality. In *Mentally abnormal offenders*, (ed. M. Craft and A. Craft), pp. 177–85. Baillière Tindall, London.

Craft, M. (1985). Low intelligence and delinquency. *Mental handicap: A multi-disciplinary approach*, (ed. M. Craft, J. Bicknell, and S. Hollins), pp. 51–7. Baillière Tindall, London.

Craissati, J. and Hodes, P. (1992). Mentally ill sex offenders—the experience of a regional secure unit. *Brit. J. Psychiat.* **161**, 846–9.

Davies, B. M. and Morgenstern, F. S. (1960). A case of cysticercosis, temporal lobe epilepsy and transvestism. *J. Neurol. Neurosurg. Psychiat.* **23**, 247–9.

Davis, G. E. and Leitenberg, H. (1987). Adolescent sex offenders. *Psychiat. Bull.* **101**, 417–27.

Day, K. (1988). A hospital-based treatment programme for male mentally handicapped offenders. *Brit. J. Psychiat.* **153**, 635–44.

Day, K. (1990). Mental retardation: clinical aspects and management. In *Principles and practice of forensic psychiatry*, (ed. R. Bluglass and P. Bowden). Churchill Livingstone, Edinburgh.

Dewhurst, K., Oliver, J. E, and McKnight, A. L. (1970). Socio-psychiatric consequences of Huntington's Disease. *Brit. J. Psychiat.* **116**, 255–8.

Di Mascio, A. (1973). The effect of benzodiazepines an aggression; reduced or increased? In *The benzodiazepines* (eds. S. Garattini, E. Mussini, and L. O. Randall). Raven Press, London.

Doctor, R. E. (1988). *Transvestites and transsexuals: Toward a theory of cross-gender behaviour*. Plenum, New York.

Dyer, C. (1988). Chemical castration controversy. *Brit. Med. J.* **297**, 640.

East, W. N. (1924). Observations on exhibitionism. *Lancet*, **2**, 370.

Elliott, M. (ed.) (1993). What survivors tell us—an overview. In *Female sexual abuse of children, the ultimate taboo*, (ed. M. Elliott), pp. 5–14. Longman, Harlow.

Epstein, A. W. (1961). Relationship of fetishism and transvestism to brain and particularly to temporal lobe dysfunction. *J. Neurol. Ment. Dis.* **133**, 247–53.

Eysenck, H. J. and Rachman, S. (1965). *The causes and cures of neuroses*. Routledge & Kegan Paul, London.

Faller, K. C. (1987). Women who sexually abuse children. In *Violence and victims*, Vol. 2, pp. 263–76. Springer Publishing Company, New York.

Fehrenbach, P. A., *et al.* (1986). Adolescent sexual offenders: offender and offence characteristics. *Am. J. Orthopsychiat.* **56**, 225–33.

Ferracuti, F. (1977). Medico-legal considerations pertaining to anti-androgens. In *Androgens and anti-androgens*, (ed. L. Martini and M. Moppa) Raven, New York.

Finkelhor, D. (1986). Abusers: special topics. *A source book on child sexual abuse*, (ed. D. Finkelhor). Sage, London.

Finkelhor, D. and Russell, D. (1984). Women as perpetrators In *Child sexual abuse: New theory and research*, (ed. D. Finkelhor), pp. 171–85. Free Press, New York.

Flor-Henry, P. (1987). Cerebral aspects of sexual deviation. In *Variant sexuality: Research and theory*, (ed. G. D. Wilson). Johns Hopkins University Press, Baltimore.

Freud, S. (1905/1953). Three essays on the theory of sexuality. In *Complete psychological works of Sigmund Freud*, (Standard edition, Vol. 7). Hogarth Press, London.

Friedrich, W., Urquiza, A., and Bielke, R. (1989). Behaviour problems in sexually abused young children *J. Paediat. Psychol.* **11**, 45–57.

Fritz, G. T., Stoller, K., and Wagner, N. (1981). A comparison of males and females who were sexually molested as children. *J. Sex. Marital Ther.* **7**, 54–9.

Fromuth, M. E. and Burkhart, B. R. (1989). Long-term psychological correlates of childhood sexual abuse in two samples of college men. *Child Abuse Negl.* **13**, 533–42.

Furby, L., Weinrott, M. R., and Blackshaw, L. (1989). Sex offender recidivism: a review *Psychol. Bull.* **105(1)**, 3–30.

Gagné, P. (1981). Treatment of sex offenders with medroxyprogesterone acetate. *Am. J. Psychiat.* **138**, 644–6.

Gibbens, T. C. N. and Robertson, G. (1983). A survey of the criminal careers of hospital order patients. *Brit. J. Psychiat.* **143**, 362–9.

Gittleson, N. L. and Levine, S. (1966). Subjective ideas of sexual change in male schizophrenics. *Brit. J. Psychiat.* **112**, 779–82.

Glasser, M. (1990). Paedophilia. In *Principles and practice of forensic psychiatry*, (ed. R. Bluglass and P. Bowden). Churchill Livingstone, Edinburgh.

Goodwin, F. K. (1971). Behavioural effects of L-dopa in man. *Seminars Psychiat.* **3**, 477–92.

Groth, A. N. (1979). Sexual trauma in the life histories of rapists and child molesters. *Victimology*, **4**, 10–16.

Grubin, D. and Gunn, J. (1990). *The imprisoned rapist and rape*. Department of Forensic Psychiatry, Institute of Psychiatry, Home Office, London.

Gunn, J. (1993). Castration is not the answer. *Brit. Med. J.* **307**, 790–791.

Haddad, P. M. and Benbow, S. M. (1993). Sexual problems associated with dementia: I. Problems and their consequences. *Int. J. Geriat. Psychiat.* **8**, 547–51.

Halleck, S. L. (1981). The ethics of antiandrogen therapy. Editorial. *Am. J. Psychiat.* **138**(5), 642–3.

Harrison, H. (1993). Female abusers—what children and young people have told Childline. In *Female sexual abuse of children, the ultimate taboo*, (ed. M. Elliot), pp. 95–8. Longman, Harlow.

Heim, N. and Hursch, C. J. (1979). Castration for sex offenders: treatment or punishment? A review and critique of recent European literature. *Arch. Sex. Behav.* **8**, 281–304.

Higgins, J. (1990). Affective psychoses. In *Principles and practice of forensic psychiatry*, (ed. R. Bluglass and P. Bowden). Churchill Livingstone, Edinburgh.

Higgs, D. C., Canavan, M. M., and Meyer, W. J. (1992). Moving from defense to offense: the development of an adolescent female sexual offender. *J. Sex. Res.* **29**(1), 131–9.

Hindman, J. (1989). *Just before dawn*. Alexandria Associates, Oregon.

Hirschfeld, M. (1936). *Sexual anomalies and perversions*, (limited edn). Frances Aldor, London.

Hoare, S. and O'Brien, G. (1991). The impact of the Mental Health (Amendment) Act 1983 on admissions to an interim regional secure unit for mentally handicapped offenders. *Psychiat. Bull.* **15**, 548–50.

Howells, K. and Hollin, C. (1991). Sex offenders and victims: overview and conclusions. In *Clinical approaches to sex offenders and their victims*, (ed. C. Hollin and K. Howells). Wiley, Chichester.

Hucker, S. (1990a). Sexual asphyxia. In *Principles and practice of forensic psychiatry*, (ed. R. Bluglass and P. Bowden). Churchill Livingstone, Edinburgh.

Hucker, S. (1990b). Necrophilia and other unusual philias. In *Principles and practice of forensic psychiatry*, (ed. R. Bluglass and P. Bowden). Churchill Livingstone, Edinburgh.

Hucker, S. and Bain, J. (1990). Androgenic hormones and sexual assault. In *Handbook of sexual assault*, (ed. W. L. Marshall, D. R. Laws, and H. E. Barbaree). Plenum, New York.

Hunter, R., Logue, V., and McMenemy, W. H. (1963). Temporal lobe epilepsy supervening on long-standing transvestism and fetishism. *Epilepsia*, **4**, 60–3.

Huws, R. Shubsachs, A. P. W., and Taylor, P. J. (1991). Hypersexuality, fetishism and multiple sclerosis. *Brit. J. Psychiat.* **158**, 280–1.

Jeffcoate, W. J., et al. (1980). The effect of cyproterone acetate on serum testosterone, LH, FSH and prolactin in male sexual offenders. *Clin. Endocrinol.* **13**, 189–95.

Jennings, K. T. (1993). Female child molesters: a review of the literature. In *Female sexual abuse of children, the ultimate taboo*, (ed. M. Elliott). Longman, Harlow.

Johnson, R. L. and Shrier, D. (1987). Past sexual victimization by females of male patients in an adolescent medicine clinic population. *Am. J. Psychiat.* **144**, 650–2.

Jones, G., Huckle, P., and Tanaghow, A. (1992). Command hallucinations, schizophrenia and sexual assaults *Irish J. Psychol. Med.* **9**, 47–9.

Jost, F. (1975). Treatment of abnormal sexual behaviour with the anti-androgen cyproterone acetate (1971–1975). *Inform. Arzt*, **3**(8), 303–9.

Kafka, M. P. (1991a). Successful antidepressant treatment of non-paraphilic sexual addictions and paraphilias in men. *J. Clin. Psychiat.* **52**, 60–5.

Kafka, M. P. (1991b). Successful treatment of paraphilic coercive disorder (a rapist) with fluoxetine hydrochloride. *Brit. J. Psychiat.* **158**, 844–7.

Kaplun, D. and Reich, R. (1976). The murdered child and his killers. *Am. J. Psychiat.* **133**, 809–13.

Kelly, J. R. and Cavanaugh, J. L. (1982). Treatment of the sexually dangerous patient. *Curr. Psychiat. Ther.* **21**, 101–11.

Kempton, T. and Forehand, R. (1992). Juvenile Sex Offenders: similar to or different from other incarcerated delinquent offenders? *Behav. Res. Ther.* **30**(5), 533–6.

Kennedy, H. G. and Grubin, D. (1992). Patterns of denial in sex offenders. *Psychol. Med.* **22**, 191–6.

Kiersch, T. A. (1990). Treatment of sex offenders with Depot Provera. *Am. Acad. Psychiat. Law*, **18**(2), 179–87.

Klaf, F. S. and Davis, C. A. (1960). Homosexuality and paranoid schizophrenia: a survey of 150 cases and controls. *Am. J. Psychiat.* **116**, 1070–5.

Klüver, H. and Bucy, P. (1939). Preliminary analysis of functions of the temporal lobes in monkeys. *Arch. Neurol. Psychiat.* **42**(6), 979–1000.

Kockott, G. (1983). Treatment of sex offences with anti-androgens. *Psychiat. Prax.* **10**, 158–64. (in German with abstract in English).

Kolarsky, A. *et al.* (1967). Male sexual deviation. *Arch. Gen. Psychiat.* **17**, 735–43.

Knopp, F. H. and Lackey, L. B. (1987). Female sexual abusers: a summary of data from 44 treatment providers. The Safer Society Program of the New York State Council of Churches, Orwell, VT.

Krugman, R. (1989). Recognition of sexual abuse in children. *Paediat. Rev.* **8**, 25–39.

Kumar, A., *et al.* (1988). Behavioural symptomatology in dementia of the Alzheimer type. *Alzheimer's Dis. Assoc. Disord.* **2**, 363–5.

Langevin, R. (1990). Inappropriate sexual behaviour in adolescent boys. *Topics Hum. Sex.* **2**, 3.

Langevin, R., *et al.* (1988). Sexual sadism: brain, blood and behavior. *Ann. N. Y. Acad. Sci.* **528**, 163–71.

Lanyon, R. I. (1991). Theories of sex offending. In *Clinical approaches to sex offenders and their victims*, (ed. C. R. Hollin and K. Howells). Wiley, Chichester.

Laschet, U. and Laschet, L. (1975) Antiandrogens in the treatment of sexual deviations of men. *J. Ster. Biochem.* **6**, 821–6.

Laws, D. R. and Marshall, W. L. (1990). A conditioning theory of the etiology and maintenance of deviant sexual preference and behaviour. In *Handbook of sexual abuse: Issues, theories and treatment of the offender*, (ed. W. L. Marshall, D. R. Laws, and H. E. Barbaree). Plenum, New York.

Lee-Evans, M. (1986). The direct assessment of sexual skills in an institutional setting. Sexual assessment: Issues and radical alternatives. In *Issues in criminological and legal psychology*, (ed. P. Pratt), **8**, 8–17.

Levine, S. B. (1982). A modern perspective on nymphomania. *J. Sex. Marital Ther.* **8**, 316–24.

Levine, M. P. and Troiden, R. R. (1988). The myth of sexual compulsivity. *Journal of Sexual Research*, **25**(3), 346–63.

Lishman, W. A. (1987). *Organic psychiatry*. The psychological consequences of cerebral disorder, (2nd edn.) Blackwell, Oxford.

Longo, R. E. and Groth, A. N. (1983). Juvenile sexual offences in the histories of adult rapists and child molesters. *Int. J. Offender Ther. Comp. Criminol.* **27**, 150–5.

MacEachron, A. E. (1979). Mentally retarded offenders: prevalence and characteristics. *Am. J. Ment. Defic.* **84**, 165–76.

Margolin, L. (1986). The effects of mother–son incest. *Lifestyles: A Journal of Changing Patterns*, **5**, 104–14.

Marshall, W. L. and Barbaree, H. E. (ed.) (1990). An integrated theory of the etiology and maintenance of sexual offending. In *Handbook of sexual assault: Issues, theories and treatment of the offender*, (ed. W. L. Marshall, D. R. Laws, and H. E. Barbaree). Plenum, New York.

Marshall, W. L., *et al.* (1991). Treatment outcome with sex offenders. *Clin. Psychol. Rev*, **11**, 465–85.

Marvasti, J. (1986). Incestuous mothers. *Am. J. Forensic Psychiat.* **7**, 63–9.

Mathis, J. (1972). *Clear thinking about sexual deviations: a new look at old problems.* Nelson-Holt, Chicago.

Matthews, K., Matthews, J., and Speltz, K. (1989). Female sexual offenders: an exploratory study. Safer Society Press, Vermont.

McCarty, L. (1986). Mother–child incest: characteristics of the offender. In *Child Welfare*, **65**, 447–58.

Mellor, C. S., Farid, N. R., and Craig, D. F. (1988). Female hypersexuality treated with cyproterone acetate. *Am. J. Psychiat.* **145**(8), 1037.

Mitchell, W., Falconer, M., and Hill, D. (1954). Epilepsy with fetishism relieved by temporal lobectomy. *Lancet*, **II**, 626–30.

Mohr, J. W., Turner, R. E., and Jerry, M. B. (1964). *Pedophilia and exhibitionism.* University of Toronto Press.

Monahan, J., Kantorowski Davis, S. (1983). Mentally disordered sex offenders. In *Mentally disordered offenders perspectives from law and social science*, (ed. J. Monahan and H. J. Steadman), pp. 191–204. Plenum, New York.

Money, J. (1986). *Lovetraps*. Irvington, New York.

Money, J. (1990). Forensic sexology: paraphilic serial rape (Biastophilia) and Lust Murder (Erotophonophilia). *Am. J. Psychother.* **XLIV**(1), 26.

Money, J. *et al.* (1975). Combined anti-androgen and counselling programme for treatment of 46 XY and 47 XYY sex offenders. In *Hormones, behaviour and psychopathology*, (ed. E. Sachar), pp.105–20. Raven, New York.

Mrazek, P. (1987). Definition and recognition of sexual child abuse. In *Sexually abused children and their families*, (ed. P. Mrazek and C. H. Kempe). Pergamon, Oxford.

Musk, H. and Gallagher, K. (1985). Sexual and physical abuse among women inmates and their families: A national survey. *Survey conducted with the support of the American Correctional Association*.

Mullen, P. and Maack, L. (1985). Jealously, pathological jealousy and aggression. In *Aggression and dangerousness*, (ed. D. P. Farrington and J. Gunn). pp. 103–26. Wiley, Chichester.

Murrey, G. J., Briggs, D., and Davis, C. (1992). Psychopathic disordered, mentally ill, and mentally handicapped sex offenders: a comparative study. *Med. Sci. Law*, **32**(4), 331–6.

Myers, S. A. (1967). The child slayer. A 25 year survey of homicides involving preadolescent victims. *Arch. Gen. Psychiat.* **17**, 211–13.

Neumann, F. and Kalmus, J. (1991). Cyproterone acetate in the treatment of sexual disorders: pharmacological base and clinical experience. *Exp. Clin. Endocrinol.* **98**(2), 71–80.

O'Connor, A. (1987). Female sexual offenders. *Brit. J. Psychiat.* **150**, 615–20.

Okami, P. (1992). Child perpetrators of sexual abuse: the emergence of a problematic deviant category *J. Sex. Res.* **29**(1), 109–30.

Perilstein, R. D., Lipper, S., and Friedman, L. J. (1991). Three cases of paraphilias responsive to fluoxetine treatment. *J. Clin. Psychiat.* **52**, 169–70.

Perkins, D. (1982). The treatment of sex offenders. In *Developments in the study of criminal behaviour.* Vol.1: *The prevention and control of offending*, (ed. P. Feldman). Wiley, Chichester.

Perkins, D. (1986). Sex offending: a psychological approach. In *Clinical approaches to criminal behaviour*, (ed. C. Hollin and K. Howells). Wiley, Chichester.

Petrovich, M. and Templer, D. I. (1984). Heterosexual molestation of children who later become rapists. *Psychol. Rep.* **54**, 810.

Pitcher, D. (1990). Fetishism In *The principles and practice of forensic psychiatry*, (ed. R. Bluglass and P. Bowden). Churchill Livingstone, Edinburgh.

Planansky, K. and Johnstone, R. (1962). The incidence and relationship of homosexual and paranoid features in schizophrenia. *J. Mental Sci.* **108**, 604–15.

Prins, H. (1990). Mental abnormality and criminality—an uncertain relationship. *Med. Sci. Law*, **30**, 247–58.

Quinsey, V. L. (1977). The assessment and treatment of child molesters. *Can. Psychol. Rev.* **18**, 204–20.

Raboch, J., Cerna, H., and Zemek, P. (1987). Sexual aggressivity and androgens. *Brit. J. Psychiat.* **151**, 398–400.

Rada, R., *et al.* (1983). Plasma androgens in violent and non-violent sex offenders. *Bull. Am. Acad. Psychiat. Law*, **11**, 149–58.

Reid, A. (1990). Mental retardation and crime. In *Principles and practice of forensic psychiatry*, (ed. R. Bluglass and P. Bowden). Churchill Livingstone, Edinburgh.

Roeder, F. D. (1966). Stereotaxic lesion in the tuber cinereum in sexual deviation. *Confin. Neurol.* **27**, 162–3.

Roeder, F. D., Orthner, H., and Müller, D. (1972). The stereotaxic treatment of paedophilic homosexuality and other sexual deviations. In *Psychosurgery*, (ed. L. Hitchcock, Laitinen, and K. Vaernet), pp. 87–111. Thomas, Springfield, IL.

Rogers, R., Gillis, J. R., Turner, R. E., and Frise-Smith, T. (1990). The clinical presentation of command hallucinations in a forensic population. *Am. J. Psychiat.* **147**, 1304–7.

Rooth, F. G. (1971). Indecent exposure and exhibitionism. *Brit. J. Hosp. Med.* **5**, 521–33.

Rothschild, B. (1970). Psychiatric–clinical experience with an anti-androgen preparation. *Schweiz. Med. Wschr.* **100**, 1918–24.

Ryle, A. (1989) *Cognitive–Analytic therapy: Active participation in change*. Wiley, Chichester.

Saba, P., *et al.* (1975). Anti-androgen treatment in sexually abnormal subjects with neuropsychiatric disorders. In *Sexual behaviour: Pharmacology and biochemistry*, (ed. M. Sandler and G. L. Gessa). Raven, New York.

Sarrel, P. M. and Masters, W. H. (1982). Sexual molestation of men by women. *Arch. Sex. Behav.* **11**(2), 117–131.

Sheldrick C (1991) Adult sequelae of child sexual abuse. *Brit. J. Psychiat.* **158**(Suppl. 10), 55–62.

Snaith, P. and Bennett, G. (1990). Exhibitionism, indecent exposure, voyeurism and frottage. In *Principles and practice of forensic psychiatry*, (ed. R. Bluglass and P. Bowden). Churchill Livingstone, Edinburgh.

Stein, D. J., *et al.* (1992). Serotonergic medications for sexual obsessions, sexual addictions and paraphilias *J. Clin. Psychiat.* **53**, 267–71.

Sterkmans, P. and Geerts, F. (1966). Is benperidol the specific drug for the treatment of excessive and disinhibited sexual behaviour? *Acta Neurol. Psychiat. Belg.* **66**, 1030–40.

Storr, A. (1990). Sadomasochism. In *Principles and practice of forensic psychiatry*, (ed. R. Bluglass and P. Bowden). Churchill Livingstone, Edinburgh.

Sturgeon, V. and Taylor, J. (1980). Report of a five-year follow-up study of mentally disordered sex offenders released from Atascadero State Hospital in 1973. *Crim. Just. J. W. State University, San Diego*, **4**, 31–64.

Stürup, G. K. (1968). Treatment of sexual offenders in Herstedvester, Denmark: the rapists. *Acta Psychiat. Scand. Suppl.* **204**(44).

Sugarman, P. *et al.* (1994). Dangerousness in exhibitionists. *J. Forensic Psychiat.* **5**(2), 287–96.

Taylor, F. H. (1947). Observations on some cases of exhibitionism. *J. Mental Sci.* **93**, 631.

Tidmarsh, D. (1990). Schizophrenia. In *Principles and practice of forensic psychiatry*, (ed. R. Bluglass and P. Bowden). Churchill Livingstone, Edinburgh.

Torpy, D. and Tomison, A. (1986). Sex offenders and cyproterone acetate—a review of clinical care. *Med. Sci. Law*, **26**(4), 1279–82.

Travin, S., Cullen, K., and Protter, B. (1990). Female sexual offenders: severe victims and victimizers. *J. Forensic Sci.* **35**, 140–50.

Wakeling, A. (1979). A general psychiatric approach to sexual deviation. In *Sexual Deviation*, (2nd edn), (ed. I. Rosen). Oxford University Press.

Walker, N. and McCabe, S. (1973). *Crime and insanity in England, new solutions and new problems*, Vol.2. Edinburgh University Press.

Watkins, B. and Bentovim, A. (1992). Male children and adolescents as victims: a review of current knowledge. In *Male victims of sexual assault*, (ed. G. C. Mezey and M. B. King). Oxford University Press.

Welldon, E. V. (1988). *Mother, madonna, whore*. Free Association Books, London.

Welldon, E. V. (1993). Women who abuse women. *Brit. Med. J.* **306**, 1206.

Wildenskov, H. O. T. (1962). A follow up of subnormals originally exhibiting severe behaviour disorders or criminality. In *Proceedings of the London Conference on the Scientific Study of Mental Deficiency*, pp. 217–22. May & Baker, Dagenham.

Wilkins, R. (1990). Women who sexually abuse children. *Brit. Med. J.* **300**, 1153–4.

Woolf, S. C. (1985). A multi-factor model of deviant sexuality. *Victimology*, **10**, 359–74.

Wolfers, O. (1993). The paradox of women who sexually abuse children. In *Female sexual abuse of children, the ultimate taboo*, (ed. M. Elliot). Longman, Harlow.

Wulach, J. S. (1983). Mania and crime: a study of 100 manic defendants. *Bull. AAPL*, **11**, 69–75.

2
Integrating the general psychoanalytical theory of perversion

Ismond Rosen

INTRODUCTION

This chapter collates current psychoanalytical research with the existing general theory of perversion. See also chapter reviews in previous editions by Gillespie (1964), Rosen (1979) and recent work by Socarides (1988) and Chapter 11, and Etchegoyen (1989).

The last fifteen years have produced many advances in the psychoanalytical understanding and treatment of perversion. Knowledge has come from a better understanding of the typologies in the paraphilias; the treatment of severe personality disorders, narcissistic and borderline states, and gender disorders; and the relationship between sex and aggression in various kinds of sexual abuse and violence. These advancements in our knowledge of the etiological factors in perversion are described in the relevant chapters. Because of the variance of approach and theoretical presentation by different schools of analytic thought, emphasis in this chapter is given to significant points of concurrence or divergence of opinion.

BRIEF HISTORICAL REVIEW OF THE CONCEPT OF PERVERSION

Freud's *Three essays on the theory of sexuality* (1905) is the basis of the psychoanalytic understanding of perversion. This work is still essential reading together with *A child is being beaten* (1919), *The economic problem in masochism* (1923), and *Splitting of the ego in the processes of defence* (1940).

Although the libido theory was only formulated in 1915, Freud (1905) described infantile sexual drives that were operative during the first four or five years of life. This was contrary to the prevailing view that sexuality began at puberty. The drives were regarded as having an aim and an object, and were linked unconsciously in pairs of opposites, such as activity and passivity, looking and touching, sadism and masochism. The object could be the child's body, or an external object such as the breast, the mother herself, or any other person, creature, or inanimate object. Infantile sexuality differed in organization from the adult and underwent a series of phase development in both sexes. These phases were the oral and anal, or preoedipal phase, followed by the genital or oedipal phase, depending on which erotogenic zone was predominant. Although particular drives were prominent during a specific phase, the other drives were also operative. Genital sensations, such as erections, were present in the oral and anal phases, while oral and excretory pleasures persisted subsequently in diminished fashion. The latency phase followed the oedipal phase, during which time sexual drives abated under various pressures. These were the unconscious influence of reaction formations, such as shame and disgust, the development of a sense of guilt, and the defences of sublimation, inhibition, regression, and repression. Freud regarded repressed sexual drives as the source of neurotic symptom formation. At puberty, biological changes occurred leading to adult sexuality. The infantile sexual drives matured and constituted an important element in adult foreplay.

Freud distinguished sexually deviant individuals from normal according to their sexual objects and aims. Those who chose as their sexual object someone of the same sex he referred to as inverts. Those with deviations concerning their sexual aim he referred to as suffering from a perversion, a term borrowed from Krafft-Ebing. In adult perversions the aim of heterosexual genital copulation was either in abeyance, secondary, or unsatisfying. The reason given for the perversion was that a hypertrophied partial infantile sexual drive had deprived the normal adult functioning of its genital primacy. Looking had turned into voyeurism; touching into frotteurism or sexual harassment; showing into exhibitionism; and sado-masochism, from being a ubiquitous ingredient of human behaviour, into a need to inflict humiliation, or cruelty, Freud pointed out the close connection between perversion and normality, where social attitudes, operating through variable attitudes of shame and disgust, determined the acceptability of sexual practices.

Freud's explanation for the quality and intensity of the hypertrophied partial drive in the perversions, was that they arose from a combination of biological and developmental factors. He conjectured that there was an interaction of body chemistry together with traumatic factors of early sexual experience such as seduction. This book continues these lines of inquiry, combining studies of biology and human psychological development.

CLINICAL FEATURES IN THE DEFINITION OF PERVERSION

Perversion differed from sexual normality not in the strength or content of the drive, but in its exclusiveness and fixation. Deviant or perverse sexuality meant a sexual preference that departed from the norm of heterosexual coitus with orgasm. It was as if sexual foreplay had grown in intensity and importance to take over the role of genitality itself.

The elements of compulsion and fixity are well known. McDougall (1972) extended their scope in her definition. 'One factor that would appear to characterize the pervert . . . is that he has no choice; his sexuality is fundamentally compulsive.' 'The erotic expression of the sexual deviant is an essential feature of his psychic stability and much of his life revolves around it.' She added that in perverse character traits there was a conscious erotization of the defences.

A distinction must be made between perverse behaviour and the pathological syndrome of perversion. In both, the sexual behaviour derives from infantile sexuality which becomes predominant, as a single component, or as alternating polymorphous perverse elements. In perversion, there is the characteristic of repetitive fixed behaviour that leads to orgasm, and which facilitates potency. Such an act or preoccupation might be the need to look at or exhibit the sexual organs, to experience or to afflict pain, as a necessity for the attainment of sexual satisfaction. The preferred sexual mode originated in some aspect of the aims and objects of an infantile component drive. The aims could be sucking, excretory, masturbation, or identification with the opposite sex. The objects could be at the level of part-object, transitional object, or whole-object, and with the same or the opposite sex. The result was that adult heterosexual genital intercourse became impossible, unsatisfying, or facilitated only by the perverse act.

Freud also drew conclusions about the relationship between perversion and neurosis. He regarded repressed infantile sexual wishes as the source of psychoneurotic symptoms. Perversions differed from neurosis in that a partial infantile sexual drive had become a consciously acceptable source of sexual satisfaction. In the neurotic, the resistances of shame, disgust, and guilt were prominent. In the perversions, in opposite fashion, these reaction formations are diminished or in abeyance, in relation to the hypertrophied infantile sexual drive. Freud therefore coined the phrase 'neuroses, are so to say, the negative of perversions'. In both perversion and neurosis, it was usual to find more than one instinct involved, in keeping with Freud's description of the polymorphous perverse nature of infantile sexuality.

Freud's theory of sexual development was that the partial instincts of earliest infancy became integrated initially under the influence of genital primacy in the phallic phase preceding latency, and permanently organized from puberty onwards. It cannot be stressed sufficiently that perversion is the interference with integrated genital sexuality by a component drive. This is revealed in maturity where one aspect of foreplay predominates in pleasure over the sexual act itself. Fenichel (1945) following Freud, postulated that perversion was due to a disturbance of genital primacy for which the partial component instinct was a substitution. He sought to determine the nature of the disturbance of genital primacy. As genital primacy commenced at the time of the phallic phase and oedipal complex, he postulated that it was the accompanying castration anxiety which undid the integrating genital primacy. Anxiety led to regression to preoedipal infantile sexuality because genital enjoyment had become too threatening and therefore impossible. The infantile component chosen was determined by previous fixations, and he largely discounted the influence of constitutional factors. Alexander (1965) thought perversion could result either from the fixation of partial drives, or be due to regression where disintegrative forces led to the genital patterns of psychic function breaking down into their components.

Balint (1965) writing on 'Perversions and genitality' pointed out that all perversions have genital pleasure as their final aim, although the perversion was usually concerned with the quality of experience gained from the object in foreplay. During coital orgasm, all persons required the capacity and the willingness to allow themselves to regress emotionally. This mature regressive capacity was the prerequisite for sexual gratification, plus the resulting tranquil contentment and sense of well-being. The achievement of this regression presupposed a well-integrated ego which had mastered castration anxiety. All perverts avoided this regression due to their ego weakness, lack of integration, faulty mastery over anxiety (especially castration anxiety), and their faulty sense of reality, which was similar to that found in neurotics but defended against in a different way.

Ostow and his group (1974) found significant differences in the role of the genitals in defining perversion, 'perverse behaviour usually occurred in two distinct phases; the specific perverse activity, followed by apparently normal intercourse in which the person's potency was augmented by the antecedent perverse behaviour'. They also believed that the occurrence of normal intercourse did not invalidate the diagnosis of perversion. In their experience it was common to find married persons with perverse patterns expressing the perverse sexuality extra-maritally, while continuing a 'lack-lustre and perfunctory' sex-life, which appeared normal, within the marriage. Such cases are known to most workers within this field. In my clinical experience, sexual excitement remains attached to the perverse object and practice, and normal intercourse may not occur, or be emotionally irrelevant, in keeping with a pseudo-genitality.

There seems general agreement that in the perversions, whatever the source of the initial erotic stimulation, which is where the height of gratification may lie, the final common pathway of sexual discharge is genital orgasm. Impotence or inadequacy of genital discharge in the absence of the perverse mechanism being exercised, is a hallmark of perversion.

The libidinal aspects of the perverse, or infantile, sexual wishes have long been stressed. Fenichel regarded the original childhood sexual fixations as having been chosen for their reassuring effect against fear, having been experienced in childhood as providing feelings of security, which warded off the anxiety of castration and therefore made genital functioning possible again. Later in the chapter we shall deal with the origins of the hyper-libidinization, or hypertrophy of the libidinal aspects of the component infantile sexual drives. The hyper-libidinization provides the intense pleasure in the practice of the perversion, which, flooding the ego, reassures against castration anxiety, and makes the perverse act realizable even at the cost of inappropriate behaviour that is out of keeping with reality.

Aggression

A growing body of evidence is now confirming the role of aggression in the aetiology of perversion. Childhood frustrations and traumas lead to an intensification of the aggressive drives in the child, which increases the sadism of the oral and anal phases, as well as the phallic castration anxiety. This will be discussed in detail later. For the clinical aspects of aggression, libido, and perversion, see Chapter 13.

Stoller has selected aggression, in the form of hatred, to be one of the major elements in his definition of perversion. In his book *Perversion: the erotic form of hatred* (1975a), he regards hostility as the primary motive in perversions, which 'takes form in a fantasy of revenge hidden in the actions that make up the perversion and serve to convert childhood trauma to adult triumph'. The trauma according to Stoller is always aimed at the sense of gender. Stoller's examination of the meaningfulness of the trauma and revenge theme in terms of the self and its narcissistic evaluation are valuable, because this theme is found in all perversions to some degree. Because of the small size of the sample of cases studied by Stoller, who were mainly gender disorders, it is doubtful if the valuation placed by him on these factors regarding aetiology is generally valid.

Ego aspects

Perversion usually implies a sexual act of some kind which is insistent and gratifying. This behaviour may be ego-syntonic, that is to say freely acceptable by the self, or, quite often after the event, ego-dystonic, experienced as unacceptable. It is frequently the threat of discovery or police arrest which makes the person request for help. Running risks introduces the element of excitement which raises self-esteem.

Object relationships

Perversion always takes as its object something representing a primary object, usually the mother. The sexual object may be some feature of the self; it may be symbolized by some material if the use of the material is necessary for sexual fulfilment; or some other person may play a carefully defined role. However, where there are strong narcissistic elements in the personality a partner may be dispensed with, and the perversion may be indulged in a solitary fashion. The function of perversion for narcissistic purposes has been stressed by Greenacre, while Rosen (1964, 1968, 1979) explored the idea of perversion as a regulator of self-esteem (see Chapter 3).

In those cases where the criteria for the presence of perversion are met, there are often additional signs of mental disturbance. Mention has been made too of the concurrence of psychosomatic disorders in homosexuality, as evidence of the early disturbances in body–ego function. See also Sperling (1968) and McDougall (1972).

Homosexuality as perversion

The question of whether homosexuality deserves to be classified as a perversion is dealt with in Chapters 9, 10, and 11.

Balint (1965) placed homosexuality among the perversions on the basis of 'the atmosphere of pretence and denial that is so characteristic of the other group of perversions'. 'This overemphasis is in order to deny—what they all know—that, without normal intercourse, there is no real contentment'.

Ostow's group considered perversion and homosexuality as two aspects of the same disorder because of their frequent association. They justified this approach on the grounds that:

(1) the developmental arrest required for one appeared to favour the other;
(2) both phenomena represented infantile fixations, with respect to the object in homosexuality and to the aim in perversion;
(3) narcissism, infantilism, and acting-out were common to both perversion and homosexuality; and
(4) homosexuality was sometimes used as a defence against other forms of sexual deviation which would become predominant in heterosexual relationships if they were permitted.

They qualified their view by the statement that homosexual behaviour need not be perverse under certain social conditions, and where there is no 'quality of compulsion and fixity'.

The importance of compulsion and fixity of homosexual behaviour would appear to be supported by the work of Limentani (1976) in his study 'Object choice and actual bisexuality'. He presented cases which revealed a protracted capacity for both heterosexual and homosexual relationships. These people commonly had borderline and narcissistic states. Their underlying psychopathology included a tendency to be caught up between anaclitic and narcissistic types of object choice. Their bisexual involvement was basically illusory, as the two objects, male and female, with whom they were involved were a cover up for splitting of the original love-object together with a severe preoedipal disturbance. (See Chapter 9)

Chasseguet-Smirgel (1991) regarded the homosexualities as a continuum. With closeness to neurosis at one end and psychosis at the other, and ranging through perversion in the middle. The chief aim of perverse homosexuality was to destroy and debase fertile genital parental intercourse.

Balint made an important point about object relationships in the perversions. Such people remained fixated in their loving to what he called 'primary love'—a partnership where only one partner may have desires, wishes, and interests. This diminished capacity for object relationship will be examined later, but it is as well to point out here that in the extreme case the fetishist may come to rely on an object that is not only symbolic but purely inanimate. Balint asserted that in perversion there was an escape from the necessity of the work of conquest with the partner, where initial indifference was changed into a co-operative genital sexual partnership. This raises important issues of classification where permissive attitudes towards sexuality may have led to increased promiscuity. Promiscuity, like the professional counterpart, prostitution, is a disorder of object relationships. The degree to which character disorder, neurosis, or sado-masochism plays a part must be determined in each case. Promiscuity as a perversion depends on the degree to which the behaviour is compulsive, necessary for the attainment of satisfactory orgasm, and fixed to a violation of cultural attitudes, plus the association of overt perverse practices which are disguised because of the sado-masochistic features.

Not all sado-masochistic relationships are perverted and therefore must be separated from true perversions. In the former, the sexual and social conquest has been made, but the relationship in its basic sexual and social meaningfulness has regressed and withered leaving the elemental battle for control over one partner, or over each other, based on emotional blackmail. Such relationships I would more properly regard as 'cruelty relationships' because of the libidinal de-cathexis of the relationship leading to hard-hearted indifference, denial of the feelings of the partner or of both, and the accent on cruel attitudes and personal gratification at the expense of the partner, who remains under subtle control and trapped in the situation. Some people cruelly use multiple objects to gratify separate urges—for sex, for domestic purposes, for comfort against loneliness. In the cruelty relationship, the aim of the sado-masochism is not sexual gratification leading to orgasm, but a raised self-esteem from controlling the object and inflicting punishment in lieu of the primary frustrating and controlling mother.

Aetiology of the perversions

In this review chapter there is an advantage in presenting the theoretical view of perversion which pertained in the early 1960s followed by an account of the evolution in psychoanalytic thinking leading to present day understanding.

Gillespie's general summary of the psychoanalytic theory of perversion (1964) was as follows.

> The essence of the theory is still to be found in Freud's *Three Essays on the Theory of Sexuality*. It is impossible to begin to understand sexual perversions without a knowledge of infantile sexuality, of its peculiar features, its development and vicissitudes, and of the transformations which it normally goes through at puberty before emerging as adult sexuality.
>
> Nevertheless, what we encounter clinically in cases of perversion is by no means, or only rarely, a simple continuation into adult life of all the elements of infantile sexuality. On the contrary, most clinical perversions are highly specialized and specific; that is, only very limited ways remain open to the adult pervert for achieving sexual excitement, discharging sexual tension and establishing a sexual object relationship. A clinical perversion of this kind has a very obvious defensive function, with the aim of warding off anxieties concerned with the Oedipus complex, and especially castration anxiety. It is, therefore, in the nature of a compromise between instinctual impulse and ego defence, and in this way closely resembles a neurotic symptom.
>
> The defences adopted in perversion involve regressions of various kinds—regression of libido to pregenital levels, and regression too in the aggressive impulse: together this leads to an increase in sadism, which gives rise to further anxieties specific to the dangers both to the object and to the self which are inherent in sadism, and to consequent defences designed to ensure the safety of both.
>
> The behaviour of the ego in perversion is especially characteristic; instead of an attitude of hostility to the instincts, dictated by super-ego pressure (as in neurosis), the ego adopts as its own one particular piece of infantile sexuality, and this helps it to oppose the rest. The result depends on a super-ego which is tolerant of this specific aspect of sexuality. Splits in the ego and in the object make possible attitudes to reality, confined to the sexual sphere, which, if more widespread, would lead to a psychosis.

Greenacre (1968) listed the areas best studied to enlarge our knowledge of the perversions:

1. Theories of aggression.
2. Studies of ego maturation and function.
3. Studies of separation and individuation.
4. Stages of object relationship.
5. Body-image development.
6. Early body–ego formation.
7. Development of self-representation.
8. Problems of identity.

Particular reference to these areas will be made in the study of the aetiology of perversion, which will be under four headings:

(a) factors contributing to the formation of the perverse drive component;
(b) early development factors;

(c) ego mechanisms and organization; and

(d) perversion as a regulator of self-esteem (see Chapter 3).

Formation of the perverse drive component

Actiological factors in perversion are best studied by examining major elements in development in isolation, and then trying to understand how they interact to produce psychic organization of structure and function. These are charted in Fig. 2.1.

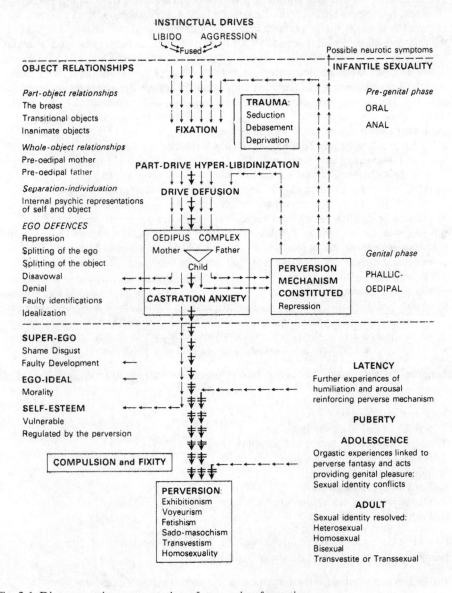

Fig. 2.1 Diagrammatic representation of perversion formation.

Infantile sexuality has a polymorphous perverse quality, which may lead to many different perverse aims being present in an organized perversion. Usually there is the intensification of only a single or partial drive which becomes the core of the perverse strivings. The drive intensification, according to the literature, stems from a combination of constitutional and environmental factors. Constitutional elements were considered by Freud: (i) as a general cause of perversion and neurosis, where both were found to occur in the same family (1905; (ii) as precursors of the weakness of the urge towards the normal sexual aim; and (iii) in the person's final attitude to sex not being determined until puberty. Bisexual tendencies were regarded as having a constitutional basis, as was the capacity for sexual pleasure from parts of the body other than the genitals.

Constitutional factors are not much better understood now, although we prefer to regard them as biological or hereditary. The biological factors underlying sexuality are dealt with in Chapters 1 and 18. On the hereditary side, there are several reports of perversions occurring within the same family—transsexualism (Hore *et al.* 1973; Hoenig and Duggan 1974), masochism (de M'Uzan 1973). Genetic factors in transsexualism were examined by Wålinder and Thuwe (1977) who studied 61 cases of transsexualism in Sweden, where excellent records exist for family relationships dating back to the 17th century. No case of cousin marriages was disclosed, although there was a normal assumption of 1–2 cousin marriages per 100 marriages in Sweden. This was against the hypothesis of recessive genes playing a part in the causation of transsexualism. Genetic influences in homosexuality have been reviewed by Bancroft (1975) for males, and Kenyon (1975) for females. The conclusions they drew were that genetic factors in some cases sensitized the individual to certain environmental influences, but did not necessarily influence the direction of the libido directly.

Isay, a gay psychoanalyst (1984, 1985, 1986, 1989, 1991, 1992) quoted by MacIntosh (1994), asserted that homosexuality was constitutional in origin, and stemmed from an independent line of normal sexual development. Any effort to change a homosexual was therefore abusive. Isay's assertion that analysts identified with society's negative attitude towards homosexuals was refuted by a survey conducted by MacIntosh in Washington, USA. 285 psychoanalysts responded to the survey and 'reported having analysed 1215 homosexual patients, resulting in 23 per cent changing to heterosexuality and 84 per cent receiving significant therapeutic benefit. Virtually all the respondents rejected the idea that a homosexual patient in analysis "can and should" change to heterosexuality, although 17 per cent had reached their opinion during the last ten years. Over a third believed that most other psychoanalysts hold this opinion even if they themselves do not. The contention of some gay activists that "traditionally trained" psychoanalysts harm and "abuse" their patient is examined and rejected.' A similarly hopeful approach to the psychotherapy of homosexuals is contained in the books edited by Socarides and Volkan (1991) and Nicolosi (1991). Rose (1994) examined homophobia among a small sample of doctors, 20 heterosexual and 8 gay. In many, their attitudes to treating homosexuals were not ethically based, but were influenced by ideology and the values of the culture. For reviews of the biological basis of homosexuality, see Bancroft (1994) and Friedman and Downey (1994). Miron Baron (1993), reviewing genetic linkage studies in male homosexual orientation, urged caution in accepting the finding of studies by Hamer *et al.* (1993) that a supposed gene for homosexuality had been located on chromosome Xq28. Methodological uncertainties hampered the results, which required repeating by others (too specialized for examination here, but discussed in Chapter 18). Bancroft (1994) makes the point that if the characteristic of homosexuality was determined solely by biological factors, it would be inconceivable that no counterpart could be found in other species. There is scant evidence in other species of sexual preference that is clearly innate and not the result of learning. He concludes that sexual orientation is a consequence of a multifactorial developmental process in which biological factors play a part, but in which psychosocial factors remain crucially important. Stoller (1975*b*) concurred that biological potentialities were subject to environmental influences for realization. Hereditary, as well as normal factors, producing variable drive intensities are discussed by Bee Brockman and Robert Bluglass in Chapter 1. In general, the effect of biology on drives and in perversion in particular remains unresolved, and clinical analysts still think in terms of a constitutional and environmental interaction producing psychic determinism.

The psychological reasons advanced for increased drive intensity in perversion are based on childhood sexual trauma due to seduction and deprivation, singly or in combination. Freud (1905) showed that seduction had both drive and object consequences. Perverse sexuality was 'an innately human characteristic in children, brought out by seduction' (p. 191). 'Seduction is confusing in that it presents children prematurely with a sexual object for which the infantile sexual instinct shows no great need'. See also Chapter 14 and 15.

In early childhood, pre-genital sexual seduction is traumatic because the intensity of the experience is beyond the infant's capacity to endure. The ego anxiety aroused by being invaded and out of control is countered by the hyper-libidinization accompanying the pleasure in the experience. The pleasure arising from the closeness and sense of togetherness of the encounters is experienced when they cease, as loneliness and loss, which contributes to the longing to repeat the experience. Actual loss is perceived as traumatic when active separation, deprivation, or rejection follows the seductions, or is interspersed with them. The inner perceptions of the self in relation to external objects are therefore somewhat distorted in the direction of a narcissistic orientation, with the pleasure–pain modality exceptionally sensitized. The ego attempts to regain mastery of these events by the compulsive repetition of traumatic aspects of pleasure and frustration and the defence of turning passive experience into activity done to others. The most important result of seduction is the hyperlibidinization or erotization, which is mobilized with the defences together with the increased aggressive feelings that are engendered. There is therefore libidinization of anxiety, ego defences, aggressive drives, as well as the accompanying affects. Libidinization of the narcissistic constellations also occurs to protect the emerging self from the traumas of being mastered, overwhelmed, and devalued, following the libidinal overvaluation from the erotic experiences.

It is generally accepted that what has been said about the aims of the drives in perversion could be equally true for neurosis. The early theoretical difference between perversion and neurosis was that the drives suffer different fates. The developmental barrier of castration anxiety led to drive repression in neurosis, but to sexual gratification of the drive in perversion. Freud's 1905 dictum, 'neurosis is the negative of perversion' is not accutate. Sachs (1923) was credited with having shown that perversion also has defensive organizational functions similar to neurosis, which was why symptoms of perversion and neurosis occur in the same person. Sachs described a mechanism in perversion, where the highly developed partial-drive with its powerful pregenital pleasure aspects was taken up into the ego and used in the repression of other wishes, aggressive and libidinal, stemming from oedipal conflicts that could not pass the castration anxiety barrier. These repressed conflicts could become linked to earlier fixations that unconsciously provided a sense of comfort and security, or they could be expressed through neurotic symptom formations. The pregenital powerful partial drive (with its object representation) passed through the Oedipus complex where it formed relationships of a special kind, which accounted for the preoedipal fixations manifesting as oedipal pathology. The manoevre whereby the perverse wish is taken up by the ego, and used in the service of repression of other unwelcome oedipal wishes, constitutes the mechanism of perversion from the point of view of the libido theory. The high degree of pleasure in the perverse infantile sexual component entering the ego is what enables it to pass the castration barrier, and to be further developed as puberty and adolescence into the full-scale perversion. (See Fig. 2.1.)

In passing it must be stressed that perversions always contain the element of conflict. Because of the apparent freedom of action and the high degree of pleasure and urge, the view has been aired that a conflict-free aspect may exist in perversion together with the traditional conflictual basis of psychic symptomatology. Some non-analysts prefer to exclude psychic conflict in perversion, because it signifies inner motivation. This approach, for example, makes it easier to attribute homosexuality to biological or social causes, which eliminates the need for treatment due to the supposed organic or statistically acceptable aetiology. This does not fit the facts found in analytical treatment situations, where perversions including homosexuality, relate to complex defence systems dealing with the unconscious conflicts of infantile sexuality, gender identity, and object relationships, especially the separation–individuation experiences and transitional object fixations. The latter phenomena are dealt with in Chapter 4 by Phyllis Greenacre, with special reference to fetishism, but they play a significant role in perversions generally. Conflict may be considered to arise from the following sources:

(a) the libidinal and aggressive drives;
(b) loving and hating affects in the relationships with parents and siblings at the pregenital as well as the oedipal level. The objects and the self must be protected from the aggressive and destructive wishes;
(c) masculine and feminine identity aims, based on biological bisexuality and the later conflicts of identification with parental figures; and
(d) castration anxiety, especially the need to protect the genitals, and in the boy, the need to maintain primacy of the penis. The analogues in the girls are discussed by McDougall (1972).

I now turn to aggression, which, in the period under review, has come very much to the fore in the study of perversion. Distinction must be made between aggression as a drive, and aggression as hostility derived from frustration (see Chapter 12). Freud regarded libido and aggression as the two basic drives normally existing together in a fused state, which gave to sexuality the impulse for mastery over the object of desire. What was fused together could conversely undergo various degrees of defusion. The sadistic aspects of the normal pregenital phases, oral and anal, were accompanied by the ambivalent loving and hating attitudes towards the same object. These disparate tendencies only became integrated later, during the phallic or genital phases. The drive regressions due to castration anxiety led, in the perversions, to an increase in instinctual defusion. The degree of defusion was reflected later in the variable intensity of sado-masochism in the perverse sexual and emotional life. Pronounced sado-masochism featuring as the major characteristic in a perversion resulted from the aggregation of several additional factors.

One case of sado-masochism reported by Ostow was described as having the aggression 'commingled' rather than completely fused with the erotic elements, so that there was no attenuation of each other. Instinctual fusion–defusion is a continuum, with the sadism of normal infantile phase development at one end, the developed sado-masochistic perversion at the centre, and at the other extreme, uncontrolled acts of violence and destruction which could be sexualized, as in rape or sexual murder. In general, the high degree of libidinization in perversion serves to bind the increased aggression and hostility, so that physical damage is rarely done to others. Danger occurs when the perversion fails, that is to say there is insufficient libido to contain the aggression, the perverse mechanisms are deficient, or there has been hyper-abundant aggression aroused by threats to the self and its preservation in reality.

In masochistic perversions, there is a conflict between the hostile wish and the placatory expiation of guilt to preserve the loved object. There appears to be a relation between the severity of the adult perversion and the severity of the traumatic experiences in childhood. The following clinical vignette exemplifies this and many other features of a perversion which will serve as an introduction to the next sections on object relationships and identification.

One patient had a lifestyle of a masochistic surrender of assets and opportunity. His sexual gratifications were perverse and required him to be beaten by prostitutes. He had idealized fantasies of loving and possessing beautiful young women, which he felt to be impossible to realize, but he was tempted to make sexual advances to very young girls which he feared would lead to his arrest. Most of his earnings went in supporting an alcoholic ex-prostitute, and he cared for her every want. He was a well-educated, mild-mannered, and softly spoken person, who lived alone. In childhood his identical twin brother died of illness. The triumph of his normal twin-rivalry death-wish was short-lived. He was present at a prestigious consultation where his parents were told he too was not expected to live—an attitude descriptive of his life thereafter in a masochistic sense. His mother who had previously been very close became withdrawn, and his oedipal conflicts and father rivalry were accentuated. He responded to all of this with passivity, unconsciously atoning and surviving by refusing to live. The aggression in the underlying conflict was turned against himself and libidinized. The masochism was also a defence against the underlying sadness and loss of the attachment to the brother. The conflicts he had experienced about actual closeness between himself, his twin, and his mother, were enacted in his symbiotic 'life-saving' dealings with the prostitute, where he reversed the roles of mother and child, turned passive into active, and exercised his primary identification with the feeding mother, and a dual identification with father and mother at the oedipal level.

This case is instructive for many reasons. It demonstrates the fact that beneath masochism there is an opposite unconscious fantasy of omnipotent mastery, which gains pleasurable gratification through suffering. The patient's sexual impulses and their being granted satisfaction in reality, signified the possibility of suffering and punishment, whether there was orgasmic relief or not. His main source of fulfilment was compliance–defiance, with his inner super-ego dominance, and a merging narcissistic submission to demands. Falling in love with a girl at work resulted in his losing his job. His basic aim in treatment was not to obtain relief, but to gain help in avoiding impulsive acts towards young girls. During treatment, aggressive impulses with masochistic aspects predominated, but were bound by the hyper-libidinization. Preoedipal fears of annihilation served to augment his castration anxiety, and a massive regression ensued. Frankly paranoid ideas emerged which supported Kohut's idea that if a great variety of polymorphous perverse acts presented in the perversion, a borderline condition lay underneath. The perversion assisted in covering the flaw in his reality sense (Glover 1964). Most of the analytical material described above was uncovered only after much treatment. Lihn (1971) has described a similar case of masochism which stresses the importance of the real preoedipal experiences of traumatic suffering and erotic experiences which were repeated in a similar pattern in adulthood. The oedipal aspects were distorted, and there were regressions to the libidinized fixations. The whole complicated picture can only be understood in all such cases as having 'a constructive function—the recovery of narcissistic integrity' (de M'Uzan 1973).

This author described a case of unusually severe masochism; the patient had a masochistic cousin, whom he married, and a father who was also masochistic. Constitutional factors were indicated in this case to explain the ego's reaction to pain, which was such as to require an escalating degree of torture for the sought-after sexual ejaculation to occur. The masochistic perverse sexual pleasure was secondary, however, to the main aim of humiliation. The self-renunciation and striving for total humiliation was to fulfil a uniquely intense fantasy, that in this way he could heal his underlying primordial narcissistic wound. This unique case was previously documented in French in the excellent publication *La sexualité perverse* (de M'Uzan 1972).

In these cases, the fantasies and passive experiences of being beaten corroborate recent findings in the literature. Most males with beating fantasies are likely to maintain an identification with a castrated mother, and this identification may obscure identification with, and a vengeful fury toward, the phallic mother. The accomodation becomes then, a solution of the oedipus complex in negative terms (Ostow). In the Novicks' (1972) study of beating fantasies in children, they found that in severely disturbed children, the beating fantasy could be called a 'fixed fantasy', because once formed it remained a relatively permanent part of the child's psychosexual life. The basis of such fixity lay in the early masochistic tie to the mother, together with severe wide-ranging masochistic pathology and accompanying ego disturbances. In their material 'the beating fantasy was not formed until the phallic-oedipal stage was reached, but the primary determinants of the beating wish which was discharged in the fantasy are pre-oedipal'.

The question of masochism in females has been reviewed by Blum (1977) in relation to female personality development and the ego-ideal. The conclusion was reached that female masochism was a residue of unresolved infantile conflict, and was neither essentially feminine nor a valuable component of mature female function and character. There was no evidence of any particular female pleasure in pain. It was important to distinguish between masochistic suffering as a goal in itself (which if it gives pleasure is a perversion), and tolerance for discomfort or deprivation in the service of the ego or ego-ideal.

In the march of psychological science, we are apt to give greater emphasis to more recent discoveries, especially with regard to their aetiological significance. This is particularly true with relevance to the importance of pre-genital versus phallic-oedipal factors in the genesis of perversion. Obviously both are important and contributory—we have to know how they interact and function on the lengthy organizational pathway a perversion must traverse before being fully formed. Bak's (1968) views are illuminating. He considered valid his 1956 observations of the over-excitation of the aggressive drive in infancy and its deleterious influence on all libidinal phases, which called attention to aggressive conflicts and the defences used against them, for example, the substitution of sexual—perverse—solutions via regression to safe-guard this object. He felt that new discoveries had tended to shift the emphasis of aetiology of the sexual perversions away from the castration complex and the phallic phase towards pregenital factors such as orality and separation–individuation. Bak still agreed with Freud that no percursors of the castration complex can diminish the importance of the phallic phase. He therefore attempted to integrate the interplay of castration anxiety, the aggressive conflict, and the early identifications, in his understanding of the perversions. Three main points were postulated:

1. Common to all perversions is the dramatized denial of castration.
2. Perverse symptoms are regressive adaptions of the ego to secure gratification without destroying the object and endangering the self which is identified with the object (Bak 1956).
3. In all perversions the dramatized or ritualized denial of castration is acted-out through the regressive revival of the fantasy of the maternal phallus. This primal fantasy constitutes the psychological core of the bisexual identification (Bak 1968).

Because of the central position of castration anxiety in the aetiology of the perversions, and its relationship to earlier traumas, a brief description of the conflicts and phenomena underlying castration anxiety now follows.

Castration anxiety

Castration anxiety, which is clearly placed in the phallic-oedipal phase, stems from certain basic fears:

1. The fantasized loss of the penis in the boy is given credence by his witnessing the female genital area, and the variable shock effect on finding the penis missing.
2. The oedipal rivalry with the father for possession of mother and for intimacy with her, is accompanied by destructive wishes to castrate the father and the fear of his retaliation. The ensuing guilt augments the castration fear as a punishment.

3. Other conflicts contributing to castration anxiety are bisexuality, expressed as identification with mother in the negative oedipal aspects, with father as the preferred partner; sadistic impulses towards the mother; the perversion of the earlier fantasy of the phallic mother and the presence of the maternal phallus.

Consideration of what provokes castration must be qualified by the factor of degree. The suddenness of any of these experiences, the shock effect, lack of understanding by the child, and the accompanying humiliation, overt fear, or anxiety, are highly productive of a traumatic response. The specific traumas of the phallic phase should be considered in the light of any possible additional cumulative trauma (Khan 1963) continuing from earlier phases. The mother, instead of acting as a protective shield, subjects the child to body–ego stresses and strains emanating from their faulty relationship.

The recent psychoanalytic literature on masochism and sado-masochism deals with developmental factors (Mollinger 1982; Grossman 1986, 1991a, 1991b; Glenn 1989; Novick and Novick 1987, 1991), character disorders (Cooper 1989, Finell 1992, and perversion (Chasseguet-Smirgel 1991; Kernberg 1991). Hanly (1993) discussed the sado-masochism in Charlotte Brontë's *Jane Eyre* (see Vols. 38 and 39, *Journal of the American Psychoanalytic Association*). Novick and Novick (1987) defined masochism as 'the active pursuit of psychic or physical pain, suffering or humiliation in the service of adaptation, defence, and instinctual gratification at oral, anal and phallic levels'. Each phase alters the masochistic impulses, so that there is no question of their origin being preoedipal or oedipal in origin. Masochistic perversions and moral masochism have this underlying fantasy structure in common, which in their opinion is the 'essence of masochism'. In a later paper (1991) Novick and Novick drew attention to a 'delusion of omnipotence' that infuses the patients' previous and current functioning. This omnipotence of thought and deed constitutes a major component of the resistance so prominent in masochistic patients. This has been a vital resistance in many of my own masochistic patients. These authors trace this omnipotence developmentally, concluding that it has survival value as it defends against feelings of total deadness. Glickhauf and Wells (1991) reviewed current conceptualizations of masochism and object relationships. They defined masochism as a self-defeating way of loving and individuating. Masochists sought fusion with a primary object with whom separation was impossible. To heal an old narcissistic injury they tried to make rejecting and critical objects love them. They tended to make relationships with borderline and narcissistic characters who fulfilled their masochistic need for an idealized symbiosis, but who recapitulated the erratic environment of the masochist's childhood.

Cooper (1989) drew attention to the masochistic character's use of every external opportunity to suffer disappointment, rejection and humiliation. This was in order to satisfy the unconscious fantasy of control over a cruel and damaging mother. In similar fashion to narcissistic character disorders, infantile omnipotent fantasies were converted into a façade of normal narcissistic strivings, which, unlike the narcissistic characters, were used in the service of masochistic strivings. The defences were extremely complex, which made their analysis of the transference very difficult.

Finell (1992) described the sadomasochistic defensive style in narcissistic and borderline characters. These types complemented each other, with one partner being exploitative, grandiose, and dominant, and the other experiencing humiliation, neediness, helplessness, and the terror of aloneness. The complementary dynamics drew on the defences of projection, enactment, and externalization, all of which were difficult to analyse.

Kernberg (1991) regarded sado-masochism as a component of infantile sexuality that was part of all the 'partial drives'. It was an essential part of normal sexual functioning, love relationships, and of the very nature of sexual excitement. Sado-masochism elements were also present in all the sexual perversions. Sado-masochistic represented a very early capacity to link aggression with the libidinal elements of sexual excitement. Sexual excitement may be considered a basic affect that overcomes primitive splitting of love and hatred. Erotic desire was a more mature form of sexual excitement. The unconscious components of sexual excitement were 'wishes for symbiotic fusion and for aggressive penetration and intermingling; prohibitions and the secretiveness of the primal scene, and to violate the boundaries of a teasing and withholding object.' 'Normal sexual excitement and erotic desire presented all the elements characteristic of perversion, such as idealization, regressive analization and regressive cannibalism in the form of the fantasied destruction of the interior of the mother's body.' What becomes specific of the perversions is the restriction of erotic desire because of oedipal prohibition and threat of castration in higher-level functioning patients. In more primitive disturbed patients, there is the threat of diffuse destructiveness—the loss of capacity for differentiated relations with a sexual object.

Kernberg also discussed the difficulties in the transference with sado-masochistic patients. Severe perverse acting-out set limits to the analyst's neutrality, while in minor cases, sado-masochistic enactment within the transference itself limited the analytic work. All patients with severe sexual inhibitions, indifference, and boredom had deep conflicts around the sado-masochistic aspects of sexual excitement; the analyst had to deal with these without becoming seductive. In the transference, after careful and otherwise successful treatment, the analyst can be accused of not helping or caring, and be forced to bear witness to perverse acting-out as a punishment. Mancia (1993) reported on a sadistic transference with a homosexual patient who regarded him as the absent father. Etchegoyen (1977, 1989) coined the term transference perversion. He suggested that the pervert does not really feel the call of sex. The instinct is transformed instead into idea, motivated by envy and guilt, so that sex is experienced not as wish but as idea. MacIntosh (1994) reported on attitudes and experiences in analysing homosexual patients.

Chasseguet-Smirgel (1991) summarized her notable writings on perversion as follows: 'Perversions, whatever their content, develop against an anal sadomasochistic backdrop. Their aim is to destroy reality'. Reality is described as the recognition of sexual and generational differences, where the child lacks procreational power, and wishes to destroy the paternal universe that is reality. Perversions sweep away adult genitality and with this the envy of the parental attributes is rejected by the regression to anal-sadism. Similarly, in moral masochism, there is the notion of disqualification of the father (the superego), which brings it closer to the perversions than to the neuroses—where guilt brings no pleasure. In the perversions, the contents are analogous to the backdrop against which they are enacted—the details of the anal sadistic regression and the phallic oedipal destructive wishes.

EARLY DEVELOPMENTAL FACTORS

Object relationships

The traumas of seduction or humiliation in childhood which seem to form the growing points of the core of the later perverse act, are produced by or in relation to the mother, the primary object. This mother is, as we know, already possessed of a character type which, especially later in relation to father's character, will influence the child in the direction of perversion (see Chapter 1). Such scope for influence exists because of the closeness in feelings which the subsequently perverse individual develops with mother in infancy. This excessive closeness, seen best in the transsexuals described by Stoller (see Chapter 5), exists in all perversion to some degree. The origin may lie in the mother's sense of bodily inadequacy, and the exaggerated use she makes of the child and its responses. to supplement the gap in her body–ego awareness. The mother's penis-envy, which includes a grossly diminished sense of self and body-self, seeks enrichment by her in a covert, highly narcissistic manner. These mothers are greedy in the manner of a temple goddess who demands continual sacrifice to her self-esteem. The child, brought up in close proximity to this already distorted maternal narcissistic system, has its growing sense of self-awareness, body adequacy, and later self-esteem deleteriously influenced. Some authors speak of the child being susceptible to the mother's unconscious needs and conflicts. In earliest childhood, the baby gives the mother satisfaction by its presence as a product she has produced. While the child is totally under her control, an extension of her self and will, there is a symbiotic flowing of the narcissistic satisfactions between mother and child, which reinforces the 'merging' experiences commonly found in adult perversion which are both longed for and feared, especially in the regression of analytic therapy. These symbiotic narcissistic satisfactions form the first intensive libidinization experiences for the child, and are proto-erotic, that is they are generalized and not yet specific as to organ, aim, and object. As the oral stage proceeds, visual experience is patterned psychically on oral phase percepts and modes. Where oral fixations occur, looking functions similarly to eating, and is subject to the same intensification and vicissitudes. Actual fixation on the nipple or breast in a compulsive-erotic way would seem, in my clinical experience to result from traumas in the oral phase which were continued into the oedipal phase and beyond, where the mother frequently exposed herself in a seductive and frustrating manner. For a more complete consideration of the development of the body ego, body image, and body awareness in the child in relation to normal and traumatic stimuli, see Chapter 4.

The child's earliest experiences of humiliation occur when some break in the intense narcissistic bodily togetherness with mother, provides a sense of devaluation to the self. Whereas this happens in all narcissistic disorders, the proto-pervert has a link established with hyper-libidinized experiences which simultaneously deal with object loss and self-devaluation on a body-ego level. Somewhere in the core of every perverse act is the notion of being looked after or the failure to be looked after. This is especially so in the masochistic elements of the perversion and in risk-taking. The perverse act in the adult is a plea for togetherness and help, and a sexualized attack for the failure to provide it, symbolically enacted in relation to the whole world, directed at the primary object once more, still on a part-object level, and with a disturbed orientation to reality as a result. By acting in the regressed manner of the perversion, the person can re-experience the narcissistic togetherness on a symbiotic level, which is the accompaniment, as I have said, of the prototype of hyper-libidinization. The success of the perversion is that it can proceed to a genital orgasm, that the individual has control over his sexual responses as well as the objects that arouse them, and is no longer under the control of the mother at a pregenital level of functioning. Post-orgastic experiences differ in perversion, varying from a sense of emptiness and guilt, to sexual gratification, triumph over and contempt for the sexual object, a sense of ego-accomplishment, and ego-ideal satisfaction. In some degree there is always a sense of failure following the perverse act. As the narcissistic pleasure level falls, the sense of separateness and inner loneliness emerges once more. The outcome depends on the prevailing emotional state. Sufferers with perversions are much more at risk emotionally during episodes of object loss or depression, and these may constitute crisis conditions, such as the acute homosexual panic following the loss of a close partner. Object loss may be defended against by hyper-activity, perverse or otherwise, whereby pain of loss, shame, and guilt are avoided. Winnicott (1935) and Klein *et al.* (1952) have conceptualized such activity as a manic defence. Because perversion necessitates action, failure to libidinize the aggressive drive may lead to substitutes involving risk, such as the suicidal attempt, the motor accident, or the loss of valuable objects, while delinquency, especially stealing, plays an ancillary role in many perversions. One transvestite would mysteriously rob his own house, and alarm the occupants, yet remain undetected. Fortunately, these manifestations are not usually of a serious nature, as the perversion protects the self as well as the object. Where open physical violence or gross sadism occurs towards the object of sexually deviant behaviour, the diagnosis must be queried whether the perpetrator basically suffers from a character disorder, or a narcissistic personality, or is a borderline psychotic. Such people are fixated at primitive oral object-relationships, and have conflicts over controlling or being controlled by the object, with resultant rage and temper tantrums. Outbursts of rage may occur early in treatment, which then contributes a threat to the therapeutic situation (Kernberg 1975).

The father plays a crucial role in the development of perversion and may fail to protect the child against the mother's anxieties and influences. From the boy's point of view, father's adequately masculine presence is essential for him to develop his own full masculinity. Whereas in both oedipal and preoedipal phases the father should be emotionally and physically available for the boy to identify with, it is particularly at the time of the Oedipus complex that the boy's future as a full functioning male is determined. 'For males, the presence of a good loving father during development is probably the best proof against homosexual development . . . . I can think of no case . . . . where such a father has been present in the early childhood years of development'. Rosen (1988) was thus quoted by Nicolosi

(1991) where this was corroborated by several authors. The underlying bisexuality of a boy and his relationships with both parents is what enables him to make relationships and identifications with both parents simultaneously. Stoller, as reported in a Panel Report (1977), described how the degree of femininity in males developed in childhood mainly under mother's influence, but in essence, the development of femininity was controlled by both parents' actions in encouraging the boy to become separate from the symbiotic relationship with his mother, and to develop his own masculinity. The degree to which masculinity was obtained was determined by a host of factors, but determined in the main by the mutual interactions of the parents with the child. Stoller (1975b) provided the basic hypotheses that the 'degree of femininity that develops in a boy and the forms it takes, will vary according to exactly (not approximately) what is done to him in earlier childhood'. Similarly, in each of the categories where a degree of effeminacy is found, transsexuals, effeminate homosexuals, transvestites, and effeminate heterosexuals, a different state of parental and personal dynamics is found. Drawing on the transsexual phenomenology Stoller postulated a very early phase in mental development which is free of conflict, during which impressions are, as it were, imprinted or conditioned on the emerging mental apparatus, which goes to form the core gender-identity, or sense of maleness of femaleness. Because of the symbiotic closeness to the mother, the boy undergoes a primitive identification with her, from which he has, in Greenson's term (1968), to 'dis-identify'. Only then can be begin to be masculine. In the transsexual, the symbiosis is maintained beyond the normal phase of separation and individuation described by Mahler (1968). No masculinity is therefore developed in the transsexual, there is no fear of castration, but rather there is a fear of loss of gender-identity. Stoller found a special interplay of family dynamics in the transsexuals. Very briefly, the marriage was empty and distant; father merely supplied the finances and was rarely around when the son was active and awake. The mother was chronically depressed, with a history of marked masculinity before puberty, and suffered severe penis-envy; the beauty these children possessed sparked off mother's reactions which led to the development of a specially intense symbiotic closeness, which was prolonged and provided a physical contact with the child in a blissful union that lasted for years. The child served the mother as the treasured phallus for which she had yearned. Such children revealed signs of femininity between the ages of one and three years, and the longer the femininity endured the less chance there was of facilitating any change towards masculinity, especially where the father had failed to disrupt the pathogenic symbiosis.

Effeminate homosexuals and fetishistic cross-dressers have conflicts concerning masculinity and femininity which preserve the underlying conflicts of the earlier experience of the wish to merge with mother at the same time as preserving themselves as separate individuals. The way the gender-identity problems, together with any actual perversion, becomes enshrined in their character structure is a vital process used by them to maintain masculinity. In both these conditions the penis is preserved as an object of gratification, existing, as it were, surrounded by a threatening femininity.

For the fetishistic cross-dresser there are intense experiences of closeness, or invariable separations from the maternal object. The important additional element is the occurrence of humiliation during the overwhelming excitement of togetherness, or the intolerable separation, or both. In the history of one such patient the mother was very attractive, narcissistic, exciting sexually to the boy but somewhat emotionally out of reach as far as he was concerned. He felt alternately excited and rejected by her, and his first discoverable act of cross-dressing occurred soon after he went to boarding school aged 8. He was discovered aged 15 squatting on the matron's bed and urinating in her knickers. Subsequently he developed a most severe and complex perversion where any frustration would lead to immediate acts of voyeurism in ladies' lavatories, stealing, and leaving erotic or shocking pictures or drawings for passers-by to see. He cross-dressed under his clothes, and was totally unable to work or form relationships. In analysis he regressed to experiences of actual baby body-ego awareness with overwhelming merging tendencies. Any separations were extremely unbearable in the transference and necessitated open access to the analyst at times. On one occasion his reality sense appeared to become altered in the direction of actual psychosis when he believed he was being penetrated, all alone in the dark in the country, spread-eagled on the bonnet of his car. In this case, the father was someone with whom there was the opportunity for masculine identification as he was successful in his job and expected his son to be likewise. Unfortunately, he was so engrossed in his work and his own problems that he failed to nurture any relationship with his son beyond that of providing for his material needs and expecting achievements from him. This patient suffered a handicap from physical illness in childhood, which further contributed to the interference with his masculinity.

The constellation of the parents in homosexuality has been described by Bieber *et al.* (1962), Socarides (1968) and in Chapter 11. In general, the mother is both seductive and threatening to the boy's unfolding masculinity, while the father is either emotionally withdrawn or openly hostile, the boy being clumsy, shy, and fearful of games (for full details see Chapters 1, 9, 10, and 11). The father's role in the aetiology of overt homosexuality is far-ranging, extending from those fathers who, in a small minority of cases, actively seduce their sons physically or who permit or encourage homosexual relationships, to the majority who are either indifferent, absent, or cruelly hostile to their sons. In such cases, the father fails the boy as an object for masculine identification, especially during the oedipal phase when castration anxiety is at its height. The boy's failure to identify with the father deprives him of full masculinity, with the result that he is forced back to an earlier imitative identification with the father; the conflict of identifying with the mother; the maintenance of castration anxiety which becomes repressed and leads to the accentuation of the phallus as an object of possession; and an increased fear of the female genitalia. Because the castration complex has not been surmounted, there remains the tendency to regress, together with the need to search for the ideal male object with whom to identify or to possess.

In my successful analysis of several patients with homosexuality, the dynamic interplay between the parents and the child from earliest infancy onwards was worked through and the patient was able to establish relationships with the father that had previously been precluded by the mother's manoeuvres in isolating the father from the child, and the father's apparent willingness to accept this. In many cases, the father had not been sufficiently strong in his own sense of masculinity to prevent this. The homosexual's close loving attachment to the mother was basically ambivalent and the violent rages stored up against her required to be worked through. One such patient treated by me was extremely religious and had intense homosexual fantasies and longings which he never revealed in any way. To further repress his tendencies he unsuccessfully tried hormone treatments followed by aversion therapy which pained him considerably and left him mildly paranoid. After a long, full analysis he married and raised a family. His inhibitions exercised a passivity derived from early oral experiences where his overwhelming mother forced food into his mouth which he refused to swallow. His father was also passive emotionally and his successful treatment lay in resolving his anger and passivity towards his mother and in his acceptance and identification with active masculinity in the transference, while mitigating his severe super-ego.

Researches based on child observation (Roiphe and Galenson 1968; Galenson and Roiphe 1974, 1976; Edgcumbe and Burgner 1975) have produced evidence for the presence of an early genital stage, occurring between the ages of 2 and 3 years in both sexes. Roiphe and Galenson showed that castration anxiety can occur in the second year of life giving rise to problems that ante-date the oedipal phase. The relevance of this material for homosexuality has been succinctly reviewed by Payne (Panel Report 1977, pp. 196–7) from which I quote.

> Recognition of this state means that we do not have to postulate a later oedipal revival of earlier developmental conflicts, or a regression from oedipal conflict to an earlier developmental phase in order to explain the coexistence of abandonment and engulfment fears with the overinvestment in and preoccupation with the genitals shown by homosexual men. Instead, the anxiety that the genitals will be lost, damaged, or defective, may occur concurrently with the fear of separation and the fear of merging with the mother. The heightened narcissistic cathexis of the genitals then plays an important role in shoring up the yet unstable structure of the representation of the body image and the development of gender identity.

The significance of the preoedipal phase is discussed further by Socarides in Chapter 11. For an account of internal object and self-representations and the development of perversion, see Chapter 3.

Individuation–separation and body-image development

It has been pointed out that the disturbances of separation–individuation occur not only in perversions but also in the more frequently found narcissistic disorders and 'border-line' personalities. Pursuing the question of what distinguishes perversion from other disorders in the area further, Greenacre suggests that disturbances of individuation in itself may occur based on the experiences the child receives in its growing awareness of anatomical sexual differences between the sexes (see Chapter 4). The boy's awareness of his genitals as part of his own body–ego identity may be influenced by the degree to which he is exposed to visual perception of female genitals, his mother's or sister's. A great deal of controversy exists concerning the influence of such experiences on later development. Freud placed emphasis on boys seeing sexual differences which contributed to the castration complex; the fantasy of the phallic mother, and the need for ego splitting to contain the two ideas of the mother with and without a penis. In a study of my own at the Hampstead Clinic, all Index cases were examined, and three boys and three girls in full analysis were discovered to have parents who had a liberal attitude towards appearing nude with their children. The children became disturbed where the parents had wittingly or otherwise introduced emotional elements into the shared nudity which became over-stimulating to the child, producing frustration rather than liberation, and led to oral regressions in some children. In some of the boys, there was premature libidinal development, or the excessive stimulation led to an enhancement of oedipal phase phenomena, an increased comparison and competitiveness with father, and a resulting feeling of inadequacy instead of a gain in masculine pride and identification. A greater bodily cathexis occurred, especially for the penis. The awareness of sexual differences and retaliatory fears produced a heightened castration anxiety and complex, which was associated with a wide range of defensive processes. These defences were characterized by regression to anal and especially to oral phases; defences against perception—denial, disavowal, perceptual distortion; and increased fantasy due to the hyper-libidinization and aggressiveness. This resulted in learning and ego inhibitions. Sublimations were initially minimal in all three boys. Inhibition of any show of aggressiveness was finally the picture in all three boys. Two latency children remained sexually active in fantasy and all three developed passive, dependent positions in relation to their fathers, the older two conforming to a passive homosexual orientation.

Greenacre considers that early exposure to the child, if repeated and almost constant, can lead to attitudes of genital interest and confusion. Any conditions which interfere with the attainment of separation will intensify this genital confusion. In my experience, compulsive questioning regarding the genitals may involve other areas. For example, one sado-masochistic patient with perverse character formation, who came to treatment for impotence, had a profound sense of the smallness of his penis. He also had a torturing preoccupation with the small size of his girl-friend's breasts, with whom he was otherwise well suited. The breast preoccupations were a substitutive regression from his castration anxiety, which linked with his exposure to the naked, seductive, and controlling mother beyond the normal breast-feeding phase. In this man's adolescence, his narcissistic mother would still ask him to admire her figure, and the continual arousal of his incestous desires sharpened his sense of physical inadequacy and the unconscious oedipal rivalry. Actual incestuous relations with a sister, who practised similar breast seductions in adolescence, were only just resisted.

However, one can also quote cases in which mothers have overwhelmed infants in prolonged feeding situations and kept them in the bathroom while they bathed for many years of childhood. Such a patient revealed in analysis actual body–ego experiences of breast proximity which were highly pleasurable, but unbearably overwhelming. However, overt features of perversion were missing except for masochistic needs and self-damage amounting to actual suicide attempts. Some ingredient appeared to be missing, which if present, would have led to homosexual perversion, but which was forbidden by the ego-ideal attitudes.

Perversions are disturbances in sexual development taking place in the area of ego development.

Greenacre (1968) has put the relationship between perversion and ego development most lucidly in her statement 'The defectively developed ego uses the pressures of the libidinal phases for its own purposes in characteristic ways because of the extreme and persistent narcissistic needs'. She has described two phases of phallic sensitivity. One related to the oedipal period in the fourth year, belonging to the accepted phallic phase of development. The other started much earlier, in the second year of life, and related to the sense of bodily exhilaration associated with better sphincter control and the assumption of the upright posture. Both phases contain a marked sensitivity to bodily trauma and increased fear of castration.

Greenacre has concluded that trauma is important as a predisposing factor in perversion if it occurs in the second and fourth year of life to children who are already unusually uncertain about their bodies, especially their genitals. This is especially pertinent if mutilation or bleeding is experienced or seen in others. Such events are commoner than is supposed, with evidences of menstruation, miscarriages, or accidents being seen by the child.

Trauma is of importance according to the degree to which the child is overwhelmed and resorts to fantasy or denial of reality in order to deal with the panic. The fetish fulfils these conditions admirably.

EGO DEFENCES

The ego defences found in perversions relate to the level of developmental fixation as well as to the use of particular mechanisms associated more with one type of disorder than another. For example, introjection–projection mechanisms predominate in early oral/anal conflicts. Splitting of the ego and of the object, together with denial, are found more commonly in fetishism. The reader is referred to the chapters on specific perversions for further details of mechanisms used.

Of greater interest in this section is the function of the personality as a whole in perversions, the character type of defences, so to speak. Various perverse manifestations may exist in layered fashion and in these persons denial is a particular feature.

Fenichel (1945, p. 328) following the Sachs mechanism, has drawn attention to the similarity between the defence mechanism of denial, perverse symptom formation, and the psychology of screen memories. 'In perversions, as in screen memories, the work of repression is apparently facilitated through something associatively connected with the repressed being consciously stressed. The fact that certain impulses, usually forbidden, remain in consciousness [the perverse drives] guarantees the repression of the oedipus and castration complexes'. A clinical example is given below, in conjunction with an examination of the role of denial in perversion.

Denial is used when the child is continually brought face to face with an unacceptable reality over which it has no control, and may defend against unwelcome drives, object-relationships or affects. While denial is common among sexual offenders at the time of assessment, it is only now being studied systematically. Denial poses real problems for the assessing clinician because denial of the sexual offence accompanies denial of severe psychopathology and the minimizing of symptoms (Grossman and

Cavanaugh 1992). This was confirmed by Haywood *et al.* (1993) who recommended the use of psychological testing in the assessment of alleged sex offenders. Kennedy and Grubin (1992) described four groups of denial in imprisoned sex offenders:

1. 'Rationalizers', who admitted their offences, but claimed to have helped their victims. Many had offended against children and were the most recidivist group.
2. 'Externalizers', male offenders against young females, whom they blamed for the offence. Their use of projective mechanisms often became persecutory in tone.
3. 'Internalizers', which included heterosexual offenders, who accepted blame and the harm to the victim, but who attributed the offence to temporary aberration of behaviour or mental state.
4. 'Absolute denial', where males were convicted of sexual offences against adult females, and in this sample, where three-quarters were from ethnic minorities.

The authors concluded that denial on its own was a poor predictor of outcome, even though assessors regarded it as an indicator of motivation for change. Two examples of the complexities of assessment and treatment follow.

An exhibitionist offender denied having exposed himself to some young girls, but the facts seemed incontrovertible, especially as he had a history of such exposures. In the light of the evidence, his denial seemed curious. The multi-faceted reasons for it were discovered much later when he reported reluctantly that he was forced to share his mother's bed from birth up until his early twenties. Using denial he tolerated his mother's nocturnal embraces, and his waking with erections in the morning. He was a love-child to whom his mother clung tenaciously. He knew his father only briefly, from a screen memory; the father came to visit twice weekly in his childhood, when he would be sent off for a walk, while the parents had intercourse. He was expected to deny his childhood awareness of these clandestine arrangements. The exhibitionism was the uppermost of a series of defensive layers. The underlying layer was of overt homosexual behaviour of mutual masturbation with strangers in cinemas, which defended against massive hostility, intense castration anxiety, and active incestuous wishes. His pubertal masturbation fantasies centred on maternal intercourse and were repressed. Hidden by the screen memory was his love for his father. Analytically speaking, this patient's narcissistic proclivity for mastery was used in the service of the cure, the aspects described being mostly resolved.

In contrast to this case, I was consulted by a lawyer accused of exhibiting himself by alleged witnesses. He denied the accusation and sought my help to determine if he possibly could have exposed himself. Nothing in his history or recent life or psychopathology fitted with the diagnosis of an exhibitionist. It was only finally in court after witnesses (including a policeman) had testified to his guilt, that suddenly a garage attendant attested that the accused was far away having his car filled with petrol at the time the offence—a near psychotic one—was committed. This case of mistaken identity could have disastrously ended his professional reputation, had he been found guilty of what in that court was a minor first offence punishable by a small fine. His strenuous legal defence preparations saved him, and there was no pathological denial in this very co-operative person. Examination of his psychopathology had shown a reliable witness, based on the absence of precipitating factors; there was positive evidence of a healthy self-esteem amply nourished by reality attainments; satisfactory whole-object relationships of a family, sexual, and social kind; good previous response to stress, and no history of childhood or infantile traumas, seductions, or perverse activities.

Ego organization

Freud in his early writings used the word 'ego' to connote the executive psychic apparatus of the mind, as well as the person's subjective experience usually known as the 'self'. Hartmann (1956) made a formal distinction between the ego apparatus and the self. He defined the term ego as 'a substructure of personality defined by its functions'. Freud had already emphasized the functions of the ego as centring around the relation to reality in his remark, the 'relation to the external world has become the decisive factor for the ego' (1932, p. 75). Hartmann regarded the ego as organizing and controlling motility and perception—perception of the outer world but probably also of the self. Self-criticism, while based on self-perception, was a separate function attributed to the super-ego. The ego therefore had to deal with the outer world, with id drives, the super-ego demands, and with the self.

Accepting the distinction between ego and the self, this section examines the way the ego develops specific perceptual modes and patterns of motility, in relation to particular external stimuli, which contribute to perversion. The self, which is more properly conceptualized as an inner mental representation of the self, is studied in the next section, on perversion as a regulator of self-esteem.

Disorders of perception

The ego defects found in perversion are fundamentally preoedipal in type. Such ego defects stem from interferences in the earliest mother–child relationships. Their exact nature depends on the fixation points which occur during the process of separation–individuation, as the child matures away from the initial symbiotic relationship with the mother (Mahler 1968). These fixation points are described differently depending on the theoretical orientation of early ego- and self-formation, see page 69 (see also Kohut 1971).

Perversions may be considered as disturbances in sexual development taking place in the sphere of a developing ego. The earliest ego perceptions appear to be that of body-ego symbiosis. Only later is there the growth of awareness of the genital body-image in the context of gender-identity—the formation of the sense of masculinity or femininity.

The clinical psychoanalytical situation provides numerous examples in perverse patients of conflicts concerning regression to early symbiotic levels. There is the conflicting wish and fear of regressing to the state of merging with the earliest part-object, the breast. This arouses defences against the fear of being overwhelmed by the actual merging experience; or against the painful loss if, in the merged state, the object suddenly disappears. The adult perverse act or character defence symbolically expresses both sides of this equation of conflict. When actual regressive experiences of a body–ego kind occur in analysis, they prove to be frightening to the patient, for example, experiencing the physical proportions of being a baby, with large head and small body: wishes and experiences in the transference of merging with the analyst in the role of the feeding mother; the anger or rage at the frustration of these wishes; or the very frightening somatic compliances symbolizing castration. Such observations, made with transvestite patients, as well as with homosexuals, bear out the contention of authors such as Socarides (1977, see Chapter 11) on the significance of merging experiences as part of early symbiotic fusion desires that are defended against in homosexuals. In Ostow (1974), Gero has elaborated on the visual aspects of merging in a homosexual patient, by which it was possible to become like his idealized athletic partner, and to possess his penis, by the patient seeing the objects of his desire. Merging through tactile experience was observed in another patient who by putting on mother's nightgown relieved the tension of separation—this went beyond the ordinary identification of wearing the mother's garment.

Apart from constitutional factors, visual sensitivity in perversion has early environmental origins. One patient was referred after a long analysis because of homicidal threats to the referring therapist at the ending of fruitless treatment. He was found to have a relative impotence, great masochistic material losses, massive perverse fantasies of a defensive kind, and an inability to look at the therapist. Resolving the perverse defences enabled the visual component to be investigated. He was unable to look at nudity and especially not at nipples. There were early traumatic sights of mother's nipples through her nightgown which overwhelmed him. The libidinization and repression of seeing nipples defended against his actual visual sensitivity which had the quality of a devouring desire which was never to be fulfilled. this formed the basis of his severely masochistic instinctual life, including the initial negative therapeutic reaction. His highly narcissistic mother deprived him orally in reality. In face to face treatment, he was persuaded to 'take in' the therapist visually, resistances against this were analysed, and a meaningful relationship became established, which led to a successful result.

Some homosexuals establish an 'eye' for beauty which becomes fixated on the phallic male and cannot delight in females to the same degree. This may be difficult to alter in treatment due to the ego-ideal and ego-syntonic factors, together with the intensity of castration anxiety that is somatized, and defended against.

The high degree of libidinal cathexis invested in these visual images and abilities probably also makes it difficult for therapists using conditioning modifications on preorgastic fantasies in homosexuality to reduce their intensity where visual merging qualities are present (see Abel and Blanchard 1974).

There is a 'literalness' or concreteness of experience and expression in such patients which not only shows the early ego derivation, but which enters into ego perceptions of later phase developments. Mention has already been made of the importance and intensity of castration anxiety in perversion. The following example illustrates how the concreteness of body–ego and self-awareness altered the quality of castration anxiety in an already intensified oedipal rivalry. This patient had homosexual preoccupations and overt adolescent encounters. His parents were those classically described in homosexuality, and in childhood there were many primal scene experiences. In analysis he relived experiences at the age of three to four years where he said, 'I was so afraid, I *became* terror'. He reported a memory of a hand at the foot of the bed which he actually felt holding his foot; the terror of the hand reaching up and taking away his penis; or his penis was felt to become his anus—a concrete body–ego elision. He would search the house, symbolically, to investigate every part of mother, where he thought his father or brothers had been. In the analysis, he re-experienced early psychosomatic complaints relating to maternal dependence and the anger at separation. In the transference, he relived his need for physical contact, including the feeling of feminine identification in the primal scene, where he experienced being underneath the analyst. His aggression emerged against the early mother: 'You're a despicable bitch and I should cut off your tits and throw them away, take out your teeth and grind them away, and there would only be a head and a body left. Where have you gone? I can't make you come back'. He felt forced to conclude that if he admitted his inadequacy in being unable to make mother come back, 'it means I am nothing. There is nothing for you to see if you don't want to come and see me'. That is, his threatened loss of self required mother's attention, in being seen. This patient set up a configuration in his world to deal with the threat of such traumatic separations whereby the representation of his mother image, was fused with his self-representation and influenced and was present at his every move. In his later fused mother–self identity he experienced the importance of seeing attractive men, or being well-dressed.

Visual concreteness or merging, deals with the threat to the self which results from the loss of the early part-object at the stage of symbiotic fusion and the literal body–ego perceptual awareness. Perversion and narcissistic character disorders share much in common due to fixations at this level. The perversions are hyper-libidinized or sexualized and therefore have a greater power of binding the aggression. In the patient described above, the sexualization derived from the stimulating, exciting narcissistic mother who would rub his anus to soothe him, yet left nursemaids to care for him.

This case illustrates the part-object need-satisfying level of relationship at which the patient remained fixated, and the mother continuing to function towards her son in a similar part-object idealized and frustrating manner. This is typical of the developed perversion. The libidinization of early mother–child experience may thus take place through actual acute seduction which is repeated, or occur as a result of the less overt maternal excitement on a narcissistic basis, but which is transmitted to the immature ego at periods of phase susceptibility. See Coopersmith (1981) who considers all forms of perverse behaviour in terms of oral and anal sadism and their effect on self and object development. The result is an ego capacity for high libidinal excitement, together with undue sensitivity to frustration and rejection, which are used defensively against the threat of loss of object, rejection of the self, and the accompanying frustration, hostility, and anger.

The early libidinization links with needs to regress to symbiotic closeness and omnipotent control of objects. The sequelae of these early conflicts are a fixation of ego structure and function. Sublimatory capacities are interfered with, and many patients enter treatment because of their inability to work or use their creative capacities. It is often such patients who lose perversions such as homosexuality, for which they had no wish to be treated, in the course of treatment.

Ego boundaries are also disturbed in perversion. In the safety of the analytic situation, patients experience loss of control of their thoughts; feelings of falling off the couch; and various other manifestations indicative to the individual that he is out of control in an overwhelming environment. These phenomena are usually defended against by fantasy, by passivity which is demeaning to the self, or by recourse to perverse action, or each in turn. The passivity–activity axis is one of the determinants of the perverse character style. Action serves to avoid the aloneness with its immobilizing passivity that links with early traumatic experiences of separation from mother or both parents. This loneliness and object-loss carries an underlying quality of intense fear of abandonment, which is temporarily removed by the libidinization in perversion. One patient libidinized the inner merged self-object, which masqueraded as a maternal image, which kept him company constantly.

During the course of psychoanalytic treatment, the patient is faced with the working through of these deep conflicts of the fears of engulfment and of abandonment, the symbiotic merging with mother and the loss of ego boundaries (Person's comments in Panel Report 1977). Primary identification with the original maternal object is maintained, increasing the bisexual conflict and the task of self-individuation. Dual identification is also a feature in any sexual or social life encounters.

The ego and motility

Because of the infantile seduction and sexualization, the adult ego is compelled to seek action in risk-taking, excitement, thrills, and orgastic discharge. The tolerance for high degrees of stimulation is exemplified by some homosexuals with a high orgastic capacity and the compulsive need for casual sexual encounters amounting to hundreds annually.

The simultaneous sensitivity to humiliation and low tolerance for frustration, induces the capacity for disparate modes of functioning which is replicated in all spheres and gives to the character a quality of contradictoriness. The underlying aggression in response to over-stimulation or frustration puts the person at risk and necessitates perverse libido to counteract it. True neutralization does not occur. Voyeurs are particularly sensitive to being over-stimulated by sexual scenes, and occasionally the aggression which is aroused may lead to violent attacks, for example, on couples petting in unfrequented places.

Ostow (1974) covers research on the basic mode of action in perversion. Action is a way of life which circumvents conflict, and is reinforced by a hyper-cathexis of perception (especially visual) at the expense of abstract thinking capacity and a tendency to seek a literal concrete experience. The perverse act occurs where fantasy gratification fails and is a repetition of childhood seduction and frustration. Based on the original object, the pleasure-giving and idealized, as well as hateful, aspects of the mother, there is a need for action as a means of solving the contradiction between the inculcated passivity and the identifications with the active stimulating, coming-and-going mother. Over-activity in childhood and infancy is reported in some perverse individuals and may be partly constitutional in origin.

The action patterns and the perverse act itself are the result of ego modifications in development, which are based on the early seduction experiences and the over-cathexis of the perceptual and motor systems, which later are used to rectify anxiety, of castration in particular, by discharging it along pathways laid down in the perverse mechanism. Perverse fantasy may be used as the initial source of gratification, but where this fails, action supervenes—the fantasy is achieved in a literal way. The final form or expressions which perverse needs may actually take are determined largely by chance external events which occur in childhood, latency, and especially in adolescence, when orgasm further fixates orgastic behavioural determinants of the perversion with regard to object, place, and sexual act.

Acting-out of perverse behaviour occurs in response to loss or the lowering of self-esteem. In some cases the patient is aware of the fused self-object manifesting internally as the mother's voice urging him towards such activities. In the ensuing sexual encounters attempts are made to reach the intensity of infantile sexual arousal before relief in orgasm or defusion occurs. Hence the need for multiple partners, exaggerated sexual behaviour, or risk taking, which nowadays may mean conscious exposure to AIDS in spite of counselling and education. Kelly (1992) reported having 'surveyed 526 homosexuals and found that 37 per cent reported that they continue to engage in unsafe practices. The strongest predictors of continued high-risk behaviour were perceptions that safer sex insistence was not an acceptable notion within one's own peer group, inaccurate underestimation of personal vulnerability, high overall levels of sex activity with multiple partners, and younger age'. In Britain, a Stonewall survey found that only 2.5 per cent of gay men had any information on AIDS and homosexuality (Peter Tatchell, personal communication 1994). See also Gala *et al.* (1993) on the psychosocial impact of HIV infection in gay men who found that any resulting stress was dependent on the previous and current lifestyle independent of HIV status.

In Britain in 1993, the public discussed the age at which male sexual orientation was finally determined. Expert opinion varied from puberty to mid-adolescence, the range obviously being wide because of individual variation. This was in connection with parliamentary debate on a motion by Edwina Currie MP, to change the law on the age of homosexual conset from 21 to 16. The legal age in many European countries varied from 12 to 16; some authorities stating that final sexual preference was established before puberty; the British Medical Association backed the proposal to change to 16 (Beecham 1993).

In a televised debate with Edwina Currie (*Kilroy*, BBC 1) I presented the view that the legal age of consent was to protect the vulnerable rather than to license the capable. Psychoanalytic theory and observation placed the maturation of sexual preference during adolescence. Many adolescents needed time to mature in their sexual orientation without undue influence. On this basis I opted for a change in the law from age 21 to 18. A similar viewpoint prevailed in the final Commons decision to lower the age of homosexual consent to 18. The danger for the adolescent experimenting with same gender sex, or caught up in a school or social situation, is that he/she may prematurely and erroneously identify him/herself as gay, or be pronounced gay by medical or other authorities to whom he/she may be referred (Rosen, Freud Memorial Lecture, 1987). Rigid attitudes and opinions about sexual identity and preference are dangerous. Dr William Owen's views (1986) could easily be used by doctors to fob off and refer as indicated below, an adolescent or the parents, seeking help, instead of providing for a proper psychosocial assessment. 'The physician can assist homosexual patients who are becoming aware of their sexual orientation ("coming out") by reassuring them that homosexuality is a normal variant rather than a medical illness and by referring them, where indicated, to the appropriate local service agencies and homosexual community organizations that have developed in recent years.'

The next section on the logic of this presentation, perversion as a regulator of self-esteem, is in Chapter 3.

REFERENCES

Abel, G. G. and Blanchard, E. B. (1974). The role of fantasy in the treatment of sexual deviation. *Arch. Gen. Psychiat.* **30**, 467.

Alexander, F. (1965). A note to the theory of perversions. In *Perversions: psychodynamics and therapy*, (ed. S. Lorand and M. Balint). Random House, New York.

Bak, R. (1956). Aggression and perversion. In *Perversions: psychodynamics and therapy*, (ed. S. Lorand and M. Balint). Random House, New York.

Bak, R. C. (1968). The phallic woman: the ubiquitous fantasy in perversions. *Psychoanal. Study Child*, **23**, 15.

Balint, M. (1965), Perversions and genitality. In *Perversions: psychodynamics and therapy*, (ed. S. Lorand and M. Balint). Random House, New York.

Bancroft, J. H. J. (1975). Homosexuality in the male. *Contemporary psychiatry*, selected reviews from the *British Journal of Hospital Medicine*, (ed. T. Silverstone and B. Barraclough). Headley Brothers, Ashford, Kent.

Bancroft, J. H. J. (1994). Homosexual orientation. *Brit. J. Psychiat.* **164**, 437–40.

Baron, M. (1993). Genetic linkage and male homosexual orientation. *Brit. Med. J.* **307**, 337–8.

Becker, J. V., *et al.* (1992). The relationship of abuse history, denial and exectile response profiles of adolescent sexual perpetrators. *Behav. Ther.* **23**, 87–97.

Beecham, L. (1993). Editorial. BMA votes to reduce age of consent for homosexual men. *Brit. Med. J.* **306**. 27 February.

Bieber, I., *et al.* (1962). *Homosexuality: A psychoanalytic study of male homosexuals*. Basic Books, New York.

Blum, H. (1977). Masochism, the ego ideal, and the psychology of women. (In supplement: Female psychology.) *J. Am. Psychoanal. Assoc.* **24**(5), 157.

Chasseguet-Smirgel, J. (1984) *Creativity and perversion*. Norton, New York.

Chasseguet-Smirgel, J. (1991). Sadomasochism in the perversions: some thoughts on the destruction of reality. *J. Am. Psychoanal. Assn.* **39**, 399–416.

Cooper, A. M. (1989). Narcissism and masochism. The narcissistic-masochistic character. *Psychiat. Clin. N. Am.* **12**, 541–52.

Coopersmith, S. E. (1981). Object-instinctual and developmental aspects of perversion. *Psychoanal. Rev.* **68**, 371–83.

Edgcumbe, R. and Burgner, M. (1975). The phallic-narcissistic phase: a differentiation between pre-oedipal and oedipal aspects of phallic development. *Psychoanal. Study Child*, **30**, 161.

Etchegoyen, R. H. (1977). Perversion de transferencia. Aspectos teoricos y tecnicos. In *Practicas psicoanaliticas comparadas en las psicosis*. ed. L. Grinberg, pp. 55–83. Paidos, Buenos Aires.

Etchegoyen, R. H. (1989). The concept of perversion in psychoanalysis. *Brit. J. Psychiat.* **154**, 81–3.

Fenichel, O. (1945). *The psychoanalytic theory of neurosis*. Norton, New York.

Finell, J. S. (1992). Sadomasochism and complementarity in the interaction of the narcissistic and borderline personality type. *Psychoanal. Rev.* **73**, 361–79.

Freud, S. (1905/1953). Three essays on the theory of sexuality. In *Complete psychological works of Sigmund Freud*, (standard edition, Vol. 7. London. Hogarth Press,

Freud, S. (1932/1964). New introductory lectures. *Complete psychological works of Sigmund Freud*, (standard edition, Vol. 22). Hogarth Press, London.

Freud, S. (1919/1955). A child is being beaten. In *Complete Psychological works of Sigmund Freud*, (standard edition, Vol. 17). Hogarth Press, London.

Freud, S. (1924/1961). The economic problem in masochism. In *Complete psychological works of Sigmund Freud*, (Standard edition, Vol. 19). Hogarth Press, London.

Freud, S. (1940/1964). Splitting of the ego in the processes of defence. In *Complete psychological works of Sigmund Freud*, (standard edition, Vol. 23). Hogarth Press, London.

Friedman, R. C, and Downey, J. I. (1994). Homosexuality. Special article. *New. Eng. J. Med.* **331**, 923–9.

Gala, C., Pergami, A., Catalan, J., Durbana, F., Musicco, M., Riccio, M., Baldeweg, T., and Invernizzi, G. (1993). The psychosocial impact of HIV infection in gay men, drug users, and heterosexuals. Controlled investigation. *Brit. J. Psychiat.*, **163**, 651–9.

Galenson, E. and Roiphe, H. (1974). The emergence of genital awareness during the second year of life. In *Sex differences in behaviour*, (ed. R. C. Friedman, R. M. Richart, and R. L. Van de Wiele). New York.

Galenson, E. and Roiphe, H. (1976). Some suggested revisions concerning early female development. (In supplement: Female psychology.) *Am. J. Psychoanal.* **24**, 5, 29.

Gillespie, W. H. (1964). The psycho-analytic theory of sexual deviation with special reference to fetishism. In *The pathology and treatment of sexual deviation*, (ed. I. Rosen). Oxford University Press.

Glenn, J. (1989). From protomasochism to masochism. *Psychoanal. Study Child.* **44**, 73–86.

Glickhauf-Hughes, C. and Wells, M. (1991). Current conceptualizations on masochism: genesis and object relations. *Am. J. Psychother.*, **xiv**, 53–68.

Glover, E. (1964). Aggression and sado-masochism. In *The pathology and treatment of sexual deviation*, (ed. I. Rosen). Oxford University Press.

Greenacre, P. (1968). Perversions: general considerations regarding their genetic and dynamic background. *Psychoanal. Study Child*, **23**, 47.

Greenson, R. (1968). Dis-identifying from mother. *Int. J. Psycho-Anal.* **49**, 370.

Grossman, L. S. and Cavanaugh, J. L. Jr. (1990). Psychopathology and denial in alleged sex offenders. *J. Nerv. Ment. Dis.* **178**, 739–44.

Grossman, W. I. (1986). Notes on masochism: a discussion of the history and development of a psychoanalytic concept. *Psychoanal. Q.*, **55**, 379–413.

Grossman, W. I. (1991a). Pain, aggression, fantasy, and concepts of sadomasochism. *Psychoanal. Quart.* **LX**, 22–52.

Hamer, D. H., Hu, S., Magnuson, V. L., Hu, N., Pattatucci, A. M. L.(1993). A linkage between DNA markers on the X chromosome and male sexual orientation. *Science*, **261**, 321–7.

Hanly, M. F. (1993). Sado-masochism in Charlotte Brontë's Jane Eyre: a ridge of lighted heath. *Int. J. Psycho-Anal.* **74**, 1049–61.

Hartmann, H. (1956/1964). The development of ego in Freud's work. In *Essays on ego psychology*, p. 267. International Universities Press, New York.

Haywood, T. W., Grossman, L. S. and Hardy, D. W. (1993). Denial and social desirability in clinical evaluations of alleged sex offenders. *J. Nerv. Ment. Dis.* **181**, 183–8.

Hoenig, J. and Duggan, E. (1974). Sexual and other abnormalities in the family of a transsexual. *Psychiatrica Clinica*, **7**, 334.

Hore, B. D., Nicolle, F. V., and Calnan, J. S. (1973). Male transsexualism: two cases in a single family. *Arch. Sex. Behav.* **2**, 317–21.

Isay, R. (1984). *On the analytic therapy of homosexual men.* Paper read to the Washington Psychoanalytic Society.

Isay, R. (1985). On the analytic therapy of homosexual men. *Psychoanal. Study Child*, **40**, 235–54.

Isay, R. (1986). Homosexuality in homosexual and heterosexual men. In *The psychology of men*, ed. G. Fogel, F. Lane and R. Liebert. Basic Books, New York.

Isay, R. (1989). *Being homosexual.* Farrar, Strauss and Giroux, New York.

Isay, R. (1991). The homosexual analyst. *Psychoanal. Study Child.*, **46**, 199–216.

Isay, R. (1992). From the president (homosexuality and psychiatry). *Psychiat. News*, **27**, 3–17.

Kelly, J. A. (1992). Psychosocial aspects of AIDS. *Curr. Op. Psychiat.* **5**, 820–4.

Kennedy, H. G. and Grubin, D. H. (1992). Patterns of denial in sex offenders. *Psychol. Med.* **22**, 191–6.

Kenyon, F. E. (1975). Homosexuality in the female. In *Contemporary psychiatry*; selected reviews from the *British Journal of Hospital Medicine*, (ed. T. Silverstone and B. Barraclough). Headley Brothers Ashford, Kent.

Kernberg, O. (1972). Early ego integration and object relations, *Ann. N. Y. Acad. Sc.* **193**, 233.

Kernberg, O. (1975). *Borderline conditions and pathological narcissism.* Jason Aronson, New York.

Kernberg, O. F. (1991). Sadomasochism, sexual excitement, and perversion. *J. Am. Psychoanal. Assn.* **39**, 333–62.

Khan, M. M. R. (1963). The concept of cumulative trauma. In *The primacy of the self* (1974). Hogarth Press, London.

Klein, M., Heimann, P., Isaacs, S., and Riviere, J. (1952). *Developments in psychoanalysis.* London.

Lihn, H. (1971). Sexual masochism: a case report. *Int. J. Psycho-Anal.* **52**, 469.

Limentani, A. (1976). Object choice and actual bisexuality. *Int. J. Psycho-Anal. Psychother.* V, 205.

McDougall, J. (1972). Primal scene and sexual perversion. *Int. J. Psycho-Anal.* **53**, 371.

Macgregor, J. R. (1991). Identification with the victim. *Psychoanal. Quart.* LX, 53–68.

MacIntosh, H. (1994). Attitudes and experiences in analyzing homosexual patients. *J. Am. Psychoanal. Assn*, **42**, 1183–207.

Mahler, M. (1968). *On human symbiosis and the vicissitudes of individuation*, Vol. 1. International University Press, New York.

Mancia, M. (1993). The absent father: his role in sexual deviations and in transference. *Int. J. Psycho-anal.* **74**, 941–50.

Mollinger, R. N. (1982). Sadomasochism and developmental stages. *Psychoanal. Rev.* **69**, 379–89.

M'Uzan, M. de (1972). Un cas de masochisme pervers. In *La sexualité perverse.* Payot, Paris.

M'Uzan, M. de. (1973). A case of masochistic perversion and an outline of a theory. *Int. J. Psycho-Anal.* **54**, 455.

Nicolosi, J. (1991). *Reparative therapy of male homosexuality.* Jason Aronson, Northvale, NJ and London.

Novick, J. and Novick, K. K. (1972). Beating fantasies in children. *Int. J. Psycho-Anal.* **53**, 237.

Novick, J. and Novick, K. K. (1987). The essence of masochism. *Psychoanal. Study Child*.
42, 353–84.

Novick, J. and Novick, K. K. (1991). Some comments on masochism and the delusion of omnipotence from a developmental point of view. *J. Am Psychoanal. Assn*, **39**, 307–32.

Ostow, M. *et al.* (ed). (1974). *Sexual deviation: a psycho-analytical approach*. Quadrangle/New York Times.

Owen, W. (1986). The clinical approach to male homosexuality. *Med. Clin. N. Am.* **70**, 499–536.

Panel Report (1977). The psychoanalytic treatment of male homosexuality. (reporter E. C. Payne) *J. Am. Psychoanal. Assoc.* **25**, 183.

Payne, E. C. (1977). See Panel Report above.

Reich, A. (1960). Pathological forms of self-esteem regulation. *Psychoanal. Study Child*. **15**, 215.

Reich, W. (1949). *Character analysis*. Orgone Institute Press, New York.

Roiphe, H. (1968). On an early genital phase. *Psychoanal. Study Child*, **23**, 348.

Rose, L. (1994). Homophobia among doctors. *Brit. Med. J.* **308**, 586–7.

Rosen, I. (1964). Exhibitionism, scopophilia, and voyeurism. In *The pathology and treatment of sexual deviation*, (ed. I. Rosen). Oxford University Press.

Rosen, I. (1965). Looking and showing. In *Sexual deviation and the law*, (ed. R. Slovenko). Charles C. Thomas, Springfield, IL.

Rosen, I. (1968). The basis of psychotherapeutic treatment of sexual deviation. *Proc. R. Soc. Med.* **61**, 793.

Rosen, I. (1977). The psychoanalytic approach to individual therapy. In *Handbook of sexology*, (ed. J. Money and H. Musaph). Excerpta Medica, New York, London.

Rosen, I. (1979). The general psychoanalytic theory of perversion: a critical and clinical study. In *Sexual deviation*, (ed. I. Rosen), 2nd edn, pp. 29–64. Oxford University Press.

Rosen, I. (1987). *Psychoanalysis and homosexuality*. Freud memorial lecture, University College London. Unpublished.

Rosen, I. (1988). Psycho-analysis and homosexuality: a critical appraisal of helpful attitudes. In *Hope for homosexuals*, ed. P. Fagan, pp. 28–45. Free Congress Research and Education, Washington, DC.

Sachs, H. (1923). Zur genese der perversionen. *Int. Z. Psycho-Anal.* **9**, 172. (English translation by Hella Freud Bernays, 1964.) Psychoanalytic Institute Library, New York.

Socarides, C. W. (1968). *The overt homosexual*. Jason Aronson, New York.

Socarides, C. W. (1977). See Panel Report above.

Socarides, C. W. (1928). *The preoedipal origin and psychoanalytic therapy of sexual perversions*. International Universities Press, Madison, CT.

Socarides, C. W. and Volkan, V. D. (1991). *The homosexualities and the therapeutic process*. International Universities Press. Madison, CT.

Sperling, M. (1968). Acting-out behaviour and psychosomatic symptoms. *Int. J. Psycho-Anal.* **49**, 250.

Stoller, R. J. (1975*a*). *Perversion: The erotic form of hatred* Pantheon, New York.

Stoller, R. J. (1975*b*). *Sex and gender*. Vol. 2: The transsexual experiment. Hogarth Press, Science House, New York.

Walinder, J. and Thuwe, I. (1977). A study of consanguinity between the parents of transsexuals. *Brit. J. Psychiat.* **131**, 73.

Wiedemann, G. (1977). See Panel Report above.

Winnicott, D. (1935/1958). The manic defence. In *Collected papers*. Through pediatrics to psychoanalysis, pp. 129–44. Basic Books, New York.

3
Perversion as a regulator of self-esteem

Ismond Rosen

INTRODUCTION

Regulation of self-esteem is a major function of the perversions. Patients seeking help for the relief of their perversions, simultaneously complain of feelings of inadequacy, with under or over self-assertion, as evidence of a disordered narcissistic economy. Perverse fantasies or actions function as a source of intense pleasure that elevates self-esteem. Conversely, following perverse acts patients may complain of feelings of shame and guilt that diminishes their self-esteem. Others report traumatic events that suddenly precipitate episodes of exhibitionism, or homosexual acts, and which were beyond their capacity to tolerate. These traumas are experienced as painful, humiliating, and accompanied by a devaluation of the self. Individuals suffering from perversions tolerate sudden low self-esteem badly, and require rapid relief in sexual action that raises self-esteem through excitement or danger. I view self-esteem regulation as a feedback mechanism, rather than a purely evaluating measuring system. The trauma may be dealt with by a surge of sexual or violent fantasy, or a combination; unconsciously defended against; or responded to with perverse sexual behaviour that raises self-esteem. The resulting responses vary according to the individual intra-psychic structural dispositions. Perverse acts may be precipitated by trauma in a susceptible person. In some people who have heavily defended unconscious conflicts, there may be little or no awareness of any organized fantasy or plan of action, and poor perception or control of their perverse enactment. Some automatic sexually deviant acts, which are often quite repetitive, may result in rapid arrest. Other people may skilfully engineer sexual serious offences and escape detection. These examples represent two extremes of sexual deviancy, the compulsively perverse and the sociopathic.

Preservation of the personality as an integrated whole is one of the functions of self-esteem. The maintenance and regulation of self-esteem are therefore essential to healthy psychic functioning. To understand the development of personality integration and how perversion regulates self-esteem, we must first examine the psychoanalytical concepts of narcissism, the self, the ego-ideal, and the super-ego.

THE DEVELOPMENT OF SELF-ESTEEM

In his 1914 paper 'On narcissism', Freud said 'We have discovered, especially clearly in people where libidinal development has suffered some disturbance, such as perverts and homosexuals, that in their later choice of love-objects they have taken as a model not their mother but their selves. They are plainly seeking themselves as a love-object, and are exhibiting a type of object-choice which must be termed "narcissistic". In this observation we have the strongest reasons which have led us to adopt the hypothesis of narcissism'. Narcissism later became defined as the libidinal investment, or cathexis, of the self-image or self-representation. Jacobson (1975) refined narcissism as the 'intra-psychic cathexis of the self-representations with more or less neutralised or deneutralised libidinous or aggressive drive energy'. Stolorow (1976) succinctly stated that it was the struggle for selfhood that lies at the heart of the phenomenon of narcissism. Primary narcissism is today regarded as an ego-state that the individual derived from the child's early symbiotic union with the mother. Deprivation or over-stimulation in early infancy can interfere with the developmental sequences of primary narcissism in relation to self- and object-relationship development. Primary narcissism also links as a precursor of the drive to human perfectibility.

The self is defined in terms of its content within the mental apparatus, as a series of self-representations (as opposed to object-representations) which are located within the ego, the id, and the super-ego. Lichtenberg (1975) integrated the views of various previous authors on the development of the self. He defined the self as self-experience, or sense of self, and distinguished between self-image referring to experiences, and self-representation referring to structures formed from the memory traces of the experience. In his view, the self develops from the earliest stage before self-differentiation. The infant enters the symbiotic relationship with the mother, and is endowed with a 'basic core of fundamental trends', 'object-relatedness, anxiety potential and libido-aggression balance' (Weil 1970). The merging state leads to a symbiotic dependency where islands of experience, or sense of self, create the formation of ego–id nuclei (Glover 1943, 1964) of body-representations. These bodily self-images later blend experientially with images of the self that have developed in relation to objects that are perceived as separate, and with images of a grandiose self associated with ideal-objects. They form a 'sense of self that has the quality of cohesion—of unity and continuity in time, space and state'. The self as an organizational structure, crucial to the maintenance of self-esteem has been discussed by Demos (1983), Ablon (1990), and Abrams (1990). Three aspects of experience are contributory (Demos): 'judgements of one's competence versus incompetence; trust in one's inner states versus mistrust; and judgements of one's relatedness to others versus one's isolation'. Ablon proposed that the mastery of developmental tasks enhanced self-esteem. This also had significance in therapy where the patient's ability to meet the challenges of conflict resolution leads to increased self-esteem.

Over-stimulation or seduction in infancy leads to fixations of the archaic and omnipotent experiences of the self. A further result is that merging processes between self and object are intensified, which makes for difficulties in the dif-ferentiation between self- and object-representations in later development, as well as in later therapy. In the perversions, the quality of self- and object-experiences are contradictory, with a sense of inferiority being supplemented by notions of omnipotence. They are sensitive to slights, while their ego-ideals impose targets impossible to satisfy or attain. The self-esteem regulatory system is unstable and liable to upset by any lowering event or influence. The individual's sense of his/her own self and perception of external reality is distorted. He or she feels isolated, although able to work and function socially due to splitting mechanisms in the ego and super-ego.

The development of the ego-ideal as the heir to primary narcissism is complicated. Freud (1914) describes how development of the ego [self] consists in a departure from primary narcissism' . . . 'brought about by means of the displacement of libido on to an ego-ideal imposed from without'. In growing-up, the ego-ideal becomes the target of self-love enjoyed by the ego and the early narcissism lost in childhood. Freud's later view of the ego-ideal, from 1923 onwards and repeated in 1933 and 1938, was that the super-ego acts as 'the vehicle of the ego ideal by which it measures itself, which it emulates, and whose demand for ever greater perfection it strives to fulfil'. (1933, p. 64). Hartmann and Loewenstein (1962) agreed with the formulation that the ego-ideal is a structure within the super-ego. Sandler *et al.* (1963) discussed the relationship between the ego ideal and the ideal self.

Milrod (1990) traces the history and current usage of the term ego-ideal. He describes four stages in the line of development from primary narcissism to the ego-ideal. Primary narcissism is the first stage, or undifferentiated phase. This state of perfection or idealization of the self, passes into the second stage where relationships are built-up with important love-objects. Self and object-representations are built-up which differntiate the child's awareness of him- or herself as separate from the environment, so that a sense of inner and outer reality develops. The child is aware of him- or herself as small, weak, and ineffectual in comparison with the primary object, usually the mother, who becomes aggrandized as being perfect, powerful, and desirable. The child's sense of perfection shifts from him- or herself to a love-object who is desirable, or the model for identification. Gratification of possession of the mother's perfection becomes possible by regression to merging of self and object within the child. Imitative identifications magically endow the child with the mother's qualities in this stage. These become inadequate as ego growth proceeds and greater reality testing is acquired. The 'ego forms a new substructure, the wished-for self-image, which contains all of the qualities and characteristics valued and admired in important idols', which the child does not yet possess. The child strives to fulfil a new model of perfection based on this structure. The final stage occurs with the formation of the super-ego, when the ego-ideal is created, perfection passing from the wished-for image to the ego-ideal. Any gratification of the ego-ideal results in a raising of self-esteem. All aspects of personality function are measured against the ego-ideal. Milrod relates the affect of shame to the experience when we fall sufficiently below the wished-for self-image;

Chasseguet-Smirgel (1974) discussed the development of the ego-ideal as the heir to primary narcissism. In perversion she considered there was a disturbance of ego-ideal development mainly assisted by mother in the oedipal courtship. The pervert idealizes the partial pregenital instincts and regards them as superior to the aims of genital primacy. The need for idealization, which is compulsive, is never directed towards objects, but only to part-objects, preferably associated with the anal-sadistic phase.

The term self-esteem dating from 1657, is defined by *The New Shorter Oxford English Dictionary* (1993) as a 'high regard for oneself, good opinion of oneself'. Freud (1914) referred to this faculty as self-regard, which was an expression of the size of the ego and derived from three main parts: (1) the residue of infantile narcissism; (2) the fulfilment of the ego-ideal; and (3) the satisfaction of actual accomplishments. Lowered self-regard, or sense of inferiority was 'due to impoverishment of the ego [self] due to the libidinal cathexes which have been withdrawn from it, due, that is to say, to the injury sustained by the ego through sexual trends which are no longer subject to control'.

Recent child studies indicate that the development of self-esteem derives from early drive satisfactions, which, together with ego accomplishments, finally link with the structural development of the super-ego, ego-ideal, and sense of self. The manner in which pleasure in achievement links with the child's instinctual life is regarded by Anna Freud (1966) as unresolved. Certain operative factors seem unmistakable, such as imitation and identification in the early mother–child relationship, the influence of the ego-ideal, the turning of passive into active as a mechanism of defence and adaptation, and the inner urge for progressive maturation.

Pleasure in achievement, linked only secondarily with object relations, is present in very young children as a latent capacity and is used in nursery school methods (Montessori) to 'afford the child the maximum increase in self-esteem and gratification by means of task completion and independent problem solving'. 'Where this source of gratification is not tapped at the same degree with the help of external arrangements, the pleasure derived from achievement in play remains more directly connected with praise and approval given by the object world, and satisfaction from the finished product takes first place at a later date only, probably as the result of internalization of external sources of self-esteem' (A. Freud 1966). Self-esteem therefore derives from many roots:

1. Accomplishment—gratification of ego capacities in which drive activity manifestations occur as an expression of forward maturity.
2. Imitation and identification in the early mother–child relationship.
3. Ego-ideal influences which develop from residues of primary narcissism and the development of a healthy attainable ego-ideal.
4. Ego-defence mechanisms as adaptational manoeuvres, for example, turning passive into active.
5. Super-ego influences, where the idealized parental images are internalized during the postoedipal and early latency phases.

However, as Jacobson (1975) has pointed out, in a fine review with reference to depression, *regulation* of self-esteem is a complicated mechanism which must be distinguished from the factors making for its development. The preservation of a healthy level of self-esteem depends on the inner narcissistic balance, that is the economy of libidinal cathexis of the self-representations with relatively conflict-free energies. Any conflicts or excessive drives provoked within the individual or derived externally will lead to a rise or fall in self-esteem.

Lichtenberg (1975) has emphasized the positive emotional states resulting from inner-regulation of drives at the toddler stage which stem from self-cohesion, and which 'serve as esteem-raising counterparts to feelings of anxiety, shame and guilt'. He traces the grandiose omnipotent self-images of childhood, which peak at 16 to 18 months, as the precursors of adult self-images with high self-esteem. The most vulnerable point for self-esteem deflation is, according to Mahler (1968), the second

18 months of life. This is the time of life when the maintenance of a sense of control is necessary to restore a sense of being worthwhile. This sensitivity is actively continued in narcissistic and perverse patients. The most pathologically deflating effect on self-esteem at this period of growth is where the mother oscillates from overwhelming closeness to cold withdrawn rejection. The child, having no control over mother's behaviour or presence, varies from sharing in her omnipotence, to feeling an emptiness of his/her self-and object-images.

Pathological regulation of self-esteem is coincident with faulty development of the drives, self- and object-representations, ego, ego-ideal, and super-ego formation. Detailed clinical studies have been made of disturbed self-esteem regulation by A. Reich (1963) who described different types; Kohut (1971) and Kernberg (1975) in narcissistic and borderline disorders; Jacobson (1975) in depression.

Before systematically examining the developmental factors which lead to disturbed self-esteem and its regulation in perversion, it would be advantageous to examine the work of Kohut and Kernberg, on the disorders of narcissism. These new concepts of narcissism have been critically discussed by Ornstein (1974), who has well summarized the comparisons between Kohut and Kernberg, and by Hanly and Masson (1976).

Kohut (1971) formulated certain stages in the development of narcissism, which when specifically disordered provide the nuclei for clinical disturbances such as perversion and the narcissistic disorders. Based on Kohut's concepts, Goldberg (1975) discussed the feasibility of a systematic classification of the perversions based on the fixation points of developing pathological narcissistic constellations and the affects which are sexualized. Unfortunately, no such systematic studies have yet been published on these early narcissistic fixations in relation to perversion. The complexities in psychopathology which make systematic studies difficult or impossible are discussed by Socarides in Chapter 11 (p. 252).

Kohut has postulated two stages of self formation. An *auto-erotic* stage where, also following Glover's notions of ego-nuclei, there are disparate self-nuclei. As growth proceeds, a *cohesive self* is formed, which gives rise to grandiose-self and idealized-parental images. The formulations are most valuable because they are based on the child's relationship to the parents, especially the mother and her handling of its narcissistic needs. Thus, if the mother, because of her lack of empathy, rejects the child's narcissistic strivings subtly or overtly, these will be repressed, leading to what Kohut terms a 'horizontal split'. In adulthood, these unfulfilled archaic demands remain split off from the adult reality ego, draining off its energies.

Clinically, this leaves the patient in his conscious self-perception, devoid of a sense of contentment, with low self-esteem, shame propensity, and a tendency to hypochondriacal brooding.

If, on the other hand, the mother attempts to enmesh the child in her own narcissistic world and use his performance for her own narcissistic satisfactions, this will lead to a side-by-side coexistence of openly displayed infantile grandiosity coupled again with low self-esteem, shame propensity, and hypochondriacal preoccupations, maintained by the mechanism of disavowal, termed by Kohut a 'vertical split'. In the vertical split, perverse behaviour resides in a split-off sector of the psyche.

Perverse activities have been defined by Kohut in terms of sexualization of pathological narcissistic constellations, and may be used to stem regression in one of many ways: as a substitute for an absent narcissistically invested self-object; as a substitute for the non-availability of a person who was being used to represent a missing part of the self; or as a source of pathological hyper-cathexis of the grandiose self.

Kohut (1970, p. 98) describes a patient's recall of long hours in childhood where voyeuristic preoccupations (the child searching through drawers in an empty house), led to his putting on his mother's clothes. These perverse activities became intelligible when they were understood not so much as sexual transgressions that were undertaken while external surveillance was lacking, but rather as attempts to supply substitutes for the idealized-parent image and its functions, by creating erotized replacements through the frantic hypercathexis of the grandiose self. 'The various perverse activities in which the child engages are the attempts to re-establish the union with the narcissistically invested lost object through visual fusion and other archaic forms of identification' (p. 99). Compare the almost identical concrete searching for mother with my case described on p. 69.

In the next case, Kohut shows how pathological sexual fantasies were used as an inner esteem-regulator, replacing a missing stable system of idealized values. This case presented for treatment because of homosexual fantasies. The fantasies were understood in the analysis as 'sexualized statements about his narcissistic disturbance' and 'stood, of course, in opposition to meaningful insight and progress since they were in the service of pleasure gain and provided an escape route from narcissistic tensions'. Kohut showed how in this case where there was no acting-out of the fantasies, the sexualization of the patient's defects was due to a moderate weakness in his basic psychic structure, resulting in an impairment of its neutralizing capacity. The fantasies themselves, which occasionally led to orgasm, were of a quasi-sadistic triumph over men of great strength and of perfect physique in which they were rendered helpless or drained of their power by him masturbating them. After the homosexual fantasies had subsided, in the analysis, Kohut used the interpretation of their meaningfulness to deal with the underlying narcissistic conflicts. This patient suffered from the 'absence of a stable system of *firmly idealized values*', one of the important sources of the internal regulation of self-esteem. He had in his sexual fantasies replaced the inner ideal with its sexualized external precursor, an athletic powerful man; and he had substituted for the enhancement of self-esteem which is experienced by living up to the example of one's idealized values and standards, by the sexualized feeling of triumph, as he robbed the external ideal of its power and perfection and thus in his fantasy acquired these qualities for himself and achieved a temporary feeling of narcissistic balance. The specific pathogenic disturbance in this patient related to the traumatic devaluation of the father-image and its idealized aspects of the beginning of latency. This occurred on an earlier basis of an assumed failure of his mother to supply proper emphatic responses to him early in life based on her unpredictability and shallowness.

According to Goldberg (1975), the object-deficits do not cause the perversion. Sexualization is used to counter the regression, as well as dealing with the over-whelming affects that accompany the lowering of self-esteem in humiliation. The sexualization itself is explained on the basis of the unavailability of the archaic object which does not allow for neutralization and produces a more primitive drive expression.

H. S. Baker and M. N. Baker (1987), in an overview of Kohut's work on self-psychology, conclude that the proper regulation of self-esteem is dependent on the development of intrapsychic structures during infancy. Failure of parental empathy to meet the child's needs produces an individual sensitively dependent on environmental sources of satisfaction with vulnerable self-esteem regulation.

Kernberg (1975) postulated four stages of development of internalized object-relations, and correlated these with the clinical manifestations of pathological arrest or fixation at each stage. Stage 3 included borderline personality organization, embracing impulse neuroses, addictions, and narcissistic personalities. Character disorders seen in severe perversion would belong here. Severe chronic frustrations in early childhood were the main causative factor. The lack of impulse control stems from the ego weakness, where there is a poor integration of the 'good' self- and object-images with their corresponding 'bad' type. The defences, mainly of splitting, act to keep apart these frightening contradictory images. Kernberg postulates that 'the integration of loving and hating feelings in the context of internalized relationships with others seems to be a major precondition for neutralization of instinctual energy'. This lack of neutralization deprives the ego of sublimatory capacity. These drive vicissitudes are all the more significant in borderline patients because premature sexualization and oedipalization of the relationships with parental figures and siblings leads only to aggressive 'contamination' of these relationships.

In stage 4 are represented the neuroses, higher levels of character pathology, and depressive-masochistic characters. The major defences are repression rather than splitting. Oedipal, genital conflicts predominate over pregenital ones. Cases with perverse behaviour mainly of oedipal type would appear to belong to this category where there is no particular pathology of internalized object-relations, with a stable self and object-representational world.

In 1975, Kernberg examined the narcissistic disorders as a spectrum of defences protecting self-esteem and the integrity of the self, which range from non-specific character traits to the specific operations of the narcissistic personality formations. He stated that pathological character traits have as one function the protection of self-esteem and, therefore, analytic efforts to modify a neurotic character structure always included the implication of a narcissistic lesion

Kernberg (1975) has linked oral aggression with a premature development of oedipal strivings resulting in a pathological condensation between pregenital and genital aims under the overriding aggressive aims. Such factors are important in the development of male homosexuality, where the father is submitted to sexually to obtain the oral gratifications missing from mother, who is viewed as a dangerous castrator. In the girl, oral deprivation from mother leads to positive oedipal strivings being developed prematurely. Pregenital aggression is projected on to the father, which increases the oedipal conflicts and penis-envy. There may be many outcomes, such as promiscuity, masochism, and homosexuality, depending on the projective–introjective use of the rage, and the internal splits and threats from the internalized mother- and father-images.

These types of perverse psychopathology are consistent with borderline personality disorder, associated with defences of splitting, primitive idealization, early forms of projection, demand, and omnipotence.

Kernberg (1975) has classified three types of male homosexuality, using a continuum that differentiates the degree of severity of pathology of internalized object-relations. The first type, which has the best prognosis, is where genital oedipal factors predominate. The oedipal self is submissive towards the oedipal domineering prohibitive father and renounces the forbidden oedipal mother. The second type, which is more severe, has 'a conflictual identification with an image of his mother and treats his homosexual objects as a representation of his own infantile self'. These men enact the emotional tie to their mothers with their homosexual partners. However, pregenital conflicts predominate over genital ones and are consistent with findings of loving but disturbed object-relationships and possible character disorders. In a third type of homosexual relation the 'homosexual partner is "loved" as an extension of the patient's own pathologicl self, and hence we find the relation, not from self to object, nor from object to self, but from [pathological grandiose] self to self'. This has the worst prognosis because the homosexuality exists in the context of narcissistic personality structure proper. This does not exclude such persons from functioning well socially.

This brief survey indicates that where there is a pathological development of narcissism there is also a disordered regulation of self-esteem, with the affects, object-relationships, ego, and super-ego functionings being simultaneously involved. Contributing particularly to such faulty self-esteem regulation are those cases where the self- and object-images retain vague boundaries or exist in a fused state. In severe perversions, early projective and introjective identifications between mother and child are finally introjected by the child to become part of the self-image, although derived from the object. At the same time, the self-object image is filled with narcissistic self-representational material which has gained an object-representational quality. This may interfere with the affects, object-relationships, ego and super-ego functioning. This distortion of the inner self-object image is facilitated by the seductions and frustrations which occur in the symbiotic and transitional object phases. One may postulate that due to weakness of the inner boundaries, the partial drive hyper-libidinization floods the undifferentiated self-object to fuse it instead of promoting maturation and separation. The excess drive becomes available for the structural part of the ego to maintain primitive splitting defences. With maturation and further cohesion of later self-and object-representations, the hyper-libidinization becomes available in the terms of Sachs' mechanism, thus transforming anxiety into pleasure by the temporary resolution of conflict, whereby the pleasure-giving self- and object-images are libidinized, and the painful aggressive and hating of the self- and object-images are either repressed, split-off or denied. This latter manocuvre includes a swing towards pleasure in the delicate libido-aggressive balance that exists intrapsychically, thus contributing to positive inner narcissistic constellations (cathexis of the self-representations with neutralized libido and aggression). The result is a heightened self-esteem that carries, in temporary accordance, the modifying influences of the ego-ideal and super-ego.

The super-ego in perversion was previously regarded as having developed 'lacunae' towards perverse behaviour based on the tolerating attitudes in the parents (Gillespie 1964). More recent work has shown that the super-ego itself develops faults in keeping with the ego, self, and internal-object disorders described above. In particular, failures of internalization of the ego-ideal, unwillingness to identify with unsuitable parents and the tendency towards merging, all militate against normal super-ego development. The type of perversion or its absence, together with the degree or quality of the perverse act, are usually determined by the demands made upon the self by the ego-ideal and super-ego.

The following clinical case study exemplifies perversion as an esteem regulator. The patient had been in treatment on and off for over fifteen years, and was first reported in some detail in Slovenko's *Sexual deviation and the law* (Rosen 1965). A compulsive voyeur and secret collector of personal pornographic material, he feared he would be discovered to his great detriment. Of use in therapy were previous drawings by a friendly prostitute of his perverse fantasies which were passive into active reversals of childhood humiliations.

The drawings were first used for masturbation and then kept locked away with a dual purpose in mind. Resource could be had to them for masturbation, and they functioned as an inanimate source of satisfaction and excitement under the patient's control. Excitement by means of seeing was a defence against the dull feelings of loss at being rejected by someone he loved, which was based on the original loss of his mother as someone of whom he had sole possession. The thought that others would be shocked at seeing the pictures made him feel audacious and raised his self-esteem. This phallic excitement defended him against his fear of regression to a state of oral dependency on the mother. Opposing this was the fear that the drawings would be discovered and he would suffer humiliation and rejection by those he loved. Although these fears and feelings were quite conscious and the risks taken were calculated ones, he was still acting under a repetition-compulsion dating back to his childhood. These drawings were analagous to a drawing he had made of a 'little penis' at the age of five, when he had secretly kept this drawing in his pocket, and both wished for and feared its discovery by his mother. Possession of the drawing made him feel he was 'bad' and independent of her, as she was against such things and had deprecated his competitive urinary games with other boys. Being a 'good' boy meant he might be overwhelmed by her love and lose his sense of identity. He further never minded his mother discovering the drawing, as he then felt revealed as a sexual partner for her. He recalled his great sexual pleasure in having his penis fondled by mother at an earlier age, but also felt she coveted it. There was also an awareness of mother's sensual pleasure, both in these acts and in the fantasied mutuality of the breast-feeding situation. The excitement associated with the possession of the 'little penis' drawing and the later ones, therefore expressed the mutuality of his and mother's physical pleasure both in the feeding situation and in bed at night. He had shared her bedroom for the first two years of life while his father was away, and he was unceremoniously ejected on the father's return.

Already formed was the core of his perverse-mechanisms as a regulator of self-esteem. The drawing of the little penis was an ego accomplishment which gave him great pride. He could draw this in relation to mother; keep it hidden from her; and experience in anticipation the thrill of discovery and possible punishment, by which means he elevated his sense of courage as opposed to his cowardliness in having to hide it. The 'little penis' stood high in relation to father's big penis and the fetishistic aspects of the female penis by virtue of its having been drawn, which led to maturing ego sublimatory capacities. This patient never drew in later life, and possibly his talents were not up to expression in the plastic arts, or they may have been inhibited by the perverse-mechanisms. He achieved success later in other verbal sublimations. One feature that he consciously retained from childhood, apart from his compulsion to keep sexually exciting pictures, was a peculiarity of speech. A highly cultivated and articulate man, he revealed that he never used words in speech with the letter *R*. As a child he could not say *R* clearly, and on being teased, he felt humiliated and resolved never to use this letter again, nor later to reveal his intricate avoidance devices. This manoeuvre went undetected by me until he confessed after years of treatment. He could neither stand the humiliation of pronouncing a babyish *R*, nor did he want to analyse and give up the esteem-raising perverse devices. This speech disorder, while fixated on phallic and latency experiences, was based on early infantile object-dependent sources. His ego-ideal had accepted this manoeuvre as a requirement he had to pursue and maintain for gratification sake. What remained perverse were the unresolved early conflictual elements which were acted-out, thought of as perverse, kept hidden, and which if discovered would repeat the humiliation, but which gave constant gratification in the exercise of his ego capacities and their underlying sexualized aspect, that is, he would remain the baby, where he was the undisputed consort of mother's sexual and emotional life. The early infantile passivity was elevated to an achieved omnipotent gratification and ideal in the perverse mechanism. The hostile elements were also mainly hidden in the patient by his excellent integrative capacities, but expresed in his fierce independence of social codes that meant acceptance. His life activities were in separate compartments maintained by splitting mechanisms, for example, a pillar of established respectability, he consorted with prostitutes all his life, and under other names was eminent in 'progressive' fields. The ability to control the blending or separateness of the contradictory areas of his life, together with his actual perverse gratifications were the major part of the patient's successful self-esteem regulation. A charming and courteous man, he had first come to treatment when his regulating system had gone out of control, and he was in danger by virtue of his voyeurism. His treatment made him capable of whole-object relationships, and therefore liable to depressions, which were his reason for later visits, following actual object loss. One feature of this case was his need for the mutuality of excitement in his perverse activities. Urinating on his penis, practised on him by his wife, left him unmoved, because she was doing it for his sake rather than for the excitement of the act, whereas his prostitutes became excited, or feigned successfully. This excitement by the object, linked with his awareness of his mother's excitement over his penis, and brought him close to the primal object, symbolized also in the drawings.

This patient demonstrates that perversions and their precursors are intimately connected with the processes of self-esteem formation and regulation. This was evident early in the mother–child emotional relationship with its intense gratifications and frustrations, which influenced the later aspects of self and ego accomplishments in both symbolic and reality activities, and his ego-ideal attainments. In this patient, as in most perverts, self-estimation became linked with gender-identity through his notions of masculinity. The vulnerable masculine self-esteem was revealed in his passive infantile humiliations, which were repeated in latency and adolescence, and which necessitated masculine-type symbolic or real perverse acts, sexual and otherwise, to raise his sense of inferiority, both at the time and in adult life. The regular boost to his self-esteem was secured by his capacity for active conscious control and manifestation of his perversion. Patients may first seek help as he did, where the ego-control is becoming unstable, or has been overwhelmed due to traumas which repeat infantile modes of reaction, regression, and uncontrolled perverse acts.

The factors which produce perversion tend towards instability of psychic function and self-esteem. The perversion is utilized by the personality as a self-esteem regulator, where the splits within the ego and the self can temporarily gain an inner representation of wholeness or narcissistic integrity.

REFERENCES

Ablon, S. T. (1990). Developmental aspects of self-esteem in the analysis of an 11–year-oid boy. *Psychoanal. Study Child* **45**, 337.

Abrams, S. (1990). Orienting perspectives on shame and self-esteem. *Psychanal. Study Child* **45**, 411.

Baker, H. S. and Baker, M. N. (1987). Heinz Kohut's self psychology: an overview. *Am. J. Psychiat.* **144**, 1.

Chasseguet-Smirgel, J. (1974). Perversion, idealization, and sublimation. *Int. J. Psycho-Anal.* **55**, 349.

Demos, E. V. (1983). A perspective from infant research on affect and self-esteem. In *The development and sustaining of self-esteem in childhood*, (ed. J. E. Mack and S. L. Ablon). International Universities Press, New York.

Freud, A. (1966). *Normality and pathology in childhood*, Assessments of development. In *The writings of Anna Freud*. International Universities Press, New York.

Freud, S. (1914/1957). On narcissism: an introduction. In *Complete psychological works of Sigmund Freud*, (standard edition, Vol. 14, p. 67). Hogarth Press, London.

Freud, S. (1923/1961). The ego and the id. In *Complete psychological works of Sigmund Freud*, (standard edition, Vol. 19). Hogarth Press, London.

Freud, S. (1933/1964). New introductory lectures on psychoanalysis. In *Complete psychological works or Sigmund Freud*, (standard edition, Vol. 23). Hogarth Press, London.

Freud, S. (1938/1964). An outline of psychoanalysis. In *Complete psychological works of Sigmund Freud*, (standard edition, Vol. 23). Hogarth Press, London.

Gillespie, W. H. (1964). The psycho-analytic theory of sexual deviation with special reference to fetishism. In *The pathology and treatment of sexual deviation*, (ed. I. Rosen). Oxford University Press.

Glover, E. (1943). The concept of dissociation. In *On the early development of mind*. Imago, London.

Glover, E. (1964). Aggression and sado-masochism. In *The pathology and treatment of sexual deviation*, (ed. I. Rosen). Oxford University Press.

Goldberg, A. (1975). A fresh look at perverse behaviour. *Int. J. Psycho-Anal.* **56**, 335.

Hanly, C. and Masson, J. (1976). A critical examination of the new narcissim. *Int. J. Psycho-Anal.* **57**, 49.

Hartmann, H. and Loewenstein, R. (1962). Notes on the superego. *Psychoanal. Study Child*, **17**, 42–81.

Jacobson, E. (1975). The regulation of self-esteem. In *Depression and human exitence*, (ed. E. J. Anthony and T. Benedek). Little Brown, Boston.

Kernberg, O. (1975). *Borderline conditions and pathological narcissism*. Jason Aronson, New York.

Kohut, H. (1970). Opening and closing remarks of the moderator in Discussion of 'The self: a contribution to its place in theory and technique'. (D. C. Levin). *Int. J. Psycho-Anal.* **51**, 176.

Kohut, H. (1971). *The analysis of the self.* International Universities Press, New York.

Lichtenberg, J. D. (1975). The development of the sense of self. *J. Am. Psychoanal. Assoc.* **23**, 453.

Mahler, M. (1968). *On human symbiosis and the vicissiludes of individuation*, Vol. 1. International Universities Press. New York.

Milrod, D. (1982). The wished-for self-image. *Psychoanal. Study Child*, **37**, 95.

Milrod, D. (1990). The ego ideal. *Psychoanal. Study Child*, **45**, 43.

Ornstein, P. H. (1974). Discussion of the paper 'Further contributions to the treatment of narcissistic personalities' by O. Kernberg. In *Int. J. Psycho-Anal.* **55**, 215, 241.

Reich, A. (1963). Pathological forms of self-esteem regulation. *Psychoanal. Study Child*, **15**, 215.

Rosen, I. (1965). Exhibitionism and voyeurism. In *Sexual Behaviour and the law* (ed. R. Slovenko). Charles C. Thomas, Springfield, IL.

Sandler, J. Holder, A., and Meers, D. (1963). The ego ideal and the ideal self. *Psychoanal. Study Child*, **18**, 139.

Stolorow, R. D. (1976). The narcissistic function of masochism (and sadism). *Int. J. Psycho-Anal.* **56**, 441.

Weil. A. (1970). The basic core. *Psychoanal. Study Child*, **25**, 442.

Yorke, C. (1990). The development and functioning of the sense of shame. *Psychoanal. Study Child*, **45**, 411.

4
Fetishism

Phyllis Greenacre

INTRODUCTION

The concept of the fetish rests on a very broad base. The term seems to have originated in the 15th century, when Portuguese explorers in West Africa applied it to carved wooden figures or stones. It was thought that the natives regarded these as having magic value, and that they might have been considered as the habitations of gods or, spirits. This interpretation may have been derived in part from the regard and worship of relics of the saints or other holy persons, already familiar to the explorers. Here the part (the relic) stood for the person, who in turn represented God, and was cherished or worshipped in a kind of eternal mourning reaction. The body might be gone, but the spirit remained attached to some memento which was, or represented, a body part, or some object immediately associated with the body, of the deceased individual.

This kind of worship was probably an indication of adoration or awe, in which there was also a fear of catastrophe or ill-luck if the belief in the holy overseer was allowed to fade and slip away. The relic served as a constant reminder. At best, it might service as an agent of an external control; in any case, it was a token or a memento, invested with various degrees of magic. This concept then became formalized in group rituals in which the original relic was replaced by a symbol. This in turn has continued in quasi-adornments of group practices in many religious or secret organizations. To lose or to destroy the symbol becomes an act of hostility or treachery to the group and risks severe punishment, from either the god(s) or the mortal representatives of divine power. With the emancipation from direct dependence on divine guidance and intervention, and with the increase in authority invested in the group, the tangible symbol may take on the significance of an amulet, a charm, and gradually become little more than a decorative bangle. Frequently, however, the hint of magic-value, bringing luck, is lurking somewhere.

Similar phenomena are frequent in our own culture and form a normal part of children's play, especially in the latter half of latency. They appear in both individual and group games where special objects, ritualistic practices, or even sayings are used as protection against bad luck. Such practices may be abandoned in puberty or converted into more socially accepted and sophisticated forms. They may also reappear in special stylistic adornment of dress or decor and in fads in adult life. While these rituals vary considerably in different locations, periods, and cultures, there are some striking similarities in the conditions which produce them. It seems to me that, in the individual life, the dependence on such interests and practices portends a struggle with hostile aggressive impulses while these are augmented by fear in anticipation of submission in sexual union, not only to the partner, but to the unique quality of helplessness in the culmination of the sexual act itself.

The specific term 'fetish', derived from the Portuguese word *fetico*, has the connotation of an object made by art and skilfully conceived, in contrast to an actual relic; thus the term is related to artefact, which also has a two-faced meaning. It is a small something, which is especially skilfully contrived, and it is also a foreign body that is objectionably intrusive and misleading in an area of investigation or study. The fetish might also be worshipped and feared as a thing in itself, not merely as a symbol or representative of an unseen power.

All these variations and shades of meaning appear in conditions of pathological fetishism, as this is encountered in individual forms (in perversions and in more-or-less normal fetishistic phenomena) in our own time and culture. My own study has been focused mainly on fetishism as a perversion, manifest in the adult psychosexual life. (See also Chalkley and Powell (1983), Wise (1985)).

CLINICAL REMARKS

In understanding the genesis of fetishism, it is useful to consider not only the fetish as it is manifested in the perversion, but also as a phenomenon of varying form and intensity in conditions which cannot be considered definitely abnormal, as it appears ubiquitously. It may indeed be part of a vivid and rich emotional life. Perhaps the most frequent normal fetishistic phenomenon of adulthood is the love-token, or memento, which enhances the courtship love-play and may find its place as a preferred, but not a necessary, contribution to the foreplay of intercourse.

Fetishism as a perversion may be described in phenomenological terms, as the *obligatory* use of some non-genital object as a part of the sexual act, without which culmination cannot be achieved. The object chosen may be some other body part, or some article of clothing, or even a seemingly impersonal object. In this latter instance however, the fetish is found to be a symbolic substitute for a body part. In most cases, the need is for the possession of the object, so that it can be seen, touched, or smelled during or in preparation for the sexual act, whether this be masturbation or some form of sexual intercourse. In some instances not only possession of the object, but its incorporation into a ritualistic performance is required (Greenacre 1953*a*).

One of the difficulties in presenting an adequate discussion of fetishism lies in the fact that the condition is by no means a clear-cut entity. The use of the fetish in one form or another and at various times in life can be detected in very many neuroses and character disorders. It is my impression that it is also to be found in some quite regressed psychotic states. And it is encountered regularly at certain developmental stages in infancy and childhood.

Indeed there is a spectrum of fetishistic manifestations, which differ both in content and in the degree of their compelling power. At one end is the hard-core perversion, in which an object is demanded which is clearly associated with and represents the genitals. It must also be immediately available, tangible, and appealing to all the senses with the possible exception of hearing—although in a few instances this is the sense most involved. In a less severely circumscribed form of fetishism, an impersonal object, actually present or insistently remembered, or a fantasy version of an old memory will suffice. In another area of the spectrum is the use of fantasy alone, sometimes in a repetitive and sterotyped fashion, to enhance sexual pleasure. Tangibility is not demanded here: in fact, the emphasis is rather on the ability to be satisfied by a private illusion.

The fetishist does not generally seek help because of his/her need for the fetish, but because of other neurotic symptoms which are consciously more disturbing. He/she is inclined to think of the use of the fetish more as an incidental personal peculiarity than a symptom. Because this state is largely ego-syntonic, its existence may be unknown to the analyst until the patient has been in treatment for some time.

The very way in which a fetish is used indicates its defensive and quasi-reparative function. It appears as a reinforcing adjunct for a penis of uncertain potency. The fetish itself may be a single object, or any one of a number of related objects, used repetitively and quickly replaced if lost. It somewhat resembles a prosthetic body part, an artificial limb or, more precisely, a crutch or a hearing aid. It does not entirely replace a lost part but serves to increase the efficiency of an organ, the penis, which does not perform well without it. While it is not actually attached to the body, it must be nearby or recently at hand to be seen, touched, or smelled in order to exert its encouraging influence. The beneficial effect of the fetish seems to result from the incorporation through the senses of the image of the fetishistic object. This can be immediately elaborated by the arousal of unconscious memories, as occurs in the process of free association. It thus gains unique significance and lends its aid as though by magic. The result appears paradoxical, in that the inert object—the fetish—is thus unconsciously animated, and can give strength to the penis.

The ability of illusion to play an activating role is further apparent in those cases, related to fetishism, in which no external tangible object is used, its place being taken by fantasy, which is often stereotyped and repetitive. Such a state may be regarded as a fetishistic phenomenon. The need for it may seem to be less essential than when an objective fetish is used; but it is difficult to assess this situation as there is an implied, but usually fallacious belief, that fantasy is more readily controlled and modified by the patient than use of a concrete external object.

The use of the actual fetish, rather than a fantasy, may be more frequent in men than in women. It was earlier thought that fetishism only occurred in men. This disparity is largely due to the influence of the anatomical differences between the sexes, which permit a woman to conceal an inadequate sexual response, from herself as well as from her mate, more readily than is possible for a man. She appears also to have less direct conflict about this hidden 'inadequacy', and it mobilizes a different set of related conflicts; whereas in the man any appreciable interference with potency is obviously and drastically crippling to sexual performance. It is well known that an illusion of having a penis may develop early in a girl child after observing the penis of a boy or a man. This illusion is related to a prefetishistic state, and if long sustained may leave a lasting influence on the child's behaviour and character. The relinquishment of such an illusion is favoured by her later development, generally decisively so with the appearance of the menses at puberty. Symptoms more directly comparable to fetishism in the male, develop only in females in whom the illusionary phallus has gained such strength as to approach the delusional. In my experience this rarely occurs except in cases in which there are other severe disturbances in the sense of reality. This is especially illustrated in cases reported by Von Hug Helmuth (1915), Sperling (1963), Zavitzianos (1971), and Richards (1990).

Fetishism is clearly associated with a very severe castration complex. This exists as an intense, prevailing fear of castration in the male and a much more complicated, though less readily recognized, set of related reactions in the female.

THE DEVELOPMENT BACKGROUND

The early psychoanalytic description of the perversion of fetishism presented this condition as essentially due to a disruption in the usual libidinal development. This was first placed at or near puberty, when the young boy was overwhelmed by the awareness that his mother lacked a penis, and dealt with this apprehension by an unconscious manoeuvre, fixating on some part of her body or its covering (clothing) which was associated with the traumatic observation of her supposed castration. The mechanism is essentially that of a beginning screening process; but differs in its further development in that the altered memory must be both further concealed and concretized. The body part (or article substituting for it) seemed thus to be a compromise defence which both indicated the mother's genital structure and gave her a 'thing' which both concealed and represented her alarming deficiency. Articles of feminine clothing, especially corsets, shoes, or panties, were recognized as the commonest fetishistic objects. Further clinical studies modified this first point of view, and recognized that the traumatic event which precipitated the manifest fetishism involved an impact on and a disturbance of ego functioning—a splitting in the ego—making it possible for two opposing reality perceptions to operate simultaneously, to make amends for the alarming demonstration of the supposedly castrated-state of the woman. The very intensity of this traumatizing observation presumed an earlier established conviction in the young boy that his mother's genital equipment was like his own. I refer here to Freud's papers (1905, 1927, 1938), and shall return to these later in dealing with the concepts of the nature of fetishism as this was influenced by and became part of the development of psychoanalytic theory as clinical investigation progressed.

We now recognize that there are disturbances in infancy, predisposing to this outcropping of fetishism, which often occurrs in anticipation of or associated with puberty. The traumatic observation of the absence of the penis undoubtedly has a powerful and specific effect on the rising castration fears of the young boy (see also Kelman 1985). But this will not by itself be sufficient to precipitate the neurosis, unless pathogenic conditions in early infancy have already impaired the sound progress of drive development and further interfered in characteristic ways with the emerging sense of reality (Greenacre 1953a, 1955, 1960a, 1968). It is now also recognized that some quite severe cases of manifest fetishism may be found in the young child and may continue uninterruptedly into adult life (Sperling 1963; Spiegel 1967; Winnicott 1953, 1971). The significance of such early appearances of fetishism will be discussed later in this chapter, in considering their relation to transitional objects and transitional phenomena.

Our psychoanalytic understanding has been enriched through an increased interest in the forerunners and early stages of ego development, with a special concern with its autonomous functions. This puts the early ego in quite a different position in our thinking from when it was regarded as a development from the id, involved chiefly with defences. It has also been necessary for us to recast our ideas of the origin, nature, and vicissitudes of aggression. Our enlightenment has been furthered by many research studies with long-term, nursery observations of infants, especially with regard to the early infant–mother relationship. This branch of psychoanalytic research furnishes an invaluable supplement to the knowledge obtained from direct analyses of children, as well as to that gained from reconstructions in analytic work with adults. It is not my intention here to attempt the considerable task of reviewing the various theoretical conceptions with their special terminologies, which have grown out of the many, and very productive, research studies.

I would rather emphasize now that while such perversions may become manifest at various times between early childhood and young adulthood, their occurrence is more frequent and sustained in adulthood. Their development in any case regularly rests on a base of severe disturbance in infancy, that is, in the first two years of life. Such disturbances may be of various kinds, but of sufficient severity and/or duration to have an impact on, and somewhat interfere with, the orderly, progressive unfolding of development, which in these early months is so impressively rapid. There is not only the increase in the actual body size of the infant; but this is involved further with changing proportions of the body parts and the internal organs in accord with maturational processes and corresponding elaborations of functions. In addition there is a reciprocal enlargement of the scope and complexity of the infant's responsiveness and developing perceptiveness of his/her surroundings, in which the mother plays a central role.

Here I must digress to explain that my picture of what normally takes place does not coincide in all respects with the psychoanalytic theories of early psychic development as these are frequently presented. For a detailed set of quotations from various authors dealing with this subject, see Edgcumbe and Burgner (1972). My views may be somewhat more congruent with many of the observational studies of infants in nurseries, in which the infant–mother relationship is especially studied by psychologists and others, who are concerned with the physiology of infancy and its interrelation with the beginning of psychic reactions. I would mention especially the study by Greene (1958), and Escalona's discussion of the phenomenon of 'contagion' (1953). Such findings have often been considered as outside the field for psychoanalytic investigation, which should limit itself to the psyche alone. Even so it seems to me that psyche and soma are never completely isolated from each other; and that early infancy is a time zone during which physiological conditions may be important determinants of significant variations in the development of beginning psychic phenomena.

The early concept of fetishism took scant account of the disturbance in the role of aggression, although it was recognized implicitly that the use of the fetish might be associated with, or take the place of, sado-masochistic fantasies (Payne 1939; Gillespie 1940, 1952; Glover 1953; Bak 1953. See also Freud's 1909 work *On the genesis of fetishism* (Rose 1988), previously unpublished.) The acting-out of such fantasies in condensed ways sometimes formed the nucleus of fetishistic rituals; or they might appear as repetitive antisocial acts in certain other forms of perversion. They were regarded as resulting from very intense castration fears of the phallic and oedipal periods, with regressive components from the anal phase. But with the further direct observation of infants and young children, it has become apparent that both penis-envy in girls and castration fears in boys arise before this time and may be clearly discerned in the second year of life (Galenson and Roiphe 1971).

This expanding knowledge of infantile development, from direct observational studies, has also brought some shift in the psychoanalytic conceptualizations of the early psychic structuring. Importantly associated with these studies was Hartmann's theoretical contribution (1939), in which, among other things, he pointed out that the ego developed from an earlier time than had been conceptualized, and that its autonomous functions of control and adaption must depend on fundamental biologic roots. From these sources, certain ideas have evolved concerning the nature and timing of the beginning of the ego, which is still a moot question. The older theoretical postulate of the duality of psychic structuring by the differentiation of the ego from a primal id, has somewhat given way to the consideration that both instinctual drives (id) and primitive regulatory controls (possibly the earliest signs of ego) arise from an 'undifferentiated state'. The term 'undifferentiated' is used in various connotative references sometimes to mean that the ego is not differentiated from the id, and sometimes that the id is not differentiated by itself from some primordial biologically determined state.

An increasing number of studies of the conditions, circumstances, and early responses of the newborn have led to various points of view regarding the beginning of aggression and of the ego. Among the most important of these are the studies of M. Mahler and her co-workers; R. Spitz; S. Escalona; S. Brody; S. Provence, and others at the Child Study Center at Yale; the Putnam Childrens Center in Boston; the recent work of Galenson and Roiphe; as well as the many reports of individual observers. Anna Freud (1965) has stated the postulations which she and her students have worked out at the Hampstead Clinic. She sees the ego as developing from the vicissitudes of the ongoing relationship of the infant to the mother—shaped according to the latter's ability or failure to meet the infant's needs. According to this conception, the infant is in 'a narcissistic unity' with the mother (or a mother figure), and there is at first (which probably means at birth) no distinction between the self and the environment. The infant leans on the parents to understand and manipulate the outer world, so that the bodily needs may be adequately met, and the parents further limit excessive drive satisfaction 'thereby initiating the child's own ego mastery of the id'. It is considered then that the parents subsequently provide patterns for identification which are necessary for the building up of an independent structure (A. Freud, 1965, p. 46). The aggressive drive is to be considered chiefly in its relation to libidinal phases (p. 62).

My own clinical experiences have led me to formulate the developmental conditions of early infancy with a somewhat different emphasis. I believe that such a complete and primary narcissistic unity does not and cannot generally exist even at birth. It seems to imply a *complete* dependence on the mother, such as used to be thought of as characteristic of the prenatal period. Certainly there is a necessary and fateful dependence on the mother (or mother substitute) for certain basic needs, especially for food and warmth. The infant will not be able adequately to supply these predominantly on his/her own initiative for some months. The *independence* of the timing of his/her own needs from the rhythm offered him/her by the mother has in fact been the basis for the development of demand-feeding schedules, and a readjustment of ideas concerning toilet training. He or she may accommodate to her timing with more or less strain, or he/she may react with aversion as though to an intrusion if the discrepancy in timing is too great.

It appears to me, however, that the infant is partially independent of and separate from the mother at, and even before, birth. It has been pointed out (Greene 1958) that the fetus has already become somewhat independent of the mother in the first month of pregnancy, when the heart begins to beat on its own, at a rate which does not coincide with the maternal beat. The fetal motor rhythms also do not uniformly coincide with those of the mother, although the unborn infant may adapt in a considerable degree to the mother's heart beat, respiratory rhythm, and walking rhythm, even when these do not coincide with his/her own rhythms (Greenacre 1960*b*). It is considered that the neonate is made comfortable by being walked-with by his mother—in her arms or on her shoulder—because he/she has already become used to this when he/she was being carried *in utero*. His own spontaneous motions *in utero*, however, are sometimes quite at variance with the maternal activities and more responsive directly to other external stimuli. Thus it would seem that the mother is only a part (Although a very important one) of the environment and not the sole mediator of it immediately after birth. This margin of prenatal autonomy does not furnish adequate protection from the influence of certain maternal illnesses. The first three months of pregnancy when organogenesis is progressing rapidly is a time of special susceptibility. The second trimester is safer and the third trimester is again somewhat hazardous.

Already *in utero* the relation of the fetus to the mother involves other elements than are implied in a condition of narcissistic unity with her. Obviously this state cannot be considered as one of psychic activity due to psychic structuring, but it may mean that some elements in the unique organization of each unborn infant may influence his/her subsequent reaction to his mother and to the immediate outer world as well, very soon after birth, and may appreciably affect the psychic structuring when and as this becomes differentiated.

If we consider that the body–ego is the basic forerunner of the psychic–ego, it becomes clear that the development of the latter arises not only through the relationship to the mother, but in part from inborn organizing and balancing forces evident in the maturation of the infant itself. I can conceive of such a special fineness of balance in the fetal organization as would sometimes permit an unusually sensitive responsiveness to the mother *and* to the external environment very early in post-natal life. This would presage a possible later capacity for early gestalt perception, and an ability for synthesizing early sensorimotor experience. It might also contribute to facilitating the later synthesizing and integrating functions of the psychic ego. These might otherwise be regarded as furthered only by good maternal 'education'. The observations of Browne (1970) strongly suggest that there are considerable variations in the degree of dependence on the mother by the newborn infant. A group of children were studied consistently from birth until the age of 8 to 9 years. The one child who appeared most outstandingly gifted had shown an extraordinary independence from the mother and nurses from the very first post-natal days. I have discussed these possibilities in other terms in a paper on 'The childhood of the artist' (1957) and in a discussion of infants' play (1969).

Facts regarding the disturbances in the fetus–mother relationship are now increasingly recognized, and it is clear that the old conception of the intra-uterine period as a nirvana, or state of bliss, is untenable. It rests on fantasy from a much later period rather than on fact. While unhealthy maternal conditions may produce disturbances in fetal growth and maturation, it also appears that the self-regulating organization of the individual fetus and the neonate is not as stable and efficient as the homeostatic system is to become in later life. But it is probable that the organically determined integrative function in the fetus is related to the later homeostatic principle, and exists in some degree even before and during the early development of the ego, when experience does not yet attain an appreciable degree of object-relatedness.

It seems that the roots of aggression also belong to the primordial undifferentiated state and rest very largely on the early maturational pressures within the infant as a developing organism. The mother feels the kicks of an unborn child as independent of herself and interprets them subjectively, probably in accord with her emotional set toward her own pregnancy. We cannot suppose that the unborn infant has any reciprocal emotional reactivity. At most we would hypothesize some central nervous system registration of the activity as part of homeostatically based developing patterns, represeting a stage in the integration of the interweaving of the progressing functional processes.

But first let us consider the significance of the term 'aggression'. This has been used in recent years with the meaning of cruelty or destructiveness (Hartmann, *et al.* 1949). In this sense, it implies an aim and an object—a condition which can only occur when there is already a sufficiently developed psychic ego capable of an appreciable degree of object-relatedness. Aggression as an instinctual drive must arise from a primitive stage of organization of the individual organism, before this degree of object-relatedness has been reached. I speak of the *forerunners of aggression*, which I would see as arising from the undifferentiated stage of development, the stage dominated by the energetic growth of the individual. The inception of aggression is coincident with the very beginning of autonomous body functioning, which will lead to the stage of body–ego development during the early months of post-natal life. This in turn leads to hostile aggression.

An older meaning of the word *aggression* was that of *approaching, going at,* or *toward.* This was usually associated with the idea of an especially energetic approach and merged into the meaning of an attack. Aggressive traits were on the whole considered desirable, indicating an individual's energetic attitude toward the struggles of life. The term seemed later to gain a stronger pejorative tone, implying, and almost limiting to, hostility, cruelty, and destructiveness. This was especially noticeable after the World Wars, perhaps with the emphasis on 'the aggressor nations' in contrast to supposedly peace-loving ones. At any rate, this older meaning of aggression, as a *going out toward* or *approaching* seems to apply to the early expansive activity which may later sometimes develop into hostility and cruelty. Such unbridled expansion may injure that which it impinges upon, but destruction is not its aim or motivating force in any psychological sense. This is the background from which the capacity for hostile aggression in the interest of self-defence must develop. But tendencies to excessive hostility in its many various forms, have deep roots in extreme frustrations of whatever source, and increase from the more complicated struggles with hostility incident to the later libidinal-phase developments, especially the anal and oedipal periods. Such struggles result in deformations and special susceptibilities of later ego- and love-relationships.

THE EMERGENCE OF THE FETISH

It is obvious from the very character of the fetish that it defends against an unusually strong castration complex—so strong that an illusion of actual castration is easily aroused. The fetish is then the makeshift remedy. This situation indicates a weakness in the formation of the body-image. As this illusion of castration becomes too real, it is met with the use of a concretized symbol of the penis, which lends to it some strength and a semblance of adequacy. The compelling need for the fetish does not become fully evident until the young person is actually anticipating or seeking intercourse, usually in adolescence or young adulthood. Looking back through the work of analytic reconstruction in individual patients, one can see the outline, sometimes shadowy and sometimes distinct, forecasting this state of affairs at different stages throughout the early life. Such a defect in the early body–ego, involving as it does the necessity for maintaining two opposite perceptions of the genitals, brings a corresponding weakness in the psychic–ego. For the infarct in the developing sense of reality which is focused in the genitals, leads at the very least to uncertainty regarding the gender identity and may, in many instances, invade other elements in the psychic functioning. This disturbance occurs the more readily against a background of incomplete separation of the *me* from the other—specifically the mother.

In considering the antecedents of the fetish, I shall focus on three special periods of childhood. In all of these, severely unfavourable conditions tend to produce disturbances and imbalances in the somato-psychic development which *may* subsequently become manifest in fetishism. These three are: the *first two* years, the *fourth year*, and the *period leading up to and including puberty*. These are all critical periods, based on decisive stages of physical development, and anticipating and initiating obligatory changes in functioning, they are accompanied by shifts in the degree of independence necessary to proceed with the affairs of life.

The first two years

For most of the first year, the infant is predominantly dependent on the mother to supply sustenance and to supplement his/her own body warmth through her ministrations (clothing and covers, and actual body contact with her). He/or she is largely dependent on his/her own autonomously directed resources to resist or eject stimulations which are pain-provoking. Relief, when necessary, is largely through motoric responses co-operating with visceral discharge mechanisms—urination, defecation, drooling, vomiting, and so on. The conditions which are most upsetting and disorganizing are those impacts which grossly exceed the infant's maturational readiness.

At this early stage, the infant is in a symbiotic relation with the mother, with development proceeding through the operation of the introjective–projective mechanism. Ideal conditions allow the infant to achieve increasing separation and independence gradually and at its own speed. Severe disturbances in the mother may result in actual deprivation of appropriate stimulation to the infant, the effect of which can be almost as disturbing as when the discomfort has arisen primarily in the infant. Generally, however, these early reactions to traumatic conditions are more diffuse and affect the quality of organization of the incipient ego, rather than laying down patterns as specific as we see sometimes in fetishists.

The second year after birth is marked by the considerable infantile achievements of walking and talking—accomplishments which indicate and implement the growing pressure for and satisfaction in independent activity. It is still a time of rapid growth as well as of change in functions and posture, which makes for significantly new and varying perceptions not only of the outer world but of the own body, both directly and in comparison to the bodies of others. The multiplicity of the perceptual variations leads to the beginning of symbol formation, at the same time that memory (not on a conditioned basis) is being established. There is a total body invigoration and responsiveness; some upsurge and awareness of genital sensations is indicated by the frequency with which infants at this time are observed touching or playing with their genitals. Castration fears and penis-envy at this period have been recognized and variously interpreted by both child and adult analysts, and by research observers of infants in day-nurseries. This concurrence of increased genital awareness with the capacity for erectability of the total body in walking, may predispose to development of a persistent body-phallus equation. This is a somatic basis for later specific symbolization.

All this is part of a period of growing object-relatedness, with increasing capacity for meaningful attachments, both loving and hostile, to persons in the infant's milieu. There is less diffusion of rage in body states, as both rage and anger can now be directed at the real or supposed offender, rather than being spent on whatever is by chance at hand, whether it be the own body or an external object. The introjective–projective mechanism is still at work, though no longer as strong and pervasive as when individuation was less advanced.

The circumstances or events of this second year which contribute to the later development of manifest fetishism are of two general types: first, traumas which are of such a nature as directly to increase fears of castration; and second, those prolonged or chronic situations which more subtly promote uncertainty or confusion concerning the anatomical genital differences between the two sexes.

There is in any case some intrinsic castration fear in the male child, since his genitals are so exposed as to look as though they might readily be pulled or scraped off. But the greatest increase in castration fear is aroused by accidents to or operative interference with the genitals, or a contiguous area, or even other parts of the body. Since the sense of the own body is not yet firmly established, and the introjective–projective mechanism is still readily available, such traumas in other parts of the own body, or in bodies of others close to the infant, may be displaced to the genitals, introjected, and felt almost as though directly experienced. In this situation, vision is probably the sense through which any severe injury to 'the other' (the 'not me' in Winnicott's terms) is taken in. This visual incorporation is associated with a sympathetic responsiveness or resonance in parts of the infant's own body, which correspond to the observed injured area of the other's body. The earlier mirroring reaction of the first year is already developing into a capacity for imitativeness which may be expressed in consciously directed forms of behaviour or in less precise sympathetic body responses.

The integration of the inner representation of the own body has progressed sufficiently that the various body parts belong to each other in a fairly consistent functional way. This is evident in, and necessarily accomplished and consolidated in, the early stages of walking and talking. Widening but precise volitional goal-directness of the body activities is in process, but is still faltering and uneven. In other words, the infant's separation from the mother and her substitutes and extensions, has progressed and is furthered by the increasing capacity for independent exploration of the outer world. During this period of increased outwardly directed maturational pressure, the body is completing the process of getting itself together into a working unit, a process with which it has been so much concerned during the first year.

Further circumstances, fortuitous but unfortunate, and often present in this second year, may tend to increase confusion in the young child concerning the configuration of his genitals. This occurs when an infant at this age, and in the succeeding few years, is consistently exposed to the sight of the genitals of another child of the opposite sex, who is close to him in age and size. This situation is relatively common in families where young children, one to three years apart in age, are regularly bathed and dressed together, sleep together, and not infrequently play together nude.[1] Something akin to a twin relationship develops. Since the own-genital-area can never be seen as clearly or as easily as that of the other, the visual incorporation of the genitals of the opposite sex may be more clearly impressed on the child than that of the own-genitals. Conflicting impressions may then arise between what the infant sees repeatedly on the other child, and would suppose belonged to himself as well, and what he feels in any manual exploration or from the rising endogenously determined genital sensations. This situation obviously contributes to the preoedipal penis-envy in the little girl and to the early fear of castration in the little boy, which have been observed and described in studies of infants in day-nurseries. Although this state of affairs is not an essential antecedent of the development of fetishism as a perversion, in my own clinical experience I have found it a not uncommon contributing factor. Naturally, the confusion of this period is increased if there has been a prolongation and intensification of the symbiotic relationship with the mother during a disturbed first year.

The fourth year and the period leading up to puberty

Two further periods of special vulnerability to castrative traumas are experienced by the child before he reaches adolescence. The first of these occurs in the fourth year, when there is regularly a definite rise in genital excitability. By this time the capacity for object-relatedness has developed and the young child is now in the beginning

---

[1] One may also question whether it may be promoted in day-nurseries or in communes where groups of infants are cared for together, and are more liberally and consistently exposed to each other in the nude than might be true in individual families.

of the oedipal era. The second period of special vulnerability is in late latency or prepuberty, when the child is anticipating puberty and some body changes may have already become apparent.

These two periods resemble each other in that both occur at times of transition from a period characterized by increased body growth—associated with expanding physical activity with sexual interest driven largely by exploratory curiosity—to a period of intense sexual feelings involving attachment to another person. Both the phallic phase and the period of prepubescence are marked by awesome expectations of the opening of a new era, engendering both eagerness and fear.

Acute traumas, such as operations on the genitals, or on body parts symbolically representing the genitals, are particularly disastrous if undertaken at these times. They seem realistically to verify the threat of castration in an explicit way and are often met with a strong and very resistant defence by denial. The tendency to deny may subsequently spread, in such a way as to distort grossly the character development. If a severe trauma occurs in the phallic-oedipal period the memory of it may be deeply repressed, and leave in its wake an amnesia for the whole period. During analysis, it reappears in dreams, night terrors, and episodes of acting-out. If it occurs in late latency or prepuberty, it may be remembered in an isolated way but the emotion associated with it is denied and displaced on to other areas. Such traumas in prepuberty do not by themselves precipitate fetishism, but contribute to its emergence if earlier experiences of infancy have paved the way. Relatively slight traumatic experiences in prepuberty may be insistently recalled and even exaggerated, but then may be used as screens for earlier severe ones.[2]

THE FETISH AND THE TRANSITIONAL OBJECT

In considering how the fetish is related to the transitional object, I shall lean very much on my own work. This developed largely from clinical investigations during the treatment of cases of overt fetishism appearing as part of a perversion. My study, beginning in the early 1950s, was first presented in a paper, published in 1953, concerning the relation of fetishism to the faulty development of the body image. It ended with two articles (1969, 1970) on the relationship between the

[2] A fuller discussion of my ideas concerning developments in these periods is contained in earlier papers on fetishism. Chapters 2, 5, 12, 17, 18, and 19 in *Emotional growth*, Vol. 1, deal specifically with fetishism. The papers on 'Prepuberty trauma', 'Screen memories', and 'Respiratory incorporation and the phallic phase' (Chapters 9, 10, and 13 in *Trauma growth and personality*, Greenacre 1952) also deal with these vulnerable preoedipal periods. The last paper concerned a case in which a definite fetishistic symptom was present in a woman. This is mentioned but not especially stressed.

The paper on 'Prepuberty trauma in girls' (Greenacre 1952) deserves a supplement as the title might imply a restriction of the significance of this trauma to the female sex. Due probably to the nature of my practice at that time, I had not observed any striking cases among males. More recently I have been greatly impressed with the extremely disturbing effects of special genital traumas in prepuberty boys, including manipulations of or operations on the genitals, undertaken ostensibly for therapeutic reasons. The post-puberty sequelae varied, but there was always a considerable distortion in the adult sexual performance, varying from overt perversion to denial through impotence. In any case, there were also marked defects in ego development. The degree of malfunction of the ego seemed to depend as well on the nature of the early mother–child relationship.

fetish and the transitional object. My conception of the fetish as a perversion has developed further and been modified by additional clinical experience, not only with fetishism but with other related neurotic conditions in which pregenital disturbances clearly played a part in intensifying the oedipal problems and in undermining sound ego development in a variety of ways. During the last three decades especially, there has been coincidentally a general awakening of interest in developments in the infant years, and observational data of co-workers have become increasingly available.

At the end of this discussion, I shall attempt to compare my own point of view with that of Winnicott, whose first paper (1953) concerning the transitional object was published in the same year as my first paper on fetishism. His subsequent work has stimulated and influenced me very much, although there are some points on which we are not in complete accord.

There are certain basic resemblances between the fetish and the transitional object. Both are inanimate objects selected and used by the individual in maintaining a psychophysical balance under conditions of actual or potential strain. On the other hand, the transitional object appears in and belongs to infancy; whereas, the fetish—at least as used in a perversion—is commonly adopted as a necessary prop, or adjunct, for adequate adult sexual performance. While the perversion of fetishism becomes manifest under the demands of adult life, there are definite roots in early disturbances in infancy as well as in prepuberty. The transitional object by contrast is almost ubiquitous and does not generally forecast abnormal neurotic development.

When we compare transitional and fetishistic phenomena, the differences are less decisive: the two conditions seem to overlap. Thus, fetishes, or less tangible substitutes for them, may be used as magic props during latency in attempts to ensure a good outcome in adventurous or competitive activities of a non-genital type. In some cases, the use of the transitional object is continued into latency, and with puberty becomes more insistent. This transitional object may then with puberty give way to a fully fledged fetish or perversion. But this situation is the exception rather than the rule.

During latency generally there seems to be little difference between the sexes in regard to the use of benign lucky pieces, rituals, prayers, and private superstitions in the hope of success. A little girl in late latency once gave me one of her good-luck pieces. She called it a 'feeling stone', because it felt so good in her hand. It had a peculiar smoothness, which somehow suggested something satiny and softer than a stone. Irregular in shape, perhaps phallic, it had been a comfort to her when carried in her pocket. She did not use it in critical or dangerous situations, but rather to ensure good feeling and to protect against loneliness. It did not seem connected with any genital activity although it may have been a reminder of some such interest in the past. This kind of thing is extremely common. It seemed related to the transitional object and perhaps to an imaginary companion, and often becomes manifest at about eight or nine years of age. Later it may be continued in a less individualized form, as a girlish decoration, a bracelet, or whatever bit of jewellery is the current junior-miss fad. It contributes to collecting hobbies in both sexes. Here certainly the fetish and the transitional object merge. However, the use of the fetish is largely limited to men. Ritualistic performances and stereotyped fantasies as obligatory accompaniments of sexual activity may occur in women as well as in men: I would consider them as belonging in the group of fetishistic phenomena. They also occur and are intermittently acted out by transvestites.[3] The difference between the sexes, in the use of the fetish to secure sexual gratification may be due to the difference in the visibility of the genitals. Any failure of genital responsiveness in the male not only interferes with his sexual gratification, but is visible to both himself and his mate. Invoking an increased narcissistic wound, it requires a more drastic remedy.

Both fetishes and transitional objects are selected by the individual. In both instances the chosen object relates to the own body as well as to that of 'the other', the not-me, basically the mother. There is a greater variability and range of objects chosen by one adult fetishist than the transitional objects chosen by one infant. A great variety of objects may be chosen, however, by *different* infants. The infant usually selects a simple object at first, and only makes substitutions in the process of relinquishment. Thus the infant, in the process of developing, needs only time-insurance for his practical security. He or she is faithful but casual in his alternate use and neglect of this chosen comforter, as he/she progressively outgrows his/her need for its help. The adult fetishist, on the other hand, suffers a permanent need for this help and must accommodate to it. He or she may accept his/her use of it, make it ego-syntonic, and regard it as his/her own peculiarity, but he/she rarely gives it up spontaneously.

Both fetish and transitional object are clearly body-related. They offer substitutes or additions to reinforce body parts or aspects which are seemingly inadequate. The fetish is characteristically something which suggests the male genitals; but has some female attributes as well. In the perversion, the fetish is generally definitely visible and durable. If it is destroyed, it can usually be replaced. It seems clearly to be a direct body-symbol which bridges the difference between male and female genitals.

The selection of the transitional object, on the other hand, occurs usually during the first year after birth, and is almost ubiquitous (Winnicott 1953). The object is clearly selected by the infant out of various objects in his/her intimate environment. It commonly is something soft which has been used in the infant's care, such as an old blanket. which is also impregnated with body odours, from both him and his/her mother. Softness, smoothness, a suggestion of warmth, a kind of polymorphous pliability combined with relative durability seem to be the appealing qualities. The presence of body odour was thought to be almost indispensable. A freshly washed transitional object, which has previously been a favourite, will be rejected. Later studies by Busch *et al.* (1973) have indicated that texture is much more important than odour, and that after a freshly laundered object has been softened by being crumpled, it is readily accepted. Qualities of enhanced visibility such as bright colour and definiteness of outline do not count for much. In the end, the specific transitional object may be gradually given up by being reduced to a mere token of its original form. For example, a piece of a blanket previously in the infant's crib may be chosen; but even a part of its satin binding may come to serve as a substitute for the blanket itself. It rarely is decisively disposed of, but its

---

[3] Here my experience is only with male transvestites. From the study of the records of female impostors, I have thought that the episodes of imposture in such women represent the acting-out of earlier compulsive masturbatory fantasies, which are essentially fetishistic phenomena. The acting-out may then be in response to a need to experience in actual reality rather than only in fantasy. This corresponds to the fetishist's need for a *concrete* object to bolster his uncertain potency.

importance fades. The gradual relinquishment of the object suggests a spontaneous self-weaning.

While I have not made systematic studies of transitional objects in infancy, in those developmental situations observed at first hand, I have not generally detected as clear a connection between the specific qualities of the relinquished original transitional comforter and those of subsequently preferred toys, as is indicated by Winnicott. While a teddy bear or other stuffed animal may be used, children very soon turn to toys which are actively played with rather than embraced for comfort. Later, a live pet may succeed to the favoured position. We may understand this gradual change from an inanimate and polymorphously pliable object, to a more clearly defined toy, and ultimately to a fully animate but cuddly pet as meeting the needs of the baby in successive stages of his own individuation. After this is well advanced, he/she can risk establishing a friendly reliance on a pet that is capable of auto-locomotion. If he/she is not sufficiently separated from 'the other', unexpected motion, not corresponding to his/her own body rhythm, is disrupting. On several occasions, I have known babies of less than one year to become terrified when an inanimate toy seemed unexpectedly to acquire independent motion. In one instance, it was a large ball which suddenly rolled toward the baby who was sprawling on the bed. In another, a usually stationary and inert toy began to perform, since its concealed mechanism was wound up and set in motion by a visitor, intending to amuse the baby, who, however, became extremely frightened. Rhythmic motion at a distance, the swaying of mobiles attached to the crib, the soft clapping of hands, or the fluttering of leaves in the breeze, may on the other hand, attract and fascinate. Such movement perceived from a distance may be simultaneously faintly stimulating and soothing, if the rhythm is relatively even and not associated with sudden changes in intensity or tempo. It is to vision what a soft lullaby is to hearing (McDonald 1970). Like the security blanket, it helps the infant to relinquish him- or herself to sleep. An even beat may have a sustaining effect perhaps because of its resemblance to the rhythms of the heartbeat and of breathing in stages of healthy equilibrium.

The transitional object represents the infant's persistent, but less demanding, relationship to the mother during the process of separation. Periodic merging with her decreases as the autonomous urges due to maturation and growth take hold; ultimately then the mother becomes part of the environment in a different way. At first the infant is concerned with the transitional object as it conveys sensual familiarities, chiefly with the upper part of her body (her breast, arms, and face; probably with a diffuse sense of her whole body). This sense of familiarity is mediated largely through touch and kinaesthetic responses. Vision is probably not as important as it becomes when separation has progressed further. The mother who has been adequate and 'good enough' for her infant gradually and increasingly becomes part of the not-me environment, and as he/she propels himself forward, the infant adopts the transitional object to keep in touch with the mother as she used to be.

In contrast, the fetish, destined to become part of a perversion, arises in response to a focused need, because of concern about the genitals. The demand for the concrete fetish characteristically emerges as a symptom later than is true of the transitional object, and is not always preceded by a transitional object. My clinical analytical observations have convinced me that the fetish, nonetheless, usually has roots in disturbances in the first 18 months after birth. There may be such conditions that the mother is not and cannot be good enough to fulfil the infant's needs adequately. It is the influence of *trauma* in these early months as well as in later situations which lays the ground for the development of a fetish, whether this may occur in infancy itself or only surfaces in a manifest form at a much later date.

Acute or chronic traumatic conditions involving the mother, or existing in other parts of the environment, or in the infant himself may contribute to the background for the later development of a fetish.[4] For example, there may be severe deprivation of maternal contact, due to the absence of the mother or to her incapacitating illness, together with the substitution of inadequate, unreliable, and frequently changing caretakers; constant fighting and violently disruptive tensions in the household, which result in acute, overwhelming stimulation to the infant; acute or chronic physical trauma in the infant due to illness, operations, or sometimes to other unavoidable but drastic therapeutic procedures: in fact any state of unmanagable pain. Such conditions may be of an intensity for which no mother can offer sufficient comfort and relief. Infantile pain, as well as massive over-stimulation from external sources, inevitably arouses engulfing excitement which must be spent in and on the own body if maternal comfort is inadequate. Such experiences also are the forerunners of later states of blind rage. In such a situation, a transitional object might not be adequate either. The later clinical history is often that of a manifest or latent character disorder, with outbursts in which anxiety carries with it a panicky fear of exploding or 'going to pieces'.

My evaluation of the importance of these early traumatic conditions differs from that of Winnicott. He did not emphasize the influence of trauma; and believed that the fetish was derived from the transitional object and could be traced back to it. He cited cases of infantile fetishism as indications of this point of view. While, in my experience, there may be a transitional object preceding the fetish, this is not generally true in cases of fetishism developing in infancy or later as part of a perversion. Nonetheless, the two objects are closely related. In most of the cases of the use of a fetish in infancy reported by Wulff (1946) and Sperling (1959), the chosen object certainly resembled a fetish more than a transitional object. These infants had clearly less than good maternal care. The need for a fetish had appeared after weaning and was more orally focused than is true in general with transitional objects. In any case, the fetish, whether of infant or young adult, generally has a quality of hardness and concreteness in contrast to the preferred softness and plasticity of the transitional object.

In years past, thumb- and finger-sucking may have occupied a place intermediate between transitional object and infantile fetish. The tendency to such the fingers or fist is frequently well established in newborns, and has been shown to have begun before birth. But a few generations ago its persistence even in early infancy was so condemned

---

[4] It is interesting that when Freud first wrote about fetishism, in his 'Three essays on the theory of sexuality' (1905), he considered that there might be some consititutional 'executive' weakness of the sexual apparatus which has been especially affected by some *trauma* (italics mine) of childhood, and that the specific nature of the trauma affected the special character of the fetish. I would suggest that the constitutional executive weakness may have been due to the disturbed conditions of early infancy, which may be so incorporated into later development as to appear functionally as part of the constitutional equipment.

that vigorous efforts to break the habit by interposing drastic physical restraints were undertaken. These undoubtedly worsened the situation by increasing the frustration developing with them. Prolonged finger-sucking often showed a highly aggressive activity. Its prolongation into childhood may have resulted from this increased aggression of frustration, as well as earlier unusual or sudden oral deprivation, until it ultimately assumed the character of infantile fetishistic behaviour. In this respect, it may resemble the cases of infantile fetishism reported by Wulff (1946) and Sperling (1959). As already mentioned, the movement from oral to early genital preoccupation is especially easy in the latter half of the first year, when the giving up of the breast and the increasing separation from the mother occur at the same time as sitting-up, and the first attempts at walking bring a new visual relationship to the own genitals, often coincident with the beginning of toilet training. I have twice seen in consultation women who remained thumb-suckers into adult life. In both cases there were unusual disturbances and privations in the first years, and the clinical history indicated a severe degree of penis-envy. The condition was clearly a form of perversion. Both women came from affluent but emotionally deprived backgrounds, with little maternal care. Later, under the pressure of obligatory and burdensome social activities, these patients suffered such shame associated with the thumb-sucking, as well as with the conditions which formed its background that the development of heterosexual interests was grossly hindered.

By and large, the effects of chronic untoward conditions in the first months are diffuse in character. There may be an increase in aggression, which is largely body-bound since it has as yet no specific aim and object. An increase in body tension with a later predisposition to anxiety reactions may also follow. If such conditions are sustained, and so severe that the total resources of the infant are called into reaction, there is a tendency to a suffusion of excitation and an overflow of discharge with premature stimulation of zonal responses for which the infant is not maturationally ready. This may result in excretory and premature genital reactions, responses under strain which do not have a true phasic significance. Such conditions contribute to distortions in the body–ego development as well as to intensification of problems of the oedipal period, which is especially burdened by persistent narcissistic elements (Greenacre 1952). These contribute to character disorders and particularly severe neuroses which are not necessarily of a perverse type.

From my own experience in analysing adult fetishists, I have concluded that specific severe traumas as well as prolonged traumatic conditions are of special significance in the determination of later fetishism. When such severe traumatic episodes occur in the first months of life, they contribute to the need for an infantile fetish, since a transitional object will not suffice. These are the situations in which the distressed infant *cannot* get any reasonable amelioration from his/her mother, or even from a soft representational substitute for her. No mother can then be 'good enough', and sometimes the infant's own body discharges cannot suffice to care for the amount of primitive aggression aroused. The body then requires something of extraordinary firmness to offer focus and limits to his explosiveness. It is in this state of affairs that an infantile fetish is adopted which is reassuringly hard, unyielding, unchanging in shape, and reliably durable. It seems probable that the introjection of such an object, which is indestructable, lends a necessary strength, a kind of spot of organization to meet the infant's otherwise bursting omnipotence, since this cannot now be lent him/her in a controlled way by maternal support.[5] It is this mechanism of projection and return introjection which continues to operate in the use of the fetish in perversions of adult life, which I detected clinically and described in my first paper on fetishism (1953a).

I have already mentioned the fear 'of going to pieces' which may recur as a later symptom in both fetishists and other individuals with impaired ego development. Winnicott (1964, p. 139) has made similar observations in regard to severe neuroses in adolescents, with a special fear of a breakdown.

> He states the breakdown which is feared, has already been. What is known as the patient's illness is a system of defences organized against this past breakdown—the original breakdown ended when new defences were organized which constitute the patient's illness pattern. The patient's fear of breakdown has one of its roots in the patient's need to remember the original breakdown. Memory can only come through re-experiencing—the original breakdown took place at a stage of dependence on parental or maternal ego support. For this reason therapeutic work is often done on a later version of the breakdown—when the patient has developed ego autonomy and a capacity to be a person having an illness. Behind such a breakdown there is always a failure of defences belonging to the individual's infancy or very early childhood. Often the environmental factor is not a single trauma but a pattern of distorting influences, the opposite in fact of the facilitating environment which allows of individual maturation.

He does not, however, mention these particular symptoms as of any special importance in the development of fetishism, whereas to me it is an important link in the genesis of the fetish.

In my differences from Winnicott there may be a semantic problem as well as some difference in the focusing on, and interpretation of, clinical observations. Winnicott sometimes mentions trauma in connection with the development of the transitional object, when he means a degree of discomfort and of mild frustration felt by the infant in the process of separation from the mother; a degree of frustration which is healthy and strengthening, rather than disturbing to the development of the 'young ego' (1971, pp. 96–7). He seems to refer to severe trauma as 'actual' traumas and does not connect them at all with the fetish, which he regards anyway as a variant of the transitional object. I believe, on the other hand, that severe trauma has an obstructive influence on autonomous development and contributes to the later adoption of a fetish which is used at first as an emergency makeshift support. The need for this may become manifest in infancy, around puberty or in adulthood. It may be given up or used less needfully for periods, but is revived, reinstated, and incorporated into the sexual activity after puberty, when sexual feelings are more urgent. But its emergence into a condition of fetishism only recurs when additional traumata have been experienced in the phallic or prepuberty periods, and have further intensified and focused the castration fears, the ground for which has been laid in the first two post-natal years.

[5] Winnicott (1964) refers to this situation as presenting the forerunner of 'unthinkable anxiety' which is kept away by the relationship to the mother who is 'good enough' to put herself in the baby's place, not so much by adequate feeding as by adequate being. In her contact, she gives the infant a brief experiece of omnipotence.

This brings us to the consideration of the effect of any severe traumatic episode (as in contrast with chronic traumatic conditions) occurring at this early time. It has been repeatedly reported by reliable clinicians that even extremely severe traumas occurring to the infant or witnessed by him as occurring to someone (mother, sibling, a pet) in a warm relationship with him, seem often to result in singularly little disturbance. For example, Winnicott has written 'Actual trauma, however, need have no ill effect as shown by the following case; what produces the ill effect is the trauma that corresponds with a punishment already fantasied'. The implication is that if the trauma occurs very early, or is of so unprecedented a nature, that the infant has no remembered previous experience which can give meaning to the event; then the immediate reaction is soon over and no unfavourable symptoms will follow. He quotes the case of a female baby of one year who was attacked by her two-year-old brother with a hot poker which he stuck in the infant's neck just below the thyroid cartilage. An intelligent and generally jolly but rambunctious child, he had done this out of spite and was probably in a fit of jealousy toward this little intruder so close on his heels. Although the baby cried at the time, and spent six weeks in the infirmary, she subsequently seemed little affected by the experience. When seen by Winnicott, at 15 months, because of a cough, she seemed healthy and happy, showed no symptoms referable to the incident, and no undue axiety when the brother snatched toys from her or provoked her in other ways (1931, p. 9). Winnicott then added that although having a hot poker put against her neck corresponded with nothing already in her mind and no ill effect could be noted, yet it was possible that when she reached a more advanced level of emotional development, anxiety might be referred back to this incident which conceivably could then appear to her as the cruel assault that it was.

Such cases may be of special significance in the background of the fetishist. I have seen the situation from a more expanded period of time than that granted to Winnicott, who was a paediatrician at the time he made this observation. I believe that such early severe traumas produce an extraordinary effect, which is not immediately evident for the very reason that they subject the infant to an experience of extreme stimulation for which he has no clear preparatory experience. In the analysis of some fetishists and one transvestite patient, I have found that such a severe trauma may remain as a submerged organization *impression* (I cannot think of a better word) which is not ordinarily available to memory but cannot be quite completely encapsulated and sealed off. There will always be some bit that will make a connection and be related to new experiences as they come along.

The deferred effects of these early traumas are of several types. At the very least, there is an increase in the anxiety connected with any new related experience. Most striking, however, are the states in which new versions of the original traumas, sometimes only slightly modified by the accretions of later experiences and fantasies, are produced in extreme nightmares, fugue-like episodes of acting-out in a panicky state, and repetitive somnambulistic behaviour. Fragments of the original traumatic events sometimes also reappear in physical symptoms.

Such a concealed *impression* of the infantile trauma is characteristically reactivated, when, as frequently happens, new traumatic experiences occur at the age of two years, as well as in the phallic and prepuberty periods. Sometimes these seem to have been produced under the influence of the continuing pressure of the disturbed earlier conditions, and sometimes they are fortuitous. But in any case, these are vulnerable sensitive periods, susceptible to the shock of accidents (either to the child him- or herself or to other closely related individuals), and to illnesses bringing about rather radical therapeutic interferences, such as tonsillectomies, delayed circumcisions, hernia operations, mastoid operations, and other active corrective procedures of one sort or another. Even the repeated use of enemas may be definitely traumatic. Such practices contribute to the undermining of the sense of the body integrity, and interfere with the developing autonomy especially increasing the castration fear. Such 'real' or 'actual' attacks require a defence which will also be a supplement. For this purpose, a fantasy may serve temporarily but a definite demonstration of phallic ability is soon demanded. Rising genital feelings initiate a period of masturbation which may become aggressively compulsive. It is often accompanied by sado-masochistic fantasies. Although begun in the search for relief, it results in an intensification of the castration fear and a general worsening of the sense of body and emotional integrity. When the young person reaches the stage of actually wanting and attempting intercourse, he finds his phallic ability wavering and uncertain especially when he is confronted with the sight of the female genitals. This situation in itself re-establishes his old uncertainty about his genital equipment. The fetish becomes the concretized substitute for the female phallus which has been intermittently believed in, earlier in life, but realistically given up. The fetish is thus a reification of a fantasy which has proved inadequate for the actual test of intercourse.

A brief account of the first years of a fetishist patient may help to illustrate the significant connections between the preoedipal disturbances and the later perverse development. The nature of these disturbances came to light largely through the work of analytic reconstruction. It was possible some years later to verify, with slight modification, the validity of our reconstructive work. The progressive series of disturbances was as follows. During his first three years, the child was exposed to violent fights between the parents as well as to sexual scenes. The marriage was breaking up in an atmosphere of jealousy and recriminations. In the latter part of this time, the mother had two abortions, the first of which was done at home while the patient was thought to be asleep in the adjoining room. The situations of these abortions had been confused in the patient's memory, as he believed that he had seen instruments being boiled up in the kitchen in preparation for the second abortion. He later learned from his mother that this abortion had been done away from home while he was being cared for by a neighbour. A little later, in the period of three to five years, he suffered three important losses: the parents separated and he did not see his father for several years; the parental grandmother, who often took care of him, died suddenly in her sleep; and a close playmate about his own age, died suddenly of polio. When he was between five and six years old, he had a tonsillectomy done in the doctor's office: the scene of the instruments being boiled up, belonged to this event rather than to the abortion. During early latency he was himself hospitalized for a febrile illness involving considerable joint pain. In the prepuberty period, after his father had rejoined the family, the mother had a third abortion, again done at home. He was thoroughly cognizant of this, and the memory served as a partial screen to the earlier one.

SUMMARY

The central core of fetishism as a perversion seems to lie in an extraordinarily severe castration complex. This ultimately results in an illusion of some actual impairment of the genitals. It has its beginning, however, in traumatically determined pregenital disturbances involving the body ego in process of formation and transition into the psychic ego. These disturbances of the first years are such as to be focused in the genital area prematurely, either because of the specific nature of the trauma or because of its extreme or prolonged severity. In any case, both aggression and genital response are mobilized under strain before adequate discharge channels have matured. This may especially be the case, if the mother is unable for one reason or another to give the infant adequate comfort.

Such early disturbances may recur later in childhood, either fortuitously or derived from the original experiences in a compulsively repetitive fashion. Their effect depends on the degree and nature of the confusion regarding the genitals, the extent of the invasion of the sense of reality, and the nature of the utilization and control of the aggression. Corresponding to the lack of confidence in the integrity of the own genitals, there is a prolongation and strengthening of the ubiquitous illusion of the maternal phallus.

The actual emergence of the obligatory need for the fetish appears when the growing boy or young man is forced to recognize that the mother, or the woman who supplants her, lacks the male genitals. The fetish then is an object usually associated with the woman but capable of representing both sexes. It serves a function analogous to, but, in my estimation, not usually continuous with or derived from the transitional object. The typical transitional object is essentially part of normal development. The two objects are, however, related. Their atypical forms, the transitional and the fetishistic phenomena, may be indistinguishable, the one from the other.

REFERENCES

Bak, R. C. (1953). Fetishism. *J. Am. Psychoanal. Assoc.* **I**, 285.

Bak, R. C. (1968). The phallic woman. The ubiquitous fantasy in perversions. *Psychoanal. Study Child*, **23**, 15.

Browne, J. (1970). Precursors of intelligence and creativity. *Merrill-Palmer Quarterly*, **16**, part 1.

Busch, F., Nagera, H., McKnight, J., and Pezzatossi, G. (1973). Primary transitional objects. *J. Am. Acad. Child Psych.* **12**, 193.

Chalkley, A. J. and Powell, G. E. (1983). The clinical description of forty-eight cases of sexual fetishism. *Brit. J. Psychiat.* **142**, 292.

Edgcumbe, R. and Burgner, M. (1972). Some problems in the conceptualization of early object relationships. *Psychoanal. Study Child*, **27**, 283.

Escalona, S. (1953). Emotional development in the first year of life. In *Problems of infancy*, (ed. M. J. E. Senn) pp. 26, 31, 46. Josiah Macy Foundation, Packinack Lake, NJ.

Freud, A. (1965). Normality and pathology in childhood, assessments of development. In *The writings of Anna Freud*, Vol. 6, pp. 46–67. International Universities Press, New York.

Freud, S. (1905/1953). Three essays on the theory of sexuality. *Complete psychological works of Sigmund Freud*, (standard edition, Vol. 7, p. 153). Hogarth Press, London.

Freud, S. (1927). Fetishism. *Complete psychological works of Sigmund Freud*, (standard edition, Vol. 21, p. 175). Hogarth Press, London.

Freud, S. (1938). Splitting of the ego in the process of defence. *Complete psychological works of Sigmund Freud*, (standard edition, Vol. 23, p. 273). Hogarth Press, London.

Galenson, E. and Roiphe, H. (1971). The impact of sexual discovery on mood, defensive organization and symbolization. *Psychoanal. Study Child*, **26**, 196.

Gillespie, W. (1940). A contribution to the study of fetishism. *Int. J. Psycho-Anal.* **21**, 401.

Gillespie, W. (1940). Sexual perversions. *Int. J. Psycho-Anal.* **33**, 397.

Glover, E. (1953/1956). The relation of perversion formation to the development of the reality sense. In *An early development of the mind*, pp. 216–39. International Universities Press. New York.

Greenacre, P. (1952). *Trauma, growth and personality*. Norton. New York. International University Press. New York.

Greenacre, P. (1953a). Certain relations between fetishism and faulty development of the body image. *Psychoanal. Study Child*, **8**, 70. [Also in (1971) *Emotional growth*, Vol. 1, pp. 9–31.]

Greenacre, P. (1953b). Prepuberty trauma in girls. *Trauma, growth, and personality*. Norton. New York.

Greenacre, P. (1955). Further considerations regarding fetishism. *Psychoanal. Study Child*, **16**, 187. [Also in (1971) *Emotional growth*, Vol. 1, pp. 58–67.]

Greenacre, P. (1957). The childhood of the artist. *Psychoanal. Study Child*, **12**, 47. [Also in (1971) *Emotional growth*, Vol. 2, pp. 479–505.]

Greenacre, P. (1960a). Further notes on fetishism. *Psychoanal. Study Child*, **15**, 191. [Also in (1971) *Emotional growth*, Vol. 1, pp. 182–99.]

Greenacre, P. (1960b). Considerations regarding the parent-infant relationship. *Int. J. Psycho-Anal.* **41**, 571.

Greenacre, P. (1968). Perversions. General considerations regarding their genetic and dynamic background. *Psychoanal. Study Child*, **23**, 47. [Also in (1971) *Emotional growth*, Vol. 1, pp. 199–225.]

Greenacre, P. (1969). Discussion of Dr Galenson's paper on 'The nature of thought in childhood play'. In (1971) *Emotional growth*, Vol. 1, p. 353. International Universities Press, New York.

Greenacre, P. (1970). The transitional object and the fetish: with special reference to the role of illusion. *Int. J. Psychoanal.* **51**, 447. [Also in (1971) *Emotional growth*, Vol. 1, p. 335.]

Greenacre, P. (1971). *Emotional growth: Psychoanalytic studies of the gifted and a great variety of other individuals*, Vol. 1. International Universities Press, New York.

Greene, W. A. (1958). Early object relations—somatic, affective and personal. An inquiry in the physiology of the mother–child unit. *J. Nerv. Ment. Dis.* **126**, 225.

Hartmann, H. (1939). *Ego psychology and the problem of adaptation*, pp. 101, 151. (1958. International Universities Press), New York.

Hartmann, H., Kris, E., and Lowenstein, R. (1949). Notes on the theory of aggression. *Psychoanal. Study Child*, **3–4**, 9–36.

Kelman, H. (1985). A fetishist's dream. *Psychoanal Quart.* **LIV**, 624.

McDonald, M. (1970). Transitional tunes and musical development. *Psychoanal. Study Child*, **25**, 503.

Payne, S. (1939). Some observations of the ego development of the fetishist. *Int. J. Psycho-Anal.* **20**, 161.

Richards, A. K. (1990). Female fetishes and female perversions. Hermine Hug-Hellmuth's 'A case of female foot or more properly boot fetishism' reconsidered. *Psychoanal. Rev.* **77**, 11.

Rose, L. (1988). Freud and fetishism: previously unpublished minutes of the Vienna Psychoanalytic Society. *Psychoanal. Quart.* **LVII**, 147.

Sperling, M. (1959). A study of deviate sexual behaviour in children by the method of simultaneous analysis of mother and child. In *Dynamic psychopathology*, 221–42. (ed. L. Jessner and E. Pavenstedt), pp. 221–42. New York.

Sperling, M. (1963). Fetishism in children. *Psychoanal. Quarterly*, **32**, 374.

Spiegel, N. T. (1967). An infantile fetish and its persistence into young womanhood. *Psychoanal. Study Child*, **22**, 402.

Von Hug Helmuth, H. (1915). Ein Fall von weiblichem fussrichtiger Stiefelfetischismus. *Int. Z. f. art. Psychoanal.* **3**, 111.

Winnicott, D. (1953). Transitional objects and transitional phenomena. *Int. J. Psycho-Anal.* **34**, 89.

Winnicott, D. (1958). *Collected papers. Through paediatrics to psychoanalysis.* pp. 9, 27–9. Tavistock, London; Basic Books, New York.

Winnicott, D. (1965). *Maturational processes and the facilitating environment*, pp. 37, 89, 97, 139, 141. Hogarth Press, London.

Winnicott, D. (1971). *Playing and reality*, pp. 80, 96–7. Tavistock, London.

Wise, T. N. (1985). Fetishism—etiology and treatment: a review from multiple perspectives. *Comp. Psychiat.* **26**, 249.

Wulff, M. (1946). Fetishism and object choice in early childhood. *Psychoanal. Quart.* **15**, 450.

Zavitzianos, G. (1971). Fetishism and exhibitionism in the female and their relationship to psychopathy and kleptomania. *Int. J. Psycho-Anal.* **52**, 297.

5
The gender disorders

Robert J. Stoller

INTRODUCTION

Most psychoanalysts, following Freud (1905), believe all psychopathology, not just the sexual deviations, results—by such mechanisms as castration anxiety and penis-envy in the oedipal conflict—from disturbances in the development of gender-identity, that is, of masculinity and femininity. This discussion, however, will be restricted to the gross aberrations of masculinity and femininity: primary and secondary transsexualism, transvestism, certain types of homosexuality, inter-sexuality, and certain aspects of psychosis.

A few introductory concepts may help. First, 'gender' (or 'gender-identity'), which, in the past, was usually synonymous with 'sex' or 'sexual', is used here only to connote masculinity and femininity. The value in using a different word for behaviour previously included in the general category 'sexual' is that it permits one to separate out areas which are otherwise blurred. For instance, there is a purely biological connotation in the word 'sex': the male sex and the female sex. But that connotation might be inappropriate when considering those aspects of sexuality we call 'masculinity' and 'femininity'. For the latter, such terms as 'gender', 'gender-identity', or 'gender-role' have been applied (Stoller 1968). If sex and gender were in a direct relationship, if masculinity and femininity were simply the result of one's sex—that is, of biological factors—then the differentiation would be pedantic. But there need be little connection between one's sex (biological) and masculinity and femininity (psychological); the latter, in humans, is produced especially by environmental and intrapsychic effects.

The second concept is that sexual aberrations can be divided into two rather different sorts of conditions, the one 'perversion', and the other 'variant' (or 'deviation'). As used here, 'perversion' implies unconscious conflict; inability to indulge a forbidden, pregenital sexual activity is resolved by using the perversion as the conscious manifestation of compromise (an example is fetishistic cross-dressing). Perversion, then, is a sexual erotic neurosis (cf. Gillespie 1964), requiring reparative activity in the cognitive aspects of the psyche, that is, ego and super-ego activities. 'Variant' ('deviation'), in contrast, is used to imply a statistical abnormality, but not a psychodynamically active, conflict-resolving state. Changes in sexual styles and customs from culture to culture and era to era can be examples of variance. Using these terms in this way frees one from labelling a person as perverse according to such external criteria as the sex of the object, the anatomy used, the standards of a culture, or prevalence rates, but rather according to the meaning the behaviour has for its owner. The definition is made intra-psychically, not by society. The idea of variance, in the above sense, expresses the belief that certain sexual practices or modes of gender behaviour may be acquired by such conflict-free mechanisms as are familiar to learning theorists; imprinting, classical and operant conditioning, and more complex forms of behaviour modification, especially in infancy and early childhood, play a part in shaping certain erotic and gender styles.

The third concept further defines 'perversion'. It is suggested that in perversion, to resolve the ever-present, unconscious conflict and to permit potency and the capacity for sexual gratification to persist, one's unconsciously desired sexual objects must be changed intra-psychically, reinvented. To do so requires disavowal, splitting, fetishization, dehumanization. This means, in simpler terms, that one's sexual object must be made less dangerous than it is imagined to be. Moreover, if we presume that the original sexual object was stronger than oneself, traumatizing, and the source of the original conflict that is now permanently internalized, one must, to restore one's sexual pleasure, triumph over the original object. Perversion remakes reality so that the victim—the perverse person—becomes the victor, while representatives of the original traumatizer—the original victor—are reduced in the perversion to being victims. (Rape grossly exemplifies these dynamics.) This process of changing trauma to triumph, however, reduces one's sexual object from an individual human into merely the representative of a class ('all females are the same'), or the parts of a human (breasts, penis), or an inanimate object whose relationship with the original human is only symbolic (clothing).

It is my thesis that only in the creation of perversion, not of variants, does this fetishization and dehumanization occur.

One last introductory concept. I distinguish a primeval stage in the development of gender-identity, called 'core gender-identity'. It starts at the beginning of life when psychic structure is first forming. The core gender-identity—preverbal, rudimentary, but fixed as an unalterable conviction—manifests itself in that behaviour reflecting the belief 'I am a male' or 'I am a female'. This is a piece of identity, a sense of self. It is not the same as being a male or female which is a biological fact, although in almost all cases, this core gender-identity depends on one's being a male or female. More precisely, it depends on one's being unequivocally *assigned* to the male or female sex. It need not depend on one's being in fact a member of the assigned sex, only that the infant, because of the anatomy of its external genitals, appears to be a boy or a girl and is so designated (see later section on intersexuality). It is rather well-fixed, unalterable, by age 3 (Money *et al.* 1957). Masculinity and femininity, however, are much more than core gender-identity and are still forming for years after core gender-identity is laid down. This later development is well known to us since Freud's explorations of the Oedipus complex. See also gender identity disorder in boys (Panel Report 1993.)

PRIMARY TRANSSEXUALISM

Male transsexualism

This person is an anatomically normal male, considered at birth to be unequivocally male, assigned to the male sex, and given a masculine name. Nonetheless, from the time gender behaviour first appears, usually somewhere around one year of age, the child behaves in a feminine manner. As speech, fantasy life, game playing, choice of clothes, and all other manifestations of psychic development progress, this boy acts as if he were a girl—even to saying in his first few years that he wishes to grow up a girl and to have a female body. There is no time, on into adulthood, when he shows masculine behaviour or desires. Although he may be forced by society to go to school dressed as a boy and to participate in activities with other males, he cannot do so successfully, no matter how severe the threats. In time, nowadays as early as adolescence, he may attempt to have his sex changed: castration of his testes and penis, creation of an artificial vagina, growth of breasts, and softening of other body contours by use of oestrogens, and electrolysis to remove facial and body hair. Usually before this, he will have passed successfully as a female, unrecognized as a male even by close acquaintances; the 'sex change' completes the process of passing, and from then on 'she' will live unremarkably as a woman accepted by everyone, even including sexual partners, as a normal female.

In this discussion, only such a person will be called a primary transsexual. By far the greater number of males requesting 'sex change' do not fit this description, though in the literature they are classified as transsexuals because they also request sex reassignment. They will be discussed below ('Secondary transsexualism').

What causes primary transsexualism? When these people are seen in childhood, adolescence, or as adults (but only these people—not those who do not fit the above description) the following conditions are found.

First, the subject is a normal male: chromosomes are male (XY); gonads are histologically normal testes that produce normal male testosterone (unless destroyed by chronic oestrogen administration); the penis and the rest of the external genitals are unremarkably male in appearance and function; internal sexual apparatuses, such as prostate, are normal; at puberty, ordinary male secondary sex characteristics develop.

Second, such a person develops from a typical constellation, in which the mothers and fathers examined so far have had in common the following personality attributes. The transsexual's mother, in her childhood, developed a gender disorder in which a powerful masculine streak is mixed into her femininity. Her own mother is a cold, distant woman, with no respect for this little girl; the girl's mother (the transsexual's grandmother) makes the girl feel that femaleness and femininity are without value. Although her father enjoys her, he encourages her to share with him his masculine interests, and so he both promotes some sense of value in her being his little daughter and at the same time encourages her in masculine directions. But even his affection disappears, before her puberty, when he removes himself from her, either by leaving the family in a separation, divorce, or death, or by turning his attention to a new child, now ignoring this girl. When that happens, she begins to develop as if she would become a female transsexual; she will only wear boys' clothes, plays only with boys as an equal, especially in athletics, wishes she were a boy, and openly states she wants a penis on her body. As opposed to the female transsexual, however, with the body changes of puberty her hopes of becoming male are crushed, and she puts on a facade of femininity. This leads in time to her getting married.

The man she marries is passive and distant, although not usually with overtly effeminate qualities. He has been dominated in his childhood by an over-aggressive mother and has not had a firm and masculine father. When these two people have chosen each other for marriage, they are able to play out their individual pathologies in a special family dynamic, in which the wife takes over the power in the household, openly scorning her husband, while he, bitter and ineffective, stays away, engrossed in his work and his hobbies.

This state of affairs is chronic, and yet transsexualism does not appear in all the children of the couple. In fact, the condition rarely occurs in more than one child; daughters, whatever neurotic problems they develop, do not become unusually masculine, and almost never are other sons in the family feminized (when they are, it is because the aetiological conditions now being described were again present).

The third factor required for male transsexualism is the contribution the newborn son will make; if he is as described below, transsexualism occurs. The necessary quality that, when added to the family's dynamics, will cause transsexualism, is the infant's appearing beautiful and graceful to his mother. When that happens, and when she finds he is a gratifying infant—happy against his mother's body—in those first days after he is born, she immediately develops an extremely intense, loving need for the infant. At that moment, the chronic sense of hopelessness and valuelessness from which she has suffered since early childhood is 'cured'. Now she has her perfect phallus, for which she yearned so long. This may well explain the puzzling fact that all these mothers give these sons very masculine names. The idea that such mothers really wanted a little girl does not hold up in these boys. This mother wants a son, that is, a male who has a penis, and she feels complete and full of rejoicing when she bears this infant and names him.

But the above factors do not *produce* the extreme femininity in the boy; they are only the necessary precursors. What is still needed is action in the three-dimensional world that will impinge on the infant's perceptions, stimuli so different from what occurs in the usual boy's experience that a rather pure form of femininity results.

The behaviour that thus influences the infant is the mother's handling of her baby; the style of which is dominated by her feeling that he is the first and only wonderful event of her life. The joy many mothers have with the infant they wanted, a joy that will be prolonged when the infant responds happily to his mother's mothering, is the normal version of the blissful symbiosis the transsexual's mother tries to establish with her beautiful son. For her, with her life-long hopelessness, the joy she receives is so gratifying that she cannot refrain from keeping her infant in her embrace—physically and psychologically—for too many hours of every day and after so many months that, in time, it is years that have passed. Her infant, by his presence, makes her finally happy, completing her former sense of anatomical and psychological incompleteness. In addition, and augmenting an already excessive closeness, she wishes to protect this beloved son from suffering at her hands even for a moment any of the unhappy feelings to which she was exposed throughout her infancy and childhood. So she does everything possible not to let her infant be frustrated by physical or emotional wants. Not surprisingly, he responds to such bliss by sensing what his mother wants and giving her more of it.

Unhappily, she needs her son to be an extension of her own body, always under her control and never separate enough to act so as to disturb her. In addition, with her envy, and therefore hatred, of males, she cannot stand behaviour that strikes her as masculine. This would be forceful, intrusive, 'dirty', 'nasty'. She is especially concerned that he should not behave in ways that reveal a desire to be emotionally separated from her. Of course, he has been self-selected already, in that he was biologically the right infant for her: he was beautiful, cuddly, graceful, and gentle. Now, as the months pass, she rewards all behaviour that holds him in this same form and discourages whatever she feels is rough or unloving, that is, masculine. So she creates this *thing*—not a separate person but a part of her own body—and we are not surprised to find that within a year or so, he, like she, does not know where his own body ends and hers begins: he believes himself to be as she is, female. He has, unfortunately, now and forever on, an insoluble problem, for although he feels female, both he and everyone else know he is unequivocally male. The rest of his life will be spent in the hopeless attempt to resolve this paradox.

Nonetheless, it is not inevitable that the boy will be totally feminized, for if the excessively close and blissful symbiosis were interrupted, however this cleavage might pain both parties, transsexualism would not result. One therefore waits to hear that the boy's father, on witnessing this feminization, will step in. He does not. He was selected long ago by this woman for his passivity and distance, for his ability to absorb endless scorn from her, and to persist nonetheless unchanged in his performance of inadequacy. And so, as his son develops, this father is not physically present. Yet he is kept forever present in the ambience of the home, for mother loses no chance to express her disgust with him and all men (precisely excluding, however, her wonderful son). But he leaves the house in the morning before his son has awakened, and busy with work, returns home after the boy is in bed. During weekends, the father is still not present, spending his time at his hobbies or watching television. The rule is that at these times he is not to be interrupted by the children, and so the little boy does not see his father. As a result, his father is not there to interrupt the symbiosis. Additionally, this man is not there to serve as a model for masculine identification. In his almost complete absence and with his wife disparaging his image, the symbiotic process runs unchecked, and the femininity increases, nurtured and encouraged by a mother who thrills to its manifestations.

Male transsexualism is an oddity, then, not only because the condition is so strange—a male who tries to change into a female—but for reasons of interest to those concerned with psychodynamic theory. This is especially true of the oedipal development in the transsexual boy. How does it compare with that of masculine boys and with that of those who have gender perversions?

The oedipal situation in primary male transsexualism is different from that of other boys, for there is no oedipal *conflict*. In order for oedipal conflict to occur in a boy, he must desire to possess his mother and have that desire thwarted by his father, with the result that a conflict between the desire and the danger is established. But the transsexual boy does not want to *possess* his mother; instead, he would *be like* his mother (Greenson 1966). There is no erotic component to the relationship. This is not just a theoretical statement but can be seen in the boys: for example, the observation is confirmed when the boys are treated; as masculinity begins to appear, they finally direct behaviour at their mothers—also reflected in their games—that expresses desire for her as a separate person. And father is, of course, no threat. We have already noted that he is not there; in his absence, he has allowed, condoned, the symbiosis to be uninterrupted. The theoretical significance of the absence of an oedipal conflict in the creation of a major piece of psychopathology will become obvious when we discuss gender perversions.

The second oddity for the theoretician is that the transsexual, despite his apparent gross distortion of reality—he says he really is a female—is not psychotic. In the first place, male transsexuals simply do not show the clinical signs and symptoms of psychosis with which we are familiar. Additionally, those who might consider the condition a psychosis, do so because of the tremendous discrepancy between the patient's body and identity; this bizarre belief, they feel, can only be explained as a delusion (Stafford-Clark 1964; Kubie and Mackie 1968; Socarides 1970). Yet, although transsexuals believe they are females within, not one, child or adult, claims to have a female body; *that* would be delusional or hallucinatory, like Freud's Schreber case (1911) of a psychotic with transsexual delusions. Instead, they insist their gender-identity is what they sense psychically, regardless of their anatomy. We know, from observing the mother–child symbiosis, that the femininity was created there, was 'imprinted' on the infant and then encouraged as he grew. Such is not the aetiology of psychosis. And when one examines the patient, instead of one's theory, the absence of clinical psychosis fits what one knows of the children: infancy is not traumatic, deprived, or conflicted. For a further description of these aetiological factors and for more clinical data see Stoller (1968, 1975a).

Treatment

Our knowledge of treatment of transsexuals is still rudimentary, as is our knowledge of the effects of treatment. If one's goal is to achieve a person whose identity is congruous with his body, then the effects of treatment so far have been dismal. If one aims for the more modest goal of a comfortable patient, then the results are better but still leave much to be desired.

At present, there is perhaps reason for hope in the treatment of children (Greenson 1966; Stoller 1975a; Rekers *et al.* 1976). See also Loeb (Chapter 6), where this hope is fulfilled. The earlier one starts, the better, for then treatment can interrupt the still-active family processes that create the femininity. In my experience, one does not get these children for treatment before four years of age, when society begins to impinge on them and their mothers, although as the public is told more about boyhood femininity, we shall begin seeing younger boys. The more the family situation approximates to that described above, the less likely the family will appear spontaneously for help; both mother and father somehow know that the transsexual boy is the focus for whatever mental stability they can maintain as a couple, and if he changes, they sense they will be affected. So neither usually spontaneously asks for help; they do not think they need help. But after a number of experiences in which strangers or teachers ask pointedly about the child's sex, or following a vigorous referral by a family physician, treatment may begin. It should encompass mother, father, and child, but it almost never does. The fathers do not co-operate, which is in keeping with what we already know of their personalities; those few who attend for evaluation do not carry through with the treatment.

Rekers *et al.* (1976) report a behaviour modification technique, described as simple, quick, and effective, that removes the femininity in feminine boys. The few follow-ups available so far indicate that the boys remain masculine. As yet unanswered is the question of whether the shift from feminine to masculine behaviour is superficial or whether it produces a more profound and permanent change in identity.

If one is committed to a more traditional, psychodynamically oriented treatment, the mothers should be treated either with psychoanalysis or analytically oriented therapy. The first goal of treatment is to help the mother through the depression that becomes manifest when she sees clearly that the treatment aims at taking from her her feminized phallus and that the bliss is to be ruined. If this issue can be managed, then she can be kept from sabotaging the treatment during the many hours of the day when she is alone with her son (Stoller 1975a). Beyond this goal, one can work with her toward character change of value to herself.

The boy's treatment in our hands has been more a re-learning experience than an insight treatment. Our research team attempts to change the child's environment (the family's interpersonal communications) rather than undo an intra-psychic conflict. And so only a masculine male therapist works with the child, and every effort is made during treatment hours to give the boy experiences in which behaviour defined as masculine becomes pleasurable. In addition, every effort is made to have the parents encourage masculine and discourage feminine behaviour at home. This is really, then, a behaviour-modification therapy. Perhaps it could be better done by those specifically trained in behaviour-modification techniques; this is an area for further research. Or perhaps the thesis is wrong and child analytic techniques should be used; since they have not as yet been tried, one cannot report how successful they might be.

Our results so far are meagre. One transsexual boy, now in his teens seems masculine (Greenson 1966). The rest of the half-dozen treated have become less committed to pure femininity; that is, they have some masculine interests and behaviour, but it is too early to predict the outcome in adult life for any of them (Green *et al.* 1971). Loeb in Chapter 6 presents two male cases who responded well to transference interpretation of their symptoms.

In treating adult male transsexuals, the general rule has been that whatever one does, it is wrong (Stoller 1968). All one can hope is to do the least harm and assuage the most pain. While the ideal would be a masculine man, it is hard to see how that can occur in a person who has never had any masculinity built into his personality from infancy. How can one create a major segment of personality *de nouveau* in the adult? A therapy based on the conviction that the transsexual can become masculine is based on the belief either that genuine pervasive masculinity can be created in adult life, or that there has been masculinity present, even if hidden, from childhood. One treatment team (Barlow *et al.* 1973) reports the ability to do just that. They have changed a primary transsexual male to heterosexual masculinity purely by behaviour-modification techniques. If follow-up shows the results have held and the patient is content, and if other workers can do the same with still more patients, then we shall finally have available a successful treatment for transsexualism.

Those who recommend analysis must recognize that there are no reports that anyone has ever succeeded in getting a primary transsexual into analysis, much less that the patient became masculine and heterosexual. There is one report of a psychoanalyst who had a patient whom he called a transsexual (in fact a paranoid effeminate homosexual) lie down in his office over a period of six months, but even in this condition, which is not transsexualism, the treatment is reported to have failed (Socarides 1970). I have been unable ever to persuade a transsexual male to enter into any but superficial (sympathetic listener and reality manipulator) psychotherapy, much less psychoanalysis. These patients wish and permit only a supportive relationship, in which one helps them with life situations.

If one grants that there are a few people whose lot improves with 'sex-change', the main problem in assisting the transsexual to change 'her' body is that of diagnosis; thousands of people these days request sex reassignment, and only a handful are primary transsexuals. Since the follow-up studies of surgical procedures are inadequate thus far, we do not know what happens when effeminate homosexuals, fetishistic cross-dressers, or paranoid schizophrenics have their genitals removed. One can suspect that there will at times be severe psychiatric complications. Until adequate follow-up studies have resolved these questions, one hesitates to promote 'sex-change'. See Volkan and Greer (Chapter 7 pp. 158–72) for diagnostic criteria of transsexualism and the relation to surgery.

But there are problems even when one carefully selects candidates for hormones and surgery. However, invariably, primary transsexuals are happier after 'sex-change' and although, invariably, they never regret their changed body compared to the former male body as the years pass (Stoller 1975a), some gradually become hopeless: they can never deny that the changes in their body are not fundamental. They not only remember they were born male, but they know (perhaps better than many who treat them) that one cannot ever truly change sex.

As the years pass, they are also burdened by complications from the surgical procedures. The vagina scars and becomes shorter and narrower. Usually further operations are required to correct this, and even so, the vagina may not remain patent for life. Bouts of cystitis are also the rule for the operated transsexual, and although each bout can be controlled with antibiotics, the next infection always threatens.

To not 'change' the transsexual's body, is to leave 'her' chronically despairing, since it is known there are medical procedures to make 'her' body more acceptable to 'her'. On the other hand, to grant the request is to give short-term relief but another sort of despair which, I fear, may lead to suicide in some operated transsexuals. Volkan and Greer report in Chapter 7 that 'transsexuals feel threatened by anything that might obstruct their defensive search for perfection through surgery' (p. 171).

Female transsexualism

I now believe female transsexualism to be a different condition from male transsex-ualism, not as, say in schizophrenia, the same condition in a different sex. The two states are comparable clinically, however. The female transsexual, like the male, is anatomically normal but wishes to have a male body and live permanently as a man. The condition starts in early childhood and, as I define it, runs uninter-rupted by episodes of femininity. In time, the patient will request and perhaps receive 'sex-change' procedures. In the female these are: bilateral mastectomy, panhysterectomy, and testosterone to produce male secondary sex-characteristics. In a few cases, with very uncertain results, the vagina has been closed and an artificial penis created by skin grafts. [For account of the tribulations and social significance of the transformation of female to male, see Bloom (1994). Cosentino *et al.* (1993), in a study of sexually abused girls aged from six to twelve years, found that sexually abused girls manifested significantly more cross-gender behaviour in the areas of gender role preference and aggression than did non-abused girls in their comparison groups. Their findings suggest that sexual abuse in pre-adolescent girls is associated with cross-gender behaviour and gender conflict. (This does not however constitute a main cause of transsexualism—Ed.)]

The aetiology of female transsexualism is unclear, but some preliminary findings can be reported. In all the cases I have studied of these most masculine of females (those for whom the term 'transsexual' seems acceptable), the following family dynamics have been present.

Neither the mother nor the father of the little girl has a gender disorder, as is the case in the male transsexual. Instead, the baleful effect seems to originate in the mother being unable to function as a mother in the first months, or year or so, of her little girl's life. In most instances, this has been because the mother was sorely depressed, though in a few families the mother–infant relationship was disrupted by the mother's paranoid attitudes or physical illness. In any case, the constant factor has been mother's absence from her expected mothering role in a situation where the child knows her mother is there (not dead or otherwise totally removed) but beyond reach. This is the opposite of the situation in the male transsexual, whose mother is so overwhelmingly present. One would expect the father to act to ease his wife's pain, to husband her at this particular time in their relationship. He fails to do so, though at other times he has been effective. Instead of himself thus ministering to his wife, he moves this daughter into the vacuum.

Had the little girl been pretty and cuddly—that is, had she at birth and in the first weeks thereafter been perceived by the family as feminine—she might not have been so used. However, these female transsexuals are reported to be vigorous, ungraceful, and unpretty in infancy. So the infant is used to 'cure' the condition that makes mother be absent. In this process, father establishes a close, firm, and happy relationship with his daughter. Unfortunately, he does this by involving her in activities that interest him, and since he is masculine, he quickly promotes masculine behaviour in his daughter. Because she already has at birth a biological tendency toward activity, aggressivity, and other psychomotor behaviour that goes well with the masculinity, the ground is all too well laid for that development.

In brief, the masculinity is created in the child's unending labours to reach her distant and unavailing mother and in her gratifying, but not heterosexual, relationship with her father, wherein identification with him and his interests is promoted. The family situation creates a little husband out of this girl, and by the age of four or five, she is already yearning to have the anatomical insignias of maleness. The situation is not the same intra-psychically, however, as in the male transsexual. The female transsexual's masculinity is born from pain and conflict, not bliss; from premature separation from mother rather than symbiosis. The female transsexual is constantly, unendingly, and hopelessly trying to reach a mother who is beyond reach. She does this in her masculinity and in her attempt to simulate her father's maleness (i.e., to have her sex changed), but she will never quite be able to do so. This mechanism makes me look on female transsexualism as a form of homosexuality. (See Khan 1964, for confirmation in a milder homosexual reaction. For a fuller description of these aetiological factors and for more clinical data, see Stoller 1968, 1975a.)

Again, as was described for the male transsexual, the long-term results of the female transsexual's changing of her body's appearance never leads to a final, quiet success. The patients forever know they only simulate or approximate maleness, and as the years pass, they too may become despairing.

Treatment

Even fewer female transsexual children have been treated than male. So far as I know, the only ones treated are by our research team. (See Chapter 7, pp. 169–70). We have had no success in four cases, if success is measured by onset of femininity. Once again the goal of treatment is to modify behaviour rather than create insight, for I believe that the masculinity is laid down so early and so permanently that insight techniques fail. Perhaps the therapist should be a feminine woman, if one wishes to create in the child a desire to be feminine. If the family can be induced to give up its need for the child as a substitute husband, then the mother and father may also come to co-operate in encouraging femininity and discouraging masculinity.

In adults, there are no reports of successful treatment that makes the female transsexual feminine. It is unknown how often this has been attempted, for there are no reports of such treatment. I have spent four years in psychotherapy with such a patient (unoperated) who, although I tried, only slightly shifted 'his' masculinity.

Following surgery and hormones, these patients are more content. Each establishes a permanent relationship with a woman and successfully holds down a job in an exclusively male profession.

SECONDARY TRANSSEXUALISM

Male secondary transsexuals

In this group are those biologically normal males, unequivocally assigned at birth to the male sex, who nonetheless develop a desire to be feminine and, in time, a desire to change their sex to female. They differ from primary transsexuals in two ways. First, the clinical picture is different. Secondary transsexuals do not appear feminine from the start of any behaviour that can be considered masculine or feminine (somewhere around one to two years of age). Instead, they develop for years in an ordinarily masculine-appearing manner. Beneath that surface—so they report in adulthood—there was, nonetheless, an impulse toward being feminine; this may or may not have been consciously experienced as a wish to be a girl. In time, usually adolescence or later, manifestations of the underlying feminine urges appear. The most obvious of these is an urge to put on women's clothes. This may be a symptom of a fetishistic perversion (transvestism), or of homosexuality. Person and Ovesey (1974a, 1974b) describe the development of these two types of secondary transsexuals, showing how the conditions develop as defensive structures from a matrix of masculinity and oedipal conflict (in contrast to the primary transsexuals).[1]

As different from most transvestites or effeminate homosexuals, however, the secondary transsexuals gradually experience transsexual impulses—the desire to be a woman—that grow in strength and last for longer periods—hours, days, and then indefinitely. These impulses do not, however, bring an end either to the fetishism in the one group or to the erotic homosexual urges in the other, nor are the masculine aspects of identity present from earliest life ever completely submerged. Because these earlier aspects of identity persist, the desire for sex change is less insistent, and the expressions of femininity less permanent and natural-appearing over time.

The second feature that differentiates primary from secondary transsexualism is the family dynamics in infancy and childhood. The constellation of forces just described for primary transsexuals has never been reported for any other of the gender aberrations, including secondary transsexuals.

Treatment

Because this is a mixed group with a variety of clinical pictures and aetiologies (Person and Ovesey 1974*a,b*), there is no way to recommend one, clear-cut approach. The treatment most discussed in the literature has been hormonal and surgical 'sex-change'. Unfortunately, because of the gross inadequacy of the reports, including follow-ups, we still do not know which patients do well and which poorly with these treatments. One can suspect, however, that the more the patient's personality is infiltrated with masculinity, the more risk he runs on subjecting his body to such radical anatomical and physiological changes. It is therefore important with secondary transsexuals that a careful and skilled—not perfunctory—evaluation of gender-identity be performed before one plans the treatment. In the presence of even occasional masculine demeanour, acceptance of having male genitals, gratifying relationships—heterosexual or homosexual—when living in roles typical for males, we probably should not recommend 'sex-change' but instead try to engage the patient in psychotherapy. At the least, such treatment gives patients a chance to examine more closely their desire to change sex and often leads to their choosing to not do so.

Female secondary transsexuals

Apart from Volkan and Masri (1989), there are no reports that describe a group of females clinically comparable to the male secondary transsexuals. The reason may lie in the fact that classification is a device that artificially orders clinical phenomena which could as well be described in terms of continua. For instance, in reality there is no dividing line to separate primary from secondary transsexualism in males, but rather there are clusters of people who fall primarily in one group or the other. One could as well, however, place patients on continua of masculinity and femininity by criteria such as degree, naturalness, time of onset, and so on. In the case of female transsexuals, then, it may be that we are looking at a continuum of degrees and styles

---

[1] They use a somewhat different classification from mine in that they describe these two types—the fetishist and the homosexual—as 'primary' and 'secondary' transsexualism and do not report on the state I have called primary transsexualism.

of masculinity, the extreme of which fits the above description for primary female transsexualism but on which fall less-marked cases of masculinity in females such as masculine homosexual women or masculine heterosexual women.

TRANSVESTISM

As used here, 'transvestism' refers only to fetishistic cross-dressing, that is, the use of clothes of the opposite sex to produce sexual excitement. The term will not refer to all cross-dressing, for this would include too many different conditions under the same rubric.

Male transvestism

Although sexual excitement caused by women's clothes may occur for the first time in boys as young as five or six years old or in men in their forties, it typically starts around puberty or in adolescence. At that first time, without prior warning, motivated, he thinks, only by curiosity, the transvestite puts on a garment of the opposite sex and immediately becomes greatly sexually excited, more than ever before in his life. He instantly recognizes this is a crucial experience and will now indulge in it either when there is opportunity or when he does not feel too guilt-laden. The condition may take three courses over time. For some men, a single garment or class of garments remains the preferred fetish; for another group, the original preference sooner or later spreads to a desire to be completely clothed in women's garments and to pretend for a period of time—minutes to hours—to be a woman; men of the third group (far fewer than in the first two), with some transsexual tendencies (the extreme being secondary transsexuals), learn to pass as women and spend extended periods living as women.

The aetiology of transvestism is not as clear as that of male primary transsexualism, but there is enough evidence to confirm that differences in the clinical picture are associated with differences in life history (Stoller 1975*a*).

No primary transsexuals are fetishistic (in this strict sense of the word, wherein fetishism means genital sexual excitement provoked by women's clothing); fetishism is the pathognomonic sign in transvestism. The primary transsexual wishes to wear women's clothes always, because he wants to be a female all his life; the transvestite wears women's clothes intermittently, usually only for a few minutes or hours but does not want to be a female. (In advanced cases, he may even wish to *pass* as a female, but he does not wish to *be* a female.) Women's clothes for the primary transsexual are no more symbolically significant than for a feminine woman; for the transvestite, the clothes have powerful unconscious meaning—as mother's embrace, skin, or phallus; as transitional object; as evidence to the transvestite he is not castrated; and so on (Fenichel 1954). The primary transsexual has been feminine since early childhood and is unremarkably feminine all the time, every moment of the day and night, awake or dreaming regardless of garments worn; the transvestite is masculine, except when cross-dressed. The primary transsexual is sexually excited exclusively by people of the same anatomical sex, but opposite gender-identity; the transvestite almost exclusively chooses women for his sexual partners. The primary transsexual wishes to become a normal female, to approximate which requires hormonal and surgical procedures; the transvestite has a male core gender-identity and wishes to be a male, and so he does not submit to 'sex-change' surgery. The crucial difference between the two is revealed in the attitude of each toward his penis: the transsexual feels the organ is a cruel mistake that blights his life, while the transvestite's life is focused on his penis, for he is a fetishist. The transsexual wishes to be a female; the transvestite wishes to be a male. The primary transsexual's aberration is (in keeping with my definitions earlier) a sexual variant; the transvestite's aberration is a perversion.

The transsexual was created in a blissful symbiosis; what are the aetiological factors in the transvestite's early life?

Let us first mark this finding: in no case of transvestism reported in the literature, and in no case seen by myself or my colleagues, has the history of the family dynamics of the male transsexual been given. Instead, something crucially different occurs in all cases where there are reports given of early childhood and in all cases investigated by our research team: rather than a lengthy period of blissful symbiosis, the transvestite-to-be is allowed to develop a male core gender-identity; he accepts himself as belonging to the male sex in the manner as do other boys. Following that stage, he also develops masculinity. In other words, whatever flaws there are in the mother–son relationship of transvestites, the boy separates from his mother's body and individuates into someone who believes himself to be a male (sex) and a boy (gender-identity and-role). This indicates that something in the range of a typical oedipal situation exists; at least the stage for an oedipal conflict has been set by the creation of a boy who values his maleness and masculinity (and therefore can be threatened by its loss). In addition, the boy, in separating psychologically from his mother, has her before him as a separate, desired, opposite-sexed object. In his childhood, therefore, he is exposed, more or less, to the temptations and threats of the oedipal conflict, essential for the development of masculinity, whether comfortable or perverse-ridden. Transvestites' mothers, from reports in the literature and from working with transvestites, their mothers, and wives, are a heterogeneous group of women (Stoller 1968). Transvestites' fathers, about whom I know less, are also mixed: some seem distant and passive, as are fathers of male primary transsexuals, while others are frightening, angry, punishing men who, although all too present, are about as unreachable as an object for love and identification, as would be a distant and passive father, (see p. 168).

In many cases, what seems to set off the process that leads to fetishistic cross-dressing is an attack on the boy's masculinity. Frequently (but not invariably) this will be a precise event: an older woman or girl—mother, sister, other female relative, or neighbour—puts women's clothes on the little boy *in order to humiliate him*. This act induces castration anxiety, or, as I prefer to look at it, a threat to one's identity: it is not just the fear of losing his genitals that frightens the boy but the significance of his genitals in fixing him as a member of the sex to which he has long since committed himself in his core gender-identity. In certain cultures and in certain eras boys may be dressed in girls' clothes. This in itself does not cause transvestism, for the purpose is not to humiliate the child. It is not the cut of the clothes but the intent of those who clothe the boy that makes the difference.

Other humiliations or other severe threats to the integrity of one's maleness and masculinity may also predispose a boy to fetishism; the work of Greenacre (1953, 1955, 1960, 1969) and Bak (1953, 1968) indicate as much (see Chapter 4).

But this, so far, is only trauma; yet perversion is pleasure. How is the latter accomplished? And where lies the conflict supposedly essential for the definition of perversion? One conflict lies, I believe, in the oedipal situation. The issue for the boy who is to become a transvestite is how he can protect his maleness, preserve his masculinity, permit his genital eroticism to develop, and to succeed in growing up to be an intact male, a man, a lover of women (who will substitute for his original desired object, mother), and a person with identity still intact—more or less. Since those are the problems confronting every growing boy (except the transsexual or maximally disrupted children such as the severely mental deficient, brain damaged, or autistic), we need to find other conflicts, specific for the transvestite.

The route via the oedipal conflict to a desired woman is additionally blocked for the transvestite by that first cross-dressing episode, a sharp, focal attack square upon his masculinity. It augments his fear of women (produced by their power to humiliate) and his hatred and envy of them (that they can be so strong and so effortlessly do so much harm), and results in a need for revenge on them (to bring the pleasure of victory to what had been traumatic). The conflicts here are between desire to harm females and fear of their strength, between wanting to have them (heterosexuality) and wanting to be one of them (identification with the aggressor), between preserving one's maleness, masculinity, and sexual potency and giving in to women's castrating attack by becoming a woman. Each of these conflicts is solved by the perversion: beneath the women's clothes and the *appearance* of being a female (no penis), the transvestite has secretly triumphed. His penis is still there and functioning. More, it is *really* there, triumphantly erect, victoriously male. By the expedient of seeming castration ('see me looking like a woman'), he escapes with his penis intact ('but I secretly still have my penis'). For a fuller description of these mechanisms, see Stoller (1975a,b).

Treatment

So far, no children who are transvestites are reported to have been treated. Although there are not, as yet, published reports on adolescents, a few have been treated by my colleagues at our medical centre. All have been seen in psychotherapy but none in analysis. Three have stopped the behaviour; the fourth stops intermittently. We are hopeful, but it is too early to presume these are cures and not just intermittent episodes of non-perverse activity as are so often found in untreated transvestities. If one judges from the literature on adults, the prognosis for giving up the behaviour is perhaps nil. At any rate, there are no reports, with careful follow-ups, of any fetishistic cross-dresser who has stopped (including not fantasizing it during intercourse and masturbation) for years, if the treatment is psychoanalysis or other psychotherapy. There are no cases in the analytic literature of a permanent shift in psychodynamics in such a patient, so that one might be assured that the underlying forces have changed enough to permit the perversion to disappear. For further discussion of the difficulties in psychotherapy with these patients see Chapter 6.

More optimistic is the work of behaviour therapists. In brief, they state—although with adequate follow-ups so far—that the more fetishistic the transvestism, the more likely is it that the symptom can be suppressed by behaviouristic techniques. The more the transsexual elements in the patient's identity, the poorer is the prognosis; that is, the more the patient wishes to pass, the longer the episodes of passing, the more fantasies the patient has of having a female body, or the more the patient wonders whether to have transsexual surgery, the less effective is behaviour modification (Gelder and Marks 1969).

Female transvestism

Fetishistic cross-dressing is essentially unheard of in women. While women cross-dress, they do not do so because the clothes excite them erotically. In all the literature (in English), there is only one report of a woman so excited (Gutheil 1930). I have had two others as patients and a third known only through letters. In all these, genital excitement came from putting on men's clothes and feeling as if a man for the moment. The individual garments were not exciting, however, until the woman anticipated wearing them. None was compelled by erotic need to cross-dress; for none was it the preferred or most intense sexual behaviour; none was fascinated by men's clothes; none lingered over the texture, style, or smell of the clothes.

HOMOSEXUALITY

Because homosexuality is taken up elsewhere in this volume, it will only be discussed briefly here and only as concerns its gender aspects.

Male homosexuality

We consider here only effeminate homosexuality, but at the start I place a caution that this is probably not a unitary condition with a relatively organized aetiology, consistent from case to case. Rather there are many homosexualities with varied aetiologies, dynamics, and clinical pictures. In the following discussion, I only emphasize features frequently found in effeminate homosexuals and leave out a presentation of variation existing in this 'condition'.

As in differentiating primary transsexualism from transvestism, I use the theoretical framework touched on in the beginning of this chapter in order to distinguish dynamics found in these different conditions. Again it will be helpful to separate out the dynamics of perversion—which I believe are generally present in the homosexualities—from those of more simple deviation (a matter of autonomous character structure, non-conflicting from the start).

Our first clue is in the clinical appearance of the effeminate homosexual as compared to the primary transsexual or transvestite. The transsexual is feminine. 'Feminine' implies a clinical picture in which the person appears, behaves, and fantasizes in a manner falling within the range of what is considered 'feminine' for that culture; most of all, the implication is that this appearance is unremarkable, normal, easy-going, natural, not an act or an effort, not a performance that would bring applause or admiration from onlookers. It is habitual and permanent. Such is not the picture in the effeminate homosexual. The term 'effeminate', in contrast to 'feminine', implies caricature, mimicry, the secret revelation of masculinity and maleness. There is something exaggerated or unnatural, a display, a sarcasm. And that is what underlies the behaviour. The effeminate homosexual does not wish to be a woman or have a female's body. Although his admiration for women may have led to considerable identification with them from childhood on, the admiration is mixed with envy, anger, a clear, even if subtle, underlining in one's behaviour that one is not a woman but a man making fun of a woman.

The source of this anger and envy is typically found in the childhood of effeminate homosexuals. It has become folklore by now, the observations having been made by so many people—one need not be an expert—that the mothers of such boys or men are over-protective (Bieber *et al.* 1962). When one observes closely the mother–child relationship described as 'over-protective', one finds that the closeness between mother and son, and the great gratifications granted by mother, come only when the boy does what she wishes. As long as he does not stir her envy and anger toward males, she will gratify him. For she is a woman who hates males. So he learns, by the system of reward and punishment she has set up, that behaviour she considers masculine will be punished but that soft, graceful, passive, 'sweet' behaviour will please her. In order to avoid her punishment—her withdrawal of love—the boy must suppress evidence of masculinity, and he can do so only with effort, pain, frustration. His feelings about his mother's 'love' are mixed. Yet to express the anger directly would be to bring her wrath down on him, and so it must go under cover. The disguise is in the effeminacy, where, in his mimicry, he subtly adds anger to his gentle, unmasculine appearance. In that way, although seeming to comply with his mother, he is secretly hostile and, in fantasy, victorious over her.

But why does he suffer when she wishes him unmanly?—the transsexual does not. The answer can be found in the histories as given by the parents and in the analyses of such homosexuals, when childhood memories are recovered. As different from the transsexual, the effeminate homosexual, like the transvestite, has had the opportunity to develop *some* masculinity during early childhood. He has a male core gender-identity on which he has built some masculinity, and especially, some capacity to see his mother as an external, heterosexually desired object. It is his masculinity, his need to reach for his mother, his entry into an oedipal situation, that sets off his mother's punishing reaction. She forces down expressions of his masculinity, but she would not do so had they not had the chance to develop. In passing, it is worth noting that severe attacks on his masculinity by his father may also push him toward the defence of homosexuality. Perhaps these attacks will not succeed in making him homosexual unless the mother fails to protect the boy from the father's attack.

If, then, we look again at the clinical picture of the effeminate homosexual, we find, as with the transvestite and in contrast to the transsexual, that the behaviour is the result of trauma, conflict, and conflict resolution. The homosexual does not wish to be a female; quite the opposite. He loves his penis and the gratifications it brings. The problem for him is that the way has been barred to gratification provided with a female.

These homosexualities, in summary, are perversions, not simply variants. The difference, as Freud has long since indicated (1905), is found in the oedipal conflict and focuses on the importance of the penis (important not only for sexual gratification but, at a more primitive level, for preservation of identity).

Female homosexuality

Rather than discussing female homosexuality, which is taken up in more detail elsewhere in this volume, and about which I know too little, I wish to discuss briefly very masculine women. There are several types I can separate off in a preliminary manner: 'butch'[2] homosexuals, mothers of male transsexuals, 'unrealized' transsexuals, transsexuals, and 'penis' women. The clinical differences between these groups are not sharp enough to make this a true classification; all, I believe, are points on a homosexual continuum.

The 'butch' homosexual believes she is a female, and while envying and identifying with males (comparably to the way effeminate male homosexuals react to females), she is militantly proud of being a female and insistes hers is a superior state to any male. She believes she understands women better than do men and can make a better lover and friend for a feminine woman. She believes herself homosexual and states she would not have it any other way.

The mother of the male primary transsexual, strongly identifying with males, has had a period in her life when she wished to become a male. Having some femininity implanted in her in childhood, she consciously gives up her desire to be a male with the onset of puberty. Unable to make a homosexual adjustment, she disguises herself as a heterosexual and lives permanently as a married woman, yet a hater of masculinity.

The 'unrealized' transsexual (secondary transsexual?) is a female who at the start believes herself a homosexual and lives as a homosexual in the homosexual community. Because she is exclusively masculine, she gradually finds herself revealing her marked masculinity; in time, she comes to feel she should be a male and fairly late in life makes mild moves toward 'sex-change'. The intensity of her transsexual drive, however, is less than in the transsexual and the length of time she needs to find her full masculinity is far greater.

The female transsexual need not be considered again, except to recall the notion above that female transsexualism may simply be the most advanced degree of the masculine female homosexual. Because in all these females, the masculinity is probably forced on the girl by painfully applied conditions in her family during childhood (balanced by undue encouragement to identify with her father), these character disorders are not comparable psychodynamically to male transsexualism.

By 'penis' women I mean an extremely small group of biologically normal females (I have only seen three) who hallucinate a penis as a permanent, three-dimensional, intra-pelvic structure. They do not hallucinate this as a symptom of a psychotic episode but rather *feel* a penis within themselves all the time, at any time of the day or month, undiminished with the passage of years, even in the absence of any other signs of clinical psychosis. Extensive study of one such patient revealed this to be, as one would expect, a homosexual defence (Stoller 1973). This condition is the extreme version of

---

[2] There is no non-slang word for indicating an exaggerated masculinity compared to (natural appearing) masculinity, which is the equivalent of 'effeminate' *vis-á-vis* 'feminine'.

the often-heard fantasy of women that they wish they had a penis or dreamed they were a man.

INTERSEXUALITY

'Intersexuality' is used here in the sense it generally has nowadays—to indicate that one or more of the major criteria for defining sex (chromosomes, gonads, external genitals, internal sexual apparatuses, hormonal state, and secondary sex characteristics) are abnormal. This is not the place for a careful discussion of the biological features or classificatory systems possible in intersexuality. It is enough here to indicate rules and hypotheses that touch on behaviour influenced by the physical abnormality. (See Chapter 18.)

Intersexuality was a fundamental concept for Freud's general theory of psychology, where he called it 'bisexuality'. Reviewing what was known from embryology and animal research in his day, he became familiar with findings that revealed aspects of both sexes in all humans (1905). This biological bisexuality he considered the 'bedrock' on which all normal and abnormal psychology is built (1937).

Time has borne out these important findings, although significantly modifying them. At present the evidence indicates that, except for the chromosomes, in all mammals including humans, all cells, tissues, and organs begin in a state of femaleness. Only if androgens are added (their production apparently controlled in the fetus by the Y chromosome) will a normal male result. In many ways, the male is an androgenized female; for instance, the penis is an androgenized clitoris, for without androgens a clitoris results in both sexes, and with enough androgens (but only at a precise stage of fetal development) a penis results in both sexes. Especially interesting are the recent studies revealing clearly in mammals that a male's masculine behaviour requires peri-natal priming of the brain (hypothalamus) by androgens during a critical period specific for each species. In the absence of masculinizing hormones, masculine behaviour does not occur, and instead the adult animal acts feminine. This rule of the primacy of femaleness is less biologically imperative, and post-natal learning more influential, the higher the species' position on an evolutionary scale. To what extent this rule holds in humans is still unclear, since one cannot perform the testing experiments on the human fetus or infant. Studies of chromosomal/endocrine disorders in man tend, however, to bear out the fundamental rule: the absence of androgens in the fetus produces varying degrees of anatomical femaleness, absence of anatomical maleness, and a tendency toward behavioural femininity in the patient, whether chromosomally female or male. On the other hand, large amounts of circulating fetal adrogens produce varying degrees of somatic masculinization (maleness) and masculine behaviour in the child and adult, whether chromosomally male or female. The literature elaborating these findings is reviewed in Gadpaille (1972) and Stoller (1975a). What makes the matter still unclear is the question of how much do post-natal, environmental (that is, interpersonal), and intra-psychic effects override these biological tendencies in man. In my opinion the rule in humans is that in gender behaviour, psychological effects *can* almost always overpower the biological. The transsexual would seem a good test of this: in the absence of any demonstrated biological abnormality in pre-or post-natal life and under the influence of a specific set of family dynamics playing on an infant male selected for his beauty, extreme femininity results. At the other extreme, there seem to be rare cases in which the biological is the overpowering influence (Money and Pollitt 1964; Stoller 1968); an unusually large number of males, hypogonadal during fetal life, have disturbances in masculinity even to the point of feeling themselves to be girls in childhood and adult life.

Hermaphrodites—those whose external genitals do not have the appearance normal for their sex—present a 'natural experiment' testing the hypothesis that in humans, the interpersonal, rather than the biological, is the greater influence in the development of masculinity and femininity (Money *et al.* 1955, 1956; Stoller 1968). In such situations, once again, family attitudes primarily determine the child's gender-identity. Regardless of the rest of the criteria for establishing sex (chromosomes, gonads, and so on), if the infant's genitals at birth look appropriately female and the infant is unequivocally assigned to the female sex, the core gender-identity will be 'I am a female', and the equivalent with males and maleness. Then, as with the completely normal female or male, on being assigned to the appropriate sex, one develops a core gender-identity consonant with the *assignment*, not the biology of one's sex. For instance, the otherwise normal female or male, but with external genitals appearing like those of the opposite sex, will be assigned to the wrong sex; if unequivocally thus reared, the child develops a clear-cut gender-identity in keeping with the assignment, not the biology. Or, a different example, when the genitals look hermaphroditic, that is, have attributes of both sexes, if the parents are uncertain of the child's sex (as, for instance, when a physician tells them that the sex is not yet determined or is unclear), then a hermaphroditic core gender-identity results (Stoller 1968). In this situation, the child grows up with an unalterable sense of either being a member of both sexes or of neither.

Treatment

We need not discuss the hormonal or surgical management of the intersexed patient; more important, anyway, are the rules of identity formation that should underlie the decisions of the surgeon or endocrinologist.

The key concept in treatment is the core gender-identity. We have noted that once the sense of belonging to a sex is established (around three years of age) it is very difficult to modify this fundamental of identity. Everyone has a permanent sense of belonging to one sex or the other, except in the unhappy situation of those with a hermaphroditic identity; these people feel they belong to a sex to which no one else belongs; they feel they are freaks.

After early childhood, then, the established core gender-identity probably cannot be changed. One should recommend that treatment in the intersexed patient who unequivocally believes himself a male or herself a female be planned around this established identity; there should be no treatment the success of which would require that the core gender-identity change (Money *et al.* 1955; Stoller 1968). Therefore, even though the anatomical and physiological condition will require more hormonal or surgical management, the body should be modified so as to best approximate to the identity. The patient, saddened by his inadequate physical state, will still be less traumatized than the boy or man suddenly told he is in fact female; or similarly in the case of a girl. For example, there is a common hermaphroditic state in otherwise biologically normal males, in which the penis is the size of a clitoris and the rest of the external genitals may also at birth have a female look. If the child is brought up a female, she may suffer from the knowledge she is sterile and needs oestrogens to maintain a feminine figure, but to tell her at age 6, or 16, or 26 that she is a male may be catastrophic. Even if the diagnosis of maleness is properly made at birth, because there is no present-day surgical technique to build a functioning penis, the child can be brought up as a girl. The surgical and hormonal problems are manageable: remove the testes (usually cryptorchid), surgically create an artificial vagina, and administer oestrogens at puberty. The result is a normal-looking female.

The case of the patient with a hermaphroditic identity confirms the rule that core gender-identity should determine mode of treatment. This is the person so often noted in the literature who can change sex with minimal distress at any time in life. For such a patient, after years of uncertainty and feeling unhuman, it is most supportive to be told by a medical authority that the uncertainty will be resolved and that he really is a male (she really is a female). The patient then gladly submits to the change of sex. Although the core gender-identity does not change, one's adjustment in the world often does. But when an intersexed patient, believing without suspicion he or she belongs to the assigned sex, is suddenly authoritatively told this was a mistake, the consequence may be the onset of psychosis (Stoller 1968) or the start of life-long despair and withdrawal from others. See also Chapter 18.

PSYCHOSIS

Gender disorders are commonly seen in psychoses. Freud used this finding as the keystone for his theory of the aetiology of paranoia. He said that the homosexuality (perhaps better termed transsexualism, for the symptom usually takes the form of ideas about one's sex changing), latent and unacceptable in the patient, becomes the core of a conflict that can only be solved by a delusion (Freud 1911).

Although ideas about sex-change are present in transsexuals and in paranoids, the two conditions need not be confused. The paranoid has the other manifestations of psychosis (such as remaking of reality other than that related to changing sex, or a thinking disorder); the transsexual does not. The paranoid is clinically paranoid (suspicious, irritable, self-referent, subject to supernatural forces), the transsexual is not. The paranoid man is not feminine nor is the paranoid woman like a man; the male transsexual's behaviour is unremarkably feminine, and, if one were not specifically told that 'her' body was male, the patient could scarcely be distinguished from another woman in regard to femininity; or comparably for the female transsexual. The paranoid feels threatened by the possibility his body might change its sex, the idea of sex change being alien, ego-dystonic; the transsexual yearns for the body to change. The paranoid believes his sex is fundamentally changing; the transsexual does not believe his sex changes but only that the external appearance of it has changed. The paranoid believes his sex-change will occur because of supernatural forces; the transsexual believes he can accomplish 'sex-change' only by his dealing with the real world. The paranoid's transsexual fantasies emerge only during the psychosis and disappear from consciousness if it ends; the transsexual's desire to be a member of the opposite sex has been conscious since the earliest childhood and has never changed, regardless of treatment or other life circumstances.[3] The paranoid states are a defence; male primary transsexualism is not.

In short, the paranoid states clinically do not look like primary transsexualism, their psychodynamics are grossly different, and they develop from aetiological factors unlike those in transsexualism.

CONCLUSIONS

Underlying the above descriptions of clinical states are rules and hypotheses that may help clarify issues of diagnosis, dynamics, and treatment.

1. The earliest stage in the development of gender-identity (masculinity and femininity) is the core gender-identity, a taken-for-granted, usually unfelt (but not dynamically unconscious) state of acceptance of oneself as a member of one's assigned sex.

2. In almost all humans, regardless of biological state, unequivocal assignment to one sex or the other and the continuing adherence to that assignment by parents in their behaviour toward their child creates core gender-identity; in humans, the biological state, to the extent it contributes, is a silent undercurrent rarely powerful enough to overcome parental influences in the opposite direction.

3. Core gender-identity, once formed, cannot be displaced.

4. Two different classes of dynamics may underlie the aberrations; the first is that of neurosis production—perversion—in which conflict, defence, and compromise formation in order to resolve conflict produce a psychodynamically unendingly active state. The other—variant—creates an aberration in which the above dynamics are not at work. The difference between the two is especially in the dynamics of hostility; in the perversion, hostility is directed to one's sexual objects, who must be demeaned, fetishized, and dehumanized, before they can be found safe enough to be approached erotically. In the variants, this dynamic of hostility is not an issue.

5. Careful observation of the patient in the present, plus careful history-taking, allows one to separate out as different conditions primary transsexualism, secondary transsexualism, transvestism, homosexuality, intersexuality, and psychosis.

6. What Freud often called 'homosexuality' and put at the centre of psychological development, both normal and pathological, might nowadays more accurately be called 'transsexual tendencies'. This adds the connotation of an impulse toward sex-change to the connotation of 'homosexuality', which focuses only on the more superficial aspect: object choice.

---

[3] I trust that no one will think, because beneath the paranoid's conscious rejection of transsexual impulses are unconscious desires, that therefore the dynamics are actually the same in the paranoid and the transsexual. That style of theorizing would throw away the gains ego psychology has brought to theory and practice.

7. The most profound aberration of gender—the earliest to form, the least likely to change by lifeexperiences or treatment—is primary transsexualism, and yet, at odds with common sense expectation, the condition is caused by atraumatic, non-conflictual learning experiences, accomplished primarily within a timeless, excessively close physical and emotional intimacy with mother.

7. If core gender-identity is so difficult to modify after childhood, then the more its presence makes up the gender disorder being considered, the poorer the prognosis for change. This suggests that we should either develop new treatment techniques for modifying core gender-identity (psychoanalysis does not), or we should design our treatments recognizing they will be limited to the extent that the pathology is a reflection of core gender-identity.

REFERENCES

Bak, R. C. (1953). Fetishism. *J. Am. Psychoanal. Assoc.* **1**, 285.

Bak, R. C. (1968). The phallic woman: the ubiquitous fantasy in perversions. *Psychoanal. Study Child.* **23**, 15.

Barlow, D. H., Reynolds, E. J., and Agras, W. S. (1973). Gender identity changes in a transsexual. *Arch. Gen. Psychiat.* **28**, 569.

Bieber, I. *et al.* (1962). *Homosexuality: A psychoanalytic study of male homosexuals*. Basic Books, New York.

Consentino, C. E., *et al.* (1993). Cross-gender behaviour and gender conflict in sexually abused girls. *J. Am. Acad. Child Adolesc. Psychiat.* **32**, 940–7.

Fenichel, O. (1954). The psychology of transvestitism. *Collected papers*. Routledge and Kegan Paul, London.

Freud, S. (1905/1953). Three essays on the theory of sexuality. *Complete psychological works of Sigmund Freud*, (standard edition, Vol. 7). Hogarth Press, London.

Freud, S. (1911/1958). Psychoanalytic notes on an autobiographical account of a case of paranoia (dementia paranoides). *Complete psychological works of Sigmund Freud*, (standard edition, Vol. 12). Hogarth Press, London.

Freud, S. (1937/1964). Analysis terminable and interminable. *Complete psychological works of Sigmund Freud*, (standard edition, Vol. 23). Hogarth Press, London.

Gadpaille, W. J. (1972). Research into the physiology of maleness and femaleness. *Arch. Gen. Psychiat.* **26**, 193.

Gelder, M. G. and Marks, I. M. (1969). Aversion treatment in transvestism and transsexualism. In *Transsexualism and sex reassignment*, (ed. R. Green and J. Money). The Johns Hopkins Press, Baltimore.

Gillespie, W. H. (1964). The psycho-analytic theory of sexual deviation with special reference to fetishism. In *The pathology and treatment of sexual deviation*, (ed. I. Rosen). Oxford University Press.

Green, R., Newman, L. E., and Stoller, R. J. (1971). Treatment of boyhood 'transsexualism'. *Arch. Gen. Psychiat.* **26**, 213.

Greenacre, P. (1953). Certain relationships between fetishism and the faulty development of the body image. *Psychoanal. Study Child.* **8**, 79.

Greenacre, P. (1955). Further considerations regarding fetishism. *Psychoanal. Study Child.* **10**, 187.

Greenacre, P. (1960). Further notes on fetishism. *Psychoanal. Study Child.* **15**, 191.

Greenacre, P. (1969). The fetish and the transitional object. *Psychoanal. Study Child.* **24**, 144.

Greenson, R. R. (1966). A transvestite boy and a hypothesis. *Int. J. Psycho-Anal.* **47**, 396.

Greenson, R. R. (1968). Disidentifying from mother. *Int. J. Psycho-Anal.* **49**, 370.

Gutheil, E. A. (1930). Quoted in *Sexual aberration*, Vol. 1, by W. Stekel. Liveright, New York.

Khan, M. M. R. (1964). The role of infantile sexuality and early object relations in female homosexuality. In *The pathology and treatment of sexual deviation*, (ed. I. Rosen). Oxford University Press.

Kubie, L. S. and Mackie, J. B. (1968). Critical issues raised by operations for gender transmutation. *J. Nerv. Ment. Dis.* **147**, 431.

Money, J., and Pollitt, E. (1964). Psychogenetic and psychosexual ambiguities: Klinefelter's Syndrome and transvestism compared. *Arch. Gen. Psychiat.* **11**, 589.

Money, J., Hampson, J. G., and Hampson, J. L. (1955). Hermaphroditism: recommendations concerning assignment of sex, change of sex and psychologic management. *Bull. Johns Hopkins Hosp.* **97**, 284.

Money, J., Hampson, J. G., and Hampson, J. L. (1956). Sexual incongruities and psychopathology: the evidence of human hermaphroditism. *Bull. Johns Hopkins Hosp.* **98**, 43.

Money, J., Hampson, J. G., and Hampson, J. L. (1957). Imprinting and the establishment of gender role. *Arch. Neurol. Psychiat.* **77**, 333.

Panel Report. Silverman, M. A. and Bernstein, P. P. (1993). Gender identity disorder in boys. *J. Am Psychoanal. Assn.* **41**, 729–42.

Person, E. and Ovesey, L. (1974a). The transsexual in males. I. Primary transsexualism. *Am. J. Psychother.* **28**, 4.

Person, E. and Ovesey, L. (1974b). The transsexual syndrome in males. II. Secondary transsexualism. *Am. J. Psychother.* **28**, 174.

Rekers, G. A., Yates, C. E., Willis, T. J., Rosen, A. C., and Taubman, M. (1976). Childhood gender identity change: operant control over sex-typed play and mannerisms. *J. Behav. Ther. Exp. Psychiat.* **7**, 51.

Socarides, C. W. (1970). A psychoanalytic study of the desire for sexual transformation ('transsexualism') : the plaster-of-paris man. *Int. J. Psycho-Anal.* **51**, 341.

Stafford-Clark, D. (1964). Essentials of the clinical approach. In *The pathology and treatment of sexual deviation*, (ed. I. Rosen) Oxford University Press.

Stoller, R. J. (1968). *Sex and gender.* Vol. 1: *On the development of masculinity and femininity.* Science House, New York.

Stoller, R. J. (1973). *Splitting.* Quadrangle, Hogarth Press, London.

Stoller, R. J. (1975a). *Sex and gender. Vol. 2: The transsexual experiment.* Hogarth Press, London. Hogarth Press, London.

Stoller, R. J. (1975b). *Perversion.* Pantheon. New York.

Volkan, V. D. and Masri, A. (1989). The development of female transsexualism. *Am. J. Psychother.* **43**, 92–127.

6
Childhood gender-identity disorders

Loretta R. Loeb

INTRODUCTION

It is important in formulating the aetiology of adult male transsexualism to know how similar symptoms develop in childhood. I have observed transsexual symptoms in two male children whom I had in psychoanalysis. I did not have to speculate retrospectively because the symptoms manifested in the transference.

REVIEW OF THE LITERATURE

From 1908 to 1927 Freud gathered material that showed the traumatic effect on male children of their first view of female genitalia. In 1908, he said that, from knowing their own bodies, boys characteristically initially assume that everyone has a penis that is dominated by excitation and pleasure. In 1910, Freud further observed that the boy's fantasy that girls have penises may not be destroyed even after he observes their genitals. He may disavow, Freud said, . . . his own sense-perceptions which showed him that the female genitals lack a penis and hold . . . fast to the contrary conviction' (Freud 1940, p. 202). The boy may then create an unconscious fantasy in which he gives the woman a penis (Freud 1927). For example, he may fantasy that a woman's penis is small, but that it will grow (Freud 1908, p. 216), or he may fantasy that a woman has her bottom in front (Freud 1918, p. 25) and a penis in back (Freud 1918, p. 84). If a boy cannot convince himself with such fantasies, he may imagine that girls' genitals are wounds that remain where their penises were cut off. In 1920, Freud (1905) said: 'The substitutes for this penis, which they [boys] find is missing in women, play a great part in determining the form taken by many perversions' (p. 195). Freud summarized: 'Probably no male human-being is spared the fright of castration at the sight of a female genital. Why some people become homosexual as a consequence of that impression, while others fend it off by creating a fetish, and the great majority surmount it, we are frankly not able to explain . . . among all the factors at work, we do not yet know those which are decisive for the rare pathological results' (1927, p. 154). Thus according to Freud (1927), young boys can develop a tendency toward perversion if they are traumatized by the sight of female genitalia.

The work of Sperling and Greenson in this area exemplifies both Anna Freud's (1965/1966) and Geleerd's (1969) contention that knowledge derived from the psychoanalysis of children leads to better understanding of adult psychopathology.

Almost all the psychoanalytic studies dealing with cross-dressing were on adults until Sperling (1963, 1964) and Greenson (1966) reported analyses of cross-dressing children. Their studies provide data on the early pathological picture and intra-psychic structure of feminine boys. While Greenson (1966) stressed the therapeutic benefit of identification with a strong masculine figure, he recognized the transference manifestations of the pathological relationship with the mother. He felt that confrontation and interpretation in his analysis of the boy improved the pathological relationship with the mother.

Stoller (1967) said that transsexuals are cross-dressers who wish to live, and be accepted as, members of the opposite sex. They complain they are females trapped in an anatomically normal male body. Stoller referred to a person's self-designation—irrespective of their anatomy—as their 'core gender-identity'. This core gender-identity is produced by environmental and intrapsychic effects. Stoller (1973) described three mechanisms that produce normal gender-identity: (1) the anatomy and physiology of external genital organs; (2) the attitudinal influences of parents, siblings, and peers; and (3) a 'biological force' which, although hidden from conscious and unconscious awareness, nonetheless seems to provide some drive energy for gender-identity.

Newman and Stoller (1971) found several highly specific factors in the early developmental histories of adult male transsexuals. Stoller (1975*b*) and Green *et al.* (1972, 1976) found these same common features in the early developmental histories of young boys with transsexual symptoms. Stoller (1973, 1975*b*) described these features as follows: By the age of 1 year, the boys showed signs of feminine gender behaviour. By age 2 or 3 they were unusually good-looking, preferred dressing and playing as girls, expressed the wish to have a female body, and were not thought to be psychotic. Stoller (1973, 1975*b*) described their mothers as follows: They had strong bisexual characteristics, took almost all their babies to bed with them, and exhibited considerable penis-envy—their sons serving as phallic substitutes. They also encouraged an unending 'blissful symbiosis' by not allowing their sons to experience frustration.[1] The fathers of transsexuals, if not physically absent, were absent psychologically. According to Stoller, the fathers neither served as models for masculine identification nor as protectors from the mother's feminizing efforts at symbiotic merger. (See Chapter 5.)

In Mahler's (Mahler *et al.* 1975) clinical experience, transsexualism is related to the mother's unconscious attitude toward her own self—especially her belief in her femininity or lack of it, her feminine self-esteem, her castration conflicts (p. 214), her penis-awe (Greenacre 1953), her penis-envy, and her defences related to all these. In summary, the discoveries made by Mahler *et al.* (1975) regarding gender-identity in boys include: (1) gender-identity in the boy asserts itself with less conflict if the mother respects and enjoys the boy's phallicity, especially in the second half of the third year. (2) Identification with the father or with an older brother facilitates a boy's male gender identity. (3) Gender identity is impeded when the mother interferes with the boy's autonomy. This is particularly

---

[1] In my two cases I did not observe any blissful symbiosis, but neither mother could not say 'no' to her son.

true if the mother is unable to relinquish to him, his body, and the ownership of his penis.

Jacobson (1964), Roiphe and Galenson (1973), and Abelin (1977) state that the failure of the father to aid the child in achieving a separate autonomy from the mother is evident in sexual perversions. Pruett and Dahl (1982) reported on the psychotherapy of three boys under six that cross-dressed and exhibited feminine behaviour. The boy's previous behavioural shaping had not helped them resolve their conflicts. Pruett and Dahl used interpretation, clarification, and the relationship with the therapist to enable the boy's egos 'to cope in more appropriate ways'.

Green (1987) studied two behaviourally different groups of feminine boys with questionnaires, psychological tests, and interviews. He based his conclusions, not on the unconscious determinants of these boys' feminine symptomatology, but on their conscious thoughts and overt behaviour. He used behaviour modification to treat these boys and their parents, and helped them adjust to society. Green said that this treatment approach showed no major impact on these boys' sexual orientation. The therapy did not interrupt their progression from 'feminine' boys to homosexual or bisexual men (1987, p. 318).

Socarides (1970) considered transsexualism to be like all other perversions: It is the outcome of intra-psychic conflict and affords both sexual release and ego survival. For Socarides, transsexualism represents a regression to an earlier phase, in which there is both desire for, and dread of, merger with the mother. This regression is fostered by a mother who has great difficulty separating from her child. She holds on to her child, preventing him from taking the developmental step of differentiating from her. This exerts a pathological, feminizing influence on her son's gender-identity. This pathological sense of feminine gender—of being feminine and linked to mother—conflicts with the child's emerging awareness of the genital aspects of his body-image and with his phase-appropriate tendencies to disidentify. This engenders a severe internalized conflict between a desire for merger with the mother and a fear of loss of sense of self. The latter blends with castration anxiety on a preoedipal level (Roiphe and Galenson 1973).

Socarides (1970), Limentani (1979), Loeb and Shane (1982), and Loeb (1992) observed that transsexuals grow up in maternal environments that conflict with their biological maleness. These observations contradict Stoller's view (1973, 1975a, 1975b) that transsexuals never had any masculinity, castration anxiety, or intra-psychic conflict.

Person and Ovesey (1974a,b) considered the transsexual wish to be the nucleus of a syndrome. They viewed transsexualism as a symptomatic compromise formation in which the threat is from early maternal abandonment and the defensive fantasy is of symbiotic merger with the mother. Thus, in the transsexual, sexuality is largely sacrificed for the security of getting needs met. Volkan and Berent (1976) found conflict around the wish for sex reassignment surgery was not expressed directly, but appeared in dreams and in the behaviour of the adult transsexuals. P. Tyson (1982) proposed that the developmental line of gender identity be seen as: (1) core gender identity; (2) gender role identity; and (3) sexual partner orientation.

The interaction of these parts produces, she said, the final 'broad sense of gender identity'.

Harrison *et al.* (1968), Meyer (1974), and Walinder and Thuwe (1975) found histories of abandonment, disregard, and abusive language, such as calling the child 'scum', rather than extraordinary symbiosis in the history. Meyer (1982) comprehensively reviewed the existing theories of transsexualism. He examined and followed-up 526 patients who wished to have their genitalia and other physical attributes modified to that of the opposite sex. He found an absence in their history of extraordinary symbiosis. Meyer did not find patients that fit Stoller's criteria for 'true' transsexualism (p. 386). Although Meyer (1982) regretted that he did not have the opportunity to psychoanalyse the patients that he evaluated, my analyses of two boys support his conclusions (Loeb 1982, 1992).

Meyer and Duplin (1985) observed 12 children who engaged in cross-gender behaviour. As much as possible, they maintained neutrality and avoided the education, explanation, and suggestion that Green *et al.* (1974) used. They tentatively concluded that gender-disturbed behaviour is due to early traumatic experiences that result in intra-psychic conflicts. The traumatic experience is reenforced by repeated assaults by the parental object, who may be a mother, sister, grandmother, or teacher. They said (p. 260): 'Failure of object constancy in these children was apparent in their object hunger, narcissistic vulnerability, and separation anxiety, and in a neediness reflected in wanting to "get things".' In none of the male children was there evidence of a 'blissful symbiosis' of the type called for in Stoller's formulations.

The wish of a 6-year-old boy treated by Sylvia Brody to be transsexual, was observed by his teachers, not his parents.

> In his early childhood, the mother said, he had clung to her exceedingly, which she had greatly deplored. In contrast she was pleased and pround of his obedience. She had always insisted on his being orderly and controlled, for she could not bear boys who were "rought or wild" She wished him to be strong, however, and so believed it best not to show him tenderness or sentiment. He had come to perceive normal phallic striving as a threat to his allegiance to her, and had sadly resigned himself to exclusion from her emotional life. The father was utterly remote from him affectively and took no interest in the child's daily experiences, but rather was devoted to pleasures with mother alone. The boy had come to feel abandoned by both parents, and to nourish the fantasy that had he been born a girl, he would have been insured against their chronic neglect of his feelings (Brody 1994 personal communication).

Coates *et al.* (1991) reported on a 3-year-old boy, Colin, with gender-identity disorder who believed that if you wore girls' clothes you could really become a girl. He did this to please his mother, repair her depression, and cause his withdrawn mother to return. On the Rorschach they found themes of dread, separation, and loss. Representations of females were idealized and valued, while representations of males were absent. Clinically, Colin's cross-gender behaviour increased when his mother was inaccessible due to separation or depression. The inaccessibility of both parents left Colin feeling abandoned. Coates *et al.* (1992) said that the cross-gender fantasy allows the child to manage traumatic levels of anxiety.

CLINICAL CASE: CARLOS[2]

Method

My first case was a 5-year-old boy, Carlos, who wished to be a girl (Loeb and Shane 1982). I saw the child when I was a child-analytic candidate and Shane supervised me. The child fitted the criteria Stoller (1973, 1975*b*) had identified for diagnosing a primary transsexual condition.

Shane and I worked psychoanalytically with this highly motivated boy using as few parameters as possible. We worked on giving him insight into the intra-psychic conflicts that had produced his psychopathology. This eventually reduced his anxiety and diminished his symptoms. Although we had to interrupt the treatment after only eight months, the patient had significantly worked through the conflict that led to his transsexual wish. Shane and I are convinced that this boy would have become an adult transsexual without our psychoanalytic intervention. This case demonstrated that conflicts can exist in a transsexual child and that psychoanalytic treatment can resolve these conflicts and lead to the cessation of symptoms (Loeb and Shane 1982).

When I began this treatment I knew little about transsexual children. Shane recommended that, instead of reading the literature, I just treat the child following a scientific psychoanalytic investigative technique. After I completed the analysis, I read the literature and was surprised to learn that Stoller (1975*b*, p. 94) had said that the pathology was preconflictual in these children.

History

Carlos, a good-looking boy of 5 years, 10 months, was brought for consultation by his 45-year-old parents, both because he wished to be his father's daughter and because he felt women were better than men. His mother became worried when he became anxious and did not want to go to school after his kindergarten classmates teased him by calling him 'Conchita'. Although she had at first encouraged his feminine behaviour, she no longer took lightly his wearing women's clothing, make-up, and jewellery, and his playing exclusively with girls. His father became upset and angry when Carlos said he wanted to be a girl and not have a penis.

Mrs N, who came from Argentina, had separated from Mr N, an American, and had returned to Argentina to live with her sister and mother to give birth to Carlos. She remained with them until Carlos was 2½ years old. Carlos walked at 10½ months, talked by 1 year, and was weaned at 2½ years. He was toilet-trained, without difficulty, at age 3. Between the ages of 1 and 2 years, Carlos pleased his mother by putting on her lingerie and lipstick, playing with her lace, and imitating her voice.

When Carlos and his mother reunited with Mr N in the United States, a male figure entered Carlos' life for the first time. Up to that time he had slept in his mother's bed because she 'could not say "no".' When he was moved out of his mother's bed into his

---

[2] A version of this case was presented at the Annual Meeting of the American Psychoanalytic Association, Atlanta, Georigia, May 1978 and then published (Loeb and Shane 1982).

own room, he screamed for hours saying that he was afraid of the dark, bodily injury, and monsters. Carlos' father tried to stop his mother both from taking Carlos to bed and from supporting his effeminate behaviour, but his mother would not change. His father then withdrew from the family and often left home. His parents continued to separate and reunite, and when father was gone, Carlos became anxious and sad, and his effeminate behaviour increased. He would put his mother's clothing on while telling her how lucky she was *not* to have a 'wiener' (sausage). His father became alarmed when, at age 3, Carlos was still dressing as a girl, pretending he had big breasts, and playing only with girls. At age 4, after his brother was born, while hiding his penis between his legs, Carlos would 'spy' on his mother while she undressed or bathed. He would say that he was ashamed of his penis and that he would like to cut it off. His parents were frightened by these thoughts and by his occasionally cutting things with scissors—such as window screens. I thought that this might mean that when he saw that his mother did not have a penis he experienced castration anxiety and turned his mother's aggression toward himself. His younger brother had shown no signs of transsexualism by age 5.

Mrs N, an attractive, although sloppily dressed, woman was anxious in our first interview. The eldest of two daughters, she and Carlos were both named after her father. Following her father's death in an accident when she was a teenager, Mrs N assumed her father's dominant position in the family. Mr N was a tall, handsome lawyer with a suave manner. His relationship to his own mother was highly ambivalent. Mr N's step-father died while his wife was pregnant with Carlos, and Mr N left his wife to care for his mother.

Diagnosis and treatment plan

After several interviews with the family, Shane and I concluded that, despite Carlos' blatant transsexual symptoms, he clearly manifested intra-psychic conflicts. We therefore decided that I would try to help him with psychoanalysis. His parents, both of whom were eager to see their child find relief from his suffering, were placed in psychotherapy with a psychoanalytically oriented social worker.

Although this chapter will focus on Carlos' treatment, it is important to note that in her own psychotherapy Mrs N developed some intellectual understanding of: (1) her degrading attitude toward her husband; (2) her feminizing, overprotective, infantilizing closeness to Carlos: and (3) her resentment toward her own father. However, she still maintained a religious conviction that her son was 'possessed' by a woman. Mr N's attendance in psychotherapy was infrequent. Nevertheless, he noticed that his son did much better when he spent more time with the family. Mr N consequently vowed not to leave them for extended periods, and more or less kept to this promise.

Eventually, each of the basic criteria cited by Stoller for diagnosing a transsexual became a major focus in the transference, just as each of these criteria had been a focal point for the development of a conflict in Carlos. Stoller's criteria include: (1) an unending desire to be with and be attached to his mother; (2) an absent father; (3) a mother who has a castrating attitude toward men; and (4) an exceptional beauty. The conflicts we saw in Carlos include: (1) his difficulty staying close to his castrating mother; (2) his father's absence, which made him conflicted about assuming his father's masculine identity; (3) his conflicted wish to be castrated, which was promoted by his mother's continuously castrating attitude toward his father and him; and (4) his 'special beauty', which facilitated both his identification with his attractive mother and her identification with him.

Course of the analysis

At the onset of the analysis, Carlos would not leave his mother to go with me into my office. He finally did so when I offered to share my soda with him. Throughout his short analysis, he periodically asked for a soda from me. This came to represent oral-closeness to me. Occasionally, even well into treatment, he would run out of my office to look for his mother.

While making feminine gestures and imitating my voice, he began his play therapy by drawing female clothes-pin figures with breasts, long hair, high heels, and black pelvic areas. He also drew his father with the same fetish-like high heels.

Through play activities Carlos worked within the developing transference relationship on his unresolved fear of being abandoned. He would play hide-and-seek; or he would tie a baby doll to a mother doll and block the windows and doors of the doll house to prevent any separation; or he would play at being the Flying Nun, who represented both his wish to identify with is phallic mother and fly toward or away from her. He also took my girl doll home with him so he could work on what he called his 'worries'. In the transference he was using my doll as a transitional object to keep me with him.

Early in the analysis Carlos would alternate between (1) getting physically close to me and acting feminine, passive, and dependent, and (2) pushing me away from him and acting more masculine, aggressive, and independent. When acting more masculine, he would make messes and order me to clean them up. At first, I just observed this alternating sequence of behaviour and did not respond to it. Eventually, I began to interpret to him that he seemed to have a conflict between wanting to be close to me—by acting like a submissive, dependent girl—and wanting to push me away—by acting aggressive, dominant, and controlling. Later, after he acknowledged this, I also began to tell him that I did not have to do everything he told me to do when he acted like an aggressive, dominant, and controlling boy. He would respond that I 'had better behave' and follow his wishes. On one such occasion, he said he would call a policeman to force me to do what he wanted me to do. I interpreted to him that this showed that he wished to have his father—who was a type of law-enforcing agent—there with him. He responded by laughingly and deliberately spilling soda on his clothing. I asked him if he was keeping his father with him by acting like his father, and I reminded him that he had told me that his mother had recently become angry with his father and had criticized him for spilling soda on his tie. I also asked him if he might be testing me to see if I—a female like his mother—would put him down for spilling soda. When I first made interpretations like this, Carlos felt I was criticizing him for wanting to be like his father. He responded by first becoming passive, acquiescent, and effeminate, and then later becoming angry and striking out at me. As we repeatedly worked on this behaviour in the transference, he gradually became more masculine and aggressive toward me, but he continued to fear that I would reject him for doing so. Eventually, he realized that he feared that I would reject him if he were aggressive or masculine with me because his mother had repeatedly rejected both him and his father if they acted aggressive or manly. As we worked on this, Carlos gradually became more masculine with me and less acquiescent or hostile toward me. Simultaneously, he was beginning to play more with boys than with girls at school.

Thus, as Carlos began to see me less as his castrating mother and more as my real self, he became less hostilely passive–dependent and effeminate and more autonomous with me. He also began to notice my actual reactions and expressed surprise when he learned that I had needs and wishes and pains distinct from his own. For example, he realized that he could be thirsty and I did not need to drink. During the middle phase of the analytic work, he would climb precariously on my furniture as if to test his capacity to be independent. Whenever I was forced to protect him by breaking his falls, he would regress. He would speak in a feminine voice, gesture like a woman, me, and call himself 'gorgeous'. This behaviour led us to realize that he did not enjoy the role of a child dependant on an adult. Instead, under these circumstances he felt threatened by me, whom he saw as his mother who was demanding that he merge with her and give up his nascent autonomy and masculinity. Once, as he was falling, I protectively caught him. As he was gathering his balance, he acted effeminate and said he was gorgeous. I disagreed (said 'no' to him) and said that I thought he was handsome and that it is usually girls who are gorgeous. The next day he gallantly brought me candy and a Valentine's Day card. He realized that it was all right with me for him to be close to me and still be a boy. After much discussion about being a handsome boy and not a gorgeous girl, he then began to aggressively renounce his feminine gender-identity. Following this insight, he stopped sharing what happened in his analysis with his mother.

Soon Carlos became phallically competitive with me in the analytic situation, and he asked to take home my pens and my string. He gave them to his father, hoping to transmit my phallic strength—as manifested in my ability to say 'no' to him—to his father. Carlos and his father used my string to fly kites. In addition, Carlos was now taking my dolls home to bed with him and using them to masturbate. These transitional objects continued to be substitutes for me. Thus, he was relinquishing his defences against his biologically determined genital desires. These desires had previously conflicted with his internalized representation of his mother and this had led him to develop his transsexual symptoms. Later, there was a second significant developmental shift for Carlos away from an identification with his mother and toward a phallic identification with his father. This was shown when Carlos began sleeping with his father's Navy torpedo pin instead of with my dolls. Carlos showed further indications that he was moving toward the phallic-oedipal stage: he told his parents that he no longer wanted to be a girl, but would rather be a boy-angel and fly. More directly, he told me he wanted to be a boy and be a pilot. Symbolically, flying combined Carlos' phallic desires with his wish to end his extreme closeness with his mother. As Carlos became more phallic, he spoke about monsters that came at night and disturbed his sleep. In his play with me, these monsters represented his projected hostile-competitive, phallic-oedipal wishes toward his father. After I interpreted his projected hostility in this phallic-aggressive play, Carlos' oedipal anxiety gradually subsided, and he again became able to sleep without fear.

Thus, we discovered that Carlos had an unconscious neurotic conflict between his biological genital feelings toward his mother and her dislike of maleness, which he had internalized. This unconscious conflict had manifested as his transsexual symptom.

Near the end of the analytic work, Carlos sat in my chair, put his feet on my desk, and said: 'You can't tell a book by its cover'. He explained that there was a child at school who dressed like a boy, played like a boy, and had a boy's name. However, she was not a boy. She did not have a penis, and that made the difference. Carlos' interpretation of this proverb showed that he was now consciously aware of, and even able to abstractly generalize about, his previously unconscious gender-identity conflict and confusion. Immediately after explaining this proverb, Carlos exchanged the dolls he had taken from me for my cars. Later that week, in an attempt to renounce his interest in being effeminate, he asked his mother to put wings—like the Flying Nun (a phallic woman) had on her nun's cap—on his baseball cap. Thus, he was relinquishing his feminine identification with me as his mother, while retaining his identification with my phallic power through my cars and by putting wings on his baseball cap.

We had to prematurely interrupt Carlos' analysis when his father obtained a job in another city. I transferred Carlos to a male analyst in that city. During the last month of the analysis, Carlos stopped competing with me and frequently climbed on my lap. He often asked me to read to him the story of the 'Magic Bus' that could go anywhere you wanted it to go and the story of the elephant whose trunk did wonderful things. Carlos' free associations to these stories showed that they represented both his desire to be able to return to see me and his phallic ambitions. In his last session, Carlos expressed sadness about our forthcoming separation by doubting that there were guardian angels. I told him that he wished that I could magically go with him as a guardian angel, but that he really knew that he would have to take his 'worries' to his new doctor. Carlos spent the rest of his final session drawing a picture of a female figure in a long dress. Unlike the earlier unisex pictures of men and women he had drawn with me, she had prominent hips and breasts and *no* high-heeled[3] shoes. He labelled the picture with my name. The picture showed that he had an awareness of me as a woman, separate and different from himself.

Follow-up of Carlos at age 13

Carlos' mother wrote that after the move, Mr N was hospitalized for hepatitis. Although Carlos continued to function well at home and at school, during the hospitalization he again began to play with the family of dolls I had given him. This enabled him to continue to work on his 'worries' until he met with his new psychoanalyst. Presumably, Carlos had responded to his father's absence with both separation and castration anxiety, but instead of defending against these anxieties and forming symptoms, he worked on them by playing with dolls—as he had done during the analysis. Carlos began his new analysis one month later.

During the subsequent four years with the new male analyst, the analytic work

---

[3] In the case to follow, high-heeled shoes represented phallic substitutes in women.

continued with minimal parameters. Carlos remained highly motivated to seek relief from his anxiety-producing conflicts and rode 20 miles each way alone on public transportation to see his new analyst. Carlos' behaviour continued slowly to become more masculine. On completion of his second analysis at age 13, his second analyst could not be certain that he would turn out to be completely heterosexual. However, Carlos was now definitely not transsexual. He still had some uncertainty about his femininity, but in a phase-appropriate way. His analyst felt that the stability of Carlos' masculine gender-identity could best be assessed later in adolescence.

CLINICAL CASE: JAMES[4]

Method

James, the second young patient with transsexual symptoms that I analysed, demonstrated our previously reported observation (Loeb and Shane 1982) that transsexual symptoms can develop out of intra-psychic conflicts and can be resolved through psychoanalysis. This case also provided further data as to the genesis of the transsexual symptom complex. In this psychoanalysis, I was abstinent and not benevolent or supportive. Both positive and negative transference feelings developed into a full-blown transference neurosis. As we analysed the transference neurosis, we learned that he was acting-out his identification with his aggressive, seductive, and castrating grandmother. When he came to understand his unconscious conflicts, we worked them through, and his transsexual symptoms vanished. At age 10, James finished his analysis. I saw him at age 15 for a follow-up.

I tape-recorded the treatment. The recorder did not inhibit spontaneity in either James or myself. Having the analysis on tape allowed both James and me to go back and trace from their inceptions the development of themes that did not at first seem relevant. Although the accuracy of my written notes could be questioned, the accuracy of a tape-recording cannot. The recorded data show that it was James' unconscious intra-psychic conflicts that led to his transsexual symptoms.

History

James, was an attractive boy, age 4 years 8 months, who, since the age of 2½ years, had wished to grow up and be a 'mommy'. He liked to pretend he had breasts and put on women's clothing and make-up. He preferred to play with girls. When he played with boys, he pretended he was a girl. He was now tired of pretending to be Wonder Woman and had intense concern about things that came apart. Recently, he had nightmares of policemen who fell on spiders and of a red crayfish monster that climbed on his mother's face and chased him.

James was adopted at birth when his adoptive parents' natural children were 6, 8, and 10 years old. His father, a financial executive, rarely spent time with James. Like James, the father had received little discipline from his parents. James'

---

[4] A version of this case was published in Loeb (1992).

paternal grandfather had a congenitally shrunken arm. His work required him to take frequent trips, so he spent little time with his son or his grandchildren. James' paternal grandmother had low self-esteem and was very critical and condescending toward others. James' father had always avoided women who dressed attractively and seductively like his own mother.

Between the ages of 1½ and 3½ years, James, unlike his siblings, spent much time with his father's attractive mother. She lived nearby, and James' mother was happy to have a willing baby-sitter. His grandmother always dressed in 'fancy', seductive, high-fashion clothing, and disrobed in front of James. He said that his 'fancy grandmother' was a 'nice lady' with a 'yucky body'. He said that ladies dressed 'fancily' to cover their 'yucky bodies'. The paternal grandmother seldom said 'no' to any of James' requests. She gave him whatever he wanted, including 'Cool Whip' for lunch. She put make-up, jewellry, and girl's clothing on him and encouraged him to wear her high-heeled shoes.

As a toddler, James began to cover his chest with a towel after taking a bath. At age 3, he became preoccupied with Barbie dolls—especially their hair and high-heeled shoes. At 3½ years, he began to put on women's clothing. His mother worried about his wanting to be a 'fancy lady'; whereas James complained that his mother dressed too plainly. She was devoted to her home and family, and although a college graduate, she had low self esteem. She regularly took James to bed with her when she found him crying after a nightmare. While sleepwalking, James went into the bathroom, flushed the toilet several times, and then went back to bed. At age 4, James was demanding; for James' parents, like his grandmother, rarely said 'no' to him. His mother's parents spent little time with him.

When James' behaviour became increasingly more feminine, and he began to put on his mother's lipstick, his father became upset, and his parents sought help. Because James' intra-psychic conflicts had interfered with his development, I started him in psychoanalysis. At this time his parents also began psychoanalytic treatment to help their troubled marriage. During James' analysis, I met with both him and his parents whenever necessary.

Course of the analysis

Intermittently, from the beginning of the analysis, James walked as though he were wearing high heels, alluringly fluttered his eyelashes, and repeated my words in an exaggerated feminine voice. After James complained that I, unlike his mother, did not try to read his thoughts and do what he wished, he turned away from me and played with two Barbie dolls. He dressed one in plain clothing and called her 'mother'. He called the other doll 'queen-grandmother' and dressed her in a 'fancy', low-cut, strapless gown, and high heels. Several times he showed how queen-grandmother's gown could slip down and expose her breasts, and he suggested that the gown should have straps. He ignored the Ken dolls. Often he asked me to take off my clothes. This was the beginning of his grandmother-transference neurosis.

Several months into the analysis, James began breaking my toys, hitting me, spitting at me, putting his 'snot' on me, and attempting to lift my skirt. He also tried to hit my eyes so I could not see what he was doing. When I asked him if he were angry at something, he would hit me again. I asked him why he could not tell me what he was angry about and told him it was all right for him to hit the doll—and we could talk about it—but he could not hit me. He then temporarily stopped this abusive behaviour. I asked him why he wanted to hurt me, and he replied that it was not he, but the monster that came in his nightmares who did these things. In one such nightmare, a half-lady, half-pinching lobster-monster chased him. He woke up from the dream when the lobsters were running out of his mother's nose. He excitedly said, 'lobsters can pinch', and he continued to try to hurt me. Eventually, I told him that we could not work on his worries if he could not stop himself from trying to hurt me. I said that, if he continued, I would have to stop our session. When he did not stop, I told him that he was unable to say 'no' to himself, and I opened the door and asked him to leave. Then, using feminine speech and mannerisms, he pleaded to be allowed to stay. His pleading did not work with me, and I insisted that he wait outside in the waiting room for his mother to pick him up. Thus, unlike his mother, who cried and ran away from his angry words and behaviour, I confronted him and did not let him manipulate me and win. I tolerated and worked on his negative, hostile impulses in the transference, but I did not let him actually act-out his angry thoughts and wishes toward me. I firmly adhered to this boundary, and this strengthened his therapeutic alliance, which was slowly evolving.

Castration themes then began to predominate in James' play. He pretended to be Dorothy in the *Wizard of Oz*, who was seeking *shoes* for herself, a *heart* for the Tin Man, a *brain* for the Straw Man, and *courage* for the Cowardly Lion—all representing power and penises. James also played that he was Cinderella, who repeatedly lost and recovered her shoe. One day I had a bandage on my foot and James became both gleeful and anxious.

Although, like his father, James had always feared dogs, in the second year of the analysis, he asked to have my large Great Dane come to a session. When I hesitatingly brought in the dog, I found James hiding in a corner. But James insisted that the dog continue to come to his sessions. Gradually, James became less frightened of the dog. After several months with the dog present, I noted that James was copying the dog's behaviour. For example, when the Dane lay with his forelegs crossed in front of him and licked his paw, James would lay on his stomach with his arms crossed and lick his wrist. James was diminishing his anxiety by identifying with, and acting like, this feared object. I told James that he seemed no longer to be afraid of the dog because he was lying next to the dog and acting just like him. Observing how he overcame his fear of the dog by imitating its behaviour helped James understand how he had overcome his fear of his penis-less, castrating grandmother by imitating her behaviour. In both instances, James was using the defence of *identification with the aggressor*.

James repeatedly disrupted his play by using the defence mechanisms of *denial*, *repression*, *doubting*, *doing and undoing*, *reaction-formation*, and *identification with the lost object*. He frequently *forgot* things he had learned. At times we would bring them back by playing the tape-recordings. Like Carlos, he would *doubt*. He would express his central conflict by saying: 'Yes, you have one; no, you don't have one. No, you don't love me because I have one; yes, you love me because I don't have one'. He would *do and undo* by changing the doll's sex from boy to girl, or her clothing from fancy to plain, or her power from strong to weak. He would call me

'Doctor Poop'; and then, employing *reaction-formation*, he would call me a 'lovely lady'. Similarly he would kick my leg and then kiss it. I interpreted his behaviour by telling him that he wanted to hurt me and then make the hurt go away. James exhibited his *identification with the aggressor* every time he unconsciously feared I might want to take his penis. At such times, beginning during the opening phase of the analysis, he imitated my feminine gestures and behaviour in an exaggerated and hostile way. This was a repetition in the transference of his identification with his grandmother who aggressively put males down in a castrating way. Eventually, as I interpreted his defences, he would laugh and say, 'only joking'. He was developing an observing ego.

Working with their individual psychotherapists, James' parents realized that they had had difficulty saying 'no' to him. Gradually, they then became able to give him appropriate limits. He then quickly became more independent and learned to tie his shoes and tell time. Although he progressively became less feminine and engaged in more masculine activities, such as playing with boys, his intra-psychic fantasies and fears of castration remained unchanged. For example, he continued to interrupt his wedding games before they consummated in thoughts of female genitalia or sexual intercourse. After I pointed out these defensive interruptions many times, James began to play that Ken was putting his penis in Barbie's vagina. Barbie would then take Ken's penis, and Ken would be left with a vagina. James would scream 'Ken lost his penis!' Often he said: 'If you dress and act like a girl, nobody will think you have a penis. Then you don't have to worry that anyone will take it'.

During the middle phase of the analysis, James' mounting hostile-aggressive transference-resistance developed into a full-blown transference neurosis. This was both disruptive to our sessions and unpleasant for me. He frequently requested that I put every one of Barbie's hairs into a bun. I always questioned why he wanted me to do this. Eventually, I told him that it was time that he tell us why he wanted me to do this, or I would not do it any more. Instead of explaining, he began to hit me with the Barbie doll. He was very anxious, and his escalating destructive behaviour eventually forced me to interrupt many sessions. I asked him if he was trying to get me to say 'no' to him because his parents seldom did. I worked on interpreting this resistance for several weeks. He finally stopped hitting me and began to put his transference wish to be told 'no' into words while simultaneously acting it out in play with the dolls. For example, instead of hitting me with Barbie, he began swinging her precariously on a circus trapeze while saying that she should have no hairs sticking-out because that would be 'even more dangerous'.

The next session, he expressed much anger at the director of a school play for *not* giving him a part. He had displaced on to the director of the play, the anger he had toward me for stopping him from hitting me—in 'play therapy'. Then, for the first time, he began to play ball with me. This masculine behaviour strongly contrasted with the girls' games, such as with dolls, that he had played with me before. Next, he began to visualize penises in my office pictures. I told him that his anger about not getting a part in the school play seemed to have led him to see penises all over. He responded, 'a penis is anger'. He said that although he would like to know what it was like to be a woman, he would still like to be a man. In the past he had told me that I was 'lucky' to be a woman; so I asked him whether his wish to be lucky like a woman had anything to do with his wish to keep all Barbie's hairs in a bun. James adamantly said, 'no hair is to stick-out, not even one'. I asked him if he worried about anything sticking-out from him. He said, 'a penis'. When I asked if having the hair all in place was like not having his penis stick-out, his play immediately reverted to the perilous trapeze act, and he threw Barbie around the room. He had her lose her shoes—which represented to him her penis and her power. James' behaviour kept getting wilder and became dangerous to himself and to me. I said 'no', he could not do that. James responded: 'Do you want me to kill you?' I replied, 'You think you're so powerful because you feel you can get away with anything with your grandmother and mother'. He then settled down and again began to play ball with me. Why my saying 'no' so greatly affected James, now became evident: he told me that it was bad to be a woman because women have four penises—two high heels and two 'boobs' make four penises. 'They can even have 25 penises', James said. 'You can have press-on nails—some on your toes, some on your hands, and a nose. It's bad . . . because men . . . can have only one penis'. James explained that a penis is something that sticks-out, and that things that stick-out—like noses and hair—are penises. I asked him about my hidden penis that he used to talk about. He said it was the one stolen from Ken—the one women get back. I asked him: '*How* do they steal penises?' He replied: 'They steal penises because they are jealous of men, and men's penises are real penises, but women just have ones that stick-out'. 'Men', James continued, 'have one real one, and women want a real one, so they make things stick-out[5] . . . Barbie needs a real one'. I asked: 'How is she going to get it?' 'Steal one', he replied. 'Women come to the men at night and steal their penises. They have pinchers. They use two of their penises. The press-on nails are their pinchers . . . But no woman will ever get mine'. He added that when you dress like a girl, these kinds of women will not know you have a penis that they would like to have. Then James confided in me; 'I had one once. . . . I mean, I once had no penis'. [He was referring to the recent past when his parents and grandmother let him get away with things. Once his parents began saying 'no' to him, he could say 'no' to himself, which meant to him that he had a penis.] I asked: 'When was that?' He answered: 'When men know how to say "no", they get their penises back. Whenever men *don't* say "no", women take their penises, and when men say "no", they get them back. That's why only some men don't have one'. [Thus, because I had not said 'no' to him, James thought I lacked power. This meant to him that, like his grandmother, I lacked a penis and, therefore, would want to steal his. So he hit me to test me and see whether I would be impotent and helpless, or powerful and say 'no' to him. After I said 'no' to him, he felt I had power. This meant to him that I had a penis and no longer needed his. So he stopped hitting me.] James went on to say that I did not have those long fingernails like his grandmother, and so how could I catch the ball. He said the ball was a penis, and he wanted me to catch it. When it dropped, he said the penis was gone. James asked to have my Great Dane at his next session.

In that session James continued to play with the ball, which he now called a penis. He occasionally threw it to the Dane to see if the dog would bite it. Afterwards he

---

[5] James had insight into the gesturing of hysterical women who seduce men with their body language, and revealing, seductive clothing.

said: 'Nothing on ladies is supposed to stick-out. Because if it did, men would know they stole penises'. He had wanted me to wear a bun and not have any hair stick-out so that I would not be like his envious grandmother who wanted to steal penises. I asked him why I would do that. He replied that women steal penises because they are jealous of men. I asked if anyone was jealous of him, and he said that I was. He added that he did not say 'no' to his wish to do what he was not supposed to do, because he did not want me to be jealous of him. If he said 'no' to himself, it would mean he had a penis—which was his power. He felt that then, like his grandmother, I would be jealous of his penis (his power) and would want to steal it from him. If, like his grandmother, I had long nails and very high heels, that would mean I wanted a real one, that is, a real penis, to stick-out. Thus, James saw me in the transference as he had seen his grandmother. He saw me as putting him down, and he felt I was envious of his penis. When I began to explicitly say 'no', in words, to his aggressive, dangerous behaviour, in his mind I gained power—that is, symbolically I gained a penis. This meant to him that I had my own strength and did not need his phallic power. He then felt safe and could verbalize why he had had to not say 'no' to himself and had had to be aggressive toward me.

When, in her own psychotherapy, James' mother learned how her reaction-formation had prevented her from appropriately saying 'no' to him, she began setting limits on him, and his fear of her diminished. He eventually realized that both with his mother and with me in the transference he was setting up situations to provoke us to say 'no' to him. This had been a repetition-compulsion.

During the first two years of the analysis James would crawl under my chair and look up to see if he could find my hidden penis. He often called me 'Doctor Poop' (faeces). He also said that my poop (my hidden penis) was powerful, and that if I would 'poop' on him, I would make him into a girl. As we now continued to play ball, James recovered a significant early memory. He told me that, when he was about three, he had seen both a baby girl being diapered and his grandmother undressing. He saw their nude, genital areas. He said that he had then thought that girls were made backward and had their 'poop holes' in front and their penises hidden at the back. He had thought that they had lost their penises and had feared that this might happen to him. He had tried to *deny* castration *in fantasy* by imagining that women had penises that were—like faeces—hidden in back. We now understood why in the middle phase of the analysis he had tried to slap my buttocks. It was to discover my 'hidden penis'. Thus, in the transference he felt more secure when he fantasized that he had given me a faecal penis. This helped maintain the therapeutic alliance. He said that he had dressed girl dolls in fancy clothing, like his grandmother's to hide their 'yucky' bottoms, which they had instead of penises.

During his analysis, in his play with Super-Women-Heros, he pretended he was a castrator rather than being castrated. He pretended he was Wonder Woman[6] restraining dolls with her powerful rope (i.e., her penis) and locking them in boxes. Then he would release the dolls and have them fly away. Next, he would pretend he was Wonder Woman removing dolls' legs so they could not run away. Then he put their legs back. He said that if Wonder Woman and the Super-Hero female characters

---

[6] The Flying Nun represented the phallic woman for Carlos as Wonder Woman did for James.

had their own powers (i.e., penises), they would not need to take the dolls' powers (i.e., their penises) away from them. James' explained that he enjoyed playing with and imitating super-hero female characters, like Wonder Woman, because they had penises and were, therefore, powerful. Unlike his grandmother, they did not need to take penises from men. He also acted out this defence of identification with the aggressor in the transference by copying my feminine gestures whenever he feared that I might castrate him. He was fascinated, but frightened, when things came apart in my office. For example, when he accidentally pulled the tassel off my cushion, he asked me to sew it back. Then he pulled it off again and asked me to sew it back again. Working on this repetitious play enabled him to recognize that it symbolized his fear that he might lose his penis and become a girl.

We, thus, learned from:(1) his play with Wonder Woman and the dolls; (2) his identification with my dog and myself; and (3) his fear of things coming apart, that he had defended himself against his fear of his aggressive, envious, and potentially castrating grandmother by identifying with her. By, thus, pretending to be a girl he concealed his penis and prevented his grandmother from envying it and trying to steal it. He also told me that he had thought that his grandmother had caused his grandfather's arm to shrivel.

When James was 9 years old, after we had done much analytic work and he had greatly improved, his grandmother returned from a two-year absence, and he relapsed. He stopped saying 'no' to his aggressive behaviour, and his feminine speech and gestures returned. He noticed that these symptoms were worse around his grandmother. In his play with me he had a storm come and destroy the doll house. Then the doll furniture became too big to fit in the doll house. We learned that this play symbolized his fear that his penis might get big when he was near his grandmother. In the next session, while demonstrating his grandmother's seductive movements, he told me that the day before his grandmother had seductively encouraged him to feel her soft, black leather pants. He had become sexually aroused, had begun to get an erection, and had become anxious. He proudly told me that this time he had said 'no'. He had refused to feel her soft pants. He remembered that when his grandmother had been seductive with him in the past, he had acted like a girl.

James' parents reported that he was again sleepwalking. He would walk to the toilet, flush it many times, and then go back to bed. During the day, when his grandmother was around, he also went to the bathroom frequently. In play with me, he had Ken and Barbie fight or run away from each other so that Barbie would not make Ken's penis feel 'special', and want to take it away from him. We learned from this play that, when he got an erect penis around his grandmother, he became anxious because unconsciously he feared that she would envy it, want it, and take it. He then became consciously aware that he had been going to the bathroom frequently to reassure himself that he still had his penis. His frequent trips to the bathroom, his feminine behaviour, and his sleepwalking then stopped.

Within and outside the analysis James gradually became more masculine. He stopped playing the role of a girl and began to enjoy climbing trees and bicycling with male friends. Boys began to invite him to their parties. At this point James' mother spoke to James and me and told us that she feared James 'might get hurt' because he was getting so 'vigorous' and active. Both James and I could see that she was trying to inhibit him and put him down. I suggested that she talk about her fears with her own therapist.

James worked-through in the transference and understood that his wish to be a girl was an attempt to resolve his conflict between his biological masculinity and his fear of his grandmother's and mother's castrating behaviour. He now rapidly progressed developmentally, and we were able to work-through and understand his triadic, oedipal relationships with his primary caregivers.

Follow-up of James at age 15

At the age of 15 James described himself as happy with a good sense of humour. He said he had the usual ups and downs. He prided himself for receiving a school award for being the friendliest student. With a smile he said that he had not been the nicest person when he was seeing me in analysis. Besides his high scholastic performance, he was active in extra-curricular activities. He participated in drama and the choir, and he competed in gymnastics and track running. He remembered that when he was young he had not accepted himself as a boy and was jealous of girls because they were what he wanted to be. He did not know if he really wanted to be a girl or if he was just not happy with himself. His grandmother, he said, created the problem by influencing him to look at and wear her clothes and wear her shoes. She didn't say 'no'. He added that his mother did not say 'no' to him either. Laughingly, he said saying 'no' was no longer a problem for him. He said his 'fancy grandmother' still looked like she was forty, and she still could not say 'no' to him or to his father. When she visited, he mostly went up to his room, but he did spend some time with her because she was his grandmother.

James no longer had nightmares and had no memory of the nightmares he had as a child. He did not remember his play with Barbie. The only time he now felt anxious was when he acted in plays. He smiled when I asked if he had any homosexual feelings and told me that he had no interest in boys. His best friend was a boy, but he had no sexual interest in him. Half his friends were girls and half were boys. He did remember that after the analysis finished his friends were mostly girls. For a few months after the analysis, he missed talking to someone, but he learned to deal with things himself. Now he enjoyed talking to his oldest brother and his friends.

Without my asking, he talked about people who—like one of his brothers—never learned to say 'no' to themselves. They had trouble with teachers. James said he has learned to tolerate people's troubles. 'No', he said, is a powerful word. James said he had no trouble saying 'no' to friends when they offered him alcohol or drugs.

Getting close to girls was not a problem. He did not want a close relationship as yet, but went to dances and looked forward to having intercourse—when the time was right. He asked me for information about female masturbation and had some hesitancy discussing his own masturbation. He concluded our talk by saying we brought back old moments and an awareness of the past. As he left he said he would never hesitate to call me if he again became anxious.

Discussion

James' transsexual symptoms, like those of Carlos, were the result of an unconscious conflict. Before the age of 3½ years, James saw both his grandmother's and a baby girl's genitals and *denied in fantasy* (Freud 1940) what he saw to reduce his fear of castration. Like Freud's Wolf Man, he fantasied that girls had their 'poop holes' in front and their penises in back (Freud 1918, p. 25). Then, when his grandmother dressed him in girls' clothing, he concretely thought that she was preparing him for eventual castration and conversion into a girl. His grandfather's shrivelled arm made this fantasized possibility seem real. Faced with a conflict between his biologically determined masculinity and his grandmother's hostile, envious, castrating behaviour, James protected his penis from her by *identifying with* her as *the aggressor* and pretending he was a girl.

James repeated this process of *identification with the aggressor* in the transference, both with my feared dog and with me. He pretended to be a dog—and not a boy with a penis—so that the dog would not 'bite off' his penis. He acted like a girl with me when in the transference he saw me as aggressive and abandoning—such as the time I told him we would have to stop our session if he did not stop trying to hurt me.[7] Thus, like Greenson's (1966), Loeb and Shane's (1982), McDevitt's (1985), and Arlow's (1987) patients, James attempted to master the traumatic threat of castration by identifying with the aggressor.

Although child analysts maintain that one should not play the parental role by saying 'no' to child patients, I had to say 'no' to James. The child analyst must not limit the child-patient's free-play, but must say 'no' when the child's behaviour becomes dangerous either to himself or the analyst. Dangerous behaviour exceeds the bounds of free-play (the equivalent of free-association) and breaks the therapeutic contract.

I said 'no' to James in the analysis for two different reasons. In the beginning of the analysis I had to say 'no' to James and stop his sessions when his behaviour went beyond play and became realistically dangerous and destructive. I told James he could hit my doll, but not me. (As I had told Carlos that he could 'fly' my doll, but not climb my furniture.) This first limit established a boundary within which the therapeutic process could safely proceed. Later in the analysis, when James' repetitive play became a transference-resistance, I limited his play by asking him to put into words what he had been acting out in play. For example, I told him that I was no longer going to put Barbie's hair in a bun unless he told me why he wanted me to do so. This second 'no' encouraged him to verbalize, and thereby make conscious, the unconscious meanings he was acting out in his play (Freud 1915). When he resisted doing this by acting-out destructively toward me, I had to apply the first limit again by telling him that either his destructive behaviour would have to stop, or I would have to end the session. Eventually, we both learned that when I said 'no' to him, it unconsciously meant to him that, unlike his grandmother and mother, I had my own power and did not need his penis.[8]

In James, what first appeared to be a prolonged symbiotic relationship with his mother turned out instead to be an identification with his aggressive grandmother. His transsexual wish was not the result of a fixation at the symbiotic phase of the separation–individuation process. Instead, it was the result of a defensive process that he found necessary for psychological survival.

---

[7] There is also a history of actual abandonment and recurrent transference theme of abandonment in an adult male transsexual that I am now seeing in analysis.

[8] I had not seen Carlos long enough to interpret his wish to have me say 'no' to him.

Because James' father was distant, and both parents were passive, James' impulses could not be kept in check by his identification with either parent. Therefore, to establish adequate super-ego control he had identified with his aggressive, castrating grandmother. In the transference-neurosis, he unconsciously perceived my 'no's' to mean that, unlike his grandmother, I had my own power (penis), and, therefore, I did not need to steal his power (penis). He also unconsciously construed my 'no's' to be those reasonable limits that he had wished for, but had not received, from his parents. As we worked through his wish to have me say 'no' to him, he became able to disregard his excessively limiting super-ego-identification with his grandmother. Then his internalized image of his weakly limiting father became more adequate. Carlos had also developed an excessively controlling super-ego by identifying with his castrating mother instead of with his absent or passive father.

GENERAL CONSIDERATIONS ABOUT TRANSSEXUALISM

Discussion of Carlos' and James' analyses

A therapist need not be male to help transsexual patients. It is past object relationships, and not the sex of the analyst, that determines what is transferred on to the analyst. Developing a masculine identification with a surrogate father figure does have therapeutic value for transsexuals, but this approach is limited because it does not address or resolve transsexuals' underlying unconscious conflicts, which in my patients related to their mothers. I did not directly encourage either boy's masculine striving. Instead, I remained neutral by accepting their penises and their actual maleness. A therapist of either sex must be able to recognize both mother and father transferences, accept them, and help the patient work them through. Therapists' failures to recognize all transference manifestations in transsexual patients of any age, including preoedipal mother transference reactions, have led to the destructive acting out of such patients' unconscious conflicts, (e.g., actual surgical castration).

Both of the transsexual boys that I analysed had come into conflict with a maternal caretaker's negative attitude toward their boy's sexuality. Each boy dealt with this conflict by internalizing it and identifying with their maternal caretaker. This resulted in a gender-identification reversal. Psychoanalysis allowed each boy to establish a realistic view of his gender-identity.

Carlos saw his mother reject his father for being masculine; and, to avoid a similar rejection (abandonment), Carlos conflictually wished for castration. He wished he had no penis and imagined he was a girl. These symptoms intensified each time Carlos saw his mother drive his father out of the house. Thus, faced with a conflict between his biologically determined masculinity and his internalized representation of his mother's aversion to masculinity, Carlos chose to renounce his masculinity so he could maintain his state of dependency on his mother.

Because James' grandmother envied men, she stimulated his masculine desires by seductively exhibiting her genitals to him, and then she hostilely thwarted his male proclivities by dressing him as a girl. This behaviour made James fear that his envious grandmother might want to take his penis away from him—just like, as he fantasized, she had shrivelled his grandfather's arm. James defended against this possibility in two principal ways. First, he *denied in fantasy* (Freud 1940) his observation that his grandmother lacked a penis by imagining that she had 25 penises; and, second, he unconsciously *identified with his aggressive* grandmother (Freud, 1936/1966) by becoming effeminate. This concealed his penis so that she would not become envious and remove it. To master his traumatic experiences with his grandmother, he subsequently repeatedly acted-out his unconscious identification with her by pretending to be a girl. When he acted out this feminine identification in his transference relationship with me, I was able to help him trace it back to his grandmother. Once he did this, he gave up his transsexual symptoms. Following his second analysis Carlos had also given up his identification with his aggressive, seductive mother.

In their analyses Carlos and James each learned that they did not have to give up either their masculine gender-identity or their autonomy to enjoy the role of a child dependent on an adult. Before their analyses, neither Carlos' nor James' father could become the 'bridge' that Roiphe and Galenson (1973) described as necessary for a boy to achieve individuation. This was fostered during the analyses when both fathers spent more time with their sons.

Carlos' and James' mothers each learned in their own psychoanalytic psychotherapy how they had pushed their sons toward feminity. Carlos' mother, had not only sought to re-experience a closeness with her own mother through Carlos, but she also had tried to prevent him from usurping her unconsciously held male position. Her hostile dependency and her bisexual conflict had clearly acted as a developmental interference for Carlos (Nagera 1966). James' mother and grandmother each frightened him with the possibility of the loss of his penis, which also acted as a developmental interference.

Both boys had been unconsciously aware of their female caregivers' dislike and envy of both their own and their fathers' masculinity. Each boy unconsciously reacted to this by wishing his penis was gone, by pretending it was not there, and by feeling and behaving like a girl. Faced with a conflict between their biologically determined masculine inclinations and their female caregivers' aversion to masculine behaviour, they both chose to renounce their masculinity so that they would not be abandoned.[9] After both boys' transference feelings of rejection and abandonment had been worked through in some detail, both boys transferred their parents' phallic qualities onto me. Then, both became more phallic, masculine, and aggressive and began to talk about monsters that came at night. Carlos' monsters were non-specific, while James had nightmares of lobsters pinching off penises. These monsters represented their projected anger and their castration fears. After their monsters were analysed, the boys' hostile behaviour toward me decreased.

The exaggerated, seductive, effeminate gesturing of my two young transsexual patients was a repetition-compulsion in which they actively instead of passively, in an effort to achieve mastery (Freud 1920), repeated their original traumatic experiences of

---

[9] Subsequently, when I analysed an adult male transsexual, I learned that he longed for his mother not because he had had a blissful symbiotic relationship with her, but because she had ignored and abandoned him both psychologically and physically.

having been threatened with symbolic castration. If these boys had not gained insight through psychoanalysis, their repetition-compulsion to get revenge on a substitute (Freud 1920 p. 17), could, in the future, have provoked others to castrate them.

Pruett and Dahl's (1982) three patients, like my two patients, saw women's shoes as phallic symbols that represented power. Their patients also had other fantasies and symptoms, similar to those of my patients. For example: while acting like *Cinderella*, Bryan, aged 3 years 9 months, told other boys to put on a dress because it looked like armour. Buddy said that it felt so good and safe to be dressed as a girl. Bruce called himself 'sister' in family drawings and, like my patient Carlos (Loeb 1982) and Arlow's patient (1987), pulled his penis down between his legs and said 'gone'.

Greenson's (1966) and McDevitt's (1985) observations of boys with transsexual symptoms were similar to mine. Like my two patients, their patients had maternal caregivers that were both overly gratifying orally and overly seductive and frustrating genitally. Lance (Greenson 1966) and Billy (McDevitt 1985), looked up under their mother's and Barbie's skirts, while my two patients not only looked under Barbie's skirt, but also tried to look up under mine. Both of my patients made a spontaneous initial transference to me when we began the analyses by imitating my feminine walk and voice. They did this to conceal their penises so I, who they felt had none, would not be tempted to steal theirs. These imitations were identifications with me as a potential aggressor. Similarly, Lance (Greenson 1966) did everything Greenson did, and Billy (McDevitt 1985) put on McDevitt's hearing aid and glasses. Their patients, like mine, also had physically or psychologically absent fathers. Greenson's conclusion was different from mine, whereas McDevitt concluded that his patient's '. . . feminine identification was determined primarily by his need to selectively identify with those traits of the maternal representation that provided him with the best compromise solution, the solution that provided libidinal and aggressive satisfaction and served defensive purposes'.

In 1985, Stoller wrote of the Carlos case: 'Of those who question . . . [my] non-conflict theory only Loeb and Shane (1982) have presented observations I would consider to the point of my argument. Other colleagues simply make generalizations, quote authorities, or give anecdotes taken from adult, non-primary transsexuals—observations that to me simply confirm the hypothesis that such people do not suffer the constellation I described.'

My cases, together with those of Brody (1994 personal communication), Person and Ovesey (1974a), and McDevitt (1985), are important because they conclusively show that transsexual psychopathology can be the consequence of unconscious conflicts, which can be resolved through psychoanalytic treatment. These psychoanalytic findings are consistent with Socarides' (1970) view that the gender-identity problem in transsexuals is due to intra-psychic conflict.

CONCLUSION

In both of my cases transsexualism developed out of unconscious conflict. In both cases this symptom complex was the result of the boy being caught between *separation anxiety* and *castration anxiety*. The boys defended against this conflict mainly by *identifying with the aggressor*.[10] Thus, when a young boy's maternal caregiver exhibits her genitals to him, and simultaneously aggressively rejects his masculinity by treating him like a girl, he becomes anxious and may protect himself from feared castration and abandonment by unconsciously identifying with this envious, seductive, hostile woman. In so doing he pretends he is a girl to conceal and protect his penis and to assure continued nurturing. Thus, each boy felt that he could either have a penis or a maternal caregiver—not both. During their analyses, Carlos' and James' major conflict—their desire to, and dread of, pleasing their castrating female caregivers—was transferred on to me. We worked to clarify and understand this conflict and their symptoms abated.

REFERENCES

Abelin, E. (1977). The role of the father in personality development. *Psychotherapy Tape Library*. Psychotherapy and Social Science Book Club, New York.

Arlow, J. A. (1987). Trauma, play and perversion. *Psychoanal. Study Child*, **42**, 31–44.

Coates, S., Friedman, R. C., and Wolfe, S. (1991). The etiology of boyhood gender identity disorder: A model for integrating temperament, development, and psychodynamics. *Psychoanalytic Dialogues*, **1**(4), 481–523.

Coates, S., Friedman, R. C., and Wolfe, S (1992). The etiology of boyhood gender identity disorder: an integrative model. In *Interface of psychoanalysis and psychology*, (ed. Barron, J. W., Eagle, M. N., and Wolitzky, D. L.), pp. 245–65. American Psychological Association, Washington, DC.

Freud, A. (1936/1966). The ego and the mechanisms of defense. In *The writings of Anna Freud*, Vol. 2, pp. 109–21. International Universities Press, New York.

Freud, A. (1965/1966). Normality and pathology in childhood: Assessments of development. In *The writings of Anna Freud*, Vol. 6, pp. 36–43. International Universities Press, New York.

Freud, S. (1905/1953). Three essays on the theory of sexuality. In *Complete psychological works of Sigmund Freud*, (standard edition, Vol. 7, pp. 125–243). Hogarth Press, London.

Freud, S. (1908). The sexual theories of children. In *Complete psychological works of Sigmund Freud*, (standard edition, Vol. 9, pp. 205–26). Hogarth Press, London.

Freud, S. (1910/1957). Leonardo da Vinci and a memory of his childhood. In *Complete psychological works of Sigmund Freud*, (standard edition, Vol. 11, pp. 59–137). Hogarth Press, London.

Freud, S. (1915/1963). The unconscious. In *Complete psychological works of Sigmund Freud*, (standard edition, Vol. 14, pp. 159–215). Hogarth Press, London.

Freud, S. (1918). From the history of an infantile neurosis. In *Complete psychological works of Sigmund Freud*, (standard edition, Vol. 17, pp. 3–143). Hogarth Press, London.

Freud, S. (1920/1955). Beyond the pleasure principle. In *Complete psychological works of Sigmund Freud*, (standard edition, Vol. 18, pp. 3–64). Hogarth Press, London.

---

[10] When each boy was caught between the danger of separation (his fear of the loss of the maternal object) and the danger of castration (his fear of the loss of his penis), he became anxious and defended himself by identifying with the aggressor (the aggressive woman) (Freud 1936/1966).

Freud, S. (1927). Fetishism. In *Complete psychological works of Sigmund Freud*, (standard edition, Vol. 21, pp. 149–57). Hogarth Press, London.

Freud, S. (1940). An outline of psycho-analysis. In *Complete psychological works of Sigmund Freud*, (standard edition, Vol. 23, pp. 141–207). Hogarth Press, London.

Geleerd, E. R. (1969). Introduction to panel on child psychoanalysis. The separation-individuation phase: Direct observations and reconstructions in analysis. *Int. J. Psycho-Anal.*, **50**, 91–5.

Green, R. (1974). *Sexual identity conflict in children and adults*. Basic Books, New York.

Green, R. (1987). *"The sissy boy syndrome" and the development* of homosexuality. Yale University Press, New York and London.

Green, R., Newman, L. E., and Stoller, R. J. (1972). Treatment of boyhood "transsexualism". *Arch. Gen. Psychiat.* **26**, 213–17.

Green, R., Newman, L. E., and Stoller, R. J. (1976). One hundred and ten feminine and masculine boys: Behavioral contrasts and demographic similarities. *Arch. Sex. Behav.* **5**(5), 425–46.

Greenacre, P. (1953). Penis awe and its relation to penis envy. In *Drives, affects, behavior*, (ed. R. M. Loewenstein), pp. 176–90. International Universities Press, New York.

Greenson, R. (1966). A transvestite boy and a hypothesis. *Int. J. Psycho-Anal.* **47**, 396–403.

Harrison, S. I., Cain, A. C., Arbor, A., and Benedek, E. (1968). The childhood of a transsexual. *Arch. Gen. Psychiat.* **19**, 28–37.

Jacobson, E. (1964). *The self and the object world*. International Universities Press, New York.

Limentani, A. (1979). The significance of transsexualism in relation to some basic psychoanalytic concepts. *Int. Rev. Psychoanal.* **6**, 139–53.

Loeb, L. (1992). Analysis of the transference neurosis in a child with transsexual symptoms. *J. Am. Psychoanal. Assoc.* **40**, 587–605.

Loeb, L. and Shane, M. (1982). The resolution of a transsexual wish in a five-year-old boy. *J. Am. Psychoanal. Assoc.* **30**, 419–34.

Mahler, M., Pine, F., & Bergman, A. (1975). *The psychological birth of the human infant*. Basic Books, New York.

McDevitt, J. B. (1985). Pre-oedipal determinants of an infantile gender disorder. Presented at the *International Symposium on Separation–Individuation*: 'Separation—individuation and the roots of internalization and identification'. To be published in *Psychoanal. Study Child.* **50** (1995).

Meyer, J. (1974). Clinical variants among applicants for sex reassignment. *Arch. Sex. Behav.* **3**, 527–668.

Meyer, J. K. (1982). The theory of gender identity disorders. *J. Am. Psychoanal. Assoc.* **30**, 381–418.

Meyer, J. K. and Duplin, C. (1985). Gender disturbance in children. *Bull. Menninger Clinic*, **49**(3), 236–69.

Nagera, H. (1966). *Early childhood disturbances, the infantile neurosis, and the adult disturbances*. Psychoanalytic study of the child. Monograph Series, Vol. 2. and International Universities Press, New York.

Newman, L. E. and Stoller, R. J. (1971). The oedipal situation in male transsexualism. *Brit. J. Med. Psychol.* **44**, 295–303.

Person, E. and Ovesey, L. (1974*a*). The transsexual syndrome in males: I. Primary transsexualism. *Am. J. Psychother.* **28**, 4–20.

Person, E. and Ovesey, L. (1974b). The transsexual syndrome in males: II. Secondary transsexualism. *Am. J. Psychother.* **28**, 174–93.

Pruett, K. D. and Dahl, E. K. (1982). Psychotherapy of gender identity conflict in young boys. *J. Am. Acad. Child Psychiat.* **21**, 65–70.

Roiphe, J. and Galenson, E. (1973). The infantile fetish. *Psychoanal. Study Child.* **28**, 147–68.

Sperling, M. (1963). Fetishism in children. *Psychoanal. Quarterly*, **32**, 374–92.

Sperling, M. (1964). The analysis of a boy with transvestite tendencies. *Psychoanal. Study Child.*, **19**, 470–93.

Socarides, C. W. (1970). A psychoanalytic study of the desire for sexual transformation ('transsexualism'): the plaster-of-paris man. *Int. J. Psycho-Anal.* **51**, 341–9.

Stoller, R. J. (1967). Gender identity and a biological force. *Psychoanal. Forum*, **2**(4), 318–49.

Stoller, R. J. (1968). *Sex and gender.* Vol. 1: *On the development of masculinity and femininity.* Science House, New York.

Stoller, R. J. (1971). The term "transvestism". *Arch. Gen. Psychiat.* **24**, 230–7.

Stoller, R. J. (1973). The male transsexual as "experiment". *Int. J. Psycho-Anal.* **54**, 215–25.

Stoller, R. J. (1975a). *Perversion.* Pantheon, New York.

Stoller, R. J. (1975b). *Sex and gender.* Vol 2: *The transsexual experiment.* Science House, New York.

Stoller, R. J. (1985). *Presentations of gender.* Yale University Press, New Haven, CT.

Tyson, P. (1982). A developmental line of gender identity, gender role, and choice of love object. *J. Am. Psychoanal. Assoc.* **30**, 61–86.

Volkan, V. and Berent, S. (1976). Psychiatric aspects of surgical treatment for problems of sexual identification (transsexualism). In *Modern perspectives in the psychiatric aspects of surgery*, (ed. J. Howells), pp. 447–67. Brunner/Mazel, New York.

Walinder, J. and Thuwe, I. (1975). A social-psychiatric follow-up study of 24 sex-reassigned transsexuals. In *Reports from the psychiatric research center*, (ed. H. Forssman). Esselte Studium, Göteborg, Sweden.

7
True transsexualism

Vamík D. Volkan and William F. Greer, Jnr.

INTRODUCTION

Among the anomalies of human sexual development, few, if any, seem more enigmatic than that of men and women who claim that they are the victims of cruel trick of nature and are imprisoned in the bodies of the wrong sex. Although they have normal anatomies for their biological sex, they, nonetheless, aver that they are 'really' a woman trapped in a man's body or a man trapped in a woman's body. So desperate are they to correct nature's alleged mistake that they often make clamorous demands for surgical and endocrinological treatments. Accepting the patients' description of their dilemma at face value has led many surgeons and other physicians to offer them a surgical and endocrinological 'cure'. It is assumed that once concordance is achieved between their bodily and physiological habitus and their perception of their core gender-identification, their intolerable predicament will be resolved. Modern medicine's achievements in the field of organ transplants and the use of prosthetic devices make the idea of surgical 'sex alteration' much less bizarre than it might have been in the past. Sex reassignment for these persons, referred to as transsexuals, is widely available throughout the world despite a lack of consensus among investigators with regard to the genesis of this condition.

This chapter examines the clinical picture of transsexualism and theoretical models that have been promulgated by researchers to explain its origin. Our own findings, especially those illuminating transsexualism from an object-relations point of view, are presented. We describe *true* transsexuals who exhibit a *special version* of borderline personality organization. True transsexuals can differentiate between the images and representations of the self and those of the object except in regard to genital body parts. Their representations of their genital body parts remain fused with the representations of their depressed mothers' genital body parts. This situation is a reflection of a psychotic core present in true transsexuals beneath their surface expression of a borderline personality organization. The psychotic core is saturated with 'bad' affects, (i.e., depression and aggression). The patients' constant and exaggerated search for surgical and medical bodily changes is their attempt to change the external world (the appearance of the body) as if this change will modify the psychotic core. The fantasy is that if the body changes and becomes idealized, 'good', and pleasurable, the inner organization will follow and find a 'fit' between it and the external world. This allows them to maintain a hope for a more pleasurable (depression- and aggression-free) 'reality'. The constant search for bodily change, therefore, is their main defence mechanism. It allows them to encapsulate and control their psychotic cores. 'Sex reassignment surgery', in the long run, does not change their inner world. Thus, these patients usually return to the utilization of their main defensive operation; they seek more surgical and medical interventions which, they wish, would lead to perfection. They become, as it were, surgical–medical addicts.

HISTORICAL OVERVIEW

The first acccount of transsexual surgery concerns one Einar Wegener, a Danish painter, who through his/her surgical transformation in 1930 became Lili Elbe. But it was not until an American man underwent sex reassignment surgery in Denmark during the early 1950s and titillated the world with his transformation into a rather attractive 'woman' called Christine Jorgensen that the subject was widely discussed. Since then, however, it is estimated that more than 15 000 Americans have undergone surgical sex change, and that another 60 000 think they need such a metamorphosis. Although at present, surgical sex change can be performed at numerous hospitals around the world, interestingly some of the medical centres known as major transsexual surgery centres have discontinued this practice. Logic suggests that transsexuals existed before the 1930s and 1950s. Most likely, they were diagnosed with different labels, such as psychotics.

The term 'transsexualism' is a relatively recent addition to our psychiatric nomenclature. It was first introduced by Cauldwell in 1949 in the Latin form, *psychopathia transexualis*. When Benjamin began to write about the phenomenon in 1953, he called it transsexualism, but his adherence to the inner Latin meaning of 'crossing over' is clear in his preservation of the *s* in *trans-* as a prefix, and the resultant spelling of the word with a double *s*. Today, the term has been adopted by the American Psychiatric Association into its official diagnostic classification system. It is rather ironic that a condition which is considered to be a psychiatric disorder is deemed best treated by surgical, as opposed to psychological, means. It would appear that sex reassignment surgery is merely another form of *psychosurgery* in the sense that a surgical procedure is performed for the sake of behavioural or emotional improvement (Kavanaugh and Volkan 1978–9). The propriety of providing a surgical 'cure' for what is essentially a psychological disorder needs further examination. Is the self-declared candidate for transsexual surgery simply searching for such bodily change in primary and secondary sexual characteristics as skillful surgery and medicine can provide—or is he/she bent on a restless and relentless search for something beyond this?

Proponents of sex reassignment surgery are sympathetic to the demands of transsexuals for it. They present their support as if it is a part of a patient's rights or even human rights or a freedom for sexual orientation issue. But one should consider whether any demand for the mutilation of a normal organ system is altogether rational.

DEFINITION OF THE SYNDROME

There is not much consensus in contemporary medical literature in regard to what constitutes transsexualism, the 'true' transsexual, or the aetiology or treatment of the condition. Investigators (Socarides 1969, 1970, 1988; Volkan 1979; Meyer 1982; Lothstein 1983) have observed considerable variation in the personality organizations of persons who demand to be transformed into a being of the opposite sex. The term transsexual has been applied to a wide range of patients without careful attention to diagnostic criteria that might help differentiate them from others with a like wish but who suffer from another disorder. The spare descriptive criteria listed in DSMIIIR does little to improve and sharpen this diagnostic category. Meyer (1974) suggested that better diagnostic discrimination could be achieved 'by using the general term "gender dysphoric syndrome", with secondary modifying terms deciding the primary feature of the clinical presentation' (p. 556). For Meyer, the most salient clinical symptom of this syndrome is the persistent conscious wish, sanctioned and pursued by the ego, for surgical sex reassignment to resolve the disjunction between the physiological and psychological selves of these patients.

Socarides (1968, 1970, 1988), in an attempt to clarify the diagnostic confusion that surrounds the term, concluded that the presence of a conscious desire to possess the bodily characteristics of the opposite sex does not, *ipso facto*, constitute a separate diagnostic entity. He believes that transsexualism is a psychiatric syndrome that may be observed to occur in conjunction with other disorders, particularly transvestitism and homosexuality. He identified four characteristics he considered pathognomonic of this syndrome: (1) an intense, insistent, and overriding desire to be transformed bodily into a person of the opposite sex; (2) a conviction of being trapped in a body of the wrong sex; (3) concomitant imitation of the behaviour of the opposite sex; (4) an insistent search for sexual transformation by means of surgery and endocrinological supplements. Transsexualism, he contends, evolves from either a homosexual or transvestitic perversion.

Conversely, Stoller (1973, 1985) differentiates what he calls 'true' transsexuals from homosexuals and transvestities on aetiological and dynamic grounds. He described a specific family constellation that is peculiar to the developmental backgrounds of the future transsexual, a background not found in the other two disorders. He readily acknowledges, however, that only a small proportion of the many who seek to secure sex-change surgery meet his very narrow diagnostic criteria. Person and Ovesey (1974*a,b*) would seem to concur with Stoller that it is, indeed, possible to separate out from among these people those who are truly transsexual from those who are homosexual or transvestities. The former they refer to as *primary* transsexuals and the latter as *secondary* transsexuals. (See Chapter 5.)

Volkan and his co-workers (Volkan 1974, 1976, 1979; Volkan and Berent 1976; Volkan and Bhatti 1973; Volkan and Masri 1989; Kavanaugh and Volkan 1978–9) found that about 300 individuals who asked for sex reassignment surgery at the University of Virginia's Gender Identity Clinic cut across the diagnostic spectrum from high-level (neurotic) personality organizations to overt psychotic organizations. The neurotic among this patient population being evaluated for surgery was a man with fairly well-structuralized conflicts who wished to submit himself to castration in masochistic compliance with severe super-ego injunctions. Most, however, evidenced much more severe psychopathology.

Volkan accepts as 'true' transsexuals only those persons who possess the four characteristics described by Socarides and who, in addition, 'have felt trapped in the wrong kind of body from early childhood—around three years of age—and when . . . their main symptom is a preoccupation with the appearance of their genitalia and a search for perfection' (Volkan 1979, p. 192). It is this relentless search for perfection that he believes to be the hallmark of the 'true' transsexual. A search for perfection through surgical means usually manifests itself during the 'second individuation' of the adolescent passage (Blos 1979). It persists for years and involves a kind of restless, insatiable desire to achieve bodily perfection of the self-representation. The derivatives of this aspiration can be observed in the verbal and behavioural expressions of the patient. One patient seen by Volkan's research team, a man about to undergo sex reassignment surgery, remarked that he expected to be 'virgin white' after he became a 'woman'. Another male transsexual commissioned an artist, at considerable personal expense, to paint a picture of an idealized woman, which he then took to his surgeon to indicate the way he wanted to look after his/her treatment was completed. Yet another who had genital surgery 18 years earlier, was about to undergo 'her' seventh surgical procedure designed to make 'her' into a more perfect woman. Similarly, the biologically female transsexual searches for perfection when she seeks to become masculine by surgical and endocrinological means. She does not just want to become a man, but a he-man, powerful and strong—a type of man created within her own idealizing imagination. A female transsexual, for example, disclosed to her therapist before undergoing sex-change surgery that if, after she had received her penis, she heard of another surgeon who could construct a better one, she would have more surgery. The transsexual, then, is not only engaged in a search for physical transformation into a being of the opposite sex, but is psychologically committed to a relentless search to become a perfect woman or man.

THREE THEORETICAL MODELS

There are currently three major theoretical models posited to explain the origins of transsexualism, each of which has its staunch adherents. They are the: (1) biological/imprint model; (2) non-conflictual identity model; and (3) conflict/defence model (Meyer 1982). The first two have been formulated to account for the transsexuals' seemingly ego-syntonic expression of their desire for transformation into a person of the opposite sex by surgical means; whereas, the third takes this expression as a symptomatic manifestation of severe unconscious conflict rooted in childhood development. Our own findings fall into the third model which offers explanations for the *meanings* of the clinical manifestations of the 'true' transsexual better than the explanations provided by the first two models.

1. Biological/imprint model

This model has grown out of experimental research with lower mammals in which sex-specific hormones were administered at critical periods producing adult sexual behaviour characteristics of the opposite sex. Gadpaille (1972) provides an exhaustive review of this research literature.

It has been shown that even the chromosomally male (XY) animal will not develop as a male nor act in a male fashion unless androgens have been present at the right time in fetal life, and the converse is true. As far as human beings are concerned, in bisexual states such as Turner's syndrome, Klinefelter's syndrome, and androgen insensitivity syndrome, it seems that hormonal influences modify the fetal brain, permanently changing gender behaviour from that expected toward that typical of the opposite sex. The degree to which hormonal influences affect gender behaviour varies, however, particularly in humans where such biological factors are subject to experiential modification. For instance, Ehrhardt *et al.* (1968*a,b*) studied early- and late-treated andrenogenital syndrome girls andrenogized *in utero* and boys born to diabetic mothers given prophylactic oestrogens to prevent fetal wastage, and found that while there was some effect on gender behaviour, it was modest. Most importantly, there was no evidence of gender disorder in these children. Gadpaille (1980) wrote that even in the presence of 'obvious biological (or experimental) disorder and massive heterotypical hormone influence . . . the sex identity effects are usually more subtle than total' (p. 7).

Money and Gaskins (1970–1) adopted the ethological concept of imprinting in the animal world to explain both normal and abnormal identity. They consider this mechanism to be decisive in the genesis of transsexualism operating through some unspecified deleterious social influences. Stoller (1975) likewise invokes this mechanism in his account of gender-identity formation. He states that something 'is impressed upon the malleable infant's unresisting proto-psyche and unfinished CNS' (p. 55). There is at this time, however, no evidence that imprinting occurs in humans (Ovesey and Person 1973). Even those researchers who are convinced that those seeking surgical sex reassignment *must* have had some constitutional diathesis or organic defect have been forced to acknowledge with Money (1974) that such patients have 'no identifiable, genetic, anatomic, or physiologic defect or abnormality that can be measured by today's techniques. The same is true both for female and male transsexuals. The most likely site where some etiologic defect might be uncovered in the future is the brain, possibly in connection with a fetal hormone effect' (p. 341). Such a possibility notwithstanding, we await definitive proof of organic etiological defect or malfunction as the cause of transsexualism.

2. Non-conflictual identity model

This model attempts to explain transsexualism without recourse to dubious constitutional and biological hypotheses. It has been expounded primarily by Stoller, whose views on male transsexualism we will examine as illustrative of this point of view.

According to him, the origin of male transsexualism lies in an unconflictual identification with a depressed, bisexual mother who, riven with intense penis-envy, views her baby as a phallic extension. Seen as a cure to the mother's life-long hopelessness, masculine strivings are discouraged. Since the fathers of these boys are distant and unavailable, there is no incentive for them to move out of an 'excessively blissful' mother/infant symbiosis. This symbiosis was believed by Stoller to be uncontaminated by the vicissitudes of the aggressive drive. In spite of the mother's exploitation of the symbiotic phase for her own narcissistic needs, the boy is, nonetheless, thought to be untraumatized by this behaviour and to have a normal separation-individuation experience except in the area of gender-identity formation. The boy's core gender-identity remains exclusively feminine and, therefore, unconflicted. Moreover, since there is no masculine identification, there is assumed to be no oedipal passage which is typical for a little boy. Any anxiety or depressive affect that does develop in the boy is believed to be secondary to the reaction of the external world to his effeminized demeanour. The designation 'true' transsexual was reserved for that narrow band of patients whose family dynamics were compatible with those described above. Patients in quest of surgical sex reassignment whose family history departed from this constellation were considered to suffer from a perversion or some other disorder.

Psychoanalytic treatment was not recommended by Stoller (1975) for these boys because, in his view, their transsexualism did not arise from intra-psychic conflict, (i.e., it had no mental content). He believed that re-educative techniques such as '. . . behaviour modification tailored with knowledge developed from understanding the family's dynamics . . .' (p. 275) were more appropriate. He recommended, in addition, that the therapists of these boys be males so that they can serve as models of masculine identification. For optimal results, the parents should be involved in treatment to alter the family dynamics. If there was not some change in these boys' core gender-identity by the age of six or so in the direction congruent with their biological sex, he felt that the maternal identification became relatively fixed and immutable.

Mahler (1975) took issue with Stoller's assumption that a mother/infant symbiosis in which the child's phase-specific developmental strivings for separation-individuation are being frustrated can occur without severe trauma or conflict. The symbiotic phase, she reminded us, does not persist beyond the fifth month of life.

Volkan also observed family backgrounds of male transsexuals which were similar to those reported by Stoller. However, his formulation as to why male transsexualism evolves does not depend on a non-conflictual model. Volkan (1979) writes:

> How . . . can a symbiotic relationship in which there is an affective flow between the partners be "blissful" with such a mother? Symbiosis as a phase of development is, in effect, dynamic, since the child experiences a maturational push to go beyond it to achieve further differentiation of self- and object-representations and to become capable of individuation. Any interference with this forward movement creates conflicts. Whenever one speaks "of prolonged symbiosis" or "endless embrace", severe psychopathology rather than a blissful state is suggested. (p. 196).

In another review and critique of Stoller's work on transsexualism, Meyer (1982) tendered alternative explanations regarding some observations by Stoller concerning the behaviour of highly effeminized boys in terms of ego-defects and defence. Their femininity, in contrast to the normal oedipal girl, is far more concerned with the appearance of the feminine role rather than the role itself. He saw this as evidence of an impairment in the capacity for object-relatedness as well as a defence against intense separation anxiety and rage rather than an expression of an ego-syntonic core feminine gender-identity. He also noted that it is difficult to square Stoller's belief that the core gender-identity of the male transsexual has been imprinted upon them by their mothers, is non-conflictual, and therefore irreversible with reports of successful insight-oriented psychotherapy with some of these children.

For example, Kavanaugh modified the transsexual aspirations of a nine-year-old boy in psychoanalytically oriented psychotherapy when the boy's mother was treated by Volkan (Volkan 1979). Loeb and Shane (1982) report the case of a five-year-old boy with a transsexual wish who was successfully treated in psychoanalysis. They stated that 'given a psychoanalytic atmosphere with, ideally, both parents in analysis or psychotherapy, the transsexual child can achieve both an individual sense of self and a sense of appropriate gender identity. Our patient suggests that pathogenic conflicts can exist in a transsexual syndrome' (p. 431).

A search of the psychoanalytic literature failed to unearth any reports of adult patients whose transsexual desires have been resolved by psychoanalysis proper. Each of the two true transsexuals reported by Socarides (1970) and Volkan (1979) respectively left their psychoanalytic work after six months. True transsexuals, as we shall discuss later, rarely, if ever, come for genuine psychological help with their problem except under authoritative directive or to demonstrate their commitment to a surgical course of treatment. There are, however, reports of psychoanalytic psychotherapy of transsexuals. For example, MacVicar (1978–9) in a valuable contribution provides additional documentation confirming the presence of severe psychopathology in a true transsexual. Meyer and Keith (1991) describe the psychoanalytic psychotherapy of a female-to-male transsexual. Although the patient had been placed on testosterone by a physician while undergoing exploration of her conflicts, she, during her first year of treatment, never made arrangements for sex reassignment surgery. It was found that the patient suffered from severe object-relations conflicts of the kind described by Volkan and Masri (1989) in their paper on female transsexualism. The patient resolved her transsexual desire sufficiently to stop her testosterone injections and live, once more, as a woman. At the time of their report, the psychotherapy was still in progress, however, so no final determination of the success of her treatment is possible at this time.

While Stoller has certainly made many contributions to our understanding of transsexualism, particularly his description of the early developmental experiences which nurture it, we do not believe that the evidence amassed so far corroborates his central thesis that the genesis of transsexualism lies in a preconflictual, ego-syntonic identification with the mother. Indeed, we fear that such an assumption has played into the hands of those who advocate sex reassignment surgery as the only rational treatment alternative for these patients.

3. Conflict/defence model

Investigators of this model share a common observation: in true transsexuals, preoedipal conflicts dominate. Such conflicts influence the nature of the oedipal issues and may later be condensed with oedipal conflicts. It is, in fact, the condensation of preoedipal anxieties with the typical anxieties of the oedipal stage that makes this period especially disruptive for the transsexual child.

Person and Ovesey (1974a,b) believed that the transsexual, because of trauma in the symbiotic and early separation-individuation phases of development, suffered from profound separation anxieties against which they defended themselves by fantasies of merger with the mother which they attempt to concretely enact through the alteration of their genitals into that of a woman. It is the nature of the defence utilized by the transsexual, such as actual castration, that differentiates them from homosexuals and transvestities who utilize transitional phenomena for this purpose. In other words, the capacity for the symbolic expression of conflict is severely impaired in the transsexual.

Person and Ovesey's contention that impaired symbolic capacities are present in the transsexual finds support in the case of a middle-aged woman treated by William Greer. This woman, as an adolescent, often thought of going to see a surgeon to get a penis constructed in the place of her vagina. Her transsexual wish was later replaced by a symptom in which she would go into her father's bedroom at night and 'steal' his glass eye from a table next to his bed as he slept. Before he awoke the next morning, she would return it to its former place. Since 'stealing' her father's glass eye/penis induced anxiety and fear of punishment, when he died she insisted that he be buried with the eye in its socket. As a young woman she replaced this symptom with another of a more permanent kind. She created a higher-level symbolic penis in the form of a 'worry stone' which she kept on her person at all times. It is clear that her transsexual symptom transforms into a higher-level symptom when she is able to use her symbolic capacities to create a substitute for the penis that she so ardently wishes to possess.

A conceptualization of the aetiology of transsexualism similar to the one suggested by Person and Ovesey was formulated by Socarides (1969, 1970, 1988). For Socarides, transsexualism is a form of perversion that shares, in common with the other sexual perversions, a nuclear conflict in the area of separation-individuation. This conflict, which he considers primary, involves both a desire for, and a dread of, merger with the mother (her representation). True transsexualism, as well as any obligatory sexual perversion, irrespective of its surface phenomenology, serves as a defence against the fantasized consequences of such a merger and a disguised gratification of it simultaneously.

Meyer (1982) hypothesized that transsexualism, both male and female, is determined at the preoedipal level. The preoedipal child is incorporated into the mother's fantasies of phallic reparation so extensively that inchoate ego development is damaged and separation-individuation cannot be successfully negotiated. In consequence, the child reaches the oedipal passage with such massive anxieties that regression to symbiotic merger with the mother becomes a welcome refuge from the dangers of genital strivings. It is not merely castration anxieties that these children fear but ego dissolution anxieties that could lead to psychotic disintegration. What distinguishes the transsexual from those persons who develop a more classical perversion is

> . . . the degree to which the split in the ego . . . and the maternal reparative fantasy can be symbolized and the degree to which they must be made concrete. The more it is possible for the child to deny symbolically both the distinction between the sexes and make reparation for the mother's sense of damage, the more likely he is to be perverse. The more his symbolic capacities fail, or more concrete restitution to mother seems inescapable, the more likely he is to have a gender identity disorder. To the extent that the girl can create or incorporate a symbolic penis, she will be perverse; to the extent that she must confirm the fantasy in action, she will be transsexual. (Meyer 1982 p. 411).

The findings of the investigators whose work we have just reviewed directly contradicts

Stoller's view that transsexuals have a non-conflictual core gender-identity and, therefore, have no intra-psychic conflict regarding it.

VOLKAN'S FORMULATIONS

In a series of papers mentioned earlier, Volkan and his colleagues presented and gradually refined their ideas about true transsexuals. Their focus was on the object relations conflicts of these individuals whose surface picture contained clues of the existence of unintegrated self and object-representations. For example, a male transsexual as a child had fantasies that the men who came to enjoy his prostitute mother's pleasures were like bees coming to a hive. As an adult he became a beekeeper, and he separated the bees in his hive into 'good' bees and 'bad' bees, developing a ritual of painting the 'good' and 'bad' queens in different colours and ceremoniously killing the 'bad' ones. It became evident that his division of one kind of bee from another symbolically represented the split in his mother's representation. We can add to Socarides' ideas of the transsexual's wish to merge with the mother's representation by stating that the true transsexual only wishes to fuse with the 'good' mother representation while he or she is active in destroying the 'bad' mother representation and the corresponding self-representation. True transsexuals can differentiate between the images and representations of the self and those of the object, except in regard to genital body parts. This is why their self- and object-relations are different from those seen in typical borderline patients.

Let us explain with a clinical vignette what we mean by fused genital representation. A male transsexual treated on the couch by one of us (Volkan) was preoccupied with thoughts of Hawaii, especially its volcanic landscape. This had a transference reference because the name Volkan means volcano. Although he had spent some time in the islands and his fixation on Hawaii thus predated his association of the names, as the analytic process unfolded his fascination came to be understood as related to his inability to differentiate the image of his genitalia from those of his mother's in spite of his intellectual awareness that they were not alike. The changing volcanic terrain, altered by eruptions and the hardening of lava flow, attracted him by its plasticity and shifting; he saw in the concept of such fluidity a way of dealing with the 'uncertainty' (Bak 1968) of genital outline. As he lay on the couch, a bulge was noticed between his legs, and in due time it was discovered he had his trouser pocket extended so that a wallet placed in it lodged between his legs, creating the bulge. On one level, this bulge represented his mother's genitalia—was a vagina or a penis there?

What is interesting here is the clinical observation that although this patient had no difficulty differentiating himself from his mother's representation, once the analysis focused on the bulge, he began making slips of the tongue in which he referred to himself and his mother interchangeably. He could separate himself from his mother in most areas, but in the genital area differentiation was not possible for him.

At first, Volkan described true transsexuals as having a special kind of borderline personality organization. What impressed him a great deal in his five year tenure as the head of the University of Virginia's Gender Identity Clinic was the true transsexual's constant and aggressive search for perfection. The study of this search led Volkan to make a new formulation as to what lies beyond the surface picture of this special variation of borderline state. He came to understand that the true transsexual has an encapsulated infantile psychotic self (Volkan 1994), which reflects the infant's fused representation with a depressed mother. The child later evolves more mature self-and object-relations, but the initial fused (psychotic) mother/infant representational unit remains encapsulated. It is saturated with 'bad' affects which as adults we call depression, rage, or helplessness. It influences the patient for the rest of his/her life. He or she is, in turn, doomed to take action without success to dissolve it and replace it with a pleasurable fused mother/infant representation.

While the transsexual syndrome responds to wishes and defences at any developmental level, its deepest unconscious aim is to control the infantile psychotic core and modify the 'bad' affects which saturate it. Symbolic efforts are simply not sufficient to accomplish this task. True transsexuals tenaciously pursue this goal as if their lives depend on it. The fantasy that underlies their behaviour is that when the external world (the body) changes, the internal change will follow, and the 'reality' of a fused mother/infant representation loaded with 'good' affects will replace the existing one loaded with 'bad' affects. The patients force others, that is surgeons, to make them into a mixture of sugar and honey—'good' child and 'good' (non-depressed) mother. Total fusion, however, will render the patient truly psychotic; therefore, the fusion occurs only in the area of genital representations. A genital fusion also exists before surgery, but it is saturated with 'bad' affects. After surgery, the hope is that it is now saturated with 'good' affects. As we will see, however, such hope is short-lived.

The battery of psychological tests given to true transsexuals (Volkan and Berent 1976) as well as a study of such patient's dreams (Volkan and Bhatti 1973) furnishes further proof that they are actually more concerned about aggression than about sexual matters. For example, a male transsexual's Rorschach responses demonstrated that the penis is a symbol of evil. For the female transsexual, the acquisition of a penis provides her with such completeness, power, and perfection that she will never again need to exhibit her aggression.

Since surgery is performed to replace the infantile psychotic self with a pleasurable one, Volkan (1979) proposed the term 'aggression reassignment surgery' for the procedure involved. The cure is illusory, however. After surgery it is typical, for example, for male transsexuals to behave as if they have become idealized and glamorous movie stars. They use props in the external world, such as limousines and garish dresses, besides the body change, to force a change within to establish an internal 'fit' to the new external world. In fact, for a while they feel rather elated and satisfied. But before long, the carefully orchestrated external edifice collapses, or they may have a dream of having a penis (evil, aggression, depression). The illusion ruptured, they embark upon a search for further surgical and medical intervention (e.g., changing their Adam's apple). Some surgeons even go along with more bizarre requests, such as shortening the patient's legs.

The male transsexual

The University of Virginia study found Stoller's description of the family background (reported earlier) of male transsexuals to be correct. We, however, disagree drastically with him in regard to how this early maternal environment influences the developing child's psychic organization. The child does not have a 'blissful symbiosis' as Stoller claims. What settles in the child's initial self-representation is a core that reflects an 'aggressive/depressive symbiosis'. As an adult the true male transsexual will strive to be a 'perfect' woman, a woman uncontaminated with aggression and depression.

An encapsulated psychotic core in the context of a kind of borderline personality organization does not necessarily result in true male transsexualism. The specific and decisive conditions that invariably converge to produce this particular disorder have, as yet, not been determined. Further research into this thorny aetiological issue is needed before a more definitive answer can be supplied. Be that as it may, however, the investigations of Volkan and his colleagues strongly suggest that superimposed on the pathogenic early mother/child relationship is a historical trauma which occurs around the oedipal age. This trauma resonates with certain unconscious fantasies active in the child's mind at that time, giving credence to them. For the clinical picture of transsexualism to crystallize, then, we believe there must be concatenation of both early mother/child pathology and actual trauma. (This is also true for the development of female transsexualism.)

Stoller and Newman (1971) were of the opinion that because the male transsexual had no masculinity, they experienced no Oedipus complex or castration anxiety. We vigorously disagree with this assertion. The patients observed by Volkan reached the oedipal level but with the primitive defences that had evolved much earlier to encapsulate a psychotic core of self- and object-representations. Therefore, neither the Oedipus complex nor super-ego development could take a normal course. Moreover, genital-level strivings appeared prematuraly in a defensive effort to move up the development ladder to escape oral-level aggression. But they were trapped in an insoluble conflict. Projection of pregenital aggression reinforces oedipal fear of the father which, in turn, reinforces pregenital aggression and fear of the 'bad' mother and the aggressive link (penis) to her.

Five male transsexual patients had witnessed the deaths of their fathers while they were at the oedipal stage of development. This extraordinarily traumatic event increased their fear of retaliation, since all fantasized being responsible, in part, for the death of the oedipal father. Many other male transsexual patients had suffered physical injury to the genitalia before reaching the oedipal stage. Such actual traumas augment castration fantasies and preoccupation with the penis, and their effects become condensed with the child's object-relations conflict to create the true transsexual syndrome.

In addition to the role of the child's unconscious fantasies, we should pay close attention to the mother's unconscious fantasies about her child (Apprey and Stein 1993). To illustrate how the maternal environment can conflict with the child's biological sex and thus interfere with normal gender-identity formation, we cite the case of a nine-year-old transsexual boy whose mother was treated by Volkan. The mother disliked men, although she had engaged in an affair with a much older man. He urged her to become pregnant, and when she did conceive she was uncertain whether the father of her child was the lover or her husband. She developed a fantasy that her son was a product of both men; she thought it physiologically possible that semen from both had fertilized her. When the child was born she wanted to name him after her lover, but, fearing that this would betray their relationship, she gave him a name different from her husband's in only one letter. She insisted: 'My son was born two people. I know it sounds like a fairy tale, but it is the truth'.

Volkan observed that she routinely put her child between her husband and herself. The child was an aggressive penis, and he clashed with her husband. When her husband was not present, however, she saw her son as the representation of her lover; she indicated in her therapy that this older man had represented her mother to her, as well as her own loving and non-aggressive penis. Sometimes she actually thought of her son as a girl.

The mother's conscious and unconscious perception of her son made part of his evolving self-representation an aggressive penis fused with the mother's 'bad' representation. This became the boy's encapsulated infantile psychotic self. His future gender-identity confusion could be seen in his mother's fantasies about him.

The female transsexual

She, like her male counterpart, has an inner mental world dominated by object-relations conflicts. She, too, has severe preoedipal conflicts with respect to intra-psychic separation from the mother. Volkan, with Masri (1989), delineated six themes shared by such patients.

1. The mother is a martyred, depressed woman with an intense sexual hunger which she unconsciously communicates to her daughter.
2. The daughter, in turn, develops intense unconscious rescue fantasies together with fantasies that if she were only male she could save her mother from depression and thus herself from maternal deprivation.
3. She then begins to enact this fantasy by placing objects between her legs that are precursors of the penis she longs to have (Q-tips, a plastic bottle, for example). These objects are presymbolic, and they link her to her mother. They reflect the fused infantile psychotic core.
4. Conversely, as a symbolic penis, these objects serve to separate the girl from the depressed mother who lacks a penis. Thus, these objects are used both to link and unlink the child's self-representation with that of the mother's, but their utilization for linking dominates.
5. When the girl arrives at the oedipal stage, she yearns to escape from the troubled but intense relationship with the mother's representation by being loved by her father. When the father fails to intervene she consoles herself by identifying with him. The inanimate object is then unconsciously experienced as the father's phallus, and this meaning condenses with its preoedipal meaning.
6. During the adolescent passage, the girl gives up her inanimate object and demands a surgically constructed penis.

The mental representation of an actual trauma organizes the six themes identified above as characteristic of the developmental background and psychodynamics of the true female transsexual. An examination of an actual trauma experienced by a female transsexual will illustrate this point. A more detailed account of this case has been presented else where by Volkan and Masri (1989).

Carla is a 17 year-old transsexual girl who called herself Carlos. When she was born her mother was living with Carla's older sister. Her father was in a distant country on military assignment. Carla's mother became depressed and sexually 'hungry' while awaiting her busband's return. To assuage her hunger she would fantasize that various male movie stars were her lovers. Before Carla's birth, Carla's mother was persuaded that her new baby would be a boy and grow up to be very different from her unloving husband. For several months after the birth of Carla, her mother referred to her infant daughter as 'he' or as a 'Martian'. She was later to say: 'This sounds silly, but is it possible that I could transmit my thoughts about this to my daughter?'

Carla slept in her mother's bed as if she were her mother's bodily extension. At times, the mother thought of Carla as a non-human entity (a penis) and treated this child as if she should not be seen in public. The mother thought that her daughter's vagina was not properly opened, so she took her to a physician who instructed her to massage it as often as possible with a prescribed cream. When Carla was three her mother obtained what must have been a speculum which she inserted into her daughter's vagina in an effort to keep it open. This practice continued until Carla was six. This intrusion was the *actual trauma* usually necessary for the specificity of true female transsexualism. It is actual trauma super imposed on depressed mother/child interactions and the unconscious fantasies of each that comprise the principal pathogenic determinants of the syndrome.

Even after he returned, Carla's father remained unavailable to his young daughter. Being unavailable, he failed to adaptively interfere with the pathological mother–child relationship, leaving his daughter to struggle with it alone. Furthermore, he was born with a cleft palate which had been surgically repaired when he was a boy. This reconstructive surgery lent support to his daughter's belief in the value of corrective surgical intervention.

Carla, like the prototypical female transsexual, felt that she was a man trapped in the body of a woman. From early childhood, she stuffed folded toilet tissue or a sock in her panties to pretend that she had a penis. Unsatisfied with such symbolic phallic substitutes, she began to yearn for a 'real' flesh-and-blood penis. At 14, she read about sex-change operations, and became obsessed with the idea that all her problems could be solved if she underwent one herself.

IMPEDIMENTS TO RESEARCH AND PSYCHOTHERAPY OF TRANSSEXUALISM

It is clear that we do not believe that surgery helps true transsexuals. After surgery, some form of adaptation can be maintained, however, if the patient can find a stable target for projection of his aggressive, 'bad core'. For instance, writing books for a cause, crusading for the claim that transsexualism is not an illness, and fighting, even in fantasy, with those who do not support one's view can assist one's 'adaptation'. After surgery, most transsexuals find partners whose main task is to reinforce on a daily basis the post-surgery patient's 'new' identity. The relationship of the transsexual with their partner is very fragile and tenuous.

In our experience, the 'adaptation' is accompanied by open or secret new symptoms. One man, for example, appeared well-adjusted to his new body. On a visit to his therapist over a year after his surgery, he spoke of a 'midget' (Volkan 1979). A midget would appear to 'her' in the middle of the night which resembled 'her' dead father. Sometimes the midget would attempt to enter 'her' body whereupon she would become extremely anxious. The midget, a symbolic representation of the amputated penis, had once more returned to haunt 'her'. In spite of 'her' efforts to externalize and permanently rid 'herself' of this aggressive weapon that linked 'her' to the depressed representation of the mother through surgical ablation, it continued to manifest itself.

While we are opposed to surgical mutilation of these patients' bodies in the name of treatment, we are well aware of the difficulties treating transsexuals with psychoanalytic psychotherapy or psychoanalysis proper. This is why these individuals' dilemmas make them so tragic.

True transsexuals feel threatened by anything that might obstruct their defensive search for perfection through surgery; therefore, psychotherapy, perceived as an obstruction, is vigorously resisted. The therapist or analyst who refuses to endorse their demands for a surgical 'cure' may be seen as dangerous or may be denigrated and his special competence denied. The patients then break off treatment and seek a therapist more sympathetic with their defensive aspirations. The severe anxieties that are being held in check by their search for perfection through surgical sex-change make for a very recalcitrant resistance. The development of a therapeutic alliance under such conditions is extremely difficult at best. The reality that surgery is available and that some caregivers, indeed, support the patient's claim drastically disturbs psychotherapeutic efforts. Volkan recalls having a male transsexual on the couch in a proper (four sessions per week) psychoanalytic position only to have the patient's surgeon perform surgery on him the day he did not have a psychoanalytic session. The surgeon's omnipotent countertransference should be taken into account in dealing with this topic. Furthermore, in clinics set up to work with transsexuals, a split may occur within the staff that corresponds to the patient's tendency to view the external world in 'good' and 'bad' terms. This externalization of their inner struggle makes collaborative, interdisciplinary work with these patients an arduous task because of the divisiveness it creates between, for example, the surgical and psychiatric staffs. It is not uncommon for the transsexual to present contrasting states of mind to these two groups of professionals on the same day. They rapidly shift their sentiments towards the two groups along 'good' and 'bad' lines, depending on which group seems most likely to assist them in their search for perfection. The physicians' or other caregivers' responses to their psychological manoeuvring, added to the unconscious omnipotent fantasies inherent in the belief that it is possible to make a man into a woman or vice versa, make for a highly charged experience. The result is that scientific work undertaken in such an atmosphere, even when it is motivated by the most honourable intentions, is fraught with difficulties. Objectivity needed for research of this kind is readily modified or even lost in the emotional states induced in the investigators by these patients. We would suggest that in any interdisciplinary endeavour involving highly charged emotions, their influence on observation and judgement be assiduously taken into account.

REFERENCES

Apprey, M. and Stein, H. F. (1993). *Intersubjectivity, projective identification, and otherness*. Duquesne University Press, Pittsburgh.

Bak, R. C. (1968). The phallic woman: the ubiquitous fantasy in perversions. *Psychoanal. Study Child*, **23**, 15–36.

Benjamin, H. (1953). Transvestism and transsexualism. *Int. J. Sexol.* **7**, 12–14.

Blos, P. (1979). *The adolescent passage: Developmental issues*. International Universities Press, New York.

Cauldwell, D. O. (1949). Psychopathic transsexualism. *Sexology*, **16**, 274–80.

Erhardt, A., Epstein, R., and Money, J. (1968*a*). Fetal androgens and female gender identity in the early treated andrenogenital syndrome. *Johns Hopkins Med. J.* **122**, 160–7.

Erhardt, A., Evers, R., and Money, J. (1968*b*). Influence of androgen on some aspects of sexually dimorphic behaviour in women with the late-treated andrenogenital syndrome. *Johns Hopkins Med. J.* **123**, 115–22.

Gadpaille, W. (1972). Research into the physiology of maleness and femaleness. *Arch. Gen. Psychiat.* **26**, 193–206.

Gadpaille, W. (1980). Biological factors in the development of human sexual identity. *Psychiat. Clin. N. Am.* **3**, 3–20.

Kavanaugh, J. C. and Volkan, V. D. (1978–9). Transsexualism and a new type of psychosurgery. *Int. J. Psycho-Anal. Psychother.* **7**, 366–72.

Loeb, L. and Shane, M. (1982). The resolution of a transsexual wish in a five-year-old boy. *J. Am. Psychoanal. Assoc.* **2**, 419–34.

Lothstein, L. N. (1983). *Female to male transsexualism*. Routledge & Kegan Paul, London.

Mahler, M. D. (1975). Discussion of 'Healthy parental influences on the earliest development of masculinity in baby boys' by R. J. Stroller. Margaret S. Mahler Symposium, Philadelphia. *Psychoanal. Forum*, **5**, 244, 247.

MacVicar, K. (1978–9). The transsexual wish in a psychotic character. *Int. J. Psycho-Anal. Psychother.* **7**, 354–71.

Meyer, J. (1974). Clinical variants among applicants for sex reassignment. *Arch. Sex. Behav.* **3**, 527–58.

Meyer, J. (1982). The theory of gender identity disorders. *J. Am. Psychoanal. Assoc.* **2**, 381–418.

Meyer, W. S. and Keith, C. R. (1991). Homosexual and preoedipal issues in the psychoanalytic psychotherapy of a female-to-male transsexual. In *Homosexualities and the therapeutic process*, (ed. C. W. Socarides and V. D. Volkan), pp. 75–96. International Universities Press, Madison, CT.

Money, J. (1974). Intersexual and transsexual behaviour and syndrome. In *The American handbook of psychiatry*, (ed. S. Arieti and E. B. Brody), Vol. 3, pp. 334–51. Basic Books, New York.

Money, J. and Gaskins, R. (1970–1). Sex reassignment. *Int. J. Psychiat.* **9**, 249–69.

Ovesey, L. and Person, E. (1973). Gender identity and psychopathology in men: A psychodynamic analysis of homosexuality, transsexualism, and transvestism. *J. Am. Acad. Psychoanal.* **1**, 53–72.

Person E. and Ovesey, L. (1974 *a*). The transsexual syndrome in males: I. Primary transsexualism. *Am. J. Psychother.* **28**, 4–20.

Person, E. and Ovesey, L. (1974*b*). The transsexual syndrome in males: II. Secondary transsexualism. *Am. J. Psychother.* **28**, 174–93.

Socarides, C. W. (1969). The desire for sexual transformation: A psychiatric evaluation of 'transsexualism' *Am. J. Psychiat.* **125**, 1419–25.

Socarides, C. W. (1970). A psychoanalytic study of the desire for sexual transformation ('transsexualism'): The plaster-of-paris man. *Int. J. Psycho-Anal.* **51**, 341–9.

Socarides, C. C. (1988). *The preoedipal origin and psychoanalytic therapy of sexual perversions*. International Universities Press, Madison, CT.

Stoller, R. J. (1973). The male transsexual as 'experiment'. *Int. J. Psycho-Anal.* **54**, 215–25.

Stoller, R. J. (1975). *Sex and gender, Vol. 2: The transsexual experiment*. Science House, New York.

Stoller, R. J. (1985). *Presentations of gender*. Yale University Press, New Haven, CT.

Stoller, R. J. and Newman, L. E. (1971). The bisexual identity of transsexuals: Two case examples. *Arch. Sex. Behav.* **1**, 17–28.

Volkan, V. D. (1974). The transsexual issue: A cautionary psychiatric insight—A clinical report. In *Marital and sexual counseling in medical practice*, (ed. D. W. Abse, L. M. Nash, and L. M. R. Louden), pp. 383–404. Harper and Row, New York.

Volkan, V. D. (1976). *Primitive internalized object relations. A clinical study of schizophrenia, borderline, and narcissistic patients*. International Universities Press, New York.

Volkan, V. D. (1979). Transsexualism: As examined from the point of view of internalized object relations. In *On sexuality: psychoanalytic observations*, (ed. T. B. Karasu and C. W. Socarides), pp. 189–221. International Universities Press, New York.

Volkan, V. D. (1994). Psychodynamic formulations of psychotherapy in schizophrenic patients. *Directions in Psychiatry*, Vol. 14, 9 March.

Volkan, V. D. and Berent, S. (1976). Psychiatric aspects of surgical treatment for problems of sexual identification (transsexualism). In *Modern perspectives in the psychiatric aspects of surgery*, (ed. J. G. Howells), pp. 447–67. Bruner/Mazell, New York.

Volkan, V. D. and Bhatti, T. H. (1973). Dreams of transsexuals awaiting surgery. *Comprehen. Psychiat.* **14**, 269–79.

Volkan, V. D. and Masri, A. (1989). The development of female transsexualism. *Am. J. Psychother.* **43**, 92–107.

8
Exhibitionism, scopophilia, and voyeurism

Ismond Rosen

EXHIBITIONISM

Definition

An exhibitionist may be defined as a person who exposes his genitals to someone of the opposite sex outside the context of the sexual act. Exhibitionism is classified in DSMIIIR as a paraphilia, a subdivision of the psychosexual disorders. Authorities in this field agree on the practical need to distinguish various levels or degrees of exhibitionism. Schorsch *et al.* (1985) distinguished four levels of intensity of paraphilic symptoms ranging from incidental to compulsive, with the majority of their patients being in the lesser levels. From a psychoanalytical point of view, when genital exposure serves as a fixed, exclusive, or major source of sexual pleasure, and is compulsive or repetitious, exhibitionism is regarded as a perversion, as distinct from occasional perverse behaviour. Van de Loo (1987) has suggested the use of the term 'male genital-exposing behaviour' to help distinguish between a paraphilia and paraphilic behaviour.

In Britain, exhibitionism is an offence, chargeable as indecent behaviour (see Chapter. 18, p. 452). Arrests usually result from the reporting by the female victim, 60 per cent of whom are girls.

Female exhibitionism

Genital exhibitionism is rare in women, which has been explained by the difference in the two sexes of the development of the castration complex, and the absence of the reassuring effect of showing a penis due to the anatomical differences in women. Eber (1977) and Kohut (1978) regarded female exhibitionism as a disorder of bodily narcissism. Cases of female exhibitionism have been reported by Hollender *et al.* (1977) and Blair and Lanyon (1981). Grob (1985) presented an unusual case of a woman who used genital exhibitionism to maintain a damaged self-esteem.

Grob's patient was emotionally deprived in childhood except when her self-esteem became boosted by a phase of becoming the focus of her father's attention through some public approbation of her. Stimulation of her bodily narcissism was further heightened by her experiences of being observed while taking a shower. In adult life she maintained her self-esteem by her professional attainments. When she lost her position at work, she resorted to genital exhibitionism which became compulsive and addictive. While driving her car at night on the motorways she would expose her breasts and genitalia to truck drivers who could illuminate her with their spotlights, and with whom she then played a game of cat-and-mouse. With psychoanalytical psychotherapy her anxiety and exhibitionism diminished and her personality improved, but she felt compelled to repeat her driving exposures during the analyst's vacations. In this case, the exhibitionism served to repeat and defend against unresolved unconscious conflicts of her broken childhood relationships and damaged self-esteem regulation system.

Male exhibitionism

Excellent clinical descriptions of exhibitionism occur in the early literature. See Lasègue (1877) and later reviews by Rooth (1976), Rosen (1979), Glasser (1978) and Schorsch *et al.* (1985) as quoted in the comprehensive review by van de Loo (1987). For an historical review see Rosen (1979).

Incidence

Exhibitionism is one of the commonest sexual deviations, according to the criminal statistics and treatment figures. van de Loo (1987), reviewing the North American and Western European, literature found that about one-third of all sexual offenders were exhibitionists. This figure has remained remarkably consistent for the past fifty years. Detailed transcultural studies comparing the incidence of exhibitionism in Guatemala and the United States (Rhoads and Borjes 1981) showed that it was the same in both countries, though it was commonly assumed that exhibitionism was rare in Latin American countries. These authors concluded that in the exhibitionist, individual psychopathology was more significant than cultural factors.

Recidivism and other criminal behaviour

Forgac *et al.* (1984) in Toledo, Ohio, examined the records of 84 men arrested for genital exposure. They found that the tendency for pure exhibitionists to repeat their exhibitionist activity was not related to the severity of their psychopathology as measured on the Minesota Multiphasic Personality Inventory (MMPI) scaled score elevation. Any increase of severity of psychopathology, measured in this way, was associated with the presence of other factors and with the total number of criminal offences. The relationship between exhibitionism and other criminal activity was thought to be based on antisocial acting-out and tension-reducing behaviour.

In several studies of series of exhibitionists, researchers have tried to separate out different distinctive groupings. Interest has been focused on distinguishing two particular groups—those who are purely exhibitionists and others who have a history of other criminal or sociopathic behaviour. (See McCreary 1975; Rader, 1977; Forgac and Michaels 1982).

Classification

Exhibitionists can be usefully classified into main groups, with gradations in between. The first is the *simple* or *regressive* type, where the exhibitionist act follows as the result of some rather obvious social or sexual trauma, disappointment or loss, or as an accompaniment to a severe mental or physical illness, including the vicissitudes of old age and alcoholism. These people tend to the rather reserved and shy with social and sexual inhibitions and fear, but their personalities are on the whole relatively good ones, as seen in their intimate associations and work records. Maclay (1952) has given an excellent account of what he calls 'compensatory types' where 'the exposure is an act of more or less normal individuals, and is in the nature of an anomalous form of the ordinary sexual advance'. These cases would fit into this group.

Personality disturbance is much more intense in the second group which is the *phobic-impulsive* type. The quality of the personality defects is usually dependent on the pattern and intensity of the infantile level of fixation and the defence mechanisms employed. Examples are given below. In this group one finds persons who regularly exhibit and become recidivists. Where the impulsive aspect predominates they are often of an amoral cast of mind, prone to other forms of character disorder and actual perversion such as transvestism and voyeurism, as well as the commission of crimes of stealing. Thus Richard, exhibiting his feminine attire, wandered on to the wrong beat and was picked up with the other girls and driven in the Black Maria to prison, where his true sex was discovered. Several of the patients were voluble sea-lawyers, two of whom gravitated towards the office of shop-steward, where they exercised a capable irresponsibility combined with a constant shiftlessness of employment. This need for frequent change of object, whether job, possessions or interests, was typical of many patients and revealed their preoedipal character fixations. Even in their arguments they usually ended up identifying and agreeing with the other side. In this group, too, could be found well-developed phobic disorders of both hysterical and obsessional type. For example, Peter, a highly intelligent patient, had constant recurring fantasies that his genitals would be bitten off by sharks in the swimming pool, bath water, and bed, which was evidence of his severe phallic castration anxiety expressed in phobic terms; while a part-time musician, of whom we had three, had to pick up all the papers in the street prior to exposing himself. This obsessional symptom was an intensification of the reaction formation of tidiness as a defence against the anal component of 'dirtiness' in the act of exposure.

From an examination of the literature and the observations made on The Portman Clinic 1964 series of patients, it seems clear that this phobic-impulsive group exists as a syndrome or entity, separate from cases where exhibitionism occurs symptomatically in the presence of other specific causes. Some controversy exists about the diagnostic classification of this syndrome; whether it belongs to the psychoneurotic compulsive group, or to the impulse neuroses or perversions, which some classify among the psychopathic personalities. Apart from the question of nomenclature, treatment is dependent on the diagnosis preferred; diagnosis should be based on the psychopathology.

Van de Loo (1987) examined 20 male adult exhibitionists and classified them as habitual or non-habitual. Van de Loo's typology resembles Rosen's classification, especially regarding the intensity of personality disturbance, but felt that the two types do not differ in their conditions of onset. Van de Loo found that the onset of genital-exposing behaviour in adolescence and adulthood related in the majority of cases to social, personal or sexual trauma, or to physical injury. The habitual type continues to expose himself independently of such crisis conditions.

In several studies of series of exhibitionists, researchers have tried to separate different distinct groupings. Interest was focused on distinguishing two particular groups—those who are purely exhibitionists and others who have a history of other criminal or sociopathic behaviour (McCreary 1975; Rader 1977; Forgac and Michaels 1982). Rader (1977) made MMPI profile studies of a court services population of exposers, rapists and assaulters. He differentiated three groups: (1) exhibitionism as a passive 'pure' sex crime involving no violence; (2) a violent crime group where no sexual offence had occurred; and (3) rapists who had both sex and violence and who were the most disturbed psychologically.

McCreary (1975) confirmed other clinical studies in exhibitionists that those with the greater number of prior offences had the most personality disturbance. Forgac and Michaels (1982) tried to assess the personality differences between those pure exhibitionists and those with other additional criminal involvement. Using objective personality data, they described two types: a conscientious, inhibited, conforming, timid, neurotic type, and an unconventional, uninhibited, antisocial type of person. To some degree, this provided objective evidence for the clinical dual typology described above by Rosen (1964), of the simple or regressive and the phobic-compulsive types. (Similar dualities were noted by other authors such as Maclay 1952; Kopp 1962; and Rickles 1980). Forgac and Michaels however, further subdivided the phobic-compulsive group into those with predominating obsessional neurotic features and those with more antisocial or criminal tendencies. In this study, the criminal group who had long histories of other antisocial behaviour, were usefully differentiated from the non-criminal exhibitionist group with regard to their personality characteristics and degree of pathology. The criminal exhibitionist group compared with the non-criminals, were more sociopathic, less well-educated, poorly as opposed to normally socialized, and less mature. In contrast, the non-criminal group were over-socialized and neurotically inhibited. No differences occurred on the self-control scale between the two groups. These findings require future study and to assess their value for prognosis and treatment.

Berah and Myers (1983) examined a series of exhibitionists to determine their dangerousness, with special reference to the possibility of their committing further violent and sexual offences. Their data suggested that while the incidence of violent crime was low, the majority could scarcely be regarded as law-abiding. The more often a man was convicted of indecent exposure, the greater the likelihood he also had convictions for other crimes.

Saunders and Awad (1991) in Toronto, examined a series of 19 male adolescent sexual offenders, and divided them into two groups: a 'hands-off' group consisting of exhibitionists and obscene telephone callers, and a 'hands-on' group of child-molesters and rapists. The great majority of cases in this series had committed numerous sexual offences and were maladjusted adolescents from multi-problem families. Half of them had a history of non-sexual delinquencies and were likely to have committed both 'hands-on' and 'hands-off' offences. The diagnosis of sexual deviance fitted a minority of them, but was difficult to make in most of these adolescents. The sexual component of their behaviour was in retrospect denied or disavowed, leading the authors to the expectation that later sexual offending would occur. In their view, the most significant indicator for predicting future sexual offence was a history where different sexual misdemeanours are committed against more than one victim. Single-act sexual offenders, even from families with sexually deviant histories, were less likely to commit future sexual offences, but many of these continued to commit other crimes. The authors suggested that DSMIIIR definitions of paraphilia be modified to accommodate these adolescents.

Phenomenology and psychopathology

The phenomenology of the exhibitionist act is a complex and fascinating one, the full understanding of which would give the clue to many processes hitherto unexplained. The pre-conditions and liability for such responses exist in childhood where desires and acts of exhibitionism are normal in both sexes and undergo a process of repression. In the exhibitionist the normal process of repression is either exaggerated, leading to severe inhibitions, both sexual and social, or is incomplete, where there has been either intense prohibition or stimulation of interest in the boy's body and his genital functions by mother. Both Rickles (1950) and Karpman (1948) blame the heightened sense of narcissism on mother's excessive attention to the boy's body and his genitals. The unrepressed exhibitionist urges serve to hold deeper sexual wishes towards the mother in unconscious control. The age of subsequent onset of exposure is highly variable and dependent on chance environmental stimuli. Two patients described games of 'look and show' with girls, many years before puberty. Thus, in these two persons the normal latency phase was seriously interfered with, or with regard to exhibitionist tendencies, failed to occur. The latency period, following the oedipal stage and lasting until just before puberty, is characterized by strong reaction formations against infantile sexuality, plus the growing sublimatory interests in boyhood pursuits. Several adolescents exposed themselves due to the intensity of sexual feeling during puberty and the teens. It is quite often the case that the youth is already in a state of sexual excitement when the sudden presence of a female causes him to objectify the experience through her. For example, boys masturbating alone in their rooms, or urinating in the country in apparent solitude, may see passers-by from a window or other vantage point, and believing themselves to be unnoticed, complete an act, or succumb to sudden impulse. Two men started in their late teens and early twenties following their only intercourse experiences, which were with prostitutes while on sevice, and which were profoundly shocking and disappointing. It was as if all their fears of inadequacy and of the damaging effect of intercourse with a woman thereby gained material proof. Commencement at later decades was usually a result of loss or frustration, which although not manifestly sexual, nevertheless symbolized a blow to their self-esteem and masculine pride, and was associated with feelings of depression. The circumstances of the first exposure experiences contribute to an habitual pattern which is set up. This template is made use of by the police to apprehend such unfortunates. The conditioning varies proportionately and is stronger in youth, although new additional patterns may be later established. Ford and Beach

(1952) state that males who have mated with females in a particular place often show signs of sexual arousal the next time they are taken to the same enclosure. There soon develops a strong tendency to approach and remain within the setting previously associated with sexual satisfaction, and to respond sexually to any other individual met there.

This capacity for conditioning seems to stem from the high degree of fused aggression and libido which, having been withdrawn from previous objects, is freely available when the penis, highly charged with narcissistic libido, is exhibited. This has significance for treatment, because where such specific habits exist, each major pattern and element of the situation, for example, the age of the victim, the place, time of day, general mood, and so on, must be worked through in therapy; otherwise a trigger mechanism may still be set off by the presence of some of these stimulus elements. Thus one patient, aged 40, in individual psychotherapy had analysed his need to exhibit to young schoolgirls on the road walking home from the station. His desire and fantasies of exposure no longer existed in that situation. He then required to work through urges to expose himself while travelling on trains, wishes not yet under full control. This man had an unresolved oedipal conflict of high intensity and had been forced from the age of 8 by schoolgirls into exposing himself. The difficulties with his father were mirrored in his reacting badly to any superiors or masculine authority. This led to a feeling of suppressed resentment at work demands, and a sense of injustice at the failure to secure promotion. Exhibitionism was a release for these feelings. Prior to psychotherapy he was treated with stilboestrol which succeeded in banishing all his sexual fantasies. On stopping this drug the urges and fantasies of exposing himself returned immediately. By means of psychotherapy he was able to have a normal sexual life with his wife and he lost the urge to expose himself. But he was still advised to avoid those situations which previously presented a source of stimulation, which it was felt could still be dangerous if he regressed when he became depressed or angry. One feature of this patient's illness was the severe social ostracism and active anonymous hostility vented on him and his family, as a result of his court appearances being reported in the newspapers. While freedom of the Press must be earnestly upheld, the publication of details of sexual offences may result in exaggerated social sanctions, or as sometimes happens in certain much publicized cases, in a false sense of heightened esteem in the offender. The wisdom of or justification for such publication should be further examined in the light of modern knowledge.

The precipitating event may therefore be primarily one of two types. The first is that of internal sexual excitement arising spontaneously as in the adolescent, or aroused in him by sexually stimulating sights. The patient, Peter, first exposed himself at his window in response to a little girl doing handstands next door. He could never resist the sight of a girl's knickers after that. In the second type, exposures occur as a result of a non-sexual tension situation which nevertheless has the symbolic meaning of loss of security or castration. Thus a young artist exposed himself in his car on two occasions when going home from the dentist. The unconscious awareness of a dental attack as symbolizing castration was quite clear. Depressions following loss of work or status were common causes. Often, there was a mixture of the two in a complex way. The act itself, however, is usually an impulsive affair, which, when the urge arises, is beyond the capacity of the individual to control. A feeling of inner tension prevails which seems similar to that described by Freud (1905) for an infantile sexual aim; it is felt as unpleasure, is centrally conditioned and then projected on to a peripheral erotogenic zone, in this case, the genitals. On exposure, the exhibitionist becomes aware of intense genital sensations and a sense of inner pleasure, in excess of anything else he has experienced, including heterosexual orgasm. There may or may not be an erection and masturbation may or may not be indulged in. The fact that neither erection nor ejaculation is necessary for the experience of specific pleasure is evidence of the hyper-libidinization of the genital area. The sexual pleasure may be short-lived or endure for a long time. Usually, however, there is a return of self-critical faculties and many, overcome by their guilt and remorse, are easily apprehended and form the bulk of the first offenders. Many patients pride themselves on their self-control and high moral standards in other spheres. Those who plan their exposures may go undetected for years. The picture is therefore one of a temporary suspension of super-ego control as far as these unconscious instinctual desires are concerned, the ego being forced to participate in the performance of an organized act, but powerless to control the timing of it. Like the infant, the exhibitionist can neither tolerate tensions, nor wait for his needs to be satisfied. Both must be dealt with immediately. Instead of thinking they pass directly into action. Glasser (1978) describes the super-ego in exhibitionists as rigid, primitive, and merciless. In the exhibitionist act there is a splitting of the super-ego, simultaneous gratification, and triumphant self-assertion, coexisting with blissful passive surrender.

The recognition that the adult exhibitionist acts out a partial aspect of instinctual behaviour normally expressed in childhood and subsequently repressed, was first adumbrated by Freud in the 'Interpretation of dreams' (1900) and later fully described in his classical 'Three essays on sexuality' (1905). This position was maintained with little change by Fenichel, who regarded exhibitionism as the 'simple over-cathexis of a partial instinct' which was a denial of or reassurance against castration anxiety and the Oedipus complex. The Oedipus complex in its positive aspect may be said to be dominated by the boy's aggressive feelings against his father and his tender wishes towards his mother. Its negative side, which is present in varying degrees in exhibitionists, is that of a wish to take mother's place with father by identifying with her. Castration anxiety is the unconscious fear of the boy's own aggressive feelings plus the fear of the father's retaliation. While Freud felt strongly about the specificity of castration anxiety as fear of loss of the genitals, he nevertheless saw it as part of a sequence of bodily loss starting with the birth process and followed by weaning and the loss of faeces.

In its intensity, castration anxiety represents all the anxieties of loss ever experienced, while the aggression felt towards the father and expected in retaliation seems to be the sum of all previous aggression, from whatever stage and source.

In animals, reaction to fear takes one of two pathways. Either there is action, in the form of fight or flight, or there is complete immobility as if transfixed. These two patterns of behaviour are seen extremely well in the exhibitionist. In Freud's description of exhibitionist dreams, the factor of sudden physical immobility is shown to be a characteristic feature; lesser degrees of inhibition are extremely common, and are discussed in detail by him, the association between the wish to exhibit sexually and inhibitions to activity of any sort are clearly linked in these dreams, much as one finds it in the everyday life of the exhibitionist. During the time of greater fear or tension, there is the sudden impulse to exposure as an aggressive act. But this act is also a safeguard against still more dangerous fighting. One patient called Bill had several previous convictions for indecent exposure, voyeurism, and stealing. He only attended the first meeting of the first group, but returned a year later having lost his wife and job, and desperately seeking help. Having stopped exposing himself, he was afraid that if he lost his temper he would murder someone. He was taken into the second group, and described his enormous powers of control which suddenly gave way if his self-esteem was threatened, or if a superior was unfair. An ex-boxer, he was a potential murderer and everyone recognized it. The group was quite subdued for two sessions when he talked at length about his difficulties. He then found a new job and social interests and became calmer. Later some members began to assail him in a subtle way, and he left the group, unable to tolerate this aggression and what he regarded as the therapist's unfairness to a particular member.

We must now try to understand what loss of love and self-esteem means, in terms of early object-relationships. This is because there is a fundamental relation between the mechanism of depression and impulse neurosis. Both depressives and impulse neurotics are greedy people, dependent on narcissistic supplies from outside. Freud laid down a timetable of libidinal development in the infant, which progresses from auto-erotism, to narcissism, to true object-relationships. Thus in the stage of narcissism, loss of an object or a reduction in the amount of love shown, leads to a withdrawal of libido from the object and its re-direction back on to the infant's own body. The part of the body participating in this narcissistic regression is dependent on the degree to which earlier fixations have occurred in the genital and pregenital phases of development. An examination of the total personality characteristics and mental associations reveals the amount and quality of these fixations; derivatives thereof colour the exhibitionist act itself. The exhibitionist regresses to the sadistic phase of childhood, where any loss of object, self-esteem or threat of rejection results in a withdrawal of libido from the object or external reality, and a subsequent investment of this libido as secondary narcissism in the infant's own body via a specific organ, his penis.

Certain exhibitionists seem to be fixated at the oral level. Thus, loquacious Dick described himself as a 'mouth in trousers'. The hostility of the oral phase, seen as biting and devouring, is projected on to the outside world and a similar retaliation is expected. It is the strength of this fixation which gives to later objects such as the female genitalia their hostile oral character. Christoffel (1936) postulated colpophobia, fear of the female genitals, as the basic fear in exhibitionism. Melitta Sperling (1947) reported the analysis of a single case of exhibitionism in which an oral fixation was the most important determinant of the condition. This operated through the unconscious equation of breast with penis. The patient could not overcome the trauma of weaning and early separation from mother.

At the stage of object-relationship, the libido is similarly withdrawn from the object, but then a mental image of the lost object is taken into the self by the process of introjection and represented therein. This leads to an identification with the lost object and is one of the mechanisms of character formation. The time sequence of these developmental phases is important and the stage of object-relationship takes place about the time biting and anal interests are becoming prominent, at about the eighth to ninth month. Winnicott (1958) has described certain phenomena of the transitional phase between oral erotism and true object-relationship. One of these transitional phenomena is the infant putting his or her thumb into the mouth, while the fingers of that hand caress the nose or face. Exactly similar behaviour occurred as a regressive phenomenon in Roger, a youth of 17. His sullenness and silence during the adolescent group mirrored his relationships generally. He treated his parents at home as complete strangers and never spoke to them. With gentle handling and time he evinced a pleasant if rough demeanour in the group and settled down to work at a new job extremely well. When the group ended, he continued in individual psychotherapy. Each session commenced with a cheery account of the week's successful happenings, then he would lapse into silence. This withdrawal became more profound in later sessions, when the thumb-sucking and face caressing would occur in a hypnoidal state from which he was hardly rousable. He lost his exhibitionist urges, but the underlying object losses which were exposed resulted in his being sent away, as he had a kleptomaniac episode of stealing from a garage he was passing. A similar hypnoidal phenomenon was seen to affect the whole second adult group on one occasion as a response to inconsequential compulsive talking by one member. Winnicott (1958) has described both pseudologia fantastica and thieving in terms of 'an individual's unconscious urge to bridge a gap in continuity of experience in respect of a transitional object'. Some exhibitionists appear to react to loss with mechanisms from this transitional phase.

When the stage of object relationship is reached with its sadistic biting and anal aspects, the individual becomes aware of himself and others as hostile and threatening. He has great difficulty in dealing with the objects he introjects. The complex mechanisms of this phase belong to the study of depressions and super-ego development. Exhibitionists tolerate loss very badly and expose themselves as a defence against the accompanying depression. One patient out of this series exposed himself one week after the death of his father. Another adult group member showed only few signs of depression when reporting a still birth to the group eagerly awaiting news of the delivery. As a group they could become more depressed over this, than he could as an individual.

Greenacre (1952) has examined the resultants of childhood stimulation which is either premature, too intense, or too frustrating. She believes that these, if early lead to an increased somatization of memories and symptoms; if severe and massive, to the utilization of all possible channels of discharge; and in states of frustration or over-stimulation, that genital arousal occurs from an early time. Also, that genital performance may be used very largely in the service of pregenital aims, yet retaining genital form and even a modicum of genital pleasure.

In many exhibitionists, although the organ involved is the genitals, the mechanisms employed from an economic point of view is that set up by the oral-sadistic phase. The importance of oral factors as components of the castration complex has been discussed by Stärcke (1921), Fenichel (1931), and de Monchy (1952).

The problem may therefore be stated as follows. Does the exhibitionist regress to the oral-sadistic phase of childhood when he meets the difficulties aroused by the Oedipus complex in the genital phase, when castration anxiety is at its height? Or are there fixations and components from the pregential phases (oral and anal) which influence both the castration complex and the Oedipus complex? The exhibitionist's relationships with his parents (and his wife) are difficult to understand in the light of the classically described Oedipus complex. Towards both parents there is an ambivalent love–hate relationship, which in its heightened state is characteristic of the pregenital preoedipal phase. This was clearly revealed in many patients during their treatment. Thus towards the mother there was love expressed in a preoedipal way via a strong feminine identification. This feminine identification was found to be present in all the patients, even in the unlikeliest member John, who was a shop manager and who, though inhibited, appeared a virile family man. It was discovered that he prided himself on being able to handle ladies' underwear better than any of his female staff. The feminine identification was also an aspect of the negative Oedipus complex, where the son is desirous of replacing mother in father's affections. This provides an obvious stimulus to a homosexual attachment and inclination, and the act of exposure to a woman is also a defence against this homosexual component and full feminine identification. The difficulties of dealing with the latter in treatment are discussed in the section on group therapy.

The erogenous pleasure gained in the act of exposure leads to a heightened self-esteem or narcissism. Freud postulated that exhibitionism remained more narcissistic than any other partial instinct because it originated in the precursor of looking at oneself. This provided the connection with another partial instinct, that of scopophilia, the sexualization of the sensations of looking. Scopophilia and exhibitionism usually exist as instinctual counterparts in the same way as sado-masochism, active–passive wishes, and masculine–feminine strivings.

Edgcumbe and Burgner (1975) described a phallic narcissistic preoedipal stage in the child, where gratification occurs mainly through the penis. In this phase, exhibitionism and narcissistic gratification depend on being admired by the mother, the major external object. This is an important phase, the main task of which is the development of a differentiated self and sexual identity. The boy's identification with his father facilitates the completion of this phase. Galenson and Roiphe (1980) observed boys at the end of the second year of life and found that their genital play and urinary games were identificatory with their fathers. Failure to negotiate this phase adequately leads to disturbances in later object-relationships that retain a phallic-narcissistic character and in which the object serves as a source of admiration or condemnation. Exhibitionists relate to their victims very much in this manner. Fixations occur at this phallic-narcissistic stage when the penis becomes libidinized and serves as the bodily source of masculine identity. See also Allen, D. W. (1980) for a psychoanalytic view of exhibitionism.

Behavioural studies

See Bond and Hutchison (1960) for description of reciprocal inhibition therapy for exhibitionism. Behavioural scientists are evaluating the riches of clinical observation and psychodyamic theory on exhibitionism, using tests and controls. Three studies used phallometric measurement responses in exhibitionists to sexually arousing stimuli. Fedora *et al.* (1986) showed a battery of 60 slides to three groups. These consisted of 14 exhibitionists, 21 normal controls, and 34 non-exhibitionist sex offenders. They found only one significant difference among the three groups. The exhibitionists responded sexually to scenes of fully clothed erotically neutral females, whereas the two other groups did not. The authors, in keeping with their social-behavioural approach concluded that culturally unapproved sexual displays acted as signals inducing cortical disinhibition.

Langevin *et al.* (1979) used phallometric tests to examine critical stimulus response processes and personality factors. They reported that exhibitionists responded most to immature females, although there was a tenuous link with paedophilia. Findings supported the psychoanalytical view that voyeurism and exhibitionism are linked. Voyeurism was more prevalent in the exhibitionists than in the control group. This study employed behavioural theory and clinical theory, which failed to provide a unitary understanding of exhibitionism. The authors suggest that the element of narcissism in exhibitionism was significant and merited investigation. Their use of narcissism relied on external rather than internal psychic processes and precluded the consideration that sexual deviation functioned as a regulator of self-esteem.

Smukler and Schiebel (1975) clinically examined the personality characteristics of exhibitionist-voyeurs in a five-year treatment programme at Harbour General Hospital, California. They concluded that exhibiting was 'a unique way of expressing unconscious strivings without provoking the retaliatory response that direct aggression might stimulate'. However, these phallometric tests and the behavioural theories employed have shed very little light on specific character types or the psychopathology in exhibitionism.

Singer (1979) described a case of exhibitionism in which the Rorschach test revealed core-emotional conflicts, disturbed object-relationships, and poor impulse controls. The author felt the findings would be helpful in making treatment recommendations in exhibitionists. As exhibitionists were usually defensive and emotionally guarded, the test could distinguish those with greater intra-psychic problems from those who were sociopathic offenders. Van de Loo (1987) comprehensively reviewed the psychodynamic literature and the application of cognitive—behavioural techniques in the understanding and treatment of exhibitionism. He recommends integrating these two approaches. Both, however, lack sufficiently tested hypotheses. He suggests testing exhibitionists in the actual life situation, with particular reference to the characteristics of genital-exposing behaviour.

SCOPOPHILIA AND VOYEURISM

Scopophilia, the pleasure in looking, can also become a perversion, which is known as voyeurism. Freud (1905) defined it was a perversion if '(a) it is restricted exclusively to the genitals or (b) if it is connected with the overriding of disgust (as in the case of *voyeurs* or people who look on at excretory functions), or (c) if, instead of being *preparatory* to the sexual aim, it supplants it. This last is markedly true of exhibitionists, who, if I may trust the findings of several analyses, exhibit their own genitals in order to obtain a reciprocal view of the genitals of the other person'. In the perversions, the presence of exhibitionism always means an associated voyeurism and vice versa, even if only present unconsciously.

Scopophilia is thus the taking in of impressions visually, and during the first year of life may be linked with the way objects are taken in via the mouth, or sensations experienced by touch; looking and touching are intimately associated. If, however, the oral incorporative experiences are unsatisfactory and come to be characterized by greed, hunger, and insatiety, with fears of the ensuing hostile aspects, then the visual functions may come to have a similar quality and be felt as devouring, compulsive, and later be defended against by complex inhibitory systems of lack of interest or learning difficulties. The visual component of castration anxiety is exemplified in the classical myth where Oedipus blinds himself as a retribution for his incestuous crimes. These visual–oral–phallic aspects are described in detail in Fenichel's paper, 'The scoptophilic instinct and identification' (1954). See also Allen (1974), '*The fear of looking*'.

It seems that the excess of aggressive energies and their lack of fusion with libidinal elements require other bodily systems to be more highly charged as a way of dealing with them. Thus, other ectodermal structures, such as the skin, participate in and express the 'unpleasure' or tensions. Several of the patients reported the active existence of skin complaints of the nature of eczema and allergy, this being a rather frequent finding in the literature. Exhibitionism, however, is mainly linked with the phallic stage of experience; the greatest investment of narcissistic libido being concentrated on this organ due to its significance for procreation. The scopophilic instinct becomes prominent again in the phallic stage when curiosity and research about sexual matters becomes intensified. Thus, from an economic point of view, libido from both the oral and phallic stages finds a common pathway for expression and, later, repression. The reaction formation against scopophilia is shyness. The earliest intimation of shyness seems to have its origins at the time in the infant's life when it is learning to distinguish between familiar figures and strangers. Work reported by Ambrose (1961) on the smiling response in infants, shows that following a peak of smiling responses to both mother and strangers, which occurs at 20 weeks with institution infants and 13 weeks with home infants, there is a decline in response-strength towards the strangers, so that by the age of 5 to 6 months the child seems able to discriminate well between mother-figure and strangers. Other observers attributed this falling off in smiling respone to a fear of strangers; Ambrose records it as also being due to factors of curiosity and exploration. This development coincides with both the oral-sadistic phase and the important time when the child comes to see its mother more as a whole person or object. She may be incorporated as a source of pleasure; the stranger however leads only to further tensions. The reaction formation of shyness occurs at the early oedipal phase at the age of three or four years, when curiosity, concept formation, and the thirst for knowledge are aroused strongly. As Freud (1905) has stated, 'in scopophilia and exhibitionism the eye corresponds to an erotogenic zone'.

Thus, disturbances in these stages of development are likely to be reflected later in specific disorders which are found in varying degrees in all exhibitionists. The difficulty in object-relationships is seen in the exhibitionist act itself, where the woman exposed to does not have the characteristics of a whole person for the exhibitionist. She is merely there to provide a narcissistic gratification and proof against castration. Most patients readily agreed that they 'would run a mile' if the woman to whom they exposed themselves were to respond. Even for those who claim the act as means of sexual stimulation, doing it to a *complete stranger* robs it of the quality of fore-pleasure as exposure before normal intercourse my be, and turns it into an aggressive act. The exhibitionist therefore reverses the childhood formula of avoiding strangers in order to perceive mother more wholly. Exposure to the stranger is still dangerous but preferable to exposing to the familiar woman who stands for mother because of the greater danger inherent in the castration complex. Many patients were extremely prudish with their wives; they took care never to let each other be seen in the nude, and their pattern of sexual behaviour in intercourse was rigidly conventional. There is general agreement in the literature on the puritanical attitude towards sex in the families of exhibitionists as well as in themselves. The highly inhibited and shy exhibitionists are therefore a result of the excessive reaction formations against scopophilia. In the group, they could not talk, as everyone was strange, and in a few cases months passed before they could be induced into making spontaneous comments. One of the commonest complaints was of having nothing to talk about. It was well known that individuals with such complaints are usually poor readers due to their difficulties in taking in visual impressions. The importance of good reading ability as expounded by Mortimer Adler in *How to read a book* is most instructive here. He points out the philogical connexion between the words 'to read' and oral behaviour. Previously 'read' was the term given to the ruminant's fourth stomach. Oral terms are also used to denote understanding, such as the 'digestion' of a passage.

One of the commonest inhibitions observed in the group was that of inability to initiate any activity. When the talkative members were absent, one was able to analyse the fears of commencement as mechanisms for controlling instinctual drives. At least two talkative persons should be in the group to balance the shy silent ones, as lengthy silences are absolutely intolerable to the latter and should be avoided. Richard (see p. 194) left the group never to return, during a silence near the end of the first group when attendances were low. Further, thre is little to talk about if there are learning difficulties and facts cannot be taken in due to a repression of curiosity. The ideas underlying their silences were a mixture of castration fear and narcissistic inferiority, namely, that what they had to say had already been said, or would be a paltry contribution, and that they would be laughed at by others. Thinking, as a mental function, was extremely difficult and no thoughts were present. This was in marked contradistinction to the compulsive talking felt by two disinhibited members, one of whom was Dick, the 'mouth in trousers'.

Glasser (1978) discusses the conflict between the ego and the super-ego in the exhibitionist. He agrees with Rooth (1976) that exhibitionists are under-achievers, and posits that the failure to reach adequate goals may be due to the passive resistance of the ego against the sadistic demands of the super-ego. Some secondary gain accrues to the ego as a result. The exhibitionistic act is a manifestation of active, compelling defiance against the super-ego; this attitude manifests itself in all spheres of psychic activity, especially those imposing moral and ethical restraints.

Treatment

The treatment of exhibitionists and voyeurs must always be made on the basis of an individual assessment. In general, the therapy of choice is some form of psychoanalytical treatment, individual or group psychotherapy, although counselling in simple inhibited adolescents may suffice. The more pronounced the accompanying personality disorder and the tendency to repeat, the greater the need for intensive transference therapy.

All patients appearing in court should have a medical report. It is to be preferred that the psychiatrist making the report should be responsible for the subsequent treatment advised either by undertaking to give the treatment personally or under his supervision, or making suitable prior arrangements elsewhere.

Some patients of the simple regressive type may respond to the shock of the court appearance, fines or imprisonment, but these have a minimal effect on the phobic-impulsive group.

The similarity of compulsivity in exhibitionists and obsessional-compulsive disorders has led psychiatrists to treat exhibitionists with fluoxetine. Bianchi (1990) reported an adult male diagnosed as schizophrenic who had a lengthy history of genital exposures with multiple arrests and many hospital admissions. Fluoxetine 40 mg, was prescribed daily in addition to his usual fluphenazine. This resulted in a significant relief of his exhibitionist urges for the first time since his early childhood. (For details of other treatments for exhibitionism see Chapter 1 for drug treatments, and Chapter 16 for behavioural and cognitive therapy.)

Group therapy for exhibitionists

The effectiveness of group therapy is reported by Witzig (1968) and Mathis and Collins (1970) and discussed on p. 211. These reports focus on the treatment programmes in service clinics, with the aim of preventing recurrences. They excluded the sociopathic offenders as unsuitable, and made progress with the neurotic aspects of their patients, helping them to achieve improved social skills, but not being able to cope with the deeper underlying psychopathology. The group served as an important source of support against re-offending. (Group therapy is reported in detail below. Such accounts are rare in the literature.)

Obscene telephone calls

Obscene telephone calls are an exhibitionist act in another medium. In Saunders and Awad (1991) study of 108 male adolescent offenders, 19 are exhibitionists and obscene telephone-call makers. All of these are 'hands-off' offenders, not liable to make physical contact with their victims. Nadler (1968) discusses the psychodynamics of obscene telephone callers.

The medium of the telephone provides a distancing that protects the caller and allows for the expression of greater aggression and more menace. Such people are poorly integrated, require immediate relief of their need for recognition by others, and are usually not physically menacing. The calls enhance the caller's feelings of grandiosity and enable him to deny his feelings of nothingness, and overcome his difficulty in getting close to anyone. In these people, there are feelings of fear and rage at women. Underlying these feelings are fantasies of symbiotic union with the woman, who is experienced as frustrating, overwhelming, and emasculating. The resulting psychic impotence and helplessness are defended against by the obscene calls. Events that lower the caller's self-esteem usually precipitate the calling. In the personality of these obscene telephone-callers, there were major disruptions in self-esteem with self-deprecation and compensatory grandiosity. Their calling represented only part of a complex defensive system.

Goldberg and Wise (1985) report on the psychodynamic treatment of a homosexual case. It was important to confront the patient and work through his denials and his masochism, and deal with his castration anxiety, low self-esteem, and separation-anxiety.

VOYEURISM: A CLINICAL CASE STUDY

Details of a case of voyeurism will now be presented. Apart from the significant psychopathology, the difficulties in dealing with this recidivist patient from a social and therapeutic point of view are salutary and reveal areas of interaction that deserve of public and professional notice.

Noel was in his middle twenties, and had eight previous convictions for 'peeping Tom' offences. These were mainly for watching women in public lavatories, the last one being combined with that of stealing for which he was sentenced to 6 months' imprisonment. He was first sent by the court for psychiatric opinion aged 20, and his progression both medically and criminally was briefly as follows. At first he was given a conditional discharge and he commenced treatment which was hypnosis. He appeared to respond, but after 2 months failed to attend. Later he was arrested for a similar offence, was put on 2 years' probation and treatment was continued in irregular unco-operative fashion. Several other court appearances soon followed, he being bound over and then being fined £25 for breach of recognizance. His attitude was one of great resentment to his parents and indifference towards the court. The diagnosis was that of immature psychopathic personality. Diagnoses by later psychiatrists who saw him aged 23 were that of immature and unstable personality with psychopathic traits, and compulsive abnormal sexual behaviour. By this time he had had a course of psychotherapy lasting a year, the results of which he was pleased with, and also a course of hormone treatment to diminish his sexual desires. He had married during this period and no further hormones were prescribed so as not to interfere with his marital sexual life. A year later the psychiatrist referring him from one of HM Prisons to The Portman Clinic thought that he was suffering from a psychoneurotic illness with obsessive compulsive features, stemming back to childhood or adolescence, and was in need of further treatment.

Noel was then treated with weekly analytic psychotherapy when the following picture slowly emerged. His problems stemmed directly from a very disturbed early family background, characterized by his subjection to intense stimulation of an aggressive and sexual kind, together with deprivation of understanding and affection, at times alternatively, at others concurrently. As a child of 8–10 years, he would get resentful with his mother and express this in cruelty to animals. He had to show off to the other boys, or be silly to gain their attention. He craved his father's attention and admiration, but the latter took all his exploits and excellent sporting abilities quite coolly.

He reported satisfaction during sexual intercourse with his wife, but disgust on completion, and was compelled to think of millions of others having intercourse at the same time, like animals. When it was interpreted to him that he then became conscious of his parents' intercourse, he associated to his first ever awareness of primal scene activities at the age of 4 years, and ever since then, because of the paper-thin walls. He was terrified, prayed they would stop, and later lay awake waiting for a repetition of the event, feeling left out and resentful. He had a similar set of fantasies about the toilet where the sounds fascinated and disgusted him. The similarity of his feelings concerning his wish to see women in lavatories and his mother in intercourse was revealed. He felt that seeing women in the toilets was a way of degrading them. By his offences and court appearances he was able to hurt his mother. Not only was his feeling of being left out by his parents a cause of intolerable loneliness, but he also had to defend himself against the wish to become like mother. Thus, artistic sensitivity to poetry and music was a source of fear as this aroused a feeling of feminine identification, and was checked by his daring exploits. But he would imitate women's toilet behaviour he had seen, by squatting and arranging his clothes. Thus, he came to do actively what was done to him passively when young. He felt humiliated at being bathed by his mother up to the age of 11 years and humiliated women in return. As an adult, he thought mother was over-sexed as she came into the bathroom at inopportune moments, and when he became angry, she would say 'You've got nothing to look at', which led to his first voyeuristic acts in public. He then admitted to conscious thoughts of intercourse with mother. He said that this was the worst kind of incest and he found such ideas quite intolerable, but that going into toilets was the next best thing to intercourse with mother. The importance of his voyeuristic acts as a defence against his intense incestuous desires for his mother, as well as an expression of them, became clear. In his teens he would try and see mother without any clothes on and was given a hiding by her for observing her at her toilet. This also linked up with memories of discovering mother's soiled sanitary towels as an adolescent and as a small child, which aroused his disgust and the thought that if father only knew about these things what he would say; the sexually arousing effect of all this was clear, and the anal-sadistic aspects emphasized. His voyeurism was therefore a compromise mechanism which prevented and yet satisfied his wish for intercourse with mother and led to severe punishments, for he would frequently be caught, as it were, on purpose. The punishments had different significant aspects; through them he could show his masculinity to mother, make up for his sense of genital inferiority, further humiliate his parents, and counter his fears of a feminine identification. He felt his parents wanted a girl instead of him, and as a child he had fantasies of being a girl. He said he would hate to be a woman, because of chaps like him frightening them in toilets, afraid of being raped or murdered. The sado-masochistic elements in this case are quite striking; one source of such satisfaction was always the publication of his name or misdemeanour in the newspapers. The merits in Press publication of details of sexual misdemeanours remain debatable, and in many countries are disallowed. Although social sanctions such as losing jobs and friends followed, the narcissistic satisfaction was enormous.

Noel gave evidence of oral sadism as well as the anal sadism described above. His boyhood cruelties were prolific. He dug tunnels in ponds and filled them with frogs, newts, eels, and adders, watched them tangling together, then would cut them to bits with a knife, or pour on oil and set them on fire. Games of torture were frequent and included fantastic 'dares'. But this sadistic approach was contradictory; he would never hurt a bird under any circumstances and was a keen ornithologist. Birds were thought of as tender; amphibians could be tortured or burned, and mammals killed. He once killed his own pet rabbit, but could not put an injured bird out of its misery. Once at school he spoiled a prize cabbage the children were growing by poking his finger through it—and when later an interpretation about his wish to damage mother's breast was given on different material, he associated back to the cabbage and said that it had to be holed exactly in the centre. This was interpreted as representing the nipple and he then talked of his fantasies which were similar to a recent murder case where the woman was bodily mutilated. He had thoughts of cutting a woman's breasts right off where they joined the rib cage, and added that he also had fantasies of cutting women's nipples out. He continued to describe how, when he was younger and was served mince meat and mash, he would mix it all up and make the food into a square, then make a ploughed field out of it with a fork, then cut the centre square and eat it, then a square on the left, right, north and south, then other squares, but could not finish it like this and had to gobble it all up. The interpretation was made that the squares were to take the breast shape away. He replied that it was very significant when people drew doodles. He drew triangles, a large one which he then bisected, added other triangles and suddenly had to do figures of eight and then put circles into the centres of the triangles.

What needs to be emphasized here is that despite his nuisance value to women in toilets, the moral suffering inflicted on his family, and a single physical altercation with his father and fights with his brother, none of these oral-sadistic fantasies were acted out with women. The perversion of voyeurism and his complex defensive mechanisms were able to keep them all at bay. This is in marked contrast to one of Hyatt Williams' (1964) cases, where almost the precise sexual fantasies were acted upon in reality. During treatment, with increasing insight his aberrant impulses were able to be resisted, and his relationships and his work level improved.

The picture of family life seen through Noel's emotions and fantasy was certainly not visible even to the trained observer. His parents were eminently respected in their neighbourhood, and presented to legal and medical authorities as well-adjusted, responsible persons who had made great personal sacrifices in order to advance their son's education. They were completely at a loss to understand his behaviour, and were responding to advice to be as tolerant as they could towards his misdemeanours.

During treatment at the clinic the patient re-lived much of the original feelings associated with the experiences described. He became extremely sensitive to loneliness and acted out his voyeurism when he became depressed, for example, when a social engagement with his wife suddenly could not be kept. His treatment could not be carried to a successful conclusion although he was making excellent progress, as he had to be transferred to a new therapist after six months. Although the changeover was carefully handled by all concerned with his full knowledge and agreement, and he liked his new female therapist, stating he preferred her to a male doctor, this provoked a fresh burst of voyeuristic activities for which he was sentenced to prison. Although it was suggested to the magistrates that treatment as an inpatient was infinitely preferable to imprisonment in view of his excellent progress and co-operation in treatment, his record was against him. The view was taken that he was morally degraded and had brought great shame on his wife and had further failed to benefit from the opportunity for treatment; he deserved punishment and could have treatment again after his prison sentence; in the meantime, society should be protected from such as him. Although he was originally referred to The Portman Clinic for outpatient treatment from prison, an earlier psychiatrist had recommended inpatient psychotherapy. In fact he really required much more intensive therapy, such as psychoanalysis, from the start, prescribed early on in his history, but the number of trained psychoanalysts working in the field of delinquency is extremely limited; their skill has to be technically diminished by having to give analytic psychotherapy instead of full analysis to make help available to a greater number of National Health Service patients.

The diagnostic differences noted above are due to varying aspects of his psycho-pathology being presented at different times. The psychopathic quality refers to the early oral elements with their impulsiveness and denial, while after a certain amount of treatment, the more compulsive anal-obsessional mechanisms were observed with their better control and improved prognosis. Magistrates have usually been found to be extremely co-operative over allowing patients who have repeated their misdemeanours during the early stages of therapy to continue with their treatment. It is clearly impossible to alter the compulsive psychological mechanisms quickly and so prevent recurrences and further legal proceedings. The emphasis should be on prescribing correct medical treatment early on, even though it may seem more intensive than warranted by the offence, but lack of facilities prompts a legal progression of discharge, probation, fine, and prison, with a corresponding psychiatric scale of medical report, superficial talks, drugs, and intensive analytic psychotherapy.

Prevention of recidivism is important. It should be possible to detect the potential repeater by the type of character structure found at the time for the first medical report, so that these cases can be referred for intensive therapy from the outset, instead of going through a process of hardening and inner despair.

GROUP THERAPY

Due to the vast amount of data and the complexity in reporting clinical material available from three different therapeutic groups, the following presentation will be made.

1. A clinical account of some treatment sessions in sequence from the first adult group, followed by the details of one session as an example.
2. A general survey of some of the technical problems and transference phenomena.

Clinical report of group therapy sessions

The following is a clinical report on sessions of the first adult group of sexual exhibitionists which met weekly for 75 minutes. It is based on the sequences of the first half of the group therapy, followed by a report of one whole session in detail. The group started with two meetings in July, before the break for the summer holidays, and met regularly thereafter until March of the following year. The members were originally eight in number. No rigid selection of criteria were used, and those awaiting psychotherapy were offered group therapy. It was extremely difficult to keep patients waiting who were in urgent need of treatment for perverse sexual impulses, and the one patient who never attended the group was seen just prior to the summer holidays, but required admission to Horton Hospital soon after, for depression and his concern about his psychic urges. He never replied when treatment was offered after his discharge.

Seven persons attended the group at any time, two of them subsequently lapsing. One, Bill, only attended the first meeting. He was over 40, an exhibitionist, voyeur, and thief, who had over a dozen convictions to his credit and was pessimistic about treatment. He returned later and was a member of the second group for a while.

To acquaint the reader with the lives and work of these patients in the group, I shall start with a thumbnail sketch of each one, referring to them by assumed Christian names. They were Tom, Peter, David, John, Richard, Michael. Patients were addressed formally in the sessions.

Tom was 25, tall, dark, and usually in working clothes. He was married with children, and was employed in a large works. His first offence for indecent exposure was at the age of 16, and a year later he was put on probation for minor stealing offences and sent to a hostel. He disliked the hostel, ran away, was sent to prison and from there to borstal. He escaped was caught and sent to prison. He decided to become a model prisoner, behaved perfectly and after a few months sought special privileges on these grounds. In a meeting before the Prison Governor he was told he had shown no improvement in behaviour. He retorted that he had been so good he had no room to improve and was perfect. The need for improvement was insisted upon, so, losing his temper, he flung a bottle of ink at them, overturned the table, and walked out. Now he could improve, and he did so, with an early release.

He had no difficulty with the law again until seven years later when he exhibited himself publicly, but for two years there had been sexual difficulties with his wife, leading to abstinence. During group treatment, and through the probation officer's valuable talks with his wife, full normal intercourse was re-established. Tom's relationship to his parents gave the key to his attitude to life. His father was an obsessional personality who was a moral coward, especially during air raids, while his mother was strong and dependable. Tom identified with her and at the age of 16 he chased his father out of the house—it was at this age that his exposures started. All his life he had been looking for a hiding. He was a very angry young man indeed, especially in the group at times. His IQ was 126.

Peter, aged 26, was an intellectual, and the brains of the group. His manner was that of an impartial pedant, always ready to lead discussion, argue in theoretical terms about psychology, and take over the role of leader in the group. He appeared to have a good deal of insight until one realized that he expressed no affect and that this was all part of an intellectual defence and that he had a similar split between a loving relationship with a woman and a sexual life. For him, the ills of society could be healed by a return to an unhibited biological sexual existence. In his family life he regarded his father as a failure, his mother as a model of perfection, and he had successful brothers several years older, one of whom seduced him into masturbating him when he was 8 years old and chagrined him by not returning the compliment. He had a fairly free sexual life, essentially got on poorly with people, and was married to a girl his intellectual inferior. They parted when his compulsive revelations about his inner fantasy disgusted her. His exhibitionism apparently started aged 19 when he watched a girl of 11 doing handstands in the garden next door, and he exposed himself in his upstairs bedroom. This subtle surreptitious game continued for a year, after which he openly showed and masturbated in parks. He was excited by the sight of little girls' knickers and was an intense voyeur. He had never been caught. His avowed intention was to excite women for masturbation or intercourse.

David was aged 24, a well-turned-out, pleasant, gentle-looking salesman. He was quiet, maintained his individuality in the group and was referred for masturbating at open toilet windows in office blocks to female staff. His father, a regular soldier, was killed on D-day. He lived with his aged, ailing mother. He had been in the army and his only experience of intercourse was during a drunken Geisha weekend in Tokyo, and was highly unsatisfactory. David had a steady girl friend whom he had known for years and planned to marry later. He treated her with utmost respect. He suffered with asthma and nervous dermatitis. He was absent for a quarter of the meetings with dermatitis and away another quarter due to work demands. He felt his troubles would be over if he could have intercourse, which he was too gentlemanly to perform. His IQ was 108.

John was aged 40, and the oldest member. He was on probation with a condition of treatment. John was pleasant, middle-aged, dressed in a neat sports coat, with a row of pens in his top pocket. He too was quiet, most attentive, and weighed his words ponderously. For some time all statements were prefaced by 'If I can put it this way', or 'How shall I say?', or 'May I say?', the following statement usually being a generalization, or a detraction to pour oil on a group difficulty, or to come to the therapist's aid if attacked. John's demeanour was blandly enthusiastic—'we're all nice chaps'. He was a manager, happily married with children, and said he came from a happy home and had none of the difficulties the others reported, especially about homosexuality. He had courted his wife during the war, by leaving camp without permission and riding to see her on his motorbike. John would exhibit himself alighting from his car on his way home to any passing women, but dreaded any contact with them. This had happened two to three times weekly for eight months. He was upset by a manager being appointed over him. However, he lost his position due to newspaper publication of the offence, but luckily secured a better post in the same trade. His IQ was 117.

Richard was aged 37, a mechanic and was married, with one child. He was the nattiest, flashiest, dresser of all, with a grey suit, blue suede shoes, and dark blue tie with glass sparklers on it. He was good-looking in an effeminate way. He had three previous convictions, although his present attendance was voluntary. The first was aged 28 for exhibitionism. The second aged 30 was most astounding; he was picked up by the police as a prostitute as he had happened to wander into the wrong area while indulging his transvestite bent. He was only discovered when he had to undress. Ever since the age of 10 he had wanted to be a girl. He was the middle of seven children, three boys and four girls, and his father, an engineer, brutally knocked the family about, in one case breaking his brother's arm by hurling a chair at him in an argument. Although his father had died 25 years previously, he seemed to have left his mark. Richard had also been induced into passive homosexual practices for the last 5 years. His last court appearance, aged 37 was for indecent exposure. He exhibited to any female in the street or parks, without erection or ejaculation, and described an 'exhilarated feeling inside' which lasted for a long time; he had regular sexual intercourse but this did not satisfy him as much. He was variable in the group, reticent about his pervert proclivities, which were only just held in check by his attendances, but he would argue and expostulate if he was sure there would be no real counter-attack. He enjoyed berating other social groups such as 'bank clerks'. His IQ was just over 100.

Michael, aged 29, who lapsed after the eighth meeting, was the most uncontrolled member of the group, like a primitive chunk of primary process. His parents separated when he was three and he shuffled thereafter between relatives and boarding schools. He was taken into care and sent to an approved school aged 14, because of passive homosexuality. He exposed himself and masturbated to girls in the dark, in cinemas and on beaches, and was excited by the sight of girls' knickers. He was convicted for indecent exposure aged 24 and 27 and was on probation with a condition of treatment. He claimed his trouble was due to his never having had sexual intercourse, though he compared himself to his father who, he said, had even made another girl pregnant when he was born. He moved around constantly, although apparently he was a good worker as a fitter, and a shop-steward. Michael sat through the first meeting sprawled out in his raincoat and hat. He would burst into meetings late, argue firmly and inconsequentially about wage rates and hold the group's attention by his imperturbable vigour even when attacked. He settled down remarkably, came neatly dressed and showed flashes of helpful insight. He claimed to be able to control his proclivities by willpower, and later reported that he had had intercourse with a young lady he had been seeing for some time, and seemed to be improved. His IQ was 96.

Bill has been described on p. 192
The first two meetings were concerned with problems of control of their perverse sexual drives. Michael said he could control his by will power, and Bill said this was not so; he had will power beyond the average and could not. He said further that even marriage made no difference, and John and Richard confirmed this, which shattered David, who saw marriage as the end to his problem. The question of punishment was raised, Michael supporting prison as a useful deterrent. But Tom and Richard

disagreed from personal experience, and John said even a police caution initially had not helped. They went on to talk of the social implications of their acts. John and Tom had both lost their jobs and their families had suffered. John brought up the question of newspaper publication of their misdemeanours and its effect on their lives. (This topic was raised on many occasions and there were newspaper cuttings later on reporting subsequent offences by Tom. Although harmed by such reports, Tom nevertheless upheld the freedom of the Press. He was getting his punishment.)

The main interpretations at this stage were that they were all different individuals united through suffering the same complaint; that exhibitionism was normal in childhood and that we needed to try and explore earlier memories as a pattern for present behaviour; that their offences were serious in so far as they offended society. The group were intrigued by the fact that women did not suffer from this complaint and it was interpreted that they exhibited themselves in other ways. Michael said he wouldn't exhibit again because he would think of what it was like for the woman, especially if she were his daughter. But he decried the way women dressed to excite men, and how he wanted to touch them.

After the summer break Peter joined the group. John asked if there was place for further members, and on being questioned related how a man had exposed himself to his (John's) daughter of 10. She had told her mother, who telephoned the police. John felt pity for the man, was prepared for him to come into the group, as he was with the same probation officer, and the group agreed. He did not think his daughter had been harmed, but all reference to his feelings about his wife's action was avoided and the therapist purposely refrained from interpreting this.

The talk ranged on the attitude of workmates, who in reality seemed to forget about the incident after a short while. One amusing aspect, however, was that to be a successful exhibitionist one seemed to need a good memory for faces. Tom did not have one, and apparently actually exposed himself to a woman working in his own, although admittedly large, department. He said he had no idea who she was, and the group laughingly suggested he approach and ask her. Sessions later, Peter reported how on his prowls he tried to pick up two young women in the street, launching forth with 'Haven't we met somewhere before?', whereupon they said 'Aren't you the chap down by the river, but you had a beard then!' These disturbances of visual memory were a result of repression of scopophilic tendencies.

Tom talked about his strong sense of morality and how it would be impossible for him to have extra-marital relations. Incidentally, his probation officer was co-operating well in dealing with his wife, and helping her to overcome her sexual difficulties. Richard then talked of how prison made one more perverted although it was supposed to be helpful, and exhibitionism was only one of his difficulties. Sex could take thousands of different forms. Peter questioned whether he was afraid of homosexual difficulties and Richard said yes. Peter then said he had never had any experiences like that, then checked himself and said yes, there was one, and that he had thoughts that he might be homosexual too. Then he said something about 'all of us coming here and exposing ourselves before you, a beautiful girl', looking at the therapist and adding 'I wonder why I said that?' The transference aspect of this remark was noted and reserved for future use. The group were taken aback and led away from this to females exhibiting themselves. It was interpreted that the group was not confined to talking about exhibitionism, but that this was only one of the types of early sexual behaviour levels one could be stuck on. The purpose here was to try and liberate their fantasy, and also to discover the extent of their difficulties; while not frightening them away with interpretations, one had to try and hold their urges in check.

At the end of the meeting. Tom reported privately that he had in fact exhibited himself again. He was encouraged to discuss it at the next meeting. This he did two weeks later, describing how his bicycle had turned into his usual haunt, 'as if of its own accord', and he had partially exhibited himself to two girls. He felt very ashamed but a new feature had appeared; he wanted to apologize and made to do so, but they ran away. This need for apology was accepted as a hopeful sign, attributed to the work of the group. Peter resented having to be interrupted in a lengthy intellectual argument about lowering the age of consent which would solve everything. Still, it was felt we had to come to Tom's aid and discuss his problems further. But Michael interposed and described his compulsive feature of having to pick up all the papers in the street before he could expose himself. This animated the group to discuss tidiness and Tom interjected aggressively, looking at the therapist, 'You seem to have rather a nice suit on but your underwear is probably filthy underneath'. He then talked about his drawers at home being untidy and Michael shouted out 'drawers' significantly, to mean underclothes. It was interpreted that being tidy or dirty were mechanisms for the discharge of tensions and were opposites such as looking and exhibiting were, both belonging to a more immature phase.

Meetings at this time tended to be dominated by Peter, either in argument with Michael or in discussion with John or the therapist. Members generally talked to the therapist or into the group as a whole, unless actually arguing with one another. But then discussion turned more and more on their relationships with each other. They decried the odd times of arrival of members, asked for more group time, and complained of the warming-up period of each session which was stressful. This was linked with their difficulties in making relationships with people, and how they denied the need for relationship in their acts of exhibitionism, which took place with complete strangers. This led to a discussion on the defiance of authority, with Tom relating his stormy past; Peter telling how he had been punished for purposeful misdemeanours at school; and Richard describing how he told lies to his wife in the evening when he wanted to go and commit an offence, but 'did not knock her about to get out'. Although Richard became very angry, she did not let him out, and he cooled off and then felt all right. This seemed a typical adolescent rebellion, and the 'not knocking his wife about' was in relation to his own father's behaviour. These were interpreted, and the description of the vicious father then emerged from him. Peter talked of his failed father and Tom angrily despised his father at length for his weakness. The therapist interpreted Tom's defiance of authority as stemming from this and he seemed thunderstruck. John talked of his happy home life and though generally silent, nodded in assent to all the proceedings. Michael said how his father went round 'giving everyone babies' and said 'I must take after him'. It was interpreted that he was really rather afraid of the opposite sex, and had little to do with them, and everyone laughed. Perhaps this fantasy indicated his fear of identification with his father. Michael left the group when it was explained that although it was a condition of treatment for him to attend, he could have individual therapy instead; the group was purely voluntary. He much later applied to come back but could not attend regularly. Much resentment was voiced against him after he left, especially by Richard.

Richard talked of how he could not show his affectionate feelings to his wife, but could to his son, and the interpretation was given that if he let his feelings go, he might beat his wife as Tom did, as all his feelings had to be kept in check. Peter said, 'If one is stopped, the other is stopped too', and went on to describe how he couldn't achieve having the ideal mother, although his wife's hair was black like his mother's. In fact, his wife was the very opposite of an intellectual. The therapist interpreted that it was not permissible to achieve one's mother in reality. Wherever possible, the therapist tried to make interpretations that would have general group validity. Subsequent interpretations of aggressive behaviour in the group, especially to the therapist, as reliving old angers about father, were most helpful. On one occasion the therapist was asked why similar interpretations were not made about John. It was replied that he had given no such material, having always maintained that his parents were happily married. But this brought up a repressed memory of how at the age of 17 he had bought a motorbike and expected to be severely chastised by his father. The latter, however, merely said how grieved he was with his actions, and John, disappointed in his father's weakness, described how he suffered a shock, and ascribed this own passive relationships with superiors to this. Later he became very active in the group, especially after his use of phrases such as 'May I say . . .?'. etc., had been interpreted. Peter noted that these phrases were always addressed to him and he interpreted his wish to treat all problems in the group as things to be overlooked, or as avoidances. John reported how he was active in public speaking at parent—teacher meetings now, and quite recently he had been challenged by an employee to a fight and had gone outside and lightly returned the first blow, which so humiliated the other fellow that he himself roared with laughter and felt triumphant. Previously he would have mediated a middle path to avoid any disturbance. How John later took over the leadership of the group by actively dislodging Peter is shown below in the description of the complete session.

Peter finally told the group about his homosexual relationship with his brother and made his feelings overt for the therapist, as the one from whom he sought a similar experience. However, he insisted that his relationship with the therapist excluded the rest of the group, and there followed discussions over many sessions about whether one came for an individual relationship with the therapist or fitted into the group. Peter would purposely use psychological jargon which the group could not understand, question others, make tentative interpretations to them, and so play the role of assistant psychiatrist. This was always interpreted as his resistance to fitting in as a member of the group, his difficulty in expressing his feelings, and his need to split feelings and intellect. He described himself as a compulsive talker and slowly began to evince his real feelings and fears; his feelings of physical inadequacy, which Richard echoed. He described his castration fantasies; of sharks being in the swimming pool and around his bed, which would bite off his genitals, and he brought up early memories of seeing little girls' genitals which had been, as it were, cut off. However, the rest of the group weren't up to this level of fantasy, and their reaction to him generally was one of growing antipathy because of the social difference and his intellectual hostilities, while they always granted him his right of leadership because of his superior education. Peter, while losing no opportunities to attack others under interpretation from the therapist, nevertheless openly started to admire Tom's moustache, and tried hard to get Richard to discuss his homosexuality and transvestism; but Richard had had a series of arguments with Tom about their respective jobs and their merits as workers. Tom seemed to come off best in these, and Richard, retiring into passivity, stated that 'he wasn't going to argue, as you never knew how far you could go with some people', meaning his fear of Tom losing control of himself in the group.

We must return to Tom because he fell deeply into trouble with the law. While on his way to the eighth session, he was arrested a block away from the clinic for exposing himself. Apparently, a woman had been exposed to and a policeman had jumped into a taxi, ridden down the road and seen Tom. He denied the charge and was brought face to face with the woman who made it. She said she was not sure if he was the man, but at the police station they told her that he had been up for this charge before, and this seemed to have confirmed her opinion. He was charged and subsequently fined, his attendance at the group probably having been instrumental in preventing his being sent to prison. Nevertheless, from his evidence it was extremely doubtful whether he actually committed this offence. He maintained his innocence throughout and on the strength of his previous truthfulness it was hard for anyone in the group to disbelieve him.

Adult exhibitionist group session

Present: *Peter, Tom, John, Richard.*

The group started late with only Peter and John. Peter commented that this evening it was rather like some committees at work. Other members of staff could go to these committees and on occasions there were more staff than committee. It seemed that here there were 'two of us, two of you' (two patients: therapist and observer). The therapist commented that perhaps Peter felt outnumbered. Peter went on that during this last week he had felt independent of the group, that he did not need the group. The therapist suggested that this was how he felt in any group, even in a twosome with a woman, and Peter agreed. The therapist commented that Peter needed to lead in the group or else he could not belong to it; there was no halfway house for him.

Richard arrived later at 7 o'clock and commented 'You started sharp tonight', and Tom came bustling in shortly after. Peter made his 'Good evening' deliberately stand out from the rest. Peter, who had again been the group leader, or had tried to be, now relapsed into the background a little. Tom was brought up to date with the evening's proceedings but he ignored this and proceeded to tell a weak joke which he had heard at work and which he felt compelled to tell: 'A man had gone into a pub for a drink and there had been only one other person in the bar, a girl in the corner. He asked what she would like to drink and she said "A pint of beer, please". Seeing the man's surprise she said, "Don't be put off by the dress, it's only for show". There was scarcely a murmur from the group. Peter did not understand and made this plain to Tom in a very castrating sort of way. He then forced a laugh and Tom explained that 'she' had been a 'he'. (In addition to this condescension towards Tom, Peter was once later in a similar attitude towards John, and on one occasion stood up to open the window for him.)

Apropos of the story, Peter asked Richard whether this was not his problem; would he not like to talk about it now? Richard shook his head, Peter went on to say, by way of reparation towards Tom, that he (Tom) also wanted to bring up this topic tonight and he thought this was Tom's way of doing it. Peter thought if they got on with the discussion of homosexuality they could then move on to other things, and he thus began to lead the group. It seemed to the observer that Peter's attitude was to curry favour with the therapist.

Tom broke in with seemingly little relevance that he had been aggressive that week. Last Friday he had gone to the pictures with his wife and their enjoyment had been spoilt by a group of Teddy boys in front. He had gone down to ask them to be quiet and was surprised to find that they were all girls. Nonetheless, there were some boys there who were making a noise in the gangway by the wall. They were calling across to their friends on the other side of the audience. Tom asked them if they would mind being quiet; he had paid to see the film and wanted to see it. One of the boys replied 'I've met your sort before', and Tom said 'Oh no you haven't. If you had, you'd never be saying that'. The boys were quiet for a while after that. This little bit was completely by passed by the group and John, picking up again the reference to homosexuality, asked Peter about masturbation. They agreed that mutual masturbation was homosexual but were not clear about self-masturbation. Peter described what he thought was normal sexual development, from self-masturbation through mutual masturbation to heterosexual mutual masturbation, and finally to a normal sexual relationship. John observed that Richard and Tom did not recognize this homosexual factor.

There was a silence, broken by John saying he wanted to bring up the discussion which had taken place last week when the group had officially ended and the therapist had gone. Tom had complained then of his frustration in the group and that he was afraid of bringing this topic up because he thought he would 'blow his top' if he did, but he gave permission for anyone else to bring it up. The therapist commented that there was tension all round this evening (this was really an understatement) and he interpreted Tom's 'joke' as an attack upon Richard, a provocation of him. But the group did not pursue this point either, and John now proceeded to attack Peter most forcefully. He drew attention to the fact that talking was difficult for him (he had a very bad attack of laryngitis that evening). He said that Peter did not lead the group because the group did not follow, and anyway, said John, wagging his finger at Peter, 'you can't ruddy well lead the group', because Peter was a patient in the group. He, John, could not lead the group for the same reason. The therapist pointed out that he *was* leading the group, and that in a sense whoever was talking at a particular time was leading the group at that point. Nevertheless, John denied his leadership role in his usual terms of 'circumstances' and by use of the word 'naturally'. He thought that Peter, by virtue of his intellect, was perhaps the one most fitted to lead the group. He reminded the group that he would have to leave soon (at the end of last week he said he would have to leave at 7.35 this evening). It seemed rather as though he were stirring things up and then leaving them. He got agitated and talked about blowing his top at work. If people were making a mess of their jobs and realized that he knew this and mended their ways he was satisfied; but what he could not stand (at this stage he was standing up and putting his coat on, very red in the face) were the apprentices who, after he had spent three weeks showing them their job and had in all spent 130 hours on each of them, still became slipshod the moment his back was turned; he had had enough of this. And he went.

There was a long silence broken by Peter, who had been considerably taken aback by this onslaught. He said it was the first time anybody had left the group except once when he had gone at 7.55, and he had wondered then what had gone on after his departure. The therapist said he wanted to bring up what happens when he goes. There were spontaneous comments from the three. Richard spoke of relaxation and Peter said things went back to man-in-the-street level and they became ordinary people. Richard said that he was sick of the word 'intellectual', which he had heard so often in the last few weeks.

Tom began talking about the conscious restraint he put on himself in the group. He was afraid that if he did not, in spite of the frustration, he would blow his top. This was related to his incident in the cinema and in previous sessions when similar interpretations had been given that he wanted to beat Peter up, and that 'the only time you can be like father is when you are beaten up by father like a man'. Tom referred to a row which had taken place between his parents when he was young. Mother had finally blown her top and thrown a plate on the floor or at father, who had gone out to the garden and stayed there. The therapist commented that mother had in fact behaved like the lad. She had become angry and aggressive and father had taken a passive role in going out and staying out. Tom went on to say that men who fight each other sometimes have the greatest respect for each other afterwards and become the greatest of friends, even though it may have been a 'blood bath'. The therapist interpreted the homosexuality in this and at this point Peter was under great stress, although by and large he enjoyed this session in which Tom was, so to speak, put in his place. Tom went on that his father, he felt, was a cissy, and Peter took up the point that 'the only person we could justifiably, and I use the word justifiably in inverted commas, call cissy in the group is Mr——' (Richard). Richard did not rise to this at all and the therapist commented to the effect that Tom and Richard were father figures to each other, that Tom provoked Richard because he wanted Richard to attack him, because Richard's passivity was the passivity of his father who had not beaten him, and this was what Tom wanted; but that Tom also stood for Richard's father in personality in that he was a man who was violent and who could, for example, break a chair over his son's arm, and hence Richard, having had experience of this sort of father, was reluctant to say anything in the group. This defence of Richard was appreciated by him and having remained silent for most of the evening he joined in a little later for almost the first time. Tom went on that he had 'got to respect' the therapist because he had done so much for him, and Peter took up this point, particularly the word 'got', and interpreted it. Tom retreated behind a plea of a poor education but the therapist pointed out that the word 'got' was used and that in fact was what Tom meant. Tom became angry and said that the therapist's interpretations angered him, that they were wrong, he had often only half finished, the words werre twisted, and so on; what were they getting at in the group on this occasion? The therapist replied, 'We are trying to get at what you mean by blowing your top'. Tom's complaining that he was getting angry with the doctor, was interpreted as his being angry as a boy with his father for being inadequate. The interpretations, though nominally rejected, were obviously in fact going home; Peter complained and attacked Tom that he (Peter) had in fact interpreted the word 'got' before the therapist, but actually the attack had been directed upon the therapist and not himself (Peter). The implication was that he wanted Tom to attack him, as part of a homosexual attack from his brother and father.

Tom went on to talk about discipline and the virtues and values of it, and how he admired the German army for this while the Japanese were pretty terrible. Richard would not have this and said the German army was bad itself, witness Buchenwald and Belsen, both of which he had seen shortly after the war ended. Tom would not allow that this was in fact a general standard of the behaviour of the German army in the last war. Tom extolled the virtues of discipline, which was interpreted by the therapist as his need for a strong father to control his aggression, and he was reminded also of an incident to which he had referred in a previous session when, as a result of this discipline in the Guards, 15 men had been unnecessarily drowned. But in his plea for greater humanity, Richard had the best of the exchange, and this marked the beginning of a change in his submissive, complementary role towards Tom (and his own father), and the establishment of a relationship in reality of equality, or even superiority, which previously existed only unconsciously in his ego-ideal.

General comments

Peter started off trying to lead the group and later made a second attempt but finally had to give up. An enormous amount of hostility and aggression was released this evening, particularly by John but also by Tom, and it may well be that this has gone as far as it safely can and that perhaps a switch to a more sexual topic rather than an aggressive topic would be in the interests of the group. Peter this evening deliberately re-introduced the use of Christian names in an attempt to lead the group.

Technical problems and transference phenomena

As will be seen in the following reports of group sessions, initial remarks in the group were usually addressed to the therapist. From the outset all these approaches were carefully directed by the therapist to the group as a whole. In this way, social relationships were encouraged rather than narcissistic gratifications. Patients were made to regard each other as possible sources of narcissistic supply, though a low estimation of their colleagues' ability to satisfy their needs for help and understanding was openly voiced. The first few sessions were devoted to a discussion of personal theories of why they exposed themselves, and how they should be punished or treated. The question of self-control was paramount and via these topics the patients described their backgrounds, personalities, and pathological behaviour. In the main, whatever topic was discussed there were always two fairly distinct poles of opinion. This polarity functioned on all topics, and interpretations were made in such a way as to include all the members of the group depending on their position along a dimension between the two poles. Thus the introduction of Bill into the second group appeared to be a successful move. He could be presented to the others as an example of pure activity and aggression, in contrast to their passivity. Much of the talk relating to aggression was applicable directly to their sexual fantasy and behaviour.

A mechanism that was operative when one had representatives of opposite poles on the same dimension, was the tendency to identify with the opposite type of behaviour 'I wish I could take a leaf out of your book'. However, the identification and envy was only partial, leading to a limited growth along the dimension rather than a complete switch from passivity to activity, such as may occur with the return of the repressed during impulsive behaviour. Further, they experienced the permissiveness of both types of behaviour in the group, with the accent on control of extremes. There was the verbalization of affect for both types; a reduction of inhibition for the repressed and a new mode of expression for the impulsive.

Talking about a 'dimension of personality', along which all members could feel suitably placed, gave them an objective correlate in the group which provided a framework for the description of dynamic past behaviour and its reliving in the group. In this sense, the transference relationship was not to the leader of the group, but to the group as a whole, where the affective reactions to any one member were described on the dimension of either communication or aggression. This led one to determine which dimensions were suitable for exposition. Those used were activity–passivity, aggression–love, control–lack of control, masculine–feminine, infantile regressive behaviour versus mature reality directed responses. Actually, the 'love' aspects were not made much of because, in an all male group, the homo-erotic element was excessively stimulated early on. The view members took instead was that of identification or support against attack in argument.

Attendance at the group was intensely discussed and in one patient absence came to symbolize exposure. An intellectual process was set up in place of impulsive action but the patient regarded the punitive aspects of the results of exposure greater than that accruing from one absent session. Thus, a more socially accepted way of acting out was provided, which could subsequently be dealt with by the group.

The next phase of the group was that of patients finding interest in other members as individual personalities rather than in their behaviour. This led to further identifications, and, more important, to differences, of a polar kind among themselves. Not only were these perceived as existing between two individuals but clear divisions among all the members occurred. This was especially notable in both adult groups with regard to the degree of inhibition and reserve felt by some members and the almost total freedom of instinctual expression in others. Members expressed the wish that the inhibited could be more liberated and that the impulsive could gain control. Thus the group set its own therapeutic aims as a social norm against which their own personalities were mirrored, and any progress assessed.

Members were encouraged to talk about their experiences of exposure and the active wishes to repeat this. Controlling these desires was vital as nearly all of them were on probation and a breach meant possible detention. It took quite some time before the urges could be brought under control and several members of all three groups exposed themselves during treatment. In three cases the magistrates in their wisdom imposed fines, and allowed them to continue treatment, but two adolescents were sent away after further repetitions.

Acting-out of exhibitionist urges appeared to cease when the patient had reached a certain level of ability to verbalize his instinctual urges and had some feelings of security in the therapeutic relationship which was set up. In the group, numerous minor symbolic exhibitionist acts occurred all the time and became interpreted by the members themselves as such. The energies released became cathected to the group situation. Patients reported how they found themselves thinking more and more about the group between sessions; some could use thoughts of the group to control urges to expose themselves.

At a later stage a group transference phenomenon called complementation was displayed, which refers to the way in which members reacted in a lock and key fashion with each other's psychopathology. Tom for instance would have lengthy provocative arguments with Richard, who was also a transvestite, and whose father had been so actively hostile as to break his brother's arm in an altereation. Richard had retreated into a feminine identification on these grounds. In the group Richard was afraid of Tom possibly losing control of himself and becoming violent, in the way that Richard's father had behaved. He would withdraw and act passively when he felt threatened, but in time learned to stand up to Tom verbally. Simultaneously, Tom could feel chastened and controlled by interpretations which revealed that he was goading Richard in much the same way as he had acted towards his own father, whom he regarded as a moral coward. Tom stopped exhibiting but acted out his wish to be beaten. He reported how he stood up in a local cinema full of cat-calling Teddy-boys and told them to shut up. To his surprise and disappointment, they did. The operation of these dimensions of activity–passivity, masculinity–femininity, aggression–love, and control–lack of control, acting through the Oedipus complex, was instructive.

One of the effects of the complementation was an intensification of the transference towards the therapist, thus incidentally allowing for further interpretation of the transference relationship and for increased therapeutic potentialities. An excellent example of this is given in the report of the full session above, where Tom, having expressed the sort of resentment already described, turned his hostility on to the therapist, allowing the same interpretations to be made in the group situation.

There are certain advantages in treating groups composed of patients with a single shared diagnosis or instinctual proclivity such as exhibitionism. These are the greater case with which polarities of identification and difference in personality traits can be delineated; the reciprocal facilitation between this delineation and complementation phenomena; an increased intensity of group transference in affective or feeling terms; and the establishment of clear group ideals of behaviour as attainable norms.

Much of the aggressive behaviour and actual exposure was also a defence against the feminine identification with mother and thus also against homosexuality. Overt homosexual feelings became prominent and were interpreted in the first group. This seemed to contribute materially to the dissolution of the group as too great anxieties were aroused. Interpretation of these feelings, although present, were studiously avoided in the second group. Both Slavson (1954, 1956) and Hadden (1958) found that homosexuals tended to create either too much disruption and anxiety in groups, or dropped out themselves because of difficulties in discussing their problems. Litman (1961) found that one or two sexual deviants could be successfully treated in a neurotic group provided that there were women present; the feminine reactions served to buffer the rest of the group against excessive anxiety about male homosexuality. In the first group, the need for women to be introduced was specifically requested by one member, Peter, at the time when homosexual anxieties were mounting, and he was openly expressing homosexual advances to the therapist in the transference based on experiences with his brother. Unfortunately, the group could not be reconstituted with female members as this would have broken the conditions of the research setting. In any case, in the group transference, feminine roles were projected on to the therapist, so that the request for female members was a resistance to the analysis of the homosexuality aroused. Thus Peter, who was highly intelligent, used defences of intellectualization and rationalized his exhibitionism as sexual advances made in a sexually inhibited abnormal society. His condition would disappear, he argued, if free love were instituted. He was a well-controlled voyeur and exhibitionist who had never been caught and came voluntarily for treatment. He used his considerable powers of argument aggressively in the group in a subtle way to maintain his superiority, leadership, and narcissism. When this was analysed by the group, he lost the leadership of the group, showed immature dependency reactions and threatened to leave. This was a repetition of his emotional relationships which had always been superficial, and which had led to an estrangement with his wife to whom he verbally exhibited his sexual difficulties in a sado-masochistic way. He gained considerable maturity, and ability to feel, through the group, and at follow-up two years later reported no overt exposures, some sexual difficulties of an immature kind, and a working towards greater maturity in relationship with women (see follow-up letter).

Strange as it may seem, it was possible to deal indirectly with their sexuality a great deal of the time by discussing the patients' aggression. *This functional equivalence of exhibitionism for the expression of aggression is noteworthy.* John attended both groups, and from being quiet and retiring in the first group later became the dominant personality. The rivalry for leadership in the group was a transference of oedipal and sibling relationships, and was analysed as such, first by the therapist and then actively by the members themselves.

The role of the therapist was emulated in patients' active attempts to help and understand each other. Thus, in the second adult group Harry, aged 21, who had never known his father and was brought up in a completely feminine environment with his mother and several aunts, formed a strong attachment to the therapist. His exposures were deliberate and the source of great pleasure. He travelled 40 miles to the group, and after treating all the members with disdain began to take an interest in helping the most inhibited members and being actively hostile to John, the family man. Both these affectionate and aggressive impulses were worked through and he became a charming and sympathetic person, who married during the course of treatment and lost all his wishes to expose himself. In his case, the therapist provided an ideal male figure on whom he could model himself and with whom he could identify, thus filling the gap of the absent father in his childhood; while John the family man was used to express his hostility towards the absent father. In his follow-up letter he described a return of urges to expose during a severe depression, but no exposures resulted.

Perhaps the greatest technical problem of an outpatient group of sexual deviant is how to keep the group alive from the point of view of membership. Immature, impulsive, pleasure-seeking individuals are notoriously irregular in any social behaviour. That the groups survived as long as they did was gratifying; and due to unceasing interpretations by the therapist, efforts on the part of the psychiatric social worker, who sat in as an observer, and due to the close contacts with the respective probation officers, and the patients' families. If a patient missed two sessions without apology, a letter was sent to him; if he missed three, a letter went to his probation officer. (For further information on the role of the probation officer in the treatment of sexual deviants, see below.) It was thought wiser to have a closed group, even though members were down to two on occasion, than a continuous open group with regular newcomers, in order to gain a sense of personality definition among the members. Further, certain patients would not continue treatment after their one-year condition of treatment was over; others had to move out of London or found it difficult to attend for a variety of reasons. Thus towards the end of both groups the numbers had dwindled. This put a great strain on those present, and was reflected in Richard's leaving the group. It was generally felt that many of the patients would have benefited from further group treatment; hence John was included in the second group, although it made for some technical difficulties. This raises the question of whether a prescribed period of one year as a condition of treatment is wise; in all groups voluntary attendance was stressed in that even if patients were on a probation order with a condition of treatment, if they did not want to attend for group therapy voluntarily, other treatment would be found for them. These issues were amongst the earliest faced in the group. What can better determine growth towards maturity than the issues of free choice in a social setting or an interpersonal relationship?

The adolescents presented the greatest difficulties, both with regard to regularity of attendance and their extremes of shyness, inhibition, or acting-out of instinctual drives. In general, when there was a good attendance for any regular period, say a few weeks, they would find the session enjoyable, talk amiably about their interests and girlfriends and gain a feeling of support from the group solidarity. But due to the small numbers of available cases, it was not possible to constitute a good regular outpatient group. It was impossible with these means for certain members under strong emotional stress to maintain control of their sexual urges, and although they were offered individual treatment two were finally sent to borstal. Acting out of exhibitionist and aggressive anti-authoritarian wishes through dangerous driving, especially on motorbikes, was noted and required interpretation to avoid serious personal injuries resulting. Certain inhibited members did extremely well, but nevertheless one is forced to conclude that outpatient group treatment for adolescent sexual offenders requires very special conditions and that individual therapy is preferable.

Many of the inhibited adolescents gained great benefit from regular personal contact with their probation officers. This would be a treatment of choice in certain cases where there is immaturity, a need for identification with a strong but helpful male figure, and relatively minor sexual behaviour of an exploratory kind in a first offender.

RESULTS

The results of treatment and follow-up in individual cases are listed together with other details of the history in Table 8.1.

Table 8.1 Results of treatment and follow-up of cases of exhibitionism treated with individual group therapy

Name and age	Marital status	I.Q.	Exhibitionism Frequency	Offences	Other symptom manifestations	Treatment Previous treatments	Portman Clinic Psychotherapy Sessions Individual	Group	Results	Follow-up Duration after treatment	Patient	Probation	Final Result
John (41)	M.	115	3 times	Indecent exposure	Nil	Nil	Nil	64	Recovered	18 months	no reply	Satisfactory work and hom conditions. No repetitions	Symptom free Personality
Donald (28)	M.		Frequently for years	Indecent behaviour	Psychopathic personality Chronic masturbation	Nil	Nil	22	Improved +	6 months	No reply		Improved
Tom (25)	M.	126		Enclosed premises Stealing. Indecent exposure × 2		Nil	Nil	24	Improved ++	16 months			Improved
Peter (30)	M.	125+	Frequently	Indecent exposure × 2	Character disorder	Nil	Nil	27	Improved ++	18 months	Greatly Improved		Improved
David (24)	S.	108	Frequently	Indecent exposure 8 previous offences	Nil	Nil	Nil	10	Improved +	36 months	Married, recovered		Recovered
Richard (37)	M.	100	Frequently	Masquerading as female prostitute Indecent exposure × 2	Transvestite. Passive homosexual	Nil	Nil	25	Improved	24 months	No reply		Improved (slightly)
Bill (36)	M.	93	Frequently	13 previous convictions 2 × indecent exposure, voyeurism 3 × stealing, assault	Uncontrolled aggression	Nil	Nil	5	Unchanged	18 months	No reply	Personality difficulties a great handicap. No further sexual exposures	Personality unchanged. Improved
Michael (29)	S.	100	Frequently	Care and Protection Indecent exposure × 2	Immature personality	Nil	Nil	6	Improved	36 months	Greatly improved. Stable at work. No repetitions		Recovered
James (29)	M.	104	Occasionally	Indecent exposure. Insulting behaviour	Nil	Nil	Nil	18	Improved + Discontinued treatment	18 months	No reply	No further contact after 1 year condition of probation and treatment	Improved

Table 8.1 (continued)

Name and age	Marital status	I.Q.	Exhibitionism Frequency	Offences	Other symptom manifestations	Previous treatments	Portman Clinic Psychotherapy Sessions Individual	Group	Results	Duration after treatment	Patient	Probation	Final Result
Eric (23)	S.	119	3 times	Indecent exposure × 2	Nil	Nil	Nil	11	Improved ++	18 months	No reply	Improved	Improved
George (23)	S.	122	Very frequently	Indecent exposure Larceny	Immature personality	Nil	Nil	32	Married.	12 months	?	Satisfactory	Improved
Harry (26)	S.	119	Frequently	Indecent exposure	Nil	Nil	Nil	20	Improved +	18 months	No reply	Satisfactory	Improved
Roger (26)	M.	99	Frequently	Indecent exposure	Nil	Sedatives	Nil	39	Improved ++	18 months	No reply	Satisfactory	Improved
Stephen (15)	S.	124	12 times in 6 months	Indecent exposure × 2	Enuresis	Nil	Nil	6	Improved	24 months	No reply	'Completely adjusted'	Greatly improved
Dennis (15)	S.	108	Frequently	Breaking and entering Indecent exposure larceny	Immature personality	Nil	Nil	34	Improved	24 months	Continued treatment at another clinic. Further minor traffic offences. Personality greatly improved	Two further episodes of masturbation in public, and, in a state of depression	Greatly improved personality. Better sexual adjustment, two offences of exposure
Jack (16)	S.	103	Once	Indecent exposure	Immature personality	Nil	Nil	23	Greatly Improved	24 months		Personality developed considerably. Satisfactory	Greatly improved
Keith (15)	S.	116	Frequently	Indecent exposure. Care Committee	Behaviour disorder	Psychotherapy	Nil	10	Committed to Approved School	36 months		Indecent exposure Shopbreaking Still in need of treatment	Unchanged
Don (16)	S.	115	Frequently	Larceny × 3	Enuresis	Nil	Nil	24	Personality Improved Larceny committed to Borstal	24 months		Made good progress at Borstal Released	Borstal. Improved
Rupert (19)	S.	109	9 times	Indecent exposure	Immature personality	Nil	11	Nil	Greatly Improved	24 months	Nil	Nil	Improved
Max (38)	W.	116	Frequently	Indecent exposure × 4 disturbed	Severely emotionally	Psychotherapy	8	Nil	Remarried. Improved				Improved

Table 8.1 (continued)

Name and age	Marital status	I.Q.	Exhibitionism Frequency	Offences	Other symptom manifestations	Treatment Previous treatments	Portman Clinic Psychotherapy Sessions Individual	Group	Portman Clinic Results	Follow-up Duration after treatment	Patient	Probation	Final Result
Robert (53)	M.	108	Twice	Indecent exposure	Nil	Nil	5	Nil	Greatly Improved	24 months	Nil	Highly satisfactory	Greatly improved
Leonard (16)	S.	106	Frequently	Indecent exposure	Immature personality	Nil	18	Nil	Greatly Improved	24 months	Nil	Satisfactory	Greatly improved
Joe (49)	M.		Frequently	Indecent exposure × 2	Uncontrollable aggression	Nil	11	Nil	I.S.Q. Indecent exposure		Admitted to hospital for in-patient psychotherapy	Improved by stay in hospital	Relapsed. In-patient treatment with improvement
Ralph (46)	M.		Frequently	Indecent exposure	Nil	Stilboestrol	23	Nil	Greatly Improved		Nil		Greatly improved

Most psychiatric follow-up studies utilize either the morbidity figures of hospital re-admissions or responses to postal enquiries. In dealing with criminal cases, assessments are usually made on a basis of subsequent convictions. In this study, wherever possible, letters were sent to both the patient and the probation officer. The follow-up date denotes responses to the last communications sent. Some of the difficulties in completing accurate follow-up studies with outpatient delinquents are as follows.

Patients who have been placed on a probation order, or treated as a condition of probation laid down by the court, often cease treatment once these terms have been complied with, and wish to put the whole experience behind them. Efforts to communicate with patients by letter or personal visits are then resented as intrusions into their personal privacy. A letter enquiring for follow-up details may be socially disastrous as it reveals past problems which may have been successfully hidden from intimates.

At the end of treatment, all patients were instructed that if they felt the danger of exhibitionistic lapses they should report for further help. In court-referred cases, with subsequent offences, the probation officer is usually made aware of this fact, or the Clinic is asked for a report of previous treatment if the case comes up in a new court. Thus, where no further communications were received from patients and probation officers were unaware of further difficulties, it was presumed that the patient had not been convicted of a further offence; although it must be admitted that in some cases urges to exhibit and even occasional acts of exhibitionism might occur in a 'satisfactory' case where supervision had ceased. Usually, however, lapses were brought to the notice of some authority.

Differences in the quality of improvement are hard to assess in a statistical manner. Thus in some cases, real personality improvements had taken place although occasional lapses in response to severe situational stress had occurred. Two patients married, and eight showed greatly improved relationships at home and at work.

The letters that follow, written by four patients and edited to preserve anonymity, are examples of the quality of improvement. The first was written as if by a therapist, 'the subject' being, in fact, himself.

1. Your letter has just been forwarded to me, and I will answer it in the form of a report on the case with which we were concerned. I expect you will agree that this is quite appropriate as we are dealing with the matter by correspondence. You will understand that the subject's feelings about the case, and many of the details, will not come across in a report of this kind.

The subject now feels that the complex of behaviour and desires with which you are familiar has become integrated into his personality in a somewhat matured form, and no longer has the dissociated compulsive character that it had before. It is matured in the sense that, (i) he no longer feels these desires towards girls of preadolescent age, (ii) he initiates a friendly relationship with girls from this age onward, whereas previously the behaviour manifested itself in a 'social vacuum', and (iii) the specific behaviour characteristic of the case now occurs, if at all, after several weeks during which the subject plays with the young girl—and her friends if she is with them—and takes the opportunity, while, for example, helping them climb trees, etc.—of fondling her in an affectionate but discreet manner. In fact, on only one occasion in the last six months, has there been anything more than this fondling, and that took the form of 'wanting to go to the toilet' in some bushes after telling the girl so that she could keep away. In fact the subject reports that the 14-year-old girl on this occasion looked covertly at him while he was semi-concealed behind a bush, and this excited him to the point of ejaculation with very little manual stimulation. The subject and the girl went on picking berries, as before, without the situation having apparently proved traumatic. After that occasion the girl was always with friends on the few occasions when the subject met her, and circumstances effectively terminated the relationship.

At present, the subject has no similar involvement, but reports that he has seen a very well-developed girl of 14 or thereabouts with whom he would like to establish the same sort of relationship.

The subject feels that this sort of emotional involvement grades into his (by social standards) 'normal' sexual desire for older females, being only modified at the lower age-levels by social sanctions against more complete physical intercourse with young girls, and by the natural and learned restraint of girls of this age, which only force or psychological compulsion on the part of the subject would overcome. As you know, neither of these expedients has the slightest appeal to this particular subject.

From economic reasons, the subject is living a rather limited social life at present, and has not yet found a woman of what he would regard as a suitable age for the kind of intimate friendship he most enjoys—a woman of about 25 years. He reports that he had just such a relationship before going abroad, though it was unfortunately brief because of that. In the past few weeks there has been an unsatisfactory affair with an 18-year-old girl: unsatisfactory because of the extreme difference of interests and the refusal of the girl to allow the natural process of foreplay leading to sexual intercourse to proceed very far. Again, before going abroad, the subject met and had coitus on one occasion with a 17-year-old girl, who was unable to respond or experience pleasure in the act because of frigidity which she said was habitual. The subject wonders whether there is some objective characteristic of the, shall we say, 15–20 age group, perhaps connected with the war, which accounts for the difficulty he has in establishing satisfactory social or sexual contact with them. He contrasts this with the rather parental, though strongly sexual, affectionate feeling he has for girls up to about 15 from puberty, and with the egalitarian affection he can feel for women over about 20, again with a sexual component, of course.

As regards his marriage, the subject reports that his wife has hardened towards him after the long separation, and there is no feeling of love or affection between them. Perhaps a divorce will be arranged eventually.

In summary, the subject feels that he is now at least a whole personality, even though social sanctions make it necessary to be discreet about one aspect of it.

2. I have received your letter and felt that I should like to write back, first I am feeling quite well at present, I have not had any treatment since my last attendance at the clinic, as regards to being any better, let's say I am not any worse, although in all fairness, I must say that in my wife's opinion she thinks I was better for the treatment, myself I would not like to say. I feel that I was not getting anywhere, at the time I was attending the group was breaking up fast. There was only two of us there, I felt very awkward to say the least, and if you remember at the time, I did not stay, and left early. At first I was not fully aware of what the treatment entailed, but I am willing to try anything, if I thought it would be to my advantage. At the time I do feel that I was not getting anywhere, but that of course is only my opinion, you people know more about these things than I do. At least I am grateful for all you have done for me, I know it must mean a lot of work. I think the best thing I can do is to leave it to you to decide which you think is best for me, I am willing to try anything. I have not had any further trouble with the basic problem, but I know myself that I am far from cured shall we say. I still

have these urges, although my wish to be feminine is far greater, I notice this in all the things I do, this seems to be my greatest problem at present. I am wondering if any of the others are still attending. However, I will leave things as they are at the moment, hoping that this will be some guide to you.

3. I'm sorry to have kept you waiting for a reply to your letter, as you know it was always one of my faults to keep postponing things and, as you can see, I haven't changed much.

I have been debating whether to write you, as about a month ago I had been going through a rather depressing period and I had the old feeling coming back. Although I never exposed myself, I thought about it several times, and only fear of the consequences saved me.

This depression was due to my wife and I having a rather upsetting period. Being rather young, she misses her work and freedom, and what with now having a baby to care for, she gets very irritable and I'm on the receiving end.

I find it very hard not to give up, and if it weren't for the baby I think I would. I am still looking for the unobtainable in life, work and women. All pretty women still attract me, and if I had the chance to be unfaithful I would. When I am out on my own I still get that wonderful sense of freedom, and its times like these when the desire to expose myself is greatest.

I think what I miss most of all is the chance to discuss these things and if there was the opportunity of joining another group, I would, willingly.

4. Many thanks for your letter dated 17th of this month.

I will answer it the best way I can, because I am no authority on the matter in question.

Incidently, did you get my phone message last Wednesday evening? If you didn't it was to inform you that all letters are answered by me on Sunday mornings only, as I am fully engaged during the week.

Now to answer your letter. You say, you hope I am feeling well, thanks a lot. I am in great form at the moment, only wish there were more than 24 hours in a day, then I could get some more of my private work attended to. But my Sect. thinks otherwise.

The treatments you are giving are causing some anxiety, so I gather from your letter, as to whether it is doing any good to people and if it has, to what extent. Well as far as I am concerned, it had little value, that is why I stopped coming along and what is more I am glad I did, because I wanted to and I succeeded in doing, conquering this whose problem on my own, I started doing it, I stopped it, and I will tell you how. When I stopped coming along to the meetings, I did so because I wanted to spend more time at music and forget the past, but build up a future, which I am still doing. Coupled with this, I have grown up mentally and act more like a man than a child. I have become hard in many ways, mixed with people (except those not connected with music) gone out with one or two girls.

If I felt like relieving myself, I lie on my bed and do so, with the aid of a picture of a half naked girl. I don't let it bother me. If I started doing it in front of girls again it most certainly would. That's all there is I can say. I am going out with my girl friend at the moment, I have never touched her because we hope to get engaged at Christmas, not only that, we are always talking about Modern Jazz.

Group treatment

Thirteen adult patients attended two groups with an average attendance of 23 sessions each. All except two patients had been before the courts. Eight could be classified as recidivists, four of whom had been convicted of additional non-sexual offences such as stealing or assault. All 13 cases were of the phobic-impulsive type, 7 were mainly phobic and 6 mainly impulsive.

Follow-up studies on these 13 cases revealed that there was an average follow-up period of 20 months after cessation of treatment, at which date no known convictions had occurred. Fitch (1962) examined men convicted of sexual offences against children. Fifty per cent of re-convictions (30 cases out of 59) for sexual and other offences took place within 19 months over a 79-month survey period. The ability of patients to remain without indictment for 20 months or more, therefore has some prognostic significance. It was thought that urges to perform exhibitionistic or other indictable acts were possibly still present in four patients, but under control. In the others, these had apparently ceased.

There is no doubt that analytical group psychotherapy is efficacious in the treatment of the adult severe phobic-compulsive exhibitionist. It was generally felt that treatment for a longer average period than six months was required.

Mathis and Collins (1970) and Truax (1970) emphasize the importance of treating in a group consisting of people with similar problems, where the shared needs and experiences can be utilized to dissolve the defence mechanisms of rationalization, isolation, and denial. A similar group approach with serious sex offenders in Broadmoor is described by Cox in Chapter 13.

Adolescent group

Five patients aged 15–16 attended the group. Attendances were irregular and the results on the whole were uneven and unsatisfactory. Two boys with inhibited personalities obtained great benefit, while the three remaining were compulsive in type and had committed other offences, although two of them showed great personality improvement as a result of later individual psychotherapy. In these three boys, there was a change in the type of offence to that of a compulsive non-sexual kind, in two of stealing, and in the other of reckless motor cylcing.

One must therefore conclude that whereas group psychotherapy can help the inhibited shy adolescent, it is of little benefit to the compulsive instinct-ridden patient. For these, intensive analytic psychotherapy and close supervision would be required. Reality difficulties with the parents are often great obstacles to treatment in these boys.

Individual analytical psychotherapy

Six patients were treated with weekly analytical psychotherapy for an average attendance of 21 sessions. All were referred by the courts and except for one patient they had exposed themselves frequently.

In all but one case they lost all urges for exposure and there have been no notifications of relapse after a two-year follow-up period. In the single case who relapsed, inpatient psychotherapy was later given with improvement.

An attempt has been made in this chapter to correlate the psychiatric and psychoanalytic approaches to this problem. Although the call is always for more research into pathology and treatment, society must keep up with the advances in knowledge that have already been made. There is now much evidence that with skilled psychotherapeutic care, many exhibitionists and voyeurs can be relieved of the torture of compulsion and avoid the shame of social sanctions and imprisonment. The costs of providing such skilled help as against the costs of custodial care and suffering to others are difficult to evaluate, but as exhibitionism has one of the highest recidivist rates of all sexual offence, medical opinion and possible therapy should be sought early. Unfortunately, not all eclectic treatment which passes for psychotherapy is of the same order, or of a level to help such persons.

REFERENCES

Allen, D. W. (1974). *The fear of looking*. University of Virginia, Bristol.

Allen, D. W. (1980). A psychoanalytic view. In *Exhibitionism: description assessment and treatment*, (ed. D. J. Cox and R. J. Daitzman), p. 59. Garland, New York.

Ambrose, J. A. (1961). The development of the smiling response in early infancy. In *Determinants of infant behaviour*, (ed. B. M. Foss). Methuen, London.

Berah, E. H. and Myers, R. G. (1983). The offense records of a sample of convicted exhibitionists. *Bull. Mn. Acad. Psychiat. Law*, **11**, 365.

Bianchi, M. D. (1990). Fluoxetine treatment of exhibitionism. Letter. *Am. J. Psychiat.* **147**, 1089–91.

Blair, C. D and Lanyon, R. I. (1981) Exhibitionism: etiology and treatment. *Psychol. Bull.* **89**, 439.

Bond, I. K. and Hutchison, H. C. (1960). Application of reciprocal inhibition therapy for exhibitionism. *Can. Med. Assoc. J.* **83**, 23.

Christoffel, H. (1936). Exhibitionism and exhibitionists. *Int. J. PsychoAnal.* **17, 321.**

de Monchy, R. (1952). Oral components of the castration complex. *Int. J. Psycho-Anal.* **33**, 450.

Eber, M. (1977). Exhibitionism or narcissism? *Lett. Amer. J. Psychiat.* **134**, 1053.

Edgcumbe, R., and Burgner, M. (1975). The phallic-narcissistic phase. *Psychoanal. Study Child*, **30**, 161.

Fedora, O., Reddon, J. R., and Yeudall L. T., (1986). Stimuli eliciting arousal in genital exhibitionists: a possible clinical explanation. *Arch. Sex. Behav.* **15**, 417.

Fenichel, O. (1931). Antecedents of the Oedipus complex. In *Collected Iapers*. London.

Fitch; J. H. (1962). Men convicted of sexual offences against children. *Brit. J. Crim.* **3**, 18.

Ford, C. S. and Beach, F. A. (1952). *Patterns of sexual behaviour*. Eyre I Spottiswoode, London.

Forgac, G. E. and Michaels, E. J. (1982). Personality characteristics of two types of male exhibitionists. *J. Abn. Psychol.* **91**, 287.

Forgac, G. E., Cassel, C. A., and Michaels, E. J., (1984). Chronicity of criminal behaviour and psychopathology in male exhibitionists. *J. Clin. Psychol.* **40**,827.

Freud, S. (1900/1953). The interpretation of dreams. *Complete psychological works of Sigmund Freud*, (standard edition, Vol. 4). Hogarth Press, London.

Freud, S. (1905/1953). Three essays on the theory of sexuality. *Complete psychological works of Sigmund Freud*, (standard edition, Vol. 7). Hogarth Press, London.

Galenson, E. and Roiphe, H., (1980). The preoedipal development of the boy. *J. Am. Psychoanal. Assoc.* **28**, 805.

Glasser, M. (1978). The role of the super-ego in exhibitionism. *Int. J. Psycho-Anal. Psychother.* **7**, 333–53.

214   *Exhibitionism, scopophilia, and voyeurism*

Goldberg, R. L. and Wise, T. N., (1985). Psychodynamic treatment for telephone scatologia. *Am. J. Psychoanal.* **45**, 291.

Greenacre, P. (1952). Pre-genital patterning. *Int. J. Psycho-Anal.* **33**, 410.

Grob, C. S. (1985). Female exhibitionism. Single case study. *J. Nerv. Ment. Dis.* **173**, 253.

Hadden, S. B. (1958). Treatment of homosexuality by individual and group psychotherapy. *Am. J. Psychiat.* **114**, 810.

Hollender, M. H., Brown, C. W., and Roback, H. B., (1977). Genital exhibitionism in women. *Am. J. Psychiat.* **134**, 436.

Karpman, B. (1948). The psychopathology of exhibitionism; review of the literature. *J. Clin. Psychopath.* **9**, 179.

Kohut, H. (1978). Forms and transformations of narcissism. In *The search for the self*, (ed. P. Ornstein). International Universities Press.

Kopp, S. B. (1962). The character structure of sex offenders. *Am. J. Psychother*, **16**, 64–70.

Langevin, R., *et al.* (1979). Experimental studies on the etiology of genital exhibitionism. *Arch. Sex. Behav.* **8**, 307.

Lasègue, C. (1877). Les exhibitionnistes. *L'Union Médicale, troisième série*, **23**, 709.

Litman, R. E. (1961). Psychotherapy of a homosexual man in a heterosexual group. *Int. J. Gr. Psychother.* **11**, 440.

MacLay, D. T. (1952). The diagnosis and treatment of compensatory types of indecent exposures. *Brit. J. Deling.* **3**, 34.

Mathis, J. L. and Collins, M. (1970). Mandatory group therapy for exhibitionists. *Am. J. Psychiat.* **126**, 1162.

McCreary, C. P. (1975). Personality profiles of persons convicted of indecent exposure. *J. Clin. Psychol.* **31**, 260.

Nadler, R. P. (1968). Approach to psychodynamics of obscene telephone calls *N. Y. State J. Med.* **68**, 521.

Rader, C. (1977). MMPI profiles of exposers, rapists and assaulters in a court service population. *J. Consul. Clin. Psychol.* **45**, 61.

Rhoads, J. M. and Borjes, P., (1981). The incidence of exhibitionism in Guatemala and the United States. *Brit. J. Psychiat.* **139**, 242.

Rickles, N. K. (1950). *Exhibitionism*. London.

Rooth, F. G. (1973). Exhibitionism, sexual violence and paedophilia. *Brit. J. Psychiat.* **122**, 705.

Rooth, F. G. (1976). Indecent exposure and exhibitionism. In *Contemporary psychiatry*. Selected reviews from the *British Journal of Hospital Medicine*, (ed. T. Silverstone and B. Barraclough). Headley Brothers, Ashford, Rent.

Rosen, I., (1964). Exhibitionism, Scopophilia and Voyeurism. In *The pathology and treatment of sexual deviation*. (ed. I. Rosen) Oxford University Press.

Rosen, I. (ed.) (1979). Exhibitionism, Scopophilia, and Voyeurism. In *Sexual deviation*, (ed. I. Rosen), pp. 139–94. Oxford University Press.

Saunders, E. B., and Awad, G. A., (1991). Male adolescent sexual offenders: exhibitionism and obscene telephone calls. *Child Psychiat. Human Dev.* **21**, 169.

Schorsch, E., Galedary, G., Haag, A., Hauch, M., and Lohse, H., (1985). *Perversion als Straftat. Dynamik and Psychotherapie*. Springer, Berlin.

Singer, B. (1979). Defensiveness in exhibitionists. *J. Pers. Assess.* **43**, 526.

Slavson, S. R. (1954). *Re-educating the delinquent, through group and community participation*. Collier Books, London.

Slavson, S. R. (1956). *Fields of group psychotherapy*. International Universities Press, New York.

Smukler, A. J. and Schiebel, D. (1975). Personality characteristics of exhibitionists. *Dis. Nerv. Syst.* **36**, 600.

Sperling, M. (1947). The analysis of an exhibitionist. *Int. J. Psycho-Anal.* **28**, 32.

Stärcke, A. (1921). The castration complex. *Int. J. Psycho-Anal.* **2**, 179.

Truax, R. A. (1970). Discussion of Mathis and Collins (1970). *Am. J. Psychiat.* **126**, 1166.

van de Loo, E. L. H. M. (1987). *Genital exposing behaviour in adult human males.* Doctoral Thesis, University of Leiden.

Wickramasekera, I. (1972). A technique for controlling a certain type of sexual exhibitionism. *Psychother. Theory Res. Pract.* **9**, 207.

Williams, A. H. (1964). The psychopathology and treatment of sexual murderers. In *The pathology and treatment of sexual deviation*, (ed. I. Rosen). Oxford University Press.

Winnicott, D. W. (1958). Transitional objects and transitional phenomena. In *Collected papers*. Basic Books, New York.

Witzig, J. S. (1968). The group treatment of male exhibitionists. *Am. J. Psychiat.* **125**, 75.

9
Clinical types of homosexuality

Adam Limentani

INTRODUCTION

In recent years there has become apparent an increasingly marked division in the attitude to homosexuality: at a time when there is a growing tendency for people in all walks of life to regard homosexuality as normal, there remain many who use the term in a derogatory and insulting manner, quite often with an implication of social menace. The view presented in this chapter is that homosexuality is a syndrome, and that it is not sufficient to regard it only as an adjustive process, as was proposed by Sullivan (1955).

With the abolition of the more restrictive of the laws touching on relationships between individuals of the same sex, and the increased permissiveness in contemporary society, it has become apparent that homosexuality remains a condition which may in certain specific instances require treatment.

When treatment is discussed among psychotherapists, opinion is sharply divided: quite apart from doubts and divergent theoretical considerations as to what constitutes homosexuality, views appear to range from unreasonable pessimism to excessive optimism. This state of affairs is particularly unwelcome in a field which demands both co-operation and a multi-lateral approach to the patient's problem, taking into account that where one form of treatment may fail, another may succeed.

Generally, psychiatrists and psychotherapists are in no position to ignore homosexuality as a syndrome, as it may quite unexpectedly appear as a complicating feature in almost any form of mental illness. For instance, it may be part of the individual's personality and character, and not in the least responsible for behavioural disorders requiring psychiatric assessment; it may be the basic underlying cause of such a condition as alcoholism, or drug addiction; or it may be a complicating factor in a case of neurotic sexual impotence, when psychotherapy will fail to make a real impact unless the homosexual elements have been thoroughly covered.

It must be appreciated, however, that clumsy and tactless attempts to bring into the light less conscious aspects of a patient's sexual orientation may prove quite damaging to the course of any form of psychiatric intervention. The nature and depth of homosexual elements, whether conscious or unconscious, should be of more than passing interest both to the psychiatrist and the psychotherapist. A thorough assessment is imperative in the case of the homosexual who wishes to be rid of the deviation.

It is entirely understandable that any diagnostic attempt in relation to so varied a condition as homosexuality may be met by considerable scepticism or frank disbelief. How could we expect to make sense of a situation where an interest in a person of the same sex (commonly referred to as *homosexuality*) is the only common feature in the cases of the paedophiliac (where the central force is likely to be a narcissistic disturbance), and the man who is pathologically jealous of his wife (who might easily be the victim of unresolved oedipal conflicts)? The psychopathology of sexual deviation is, as has been pointed out in previous chapters, extremely complex, and the aetiology of the homosexual syndrome is unquestionably multifactorial. Readers of the relevant literature, not necessarily psychoanalytical, will be impressed by the fact that each writer tends to have a definite view, and in the end the impression is created of an almost limitless number of clinical conditions. In this presentation, an attempt is made to individuate the more recognizable of such clinical types by using both the psychoanalytic and psychiatric models.

SOME CLINICAL TYPES OF HOMOSEXUALITY AND THEIR SPECIFIC PSYCHOPATHOLOGY

In purely descriptive terms homosexuality can be repressed, sublimated, fantasied, or manifest. Each subdivision carries its own specific symptomatology, capable of influencing the individual's state of mind, his interpersonal relationships, and his role in society. Repression plays an extremely important role. For instance, repressed homosexual impulses and conflicts may represent the main aetiological factor in sexual impotence and frigidity. When repression is excessive, sublimatory activities will be impaired. When it is ineffective, the deviation may still not be manifest, but derivative patterns of behaviour will appear. Pathological jealousy is a classical example of this, and is well matched by the opposite, that is the wish to share or exchange partners.

The relation of the ineffective repression of homosexual impulses to paranoia was first described by Freud (1911), linking it with the turning of love into hate. It is important to emphasize that Freud indicated that the whole process is latent (unconscious). A criticism of this important psychoanalytic finding disregards its unconscious nature by adducing evidence that a great many persons are paranoid without becoming homosexually orientated (Friedman *et al.* 1972). This criticism also emphasizes that the majority of homosexuals do not develop paranoid delusions. It is, however, the central point of the thesis put forward in this chapter that the development of homosexual impulses and attitudes can be and often are used as a defence against neurotic and psychotic processes.

Little needs to be said about those cases where homosexual fantasies have broken into consciousness with much suffering and discomfort, but it should never be assumed that this is an indication of confirmed sexual deviation. On the contrary, such fantasies are often a last line of defence against heterosexuality which appears dangerous owing to its association with strong aggressive impulses, and particularly incestuous wishes. The patient's fantasies are a good indication of the effectiveness or failure in all methods of treatment (Marks *et al.* 1970). Studies which ignore fantasies (Randell 1959) will give an entirely different exposition of the psychopathology of transsexuals, as compared with those studies which have taken them into account (Hoenig *et al.* 1970), when they will show the importance of the homosexual element.

In manifest homosexuality, all defensive barriers against the acting-out of deviant impulses have broken down. It is in these cases that accurate assessment becomes a matter of the utmost urgency and importance, as it will guide us towards appropriate treatment or masterly inactivity, as the case may be. The innumerable types of deviation met in the literature, and in clinical practice, can be divided into three ill-defined, yet clearly recognizable groups.

Group I

In this group, manifest deviant behaviour, often associated with compulsive related day-dreaming, aims at preventing the emergence of heterosexuality, as is the presenting symptom in a large number of individuals who are basically latent heterosexuals. Some writers refer to these as pseudo-homosexuals, an unsatisfactory term as it implies a falseness in their state of mind which is not reflected by their feelings. Attachment to members of the same sex is linked with the flight from the opposite sex, which is perceived as being dangerous, threatening, and domineering. Oddly enough, the attempt to deny the very existence of the opposite sex is frequently a sign that one is dealing with latent heterosexuality rather than true deviation. A guideline in differentiating them further from 'true' deviants is guilt, which is almost always present, particularly in those who seek guidance or help. It is necessary to distinguish the guilt derived from external circumstances, social or moral influences, from that derived from unconscious psychopathology, whether it is related to the residual heterosexual conflicts at the root of the deviation, or to the homosexual activity itself.

In early papers, Freud (1905a) recognized that psychoneuroses could exist side by side with manifest perversions, and suggested that heterosexuality had been totally repressed in such cases. The psychopathology will be that of a psychoneurosis; the homosexuality indicates the persistence of a particularly severe oedipal conflict and castration anxiety. The dangers related to the expression of heterosexual impulses are obviously of such a nature that it is not sufficient to rely on the usual neurotic defence mechanisms to ward off fears rooted in the subject's internal world and object-relations; the deviation is there to create a citadel, which in practice becomes a prison which affords a degree of security.

Anxious, hysterical, or obsessional personalities are common in this clinical type. It is particularly the association of homosexuality and obsessional traits which is likely to produce a picture of shallowness of affect, ruthlessness, and compulsive behaviour, consisting of a constant search for a partner, and rare engagement in sustained or deep relationships. Any attempt at controlling or curtailing the sexual acting-out is followed by an outbreak of anxiety and depression. The depth of character and personality disturbance needs to be assessed carefully as it may affect the outcome of the treatment. The presence of serious obsessive compulsive traits may defeat all therapeutic efforts.

The following case is fairly representative of a clinical picture with a good prognosis encountered in this groups. An intelligent young man with mildly obsessional personality traits had become seriously depressed and suicidal whilst still at university, following disappointment in a homosexual love affair. At the age of 3 1/2 years, he had been separated from his parents, when he was sent to a wartime nursery in England. This was a severe traumatic incident which coloured all his subsequent relationships, as all human beings were regarded as unfaithful and untrustworthy. He was totally impotent when he first approached a girl, and soon after he became involved with a male homosexual friend. He felt extremely guilty about his sexual activities and agonized over them, but he relentlessly continued to importune his friend who eventually showed little interest in and no affection for him. He reponded well to psychoanalysis and after it was ended he married, had children, and had a very successful career. After 10 years there has been no recurrence of homosexual interests. It is worth noting here that once the homosexual attachment could be analysed and understood within the transference relationship, his condition did not differ from that of a classical straightforward psychoneurosis capable of responding well to psychotherapy.

The occurrence of homosexual behaviour as a substitute symptom has been described in the literature (Thorner 1949), and is of considerable clinical interest when the possibility of removing it is a real one. This writer reports that in the course of treatment, and concurrent with a period of sexual abstinence, a young patient developed a status asthmaticus. This symptom was linked with conflicts over aggression and was quite troublesome, until he convinced himself that he was homosexual and acted on that belief. Many observers have reported on the occurrence of haemorrhoids quite suddenly in the midst of a homosexual conflict in patients being treated for a variety of conditions.

Group II

This group includes all cases of 'true' perversion when the disturbance is deep, and the defence against heterosexuality seems almost of secondary importance. Depression is a common presenting symptom with or without periodicity, but conscious guilt is generally absent. Careful investigation will readily show that the homosexuality is employed as a massive defence mechanism, aimed at warding off overwhelming separation and psychotic anxieties, a dread of mutilation and even disintegration. Bizarre acting-out, marked identification with the opposite sex, promiscuity, and a preference for very brief contacts with partners, associated with a tendency to congregate in public lavatories, is sometimes suggestive of a prepsychotic condition or even psychosis. 'True' deviants seek treatment for reasons such as difficulties arising at work or in personal relationships, and occasionally because of some offence which has involved them in Court proceedings. They specifically ask that nothing be done to change their sexual orientation. Focal therapy may appear indicated, but in practice it is difficult to carry out because of the interaction between the sexual maladjustment and other ego disturbances. It is therefore essential that, before undertaking any form of treatment, due notice be taken of the value attached by the patient to the deviation in fighting off loneliness, isolation, alienation, and aggressiveness. There are three identifiable clinical types:

Narcissistic disorders of character and personality

are very commonly found in homosexuals of both sexes included in this group, where paedophiliacs are largely represented. The history will often show the presence of psychological disturbance in the parents, severe deprivation, and traumatic experiences. There is a tendency to seek partners, younger or of a similar age, but frequently the need to protect and to be protected, to nurse and to be nursed is the primal force in these associations (Freud 1910). The search for a narcissistic love-object may even induce a man to look for a partner who is overtly antagonistic to homosexuality, as he may also be (Khan 1970,1979). Phallic overvaluation is the rule, with loss of self-esteem and a readiness to feel hurt and injured. A double deviation is present when a man is both homosexual and paedophiliac.

Homosexuality as a defence against severe depressive states

is probably much more common than is generally recognized. The diagnosis is difficult as the presence of reactive depression, which responds to superficial intervention, hides the true nature of the problem. Early traumas, sudden deaths in the family, or separation and divorce of parents in infancy are valuable diagnostic pointers. Some writers see the behaviour of homosexuals who struggle with the threat of severe depression as a solution of the past conflict over weaning, which is felt as not only a narcissistic injury, but also a blow to the infantile omnipotence (Bergler 1951).

In the male, unbearable depressive thoughts and feelings, probably originating in very early infancy, make it impossible for him to have physical contact with any woman as the penis is experienced as a thoroughly bad part of his body (Rosenfeld 1949). Marked passivity in sexual relations serves the purpose of recovering the lost potency and acquiring something good. At times, the only safeguard against psychotic depression, apathy and despair is to become and act the part of the good mother to the partner (Khan 1970, 1979).

The serious consequence arising from the sudden failure of the homosexual solution aimed at alleviating depressive feelings can be seen in the following case history. A young woman was referred because of violent rages, in the course of which she was dangerous both to herself and a woman companion. The destructive outbursts of violence had begun after the breakdown of a long-standing lesbian relationship. She had suffered from recurrent depressive attacks for many years and had been very promiscuous. In the course of extended assessment interviews she recognized that she had used her compulsive lesbian activities as the 'cure' for her unbearable depression, as she could rely on sliding into a state of mild euphoria after successful sexual exploits. At the time of the referral she longed for the woman who had jilted her to come back, and her woman companion (a non-practising lesbian) was gradually becoming the object of her hatred and murderous feelings. Admission to hospital was the only solution.

Homosexuality as a defence against paranoid anxieties and related states

The turning of hatred into love can be found in early and late psychoanalytic writings (Freud 1923; Nunberg 1938). Glover (1933) has also noted that a perversion will involve the use of libidinization and idealization of the object as a defence against aggression and anxiety, whilst Freeman (1955) has drawn attention to the psychotic quality of the fears and the castration anxiety experienced by the true homosexual in relation to men and women alike. Projection dominates the emotional life of a certain type of homosexual, bringing some relief but much confusion. This defence mechanism implies the throwing out of unwanted or dangerous parts of oneself, which will fill the environment with a host of threatening and persecutory objects to be dealt with by the appeasement implicit in homosexual acts and relationships (Klein 1975; Rosenfeld 1949). In certain cases, it is clear that behind the phallic preoccupation and castration anxiety there is a marked fear of the loss of individual identity and of total disintegration. In cases where severe paranoid anxiety is hidden beneath a manifest homosexuality, hostile and greedy oral impulses are directed against authority figures and partners, turning them into retaliatory figures. On the other hand, these men will appease by submitting to anal intercourse and reassure themselves by fellatio about the destructiveness of their biting and devouring impulses.

Not infrequently, the deviation which presents as a simple neurosis or as a sexual disorder attributable to biological forces, conceals a fully fledged paranoid schizophrenia (Socarides 1970). Even when paranoid anxieties have erupted into florid schizophrenia, in spite of manifest homosexual activities, the perversion acts as a brake on the threatened acting-out of murderous impulses. This was seen very clearly in the following case. A 24-year-old man had been a compulsive homosexual for as long as he could remember. He would roam the streets at night looking for a 'victim', someone who could tolerate his castrating anus. He came for treatment because of his uncontrollable rages at work, where he would break furniture or get involved in violent fights with fellow workers. At intervals he would experience vivid auditory hallucinations associated with his homosexual 'victims'. During the hallucinatory episodes, he would seek hospital care voluntarily, as he would no longer trust his homosexual acting-out to protect him against killing someone. It is difficult not to believe that this might well have happened in the absence of such an outlet.

Group III: Bisexuality

Under this heading I shall deal with all those case of actual bisexuality as I first described it (Limentani 1976). There, I suggested that actual bisexuality is to be distinguished from homosexuality in a latent state and from conscious bisexual fantasies, which are not acted out, in so far as the capacity to engage in active sexual activities with both sexes concurrently would seem to involve only a limited number of male individuals, whereas women seem to be more able to deal with such situations.

A great deal has been written about bisexuality in recent years, mostly under the correct assumption that human beings are bisexual in the sense of containing masculine and feminine elements in their character structures. This interest in bisexuality has been enhanced by the fact that it is not related to a biological entity. In the course of development any individual will be exposed to the possibility of becoming identified with someone of his own or the opposite sex. The capacity for a double identification, leading to bisexual behaviour, is acknowledged as having its value in terms of facilitating the capacity to relate to others and to be creative. On the other hand, all therapists are familiar with those individuals who display a difficulty in personal relationships, social activities, or work problems due to the fact that they attempt to suppress either the femininity or the masculinity which are experienced as a threat or a danger to their way of behaving in a social context.

Some cases are described in the literature under the heading of bisexuality when women (or men) are leading a very active homosexual life while making full use of their masculine or feminine identification in other respects (see McDougall 1989). It is the absence of active concurrent heterosexual engagement in such cases that would make me reluctant to regard it as actual bisexuality in accordance with my definition of it.

The sudden occurrence of homosexual activities in the heterosexual population often occur in situations of stress, prison, or special cultural surroundings and are often dismissed by psychiatrists as abnormal behaviour, merely the result of contingency. In my view all such cases should be taken as indicative of harbouring a sexual maladjustment which emerges only when there is some justification for it, such as prison life, etc. On the other hand, a sudden homosexual experience, as can occur in some young person, can be easily shown to have been a true accident, so long as the experience was dystonic, with no desire for repetition.

I must admit, however, that my past insistence on the concurrent experiences of sexual behaviour with both sexes as evidence of actual bisexuality may have led me to believe that the condition was rather uncommon. The gathering of further information in recent years, and the willingness of many individuals to be forthcoming in their revelations of sexual activities, leads me to reconsider my view about the frequency of the condition.

Two major events have caused me to review my position. The general relaxation of moral attitudes has been associated with increased opportunities for individuals of both sexes to 'experiment' with a change of sexual partners and orientations in a less than casual way. The other important reason is the incidence of bisexuality related to cases of AIDS and drug abuse that are seen at clinics all over the world. It is correct to isolate here those instances of some young, and even middle-aged, persons who will admit that they have indulged in some homosexual acts, allegedly in search of new experiences. This type of enactment is promoted by a variety of causes but it will be of no consequence if the experience turned out to be wholly dystonic.

In all other cases to be considered under my classification of actual bisexuality, psychopathic disturbances are prevalent in the male whilst immaturity is a dominant feature in the female. Both sexes will exhibit a severe dissociation between the female and male parts of the personality, aggravated by a tendency to projection, splitting processes, and multiple identifications. Many studies tend to concentrate on the examination of the perversion, taking the heterosexuality for granted, in spite of the obvious lack of gratification and serious disturbances present in this particular area. In my view all these cases are to be considered basically homosexual when the heterosexuality is there as social cover or as *force majeur* in view of a threat to the self-esteem of the individual, something which is, of course, always more applicable to men than women. It seems natural to assume that in female development the early attachment to mother, with all its conflicts, fears, and ambivalence, provides fair ground for later experimentations and enactments in later life.

When writing on this subject in my 1976 paper, I stressed that most of the cases that had come to my notice seemed to have been exposed to direct influences in their environment which had resulted in an imperfect super-ego formation. Investigations had often revealed that either a parent, a teacher, or a person in a position of authority had actually encouraged or ignored the occurrence of feelings and actual sexual acts with persons of both sexes.

But those must be considered only aggravating factors because in my view the condition is usually occurring on the background of severe narcissistic disorders of character and personality, often in the setting of borderline states. An ineffectual or absent father is of considerable importance but a cold, remote, inaccessible mother figure is not at all uncommon. Actively bisexual individuals can create a very striking impression of being unable to choose between a heterosexual and a homosexual object. However, a careful analysis of all that is involved will reveal that whilst longing for an idealized father to rescue them from a predicament in their dealings with their (primary) love attachments, these men and women seek to re-enact an anaclitic and narcissistic type of object-relation (Limentani 1976). The sudden removal or unavailability of either sexual outlet is known to cause severe depression and to have precipitated suicidal acts.

In many cases when I was able to observe the patients over long periods, I was struck by the occurrence of frantic movements from a partner who would fit into a narcissistic object choice when the cathexis would be directed at self-representation to another partner who would provide an opportunity for object-representation. This was apparent in the case of a man who would have a rewarding but utterly depleting sexual experience with his wife, after which he would then rush to his male friend with whom he could cuddle up for the rest of the night, having masturbated himself to sleep (Limentani 1976).

A sudden outbreak of irresistible homosexual impulses associated with serious aggressive behaviour towards the male partners occurred in a man in response to his wife's pregnancy. In the transference the initial aggressiveness towards the analyst in due course evolved into a deep passive attachment to the analyst in a maternal role, prefacing his feelings of rivalry and competition with the arrival of a child.

There is no doubt that in the transference of bisexual patients we may at times be confronted by very challenging situations, easily brought out by the very nature of the complaint. Some of the more serious difficulties in the transference will be experienced if the analyst confronts the patient about the denial of the importance of the homosexual encounters or attachments. This was clearly brought out in the case of Mr X, a married man with children, who indulged in sexual activities with male transvestites whom he failed at first to recognize as such, as well as his preference for engaging in sexual activities with transsexuals who had been operated on. The analyst, impressed by the significance of his activities and the depth of his homosexual involvements, also revealed in the transference, attempted to deal directly with the situation but the patient promptly abandoned his analysis.

In this brief account I have only attempted to convey the nature and size of the problem as it seems to have developed over the last few years. In my view the bisexual is trying to achieve the impossible, that is, the separation of his original two types of object choice, the anaclitic and the narcissistic. A careful assessment of the heterosexuality in these cases will soon reveal that there is little depth to it. In general, the high degree of satisfaction reported by these patients is simply due to a projection of their femininity or masculinity, as the case may be, into their partners. In a sense, we must regard the homosexuality as an attempt to mend the split-off bodily and feeling experiences. (Khan 1964). The illusion that we are dealing with two objects, as some patients would like us to believe, could remain unaffected by therapy if we do not realize that we are only dealing with one (the original) object. The pursuit of oedipal conflicts as an explanation for the clinical facts observed can therefore prove profoundly disappointing. This possible therapeutic mistake is easily accounted for by the fact that patients would create the impression of living-out an impossible oedipal nightmare, a desire for both father and mother but in my view, as the therapy progresses, this would prove to be nothing more than a distracting, socially acceptable explanation to the patient. I am firmly of the opinion that these patients can be approached through the transference in its positive and negative aspects, without necessarily taking recourse to an excessive use of parameters.

In conclusion, I believe that only an extensive, profound understanding of homosexuality, will allow for a full appraisal of the significance of bisexuality. It will also deprive it of all its glamourous implications as well as the false belief that it is a normal activity to be expected in all human beings.

DISCUSSION

The homosexual syndrome, as it has been described in relation to certain clinical types, is seen as part of a defensive movement directed at lessening anxiety or at creating barriers against the eruption of unbearable conflicts, and quite often simply at ensuring survival. In this context, the defence includes all the techniques used by the ego to dominate, control, and channel forces which might lead to neurosis or psychosis. It follows that the homosexual solution is a defence which, when encountered, should be treated with the utmost caution, especially in those cases where its removal is under consideration. It is necessary to stress that whenever homosexual inclinations are predominant, as may occur in some cases of bisexuality, treatment of any psychological disturbance may disturb the delicate balance in the sexual sphere. Attempts to treat all kinds of homosexual behaviour indiscriminately, without reference to personality, character, and associated psychological disorders, must be held responsible for the excessive and unnecessary gloom shared by psychiatrist and public at large with regard to the likelihood of influencing the course of this condition.

There is considerable danger in attempting to classify clinical types by forcing them into diagnostic categories. Provided, however, that the classification is not applied rigidly, it may prove of value in deciding the most suitable treatment, bearing in mind a number of eventualities. For instance, some neurotic patients included in the latent heterosexual group will occasionally show the familiar picture of phobic anxiety or of a compulsive symptom covering up a psychotic illness. Equally, the homosexuality linked with a depressive illness might turn out to be an excellent psychotherapeutic proposition.

In general, all cases considered to belong to the latent heterosexual group should be offered psychoanalysis or psychotherapy over an extended period if at all possible. Careful selection will be rewarded by good therapeutic results. In the case of the true homosexual, all forms of psychotherapy may prove disappointing in terms of a change of sexual orientation, which is seldom requested. In response to a demand for help, an extensive assessment of the motivation for such request, as well an appraisal of the mental distress present, will be invaluable. During the last few years many true homosexuals have been seeking therapy with increased frequency as a result of anxiety about AIDS, HIV, and a concealed dissatisfaction with the homosexual solution and their position in society. Many suffer greatly through the loss of close friends and associates. With regard to bisexuality, it would seem that there are no great obstacles towards being accepted for treatment. Nevertheless, I would urge that the patient's motivation for change be subjected to careful evaluation. Far too many cases show little improvement in spite of serious efforts on the part of the therapist.

In this paper I set out to show that it is worthwhile to reconsider our position with regard to many individuals previously regarded as untreatable. Even if a change in sexual orientation is not forthcoming it will be, in my view, very rewarding to help some of these unhappy people to lead a better life and, in some instances, even a happy life.

REFERENCES

Bergler, E. (1951. *Neurotic counterfeit sex*. Grune & Stratton, New York.

Freeman, T. (1955). Clinical and theoretical observation on male homosexuality. *Int. J. Psycho-Anal.* **36**, 335–48.

Friedman, A. M., Kaplan, H. I., and Sadock, B. J. (1972). *Modern synopsis of psychiatry*, Ch. 14, p. 250. Williams & Wilkins, Baltimore, MD.

Freud, S. (1905a/1953). Three essays on the theory of sexuality. In *Complete psychological works of Sigmund Freud*, (standard edition, Vol. 7, pp. 125–231. Hogarth Press, London.

Freud, S. (1905b/1953). As above, footnote on p. 146.

Freud, S. (1910/1957). Leonardo da Vinci and a memory of his childhood. In *Complete psychological works of Sigmund Freud*, (standard edition, Vol. 11, pp. 59–137). Hogarth Press, London.

Freud, S. (1911). Psycho-analytic notes upon an autobiographical account of a case of paranoia (*Dementia Paranoides*). In *Complete psychological works of Sigmund Freud*, (standard edition, Vol. 12, pp. 3–80). Hogarth Press, London.

Freud, S. (1923/1961). The ego and the id. (standard edition, Vol 19, pp. 3–68). Hogarth Press, London.

Glover, E. (1933/1956). The relation of perversion-formation to the development of reality sense. *Int. J. Psycho-Anal.* **14**, 486–563. In *On the early development of mind*. Imago Publishing Co., London.

Hoenig, J., Kenna, J., and Youd, A. (1970). Social and economic aspects of transsexualism. *Brit. J. Psychiat.* **117**, 163–72.

Khan, M. M. R. (1964). The role of infantile sexuality and early object relations in female homosexuality. In *The pathology and treatment of sexual deviation* (ed. I. Rosen), Oxford University Press.

Khan, M. M. R. (1970). Lafétichisme comme négation de soi—Fétichisme de prépuce chez un homosexual: notes clinique. *Nouv. Rev. Psychoanal.* **11**, 77.

Khan, M. M. R. (1979). Fetish as negation of the self. Clinical notes on foreskin fetishism in a male homosexual. In *Alienation in perversions*, (ed. M. M. R. Khan). Hogarth Press, London.

Klein, M. (1975). The psychoanalysis of children. In *The writings of M. Klein*, Vol. II, Ch. 12. Hogarth Press, London.

Limentani, A. (1976). Object choice and actual bisexuality. *Int. J. Psycho-Anal. Psychother*, **5**, 205–17.

McDougall, J. (1989). The dead father—an early psychic trauma and its relation to disturbance in sexual identity and in creative activity. *Int. J. Psycho-Anal.* **70**, 205–20.

Marks, I., Gelder, M., and Bancroft, J. (1970). Sexual deviants two years after electrical aversion. *Brit. J. Psychiat.* **117**, 173–85.

Nunberg, H. (1938). Homosexuality, magic and aggression. *Int. J. Psycho-Anal.* **19**, 1–16.

Randell, J. B. (1959). Transvestism and transsexualism. *Brit. Med. J.* **2**, 1448–52.

Rosenfeld, H. (1949). Remarks on the relation of male homosexuality to paranoia, paranoid anxiety and narcissism. *Int. J. Psycho-Anal.* **30**, 36–45.

Socarides, C. W. (1970). A psychoanalytic study of the desire for sexual transformation. ('Transsexualism'): the plaster-of-paris man. *Int. J. Psycho-Anal.* **51**, 341–9.

Sullivan, H. S. (1955). *Conceptions of modern psychiatry*, p. 85. Tavistock, London.

Thorner, H. A. (1949). Notes of a case of male homosexuality. *Int. J. Psycho-Anal.* **30**, 31–45.

10
Reflections on homosexuality in women

Joyce McDougall

INTRODUCTION

Freud and female sexuality

Freud's revolutionary discoveries concerning the psychology and the dynamic importance of human sexuality in child and adult life are now almost a century old. They are so much an established part of Western thought today that we take them for granted and are highly critical of Freud's conceptual limitations, above all his theories on female sexuality. This is, in fact, an area of research in which Freud is particularly vulnerable. However, it is interesting to recall that Freud owed to women the initial insights that led him to the concept of the 'unconscious'. Anna O. Lucy R. Irma, Emmy von N. Dora, and Katarina, and many others were the fountainhead of his inspiration. It is equally remarkable that he actually *listened* to them and found everything they had to tell significant and important. In Freud's dominantly phallocratic day, this in itself was revolutionary. Obviously he was fascinated by the mystery of femininity and by the female sex itself (a characteristic, as he claimed, that he shared with men of all centuries). But Freud was also a little afraid of the objects of his fascination. His metaphors constantly reveal a representation of the female genitals as a void, a lack, a dark and disquieting continent where no one can see what is going on. There be lions, perhaps? He also insisted that in this line of research he was obliged to proceed from his knowledge of male sexuality. With this refracting telescope in hand, he was clearly going to be bemused by the absence of a penis and suppose the little girl's envy of the boy's visible and interesting organ, and her desire to possess a penis of her own.

But it was also Freud himself who first avowed deep feelings of dissatisfaction and uncertainty with regard to his theories about women and the nature of their sexual desires. In fact, he waited until 1931 to publish 'Female sexuality', his first paper on the subject. He was then 75 years old! In his second celebrated and much criticized paper, 'Femininity' (1933), published two years later, he writes: '. . . psychology. . . is unable to solve the riddle of femininity' and further on, '. . . the development of a little girl into a normal woman is more difficult and more complicated, since it includes two extra tasks, to which there is nothing corresponding in the development of a man' (Freud 1933, pp. 116, 117). The 'tasks' in question refer to Freud's two major conceptions of the difficulties in becoming a woman. First, she must come to terms with her anatomical configuration and effect a change of organ—from clitoris to vagina. Second, she must effect a change of object—when and why does she give up her fixation to her mother in favour of her father?

I shall discuss these two concepts under the following headings: the change of organ hypothesis, or 'Anatomy as destiny?'; and the change of object hypothesis, or 'How to eat your mother and have her too'. It will be seen that while I agree with Freud that these two dimensions do present genuine difficulties in the attainment of adult femininity and sexual functioning, I express points of view that differ considerably from those of the founder of psychoanalysis. (See also Panel Report: Contemporary theories of female sexuality. 1994.)

Anatomy as destiny?

I think most analysts would agree today that envy of her father's penis is but a partial explanation of the difficulties encountered by the little girl on her path to mature sexuality, and indeed is not specific to the young female. Boys, too, suffer from their own characteristic form of penis-envy; they invariably find their penises too small in comparison with their fathers'. If the belief persists into adult life that one's penis is smaller than it should be, based on the unconscious fantasy that the only adequate sex is the paternal one, this precipitates neurotic symptoms and anxieties that occur as frequently as those arising in the sexual life of the girl who still clings in unconscious fantasy to the fear that she is a castrated boy. Clinical experience also confirms that the boy's envy and admiration of his mother's body and sexuality is similar to the girl's envy and admiration of her father's penis; the mother embodies the magical power to attract the father's penis and make the babies that both parents desire. Thus the *phallus* (which in ancient Greek rites was always presented as the *erect penis* symbolically representing fertility, narcissistic completion, and sexual desire) becomes the fundamental signifier of human desire for children of both sexes. Each possesses half of what is required to complete the symbol.[1]

In point of fact, every child wants to possess the mysterious sexual organs and fantasized power of *both* parents. And indeed why not? Whether we are male or female, one of the greatest narcissistic wounds of childhood is inflicted by the obligation to come to terms with our ineluctable monosexuality—its scar, of course, being the problem of what to do with our psychic bisexuality. (This question will be addressed in the section on the female analysand.) Suffice it to say that the discovery of the sexual difference is matched in traumatic quality only by the early discovery of Otherness and the later revelation of the inevitability of death. Some people never accept any of these universal traumata, and most of us deny them in the deeper recesses of our minds. In the world of dreams we are all magical, bisexual, and immortal!

While many would concede that the little girl's anatomical configuration presents her with particular problems in her psychosexual development, envy of the boy's penis is but one aspect of her sexual preoccupations. Psychoanalytic research had to wait for the work of women analysts, in particular, the seminal research of Melanie Klein (1945), to highlight additional complications for the young female.

---

[1] The word *symbol* comes from the Greek *symbolon* which originally meant an object cut in two that serves as a sign of recognition when two persons, each carrying a part of the whole, meet and recognize each other in this manner.

Klein was the first to formulate the notion that the possession of a penis is narcissistically reassuring to the little boy because it is visible and mentally representable, whereas the little girl tends to see her sex as something missing and must wait till puberty to gain equivalent narcissistic confirmation, through the appearance of her breasts and periods, of her own unique sexual conformation and identity, and the assurance that she will one day be able to make babies. (A further landmark in psychoanalytic research concerning female sexuality is Kestenberg's (1968) paper on sexual differences.)

Other difficulties inherent in the girl-child's development of gender identity also have their roots in her anatomical destiny. Since the interiority of her sex is a door into her body, the vagina is destined to be equated in the unconscious with anus, mouth, and urethra, and thereby liable to be invested with the sado-masochistic libidinal fantasies that these zones carry. Added to the fact that there is no visible organ that can be controlled and verified, the little girl and the woman-to-be, are more likely to fear that their bodies may be regarded in some way as dirty or dangerous because of these zonal confusions. For a woman, too, her body often represents a dark continent in which anal and oral monsters lurk. Much of her unconscious representation of her body and her genitals will depend on the way in which her own mother invested with libidinal meaning her daughter's physical and psychological self, and the extent to which she may have transmitted to her girl-child conscious or unconscious fears concerning her own body and sexuality. Early bodily, and subsequent verbal communications between mother and daughter determine, in large part, whether oral erotism triumphs over oral aggression and whether anal-erotic impulses become more important than anal-sadistic ones.

This brings us to a third aspect of feminine anatomical destiny. Since the little girl cannot visually verify her genitals nor create other than a vague or zonally condensed psychic representation of them, she has difficulty in locating the sexual sensations of which she has been aware since early infancy. Clitoral, vaginal, urethral, and other internal sensations tend to be confused. This has important repercussions, for example, on her fantasies concerning masturbation. Although masturbation is the normal sexual expression of small children, it will eventually be interfered with by the parents. All children learn that it is not permissible to defecate, urinate, or masturbate in public. Even when these restrictions are imposed with kindness and understanding, they leave their imprint on unconscious fantasy life. When they are dealt with harshly because of the parents' own internal anxieties (and a subsequent attempt to control these through their children's bodies) the risk of later neurotic problems is notably increased.

The little boy told to give up masturbating publicly is apt to imagine that his father will attack his penis because of his sexual feelings towards his mother and his ambivalent feelings to his father. The little girl in the same phase of oedipal reorganization is more likely to fear that her mother will attack and destroy the whole inside of her body as a fantasized punishment for the child's wish to take her mother's place, to play erotic games with her father, and make a baby with him. Thus, for the boy, the feared punishment for sexual wishes and masturbation is castration, whereas for the girl-child masturbation and sexual desire are frequently equated with death.

More could be said on this aspect of female sexuality, but I shall limit myself to a brief and typical clinical example. A young woman psychiatrist, highly intelligent and intellectually informed on psychoanalytic theory, claimed that she had never masturbated as a child nor in adult life. It was two years before she could even pronounce the word masturbation, finding the idea of auto-erotic activity dirty and expressing doubts that it could truly form an inevitable part of infantile experience. Although she had no apparent sexual difficulties, she suffered from a large array of psychosomatic manifestations that seemed on many occasions to be linked to tense states of sexual anxiety.

A delicately built and pretty woman, she experienced her body as shapeless, large, and dirty. When she had her periods she would cry, saying she feared I would find her presence distasteful. In the fourth year of her analysis, she brought the following dream: 'I was picking flowers in the garden outside the house where I lived as a child. I was dancing with delight, when suddenly my cousin Pierre appeared in the doorway and I woke up with a scream'.

Since this was the first time cousin Pierre had ever appeared on the psychoanalytic stage, I asked her to tell me more about him. She sighed and said, 'I suppose I've never wanted to mention him. He was much older than me and he once played with me sexually when I was little. Then, when he was twenty and I was about twelve, he was electrocuted in his bath. At least that's what we were told'.

Because she seemed to question this version of the facts, I asked, 'What did *you* think about it?' With great difficulty, she admitted that she believed he had died because he was playing with his penis in the bath. After all, she had known since childhood that he was a bad 'sexual' boy. She then began to cry. I asked her to tell me what she was feeling at that moment and she said, 'you know my husband's been away for three weeks, and I'm so afraid you might think I've been masturbating. But I swear it isn't so . . . I'm sure you don't believe me!' I replied, 'Of course, I believe you—otherwise you'd be dead!'

For the first time she was able to laugh over her sexual fears and fantasies, but we still needed many months to reconstruct, beyond significant elements such as 'electricity', 'picking flowers', and 'dancing', all the long repressed memories of a little girl's spontaneous sexual sensations and masturbation fantasies. As was to be expected, my patient's erotic life with her husband then became fuller and considerably more satisfying to her. However, another interesting fact for which I can offer no conclusive theoretical explanation is that the majority of her psychosomatic symptoms also disappeared. For many years she had suffered from recurring digestive and arthritic pain, bronchial asthma and rhinitis, and a constant septic throat condition. These all cleared up and, with the exception of one mild asthmatic sensitivity (associated by my analysand with cat fur), none of these symptoms returned in the remaining three years of her analysis with me.

How to eat your mother and have her too

I come now to the second area of difficulty specific to female sexuality, that is, the integration of the profound homo-erotic tie to one's mother. From birth, babies of both sexes begin to weave strong libidinal and sensuous ties to both parents—provided both are tender, sensual, and loving with them. In its mother's arms every infant is experiencing the earliest blueprint, or perhaps an imprint, of sexual and love relationships to come. The father's attitude is equally vital in this transmission of early libidinal investments, for a father who is absent or uninterested in his tiny offspring, or who is treated by the mother as a nonentity (and accepts this exclusion), runs the risk of leaving his children to fulfil a role arising from the mother's unconscious problems. A mother who regards her baby as a narcissistic extension of herself, or who takes as her love-objects her children instead of their father, may be laying the cornerstone for future pathological relationships. It should be noted that a mother who brings her children up singlehandedly does not necessarily incur these risks if she does not regard her relationship with them as a substitute for an adult love relationship. From infancy on, if children see their parents as a loving couple , who sexually desire and respect each other, and if children observe also that even fierce quarrelling does no lasting harm (that is, they learn that aggression is not dangerous when love is stronger than hate) children will tend to carry these attitudes into their adult lives, following the parental model. The little girl will then identify with her mother not only as mother but also as lover and will day-dream about the man (modelled after the image of her own father) who will one day be her husband and the father of her children.

In their primordial beginnings, the infant's libidinal and object-seeking drives are deeply intertwined with the desire to live, and it is part of the mother's task to induce her child to want to live. This privileged relationship, which every infant shares with its mother in the first months of life, provides the baby girl with a double identification. The somato-psychic images that will become mental representations of her feminine body and its erogenous zones are already being formed. It is at this early stage of the construction of the erogenic body-image that mouth and vagina become linked and other internal sensations of an erogenous kind are experienced. To these we must add the clitoral sensations stimulated by the mother's physical handling and cleaning of her baby. (The latter were the only early erogenous links to which Freud gave much emphasis in his theorization concerning the development of feminine erotism.)

This early psychosexual structure provides the primitive foundation of the little girl's future love life. Upon it will be grafted the basic elements of the heterosexual model mentioned earlier, namely, a relationship with each parent that is physically and psychically loving and sensual, in addition to the model of a parental couple who love each other, who enjoy their sexual relationship, and who do not seek to give the child the impression that she is their chosen object for erotic or narcissistic completion.

Furthermore, the little girl needs to hear that the mother herself values and respects the father and men in general and that she values her sexual and social life as a woman. A girl who is told that men are selfish pigs, out to profit from women, seeking to seduce or dominate them, and the like, will certainly have difficulty, both in being prepared to like people of the opposite sex and in being able to separate from her mother.

So much for the factors that prepare the way for heterosexual identifications. Nevertheless, these do not entirely liquidate the strong libidinal tie to the mother. Freud's question remains pertinent: how does the little girl detach herself from her mother and integrate the profound erotic tie to her? Where is this vital homosexual component invested in her adult life? Freud's theory in this respect may be summarized as follows: the little girl's first desire is for her mother; she then replaces this with the desire for a penis, then for a child from her father, finally for a male child of her own. Included in the apparently implacable logic of this chain of signifiers is the implication that the girl's desire for a baby is merely a substitute for the penis she does not possess, and her love for her father a mere consequence of penis-envy. These fantasies and desires are certainly frequent in women patients, but they are far from being the only factors or even the dominant ones among the complexities that contribute to each woman's image of femininity or motherhood. In addition, Freud's concept of these object-substitutions implies that homosexual ties are eliminated through penis-envy.

Homosexual libido

First of all, what is meant by 'homosexual' libido? The term is inexact. As we know, libido was the name given by Freud to include all aspects of instinctual sexual energy in human beings. The homosexual component, therefore, designates, in the first instance, that part of the libidinal impulses directed to the same-sex parent. Homosexual desires in children of both sexes always have a double aim. One is the desire to *possess*, in the most concrete fashion, the parent of the same sex, and the second is the desire to *be* the opposite sex and to possess all the privileges and prerogatives with which the opposite-sex parent is felt to be endowed. Although it is important to differentiate between these two complementary homosexual desires, they coexist in every small child—and in the unconscious of every adult! Thus, the little girl not only wants to possess her mother sexually, create children with her, and be uniquely loved by her in a world from which all men are excluded; she also desires just as ardently to be a man like her father, to have his genitals as well as the power and other qualities she attributes to him. Since these various homosexual components are destined to remain unfulfilled, they frequently become associated with strong feelings of jealousy and aggression. Thus, to the deep attachment to both parents are added fierce and envious wishes; that is to say, the homosexual components are both tender and aggressive at the same time.

The little girl's problem is manifestly more difficult than that of her brothers. How does the small female extricate herself from this doubly complex situation with her mother? In face of the incitement and, indeed, strong erotic attraction to the father, girl-children seek to introject, very early on, all aspects of the mother's image. These will, in turn, coalesce to form a fundamental figure of identification affecting all future feminine development.

But at this point there are a number of different 'internal mothers' in our psychic world. One of these maternal introjects is adored, another desired, another resented, another deeply feared. The small girl needs to wrest from her mother the right to be her through identifying with her as an internal object, but she also needs her externally as a guide, comforter, and helper for some years to come. After the turmoil of adolescence, when she frequently rejects her mother in almost every way, she will often turn to her with renewed attachment when she herself becomes a mother. It is perhaps at this point that many girls finally forgive their mothers for all the infantile resentments they harbour against her, and they then become close adult friends.

Just as every child she bears represents, in woman's unconscious fantasy, a baby she has made with her father, so too her babies are often felt to be a gift to the mother. These factors may cause psychic pain and conflict, or they may add to the immense joy of each new birth. Other women may identify with their mothers as sexual partners in love-relations but do not themselves desire children. They sometimes regard their professional, intellectual, or artistic productions as symbolic children. Here again specific feminine problems may arise. Some women in analysis reveal the fear that they are obliged to choose between being lovers and mothers, or again they feel they must choose between both of these roles and being professionally competent people. The articulation of these three distinct feminine desires—the sexual, the maternal, and the professional—requires a delicate balance, and women often feel impelled to sacrifice their own narcissistic and libidinal needs in one or another area.

These considerations concerning woman's love life, social life, work life, and motherhood bring me back to question of feminine homosexual libido in adult life. How and where is it invested?

My reflections on myself, as well as on all that my women patients have taught me during thirty years of psychoanalytic practice, have led me to the following conclusions:

1. Our homosexual libido serves first of all to enrich and stabilize our narcissistic self-image. In other words, every little girl needs to be able to give to herself some of that early love and appreciation of the mother and her body, in order to have affection and esteem for her feminine self and sex organs. She is then free to offer to the other sex her own erogenous zones and to accept with longing, that which she herself does not possess, (since the sexual difference is the fundamental factor that leads each to become the object of the other's desire). In other words, the young girl gives up wanting to have the woman in order to be the woman and in this same psychic movement, her envy of the penis is transmuted into desire for it.

2. The profound wish to be the other sex (if and when it is relinquished) finds an important investment in woman's love life, particularly in the sexual relationship itself, in which identification with her partner's desire and pleasure adds to her own erotic enjoyment. For it is in love-making that we can best recreate the illusion of being both sexes and losing, even if momentarily, the narcissistic limits that monosexuality imposes on us.

3. I believe that our relationship to our children offers a treasure trove of homosexual riches. I can still remember my overwhelming pleasure in having given birth to a son and the feeling that his penis was also mine. I well remember too, when my daughter was born some two years later, my narcissistic wish that she would achieve all I had failed in, to which was added the complex and somewhat ambivalent relationship we had throughout her adolescence. All these memories leave me with little doubt today as to the importance of the homosexual dimension to my maternal feelings in both their pleasurable and their conflictual aspects.

4. It has always seemed to me that the pleasure experienced in intellectual and artistic achievements is pregnant with considerable narcissistic and homosexual fantasy since in such production, every person is both man and woman at the same time. Our intellectual and artistic creations are, in a sense, parthenogenetically created children. Further more, clinical experience has taught me that conflicts over either of the two poles of feminine homosexual wishes, that is, the wish to possess the mother's creative power as well as the father's fertile penis, may create serious inhibition or even total sterility in their capacity to 'put forth' symbolic children.

5. Finally, the homosexual investment, usually divested of its conscious sexual aim, gives warmth and richness to the affectionate and essential friendships we maintain with other women.[2]

The foregoing is, of course, something of an ideal description of the way in which narcissistic and bisexual wishes may be invested in sexual life, and in social and professional activities. Leaving aside the question of manifest homosexuality, with which I have dealt extensively elsewhere (McDougall 1970, 1979), we find in analytic work innumerable signs of profoundly unconscious homosexual conflict that may express itself in any of the fields of investment already mentioned. Endless domestic scenes, sexual problems, difficulties with children, with colleagues, with friends or with creative pursuits, are liable to reveal, in analysis, their unconscious homosexual counterpart.

And what of the therapeutic relationships itself? How often are homosexual fears, wishes, and projections overlooked? And whose unconscious homosexuality is causing an obstruction to the analytic process? The unrecognized homosexuality of the analysand? Or of the analyst? We shall explore this question further by means of a clinical illustration.

THE FEMALE ANALYSAND AND THE FEMALE ANALYST

I should now like to give a brief vignette from the analysis of one of my patients. An important during point in her analytic voyage came about as the result of a dream that she brought in the second year of our work together. I shall also recount a dream of my own that occurred on the night following her session; its dream theme was related to the fact that certain unconscious homosexual fantasies of my own had been stirred up by those of my patient.

Madame Marie-Josée T, 35 years of age, first came to see me because of a number of crippling phobias that had caused her intense suffering since childhood. She was claustrophobic as well as agoraphobic; she was unable to take a plane (particularly if she had to cross water), without heavy medication; a lover of opera and theatre, she suffered in advance of each performance at the thought of being unable to escape should an anxiety attack suddenly arise. An impending appointment with a stranger filled her with anticipatory panic; staying alone at night brought her a thousand tortures. In all these threatening circumstances she regularly had recourse to psychiatric drugs. She had no children and felt too disturbed within herself to contemplate motherhood.

Marie-Josée went on to tell me that the phobia which caused her the greatest suffering occurred when she was obliged to stay alone because of her husband's frequent absences in the course of his work. She would become overwhelmed with feelings of terror as well as a conviction of impending danger. Once in bed she was unable to sleep or would wake up many times throughout the night. Marie-Josée added that she had no difficulty in sleeping when her husband, to whom she was

---

[2] Despite the important differences between male and female sexualities, it should be noted that the above investments of the bisexual wishes of infancy apply to males and females alike.

'deeply attached', was at home. To combat her insomnia she would drug herself with sleeping-pills or, as a last resort, would go back to her parents' home until her husband returned.

She was an only child, loved and admired by her father, but he, like her own husband, was remembered as being more often absent then present. She described her mother as a classical example of 'smother-love', and expressed irritation about her 'over-protectiveness'. She claimed that she returned home, during her husband's lengthy absences, largely at the insistence of her mother and hinted that she thought her mother was profiting from her phobic fragility.

At our second preliminary interview, Marie-Josée spoke in passing of another symptom, but took pains to tell me that this was the least of her problems: she had to urinate many times a day and was constantly concerned that she might have the urge to urinate at in appropriate moments. Two eminent urologists had both confirmed that there was no physiological cause for her urinary frequency. I asked her what she thought might be the cause and she replied, 'Oh, it's not a psychological problem; it's just that my bladder is smaller than other women's bladders'.

In my notes following this interview I had written that this symptom, of which she appeared to make light, might well be an indication of an essential psychological conflict but one that was perhaps more difficult for her to accept. Thinking of her assertion that 'her bladder was smaller than other women's', I had written 'Does she think she has a little girl's bladder and not a grown woman's one?'

For the purposes of this illustration I shall refer only to my patient's phobia of being alone at night and her symptom of urinary frequency, since these elements were essential to understanding the infantile longings that underlay the content of the dream.

Marie-Josée spent many sessions describing her nocturnal dread when alone in her home. As time went on, we learned that her anxiety became uncontrollable only at the moment she was preparing to go bed. In her lighted kitchen, she was uneasy but able to cope. With my encouragement she tried to find a scenario capable of arousing such strong emotion.

MJ: 'Well, when I come to think of it, I do know what I'm afraid of-someone is trying to force an entry through my bedroom window.'
JM: Can you tell me more about this person?
MJ: It would be a man of course.
JM: What's he doing there?
MJ: Oh it's obvious! He'll try to rape me. And of course I won't allow that so it's quite likely that he would kill me.

It required sometime for Marie-Josée to accept that she was the author of this nightmarish script and that the rapist-killer was also a personal creation. She proceeded to search for proof that my interpretations were erroneous and supported her contention by meticulous gleaning of the daily news for evidence that women were constantly in danger of sexual attack by unknown men. Her insistence impelled me to tell her the well-known story of the woman who dreamed that a tall black man with a strange light in his eyes was approaching her bed. The woman cries, 'What are you going to do to me?' and the handsome black man replies, 'I don't know yet. It's *your* dream!' In spite of the uncertain outcome of such interventions, Marie-Josée's terror of nocturnal solitude eventually disappeared. It was replaced, interestingly enough, by masturbation. This now became the condition that allowed her to sleep peacefully through the night without medication. She complained, however, that there was a compulsive dimension to her auto-erotism. It had become somewhat addictive, replacing the once indispensable sleeping-tablets, and she also felt compelled to masturbate whether she wanted to or not.

Another equally important part of her discourse at this point in her analysis centred on the overwhelming maternal solicitude by which she clamed to be persecuted. According to my analysand, Madame X, her mother, would seize any slim pretext to get her daughter home, as though she were constantly replaiting the umbilical cord in a symbolic attempt to draw her phobic child back into her womb. Invitations to dine, to stay for the weekend, or to accompany the parents to the theatre were rained upon Marie-Josée. 'A real cannibal mother', I thought to myself, 'and perverse as well! Not only does she complain that her daughter has been neurotically crippled for the past thirty years, but she also does everything in her power to keep her in this state!' Although I kept telling myself that this was merely one version of Marie-Josée's internal representation of her mother and that she needed to maintain in a persecutory role, I found myself violently disliking this mother as a threatening external object who was preventing her daughter—my patient—from getting well.

The session from which I wish to quote came at the end of our second year of analytic work.]

MJ: I had a frightening dream last night. I was swimming around in a tumultuous sea and I feared I might drown although I noticed that the water and the scenery were rather pretty. I had a feeling that I'd been there before. The waves grew larger and I said to myself 'I'll have to find something to cling to or I shall die in this water'. At that moment I saw one of those hitching posts that are used to attach boats. I reached out to grasp it. It was made of stone. I can't remember what they're called. Anyway, I woke up in a state of panic.

[My own free-floating associations led me to feel that the dream was connected to Marie-Josée's feelings about being smothered or drowned by her mother's solicitude (particularly since the words for 'mother' and 'sea' sound identical. But I wondered about the 'hitching post' whose name escaped her memory, as well as the detail that it was 'made in stone' which in French is *pierre* (and her father's name is Pierre-Joseph).]

MJ: I don't think there's anything new in this dream; its just the panic that I always feel when I have to go out anywhere—and it's all got to do with my mother. She's everywhere threatening to possess me.

JM: What about the hitching post?
MJ: Oh, I know what it's called, it's a *'bitte a amarrer'* or is it *'une bitte de mouillage'*?

[These vertical posts are called bollards in English; the first refers to a bollard placed on a boat and the second to that on the wharf. But I must here explain a play on words in French: '*Bite*', although it is not spelled in the same way, is the popular slang word for the male sex organ and '*mouiller*' is a slang term to describe a woman's genitals when she is experiencing sexual desire. The word '*amarrer*' means to tie something up safely or to moor a boat. The term 'hitching post' which Marie-Josée had put in the place of the term '*bitte*' refers to a post used only on land for tethering horses. It seems that Marie-Josée wishes to repress the underlying significance of these words by confusing or forgetting them. However, she herself saw the connection between '*bitte*' and '*bite*'.]

MJ: "Oh, this has something to do with my father—my memory of seeing his penis that day in the bathroom, when I was about four, and I was sure my mother would be angry with me for having spied on him with such excitement. Perhaps that's why I woke up in such panic.

[She insisted once again that the dream had no real interest, that it was the same old problem. I myself hesitated, in view of her resistance to exploring over and beyond the oedipal reference the underlying homosexual content, to push her to associate to the '*bitte de mouillage*', as well as to seek some link between her continuing urinary problem and the wild sea-dream (*la mère*) that had threatened to engulf her. It had occurred to me that one underlying meaning to her symptom might well be the wish to drown her mother in her urine, and thus it would be comprehensible that in the dream-scene she might reverse the situation and fear that her mother would drown her in a vengeful sea of urine. Her only recourse would be to turn to her father, the '*bitte à amarrer*', which would come to signify 'the penis that gives security'; this phallic symbol would presumably secure her against being wrecked by her overwhelming mother, but also against her wish to maintain her angry infantile love–hate tie to her mother.

In her flight from the dream Marie-Josée turned her attention to our work and its lack of progress. I had become the bad mother who was not helping her find her way out of this maze of frightening fantasy.]

MJ: It's all very well that my panic about being alone at night has disappeared, but my daytime terrors are as strong as ever, and I feel more and more ashamed of them. I'm not getting anywhere in this analysis. Let me just tell you what happened yesterday. I had promised to have tea with old Suzanne who's a good friend of my mother's and I love her dearly. But as usual I couldn't find a parking place anywhere near her house. She lives in a little one-way steeet and the only possible parking spot was on the other side of the Boulevard Foch. There wasn't a soul in sight and the thought of crossing that empty boulevard almost made my heart stop beating. I just couldn't do it. Suddenly I had the brilliant idea of driving backwards into the one-way street, though I was really scared of getting caught by a cop. When I arrived about half an hour later than the agreed time Suzanne said 'I thought you weren't coming; you're rather late you know'. I was too ashamed to tell her why.

[Marie-Josée then proceeded to give numerous associations to her daytime panic, drawing on everything we had understood together during the past two years. Her transference feelings, as well as most of her personal relationships, had led us to conclude that she spent her life trying to escape any situation, or any relationship, that was apt to represent an archaic image of her mother as an omnipotent and omnipresent being seeking to devour her. In particular, she was compelled to avoid situations such as open spaces, heights, balconies, and open windows where it might be suspected that she was still awaiting the amorous approach of her father, disguised as the rapist-killer of her phobic fantasy-construction. Marie-Josée herself acknowledged that her own childhood wishes had once again pushed her to agoraphobic terror; that she alone was the script-writer and director of this infernal play; and that she apparently continued to endow her mother with environmental omnipotence, which she experienced as her mother's wish 'to possess her body and soul'.]

At the end of this session I had a feeling of dissatisfaction. We were treading familiar ground and had had many sessions with similar content. I was convinced there must be a link between Marie-Josée's terrifying night-dream and her daytime nightmare (expressed through the resurgence of her phobic symptom on the way to visit her friend) but could not see further into this connection although I suspected that both experiences had to do with frightening fantasies about her mother. However, I had completely overlooked the fact that Suzanne was a mother-figure for whom she expressed feelings of love rather than resentment and that in her predicament over parking her car, she was only able to reach her friend by taking a forbidden, one-way street. In the same vein I had paid scant attention that some part of Marie-Josée *wished* to be engulfed in the tumultuous maternal sea. Furthermore, I had paid little heed to the play on words contained in my patient's grasping at a stone bollard which recalled her father and in addition a masculine part of her own name. These, then, were the daytime residues I used to make a dream that surprised me by its manifest theme. The latter was so intense that it awoke me in the middle of the night and created a strange impression that I have never forgotten. A further significant detail is that due to a dispute with the most important man in my life, I too was sleeping alone in my bed that night.

Here is the dream:

> I am to meet someone in a certain district in Paris, that is, in fact, little known to me and which has the reputation of being dangerous at night, particularly in the underground railway in that area. As I approach the house, I am permeated with the sense of something uncanny yet vaguely familiar at the same time. Several people get in my way but I hurry on, asking them to step aside. Suddenly I find myself in the presence of an attractive oriental woman, dressed in a provocative, sexy style. She looks at her watch as though to say, 'You're rather late you know!' I stammer out some sort of excuse and reach forward to caress the silken material of her dress, with the impression of being forgiven by being seductive to her. It becomes evident at that moment that I am to share some kind of erotic relationship with this mysterious stranger. I feel embarrassed, because I am not sure what is expected of me. I decide that I have no choice: I must renounce all willpower and submit passively to whatever this exotic woman wants. The anxiety, no doubt mingled with excitement, aroused by this disquietingly erotic situation woke me suddenly with the feeling that my life was in danger.

Unable to return to sleep, I had plenty of time to ponder on the potential significance of this manifestly homosexual dream. This led me to reflect that my two analysts, both men, had hardly ever interpreted any genuinely homosexual material (no doubt because I had not furnished the necessary associations to allow of this!) So here I was, in the dead of night, left to fathom this complicated problem alone.

The first association that came to mind was Marie-Josée's session, through the verbal link of 'being late' for an appointment. Why had I followed in my patient's footsteps? Yet my appointment was not with an elderly mother-substitute but a langorous and erotic oriental? Slowly there came back the memory of an oriental patient who had once come to consult me several years earlier. I must have seen her in all, five or six times. The nature of her therapeutic demand had completely disappeared from my mind. What I did remember was that her father had had three legal wives, her mother being the third. I then remembered that she had said of her mother, 'she was more a big sister than a mother to me. We would play games together and we shared secrets about the other members of the household'. I recalled her disappointment at having a 'mother-sister' rather that the 'real' one, the first wife, who ruled over the household. Why, I wonder, had it not occurred to me that even if the little girl were jealous of her father's first wife and wished she had been their child, it could also be highly agreeable to have a 'mother-sister' in complicity with her daughter and always there to play games with you? For some obscure reason I then felt it was important to recall the name of this patient. After groping around in my memory her first name came back to me in a flash: She was called 'Lili'. I could no longer deny the unconscious significance of the glamorous oriental of my dream. My mother, who in no way resembles an exotic and beautiful oriental, is called Lillian!

Then I remembered one evening when I was about eight or nine, in which my mother came in to say goodnight to my sister and myself because she and my father were going to a party. She was wearing a dress of shimmering silky material which seemed to change colour as she walked. She told me it was called 'shot silk' and that it came from China. I thought I had never seen anything so beautiful in my life. My first interpretation to myself was that I was almost certainly jealous because my father was taking her out instead of me. But in the light of my dream I began to wonder if I perhaps wished that my mother would take me rather then father to the party—and perhaps I too would be dressed in shimmering shot silk. Was this the 'mother-sister' whom I had never known? Whom perhaps I had longed for?

I then began to explore and to understand other obscure references in the dream-theme; these in turn led to further latent thoughts, embedded in the dream's manifest content, leading from nostalgic longings for a barely remembered past to primitive feelings of love and hate with erotic overtones. These in turn gave way to childhood fears of death—my own or my mother's, or both. As for my father, the little girl in me believed him to be immortal. Only he could save my mother and myself from some kind of fusional death!

After some time of reflection I began to wonder what my dream had to do with Marie-Josée's analysis. I allowed myself to recognize, for the first time, that my own mother was, in many ways the opposite of the mother described by Marie-Josée. My mother's days were occupied with social activities; she worked devotedly for the church to which we belonged; she was an enthusiastic player of croquet and golf; she took singing lessons and would practise playing on her violin in her spare moments when she was not cooking for the family or sewing elegant little dresses for my sister and myself. Thus, she was not demanding of our presence like the mother of my patient. In fact I considered myself lucky in comparison with some of my schoolmates, who had envied my liberty. Of course, I had spent several years on the analytic couch, lamenting my mother's failings on almost every conceivable plane and complaining of my father's blind devotion to her in spite of her obvious faults. I had analysed so carefully, in both Marie-Josée and myself, the hostile feelings attached to the internal mother-image, but had I not, at the same time, overlooked the importance of the unconscious homo-erotic ties? This oversight with regard to my patient was clearly influenced, among other possible aspects, by my need to maintain in repression *my* infantile wish to be the chosen object of my mother's love! To have waited so many years for a dream to reveal the wish-fulfilment of a totally unconscious desire confirmed that I was, effectively, 'rather late' in recognizing the primary homosexual wishes of the past.

What was even more disquieting was the realization that, up until now, I had not been listening to Marie-Josée's denied wish either. I had taken her complaints at face-value!

At our next session Marie-Josée's continuing complaints about her mother offered me the occasion to ask her if, behind all her expressed dissatisfaction with her demanding mother, there might also be a wish to prove to me and to herself just how much she was loved by her mother and perhaps a secret pleasure on her part in complying with these maternal demands. My intervention was received in tense silence followed by an embarrassed confession.

MJ: Well it could be that I am more demanding than I realized. The other day when I rang to ask if I could spend the weekend with my parents as I will be a bit lonely without my husband for a few days my mother made it clear that she and my father were a little tired of 'baby-sitting' me every time my husband went abroad. I just couldn't believe my ears.
[She began to cry quietly and after a short while continued through her tears:]
MJ: "She . . . er . . . well she even said that they were planning to go away alone for a few days and they didn't want to be constantly worried about how I was doing back in Paris . . ."
[Tears again interrupted her sentence but she managed to stammer out]
MJ: . . . and Mother said they actually dreaded my phone calls at such times.

[I was struck silent by this revelation. Although I had few doubts about the complicity of Marie-Josée's mother in their interdependent relationship, it was above all my own unconscious complicity that had prevented Marie-Josée's becoming conscious more rapidly of her positive desire to be the object of her mother's love and to put her mother in the place of her husband whenever the opportunity arose.

As a consequence of elaborating more fully my countertransference in this analytic relationship, I was now able to turn to another 'late' area in my understanding of Marie-Josée's complex tie to her mother. Why I had shown little interest in Marie-Josée's masturbation fantasies, especially since her nightly auto-erotic activity had taken the place of her old nocturnal phobia and her fantasy of the rapist-killer. Would the hidden erotic link to her mother be revealed in her auto-erotic fantasies?

My newly acquired receptivity bore immediate fruit, and furthermore, uncovered a fundamental element that contributed to her symptom of urinary frequence. This occurred in a session some weeks later, in which my patient referred once again to her old nocturnal anguish; I pointed out that she seemed to avoid talking about what had taken its place—the compulsive nightly masturbation.]

MJ: Yes, it's very difficult for me to talk about.

JM: You remember that when you were so afraid of being alone at nights we found this was linked to some violent sexual ideas and a buried fantasy of your father as the rapist-killer. If your sexual fantasies include some of the same ideas you might have difficulty in talking about them–like the difficulty in talking of the feelings of attachment to your mother.

MJ: Well it isn't difficult for me to tell you what I imagine. There are both men and women in my sexual day-dreams. But what is painful for me to say is . . . er . . . the way in which I do this sexual thing. OK, I must say it. I stimulate myself with an electric water-jet apparatus for cleaning teeth.

JM: Can you tell me more about this apparatus?

MJ: Oh it was a present my mother gave me. But I haven't used it in the way she intended.

JM: So maybe it's a way of making love with your mother?

[Marie-Josée then laughed, and seemed visibly relaxed.]

MJ: Yes I'm sure you're right. It's that little girl again who's still longing to be her mother's erotic treasure! And perhaps as you said the other day, it's my need to be able to identify with her as a sexual woman, so that the little girl in me can grow into a woman also.

Following this session we were able to bring to light multiple unconscious meanings associated to the little apparatus and its erotic jet of water. We turned back to the dream of the tumultuous sea and this brought common childhood sexual fantasies to come to the fore, in particular, urinary fantasies of parental coitus. These could now be explored in both their sadistic and their erotic dimensions. We were also able to understand the the 'window intruder' of the past was a thoroughly *bisexual* figure. Marie-Jasée recalled that she had experienced her mother as an implosive intruder because of her concern over her daughter's toilet training. I learned that my patient had eroticized traumatic incidents of this kind from the past. She recalled, among other anxiety-arousing memories, her terror of bed-wetting in childhood.

My countertransference deafness and my own repressed fantasies had functioned like an opaque screen, hiding not only the analytic exploration of Marie-Josée's unsatisfactory adult sex-life, but more specifically the dominant element in her partial frigidity, namely the hitherto unconscious homosexual wishes.

The latter could now be verbalized, allowing insight into Marie-Josée's hitherto unacknowledged attitude of envy of her mother and her mother's sex, and her childhood longing to be her mother's sexual partner in order to be a mother and a woman in her own right. This now gave access to the significance of Marie-Josée's radical rejection, up to this point in her analysis, of the wish for a child of her own; she was still the child with a little girl's genitals and a little girl's bladder, and was subsequently able to tell me about her feeling of hatred for her body, which she experienced not only as incomplete and unclean, but also as dangerous should it become sexually alive in relation to a man.

Through the medium of the electric apparatus, she had been able to maintain a certain distance from her sex, yet at the same time act out her childlike wish to have imaginary erotic contact with her mother and thereby absorb some of the idealized qualities she attributed to her. This was a halfway step to a fuller feminine identification. But much analytic work still lay ahead before this 'transitional' erotic-object gave way to a genuine identification with the adult woman and genital mother that Marie-Josée believed her mother to be. With these new insights the urge to urinary frequency diminished and, with the exception of certain stressful situations, finally disappeared.

As we can see from this fragment of Marie-Josée's analytic voyage, the path from infancy to adult femininity is infinitely more complex than Freud envisaged in his 'change of zone' and 'change of object' concepts. Not only are the roots of feminine erotism laid down in early infancy, giving rise to a multiplicity of zonal confusions, but the identification to the genital mother, even when the object change to heterosexuality has been adequately achieved, still leaves in its wake many problems regarding the integration of feminine homosexual libido.

TRAUMA, BISEXUALITY, AND CREATIVITY

In the introduction to this chapter I had proposed that the universal bisexual wishes of childhood play a cardinal role in promoting creativity and that creative work in any field requires the integration of both the masculine and feminine identifications of each individual. Moreover, failure to identify with the potential fertility of both parents due to impediments in this integration is a frequent cause of serious intellectual and creative inhibition. With the aid of a clinical illustration I shall explore the unconscious significance of bodily trauma when it affects the representation of one's sexual self, and its subsequent regressive effects on the creative process.

Clinical vignette[3]

For this purpose I have chosen a vignette of three consecutive sessions from the analysis of a woman (whom I shall call Benedicte) who initially sought analytic help because of a severe writing block as well as a conflictual relationship with her lesbian lover Frédérique.

Benedicte's father died of a rectal cancer at the age of 40 when she was 15 months old. When Benedicte first came to analysis she claimed that her father had played no role whatsoever in her psychic life. In a sense this feeling arose from an aspect of her

---

[3] An account of the early part of this analysis was given in 'The Dead Father: on early psychic trauma and its relation to disturbance in sexual identity and in creative activity' (McDougall 1989, p. 205).

personal history. After the father's death Benedicte's mother lied to the little girl. In reply to her continual questioning she answered: 'You can't see your father. He's in the hospital'. His death was kept a secret, at the mother's insistence, by all members of the family. Quite by accident Benedicte learned the truth from a neighbour when she was five years old.

In the course of her analysis Benedicte was to discover that not only had her father been extremely devoted to his only child but he had also played a maternal role, caring for her physically when the mother's phobias inhibited her in her caretaking functions. As the dead father slowly came alive in Benedicte's mind we were able to understand that both her homosexuality and her writing career were paths of identification with him, unconscious monuments to her forgotten love of and need for him. Within two years her writing block was successfully overcome and Benedicte became a respected and published author. As the analysis progressed many other inhibitions and anxieties also disappeared. In the sixth year of treatment Benedicte put forth a vague project of termination. Before the year was up a massive endometriosis led to her undergoing an ovarectomy.

This mutilating operation precipitated a return of her writing block, and a decision on both our parts that the analysis was far from finished. Benedicte was relieved and we were able to understand that the termination which she herself had proposed was a way of ending the treatment on her own initiative since she feared I might decide that our work together could now come to an end.

In this vignette (noted a month after Benedicte's return to analysis), I shall concentrate on the period following the dramatic surgical intervention in order to highlight the intimate relationship between bisexual identifications, body-schema fantasies, and the creative process.

14 June

B: My operation is another hideous secret like my father's death.

[She then goes on to make a link between her surgery and her father's operation for rectal cancer. A childlike part of her holds her mother responsible for his death. Through this bodily and death-like link, as we shall see, she now reveals an unconscious fantasy that her mother is also responsible for her ovarectomy. In her associations it becomes clear that this aspect of the internalized mother is now fantasized as having attacked her sexuality and destroyed her capacity to bear children.

Benedicte is very concerned about the novel on which she is presently 'stuck', to which she cannot 'give birth'. It's provisional title, 'Criminal in search of a crime' has, in the past few sessions, led me to number of free-floating hypotheses with regard to the nature of Benedicte's 'crime'. For example, in typically childlike and megalomaniac fashion she (like many an only child, and in addition, with a dead father) may unconsciously believe that she is responsible for having destroyed the parents' possibility of ever making another baby. As a result, it may well be the small criminal Benedicte who can now no longer produce either babies or books.

Benedicte now recalls yesterday's dream: 'a woman who has apparatuses where one might have expected legs is trying to get down from a train; they're not yet attached although it's clear they're intended eventually to be used as legs. They're laced like the corsets my grandmother wore.'

Her associations to this dream are all related to men who are dead . . . her father, her grandfather, the husband of her lover Frédérique, etc.]

B: Yes, they're all men . . . perhaps those apparatuses are men? Or penises? As though women need some artificial support if they have no men. Of course that's the message I got from my mother.
[She then recounted the story of a male friend who had his leg amputated and weaves her way through the underlying associative links: legs–penises–amputation–castration. This then recalls her operation along with the poignant feelings and anxieties it has aroused.]

B: I too am amputated.
[Benedicte now brings up a detail from her past that she has never mentioned in seven years of analysis and which reveals her deep longing for a child that had to be denied.]

B: Did I ever tell you about my only 'baby'? It was a mere promise of one just before I came to Paris, after my short love affair with Adam. My periods stopped throughout the summer. There was every chance I was pregnant yet I never gave it a thought. Crazy. The truth was I didn't believe I could become pregnant because I'm not real in that way.
J: Martians don't have babies?
[I had proposed the 'Martian' metaphor some years ago in response to Benedicte's frequent assertion that she was neither male nor female, nor even sure she truly belonged to the human race. She considered herself a failure in all these respects. . . . To my asking if Martians could have babies she replied:]
B: Of course not! (Long pause) They showed me the X-rays of my two ovaries. I have a fantasy that in one there was Adam's son and in the other his daughter. They had to be taken away from me of course!
J: The twin dolls?
[This refers to a childhood memory: Benedicte had been given twin dolls, a boy and a girl, for her birthday and played exclusively with the boy. One day her mother declared the dolls had to go to 'the hospital'. When they came back they were both girls.]

B: You know, that's what she did to me—she never ever wanted a daugher. All she wanted was a girl *doll*.
[Benedicte's mother now appears as a little girl with doll-babies who might well be expected to attack Benedicte's womanly self and her wish for babies of her own. Whatever her mother's pathology may have been, there is certainly an element of projection here, in that it is the little girl who tends to imagine getting inside her mother's body to take away all her treasures: the babies, the father and his penis. This common fantasy is now transformed in Benedicte's mind into the avenging mother who has destroyed her ovaries so that she may not bear Adam's babies.]

B: I have two novels waiting to be born . . . so desperate . . . I can't get on with either of them.
J: So you're holding on to your babies?
B: Huh! Guess I think I'm immortal, that there'll always be time. One can wait

too long to produce anything! Maybe you're right. I'm holding on . . . then again I often have the feeling that if I put forth all my fantasies and day-dreams there'll be nothing left.

[Here we find a further elaboration of the fantasy that her creativity has been destroyed by the internalized mother. The metaphor now suggests a primitive faecal fantasy. Benedicte remembers with irritation her mother's endless concern over bowel-functioning, her own and Benedicte's, throughout her childhood. Her fantasy that 'there'll be nothing left' if she allows all her stories to come out suggests that it is no longer a question of her right to sexual and childbearing fulfilments but a regressive version of these, the fantasy of being emptied out faecally by the anxious mother of childhood. She once again fears the loss of all her precious contents. In her projection of this unconscious fantasy it is now her 'public' that will empty her out.]

J: Is this a refusal to give freely? It's as though you're *constipated* with this novel?.

[This was a loaded remark not only because Benedicte's mother displayed such concern about defecation but her father's death from rectal cancer is also implied.]

B: I don't really want to talk about what's on my mind . . . well . . . Fédérique gave me her comments on the few pages I've managed to squeeze out—or down. Made me feel that what I've written, the whole story, is just a lot of shit. Frédérique said: 'It's too tight, too fast . . . you make it too hard for the reader'.

[It is interesting to speculate on the many aspects that the anonymous 'public' may unconsciously represent for a writer. If Benedicte's books are unconsciously equated with either children or faeces, we are not surprised to discover that her public is felt to incorporate the negative aspects of her representation of her mother as the one who will destroy all her inner contents.]

B: If I've started this last book the way I started my life, then of course I don't want my construction to stand. It has to fall down. *I'm not supposed to create!* Like the way I had to lose my ovaries. I love taking my endless notes but when it comes to giving birth then I have to abort. Am I being my own mother when she destroyed the first piece of writing I ever did? Must I destroy to fulfil my destiny? What else is missing?

[Benedicte herself supplied the associations that tended to confirm my unspoken hypothesis: that her inability to create anything at the present moment is in large part due to her projection of destructive tendencies onto the internal mother—as though she were in no way responsible for her attack on her own productivity. Whatever the pathology of Benedicte's mother may have been, I wonder to what extent her destructiveness is a reflection of her own childhood envy. Although her mother's problems would appear to lend themselves to such projective fantasies, our analytic exploration can deal only with Benedicte's own unconscious childhood motives.

These ruminations now give rise to further free-floating thoughts in my mind about the unconscious reasons for Benedicte's constant attacks on her creative potential and its link with her physical trauma: if she puts forth her present brain-child, does she fear she will destroy her own child-self? The one who was destined to fail, to fall down, to be aborted? And thus lose her masochistic tie to the angry but profoundly important relationship with her mother? Does she feel guilty not only for believing herself to be responsible for her mother's widowhood and single child status, but also for having reduced her mother to the 'unreal' person she always claims her to be?

To create artistic or intellectual 'children' one must unconsciously assume the reproductive role of both parents, be both the fertile womb and the fertilizing penis. Perhaps these fantasized transgressions contribute to the suffering that many writers and artists endure? The creative act always runs the risk of being experienced, unconsciously, as a crime against the parents: the theft of their sexual organs and generative powers.

Benedicte's associations tend to reveal this fantasy but include also the metaphor of her productions 'just a lot of shit', leading to the fear of the irrevocable loss of all her stories and characters. The 'crime' will be detected through 'soiling the page' and displaying this to the whole world.

She then elaborates on her belief that it was forbidden to take pleasure in anything that was not fundamentally her mother's pleasure. To do or be anything on her own constituted a serious transgression. Since any independence such as spontaneous creative activity represented a narcissistic threat to her mother, her own integrity was also threatened.

This symptomatic area is at the same time closely connected with a measure of breakdown in the maturation of 'transitional phenomena', as defined by Winnicott. If a small child dare not play on its own, in its mother's presence, because it fears that mother will withdraw interest from the infant's play and disappear or, on the contrary, take the game over, then any thrust toward creative independence will be fraught with danger. To create is to claim one's right to separate existence and individual identity. Benedicte and I had worked many a time on her belief that in writing she was being disloyal to her mother. Her destiny, as she interpreted it, had been to repair her mother through being a narcissistic prolongation of her.

Rather than accept such a fate Benedicte refused from early childhood to be the 'girl-doll' she felt her mother demanded, and indeed fought violently against conforming to anything her mother was felt to expect from her. To have complied would have meant 'to be nothing', the equivalent of psychic death. However, she did fulfil the goal of being reparative in the two important relationships she has had with women lovers. She acted toward them as she believed she should have acted in regard to her mother. In both love-relationships she had in fact replaced a dead husband.

Benedicte now struggles with a transference thought that she claims is difficult to reveal.]

B: I'm worried about you. You remember your paper-weight was holding down a stack of urgent mail when I came in yesterday and I asked if things were going badly.
[In reply to Benedicte's query at the end of the session I had said, echoing her question, 'So things are looking bad?]
B: And I see all those books and papers stacked up under the window. As though you can't cope with everything you have to do. The difficult thought is this: you no longer have a man in your life. So you're all alone, broken up inside, because you just can't do everything by yourself.
J: Like Frédérique and Marie-Christine whose men are dead? You killed them magically along with your father. Maybe it's my turn?

[This interpretation took her totally by surprise. After the session I noted that we have analyzed many versions of her killer-fantasy with regard to the husbands, but I wonder now if there isn't an added dimension. Does she imagine she's carrying her dead father within her? Or a dead baby she has had with him? Perhaps the 'son and daughter petrified in her ovaries' stand also for some part of herself that is felt to be dead?

In addition, she often presents her mother as not being truly alive in relation to others. Did she feel that she was responsible for paralysing the life-force in her mother too? If she brings this novel to life as a result of our analytic work, not only will the crime be revealed but she may suffer once more, as in childhood, from overpowering guilt and fear as a consequence of her dangerous acts. To bring forth her novel may then confirm that the story is not a fantasy; that she is indeed the author of a real crime. If her novel were not fiction but truth this might contribute to the reasons for which it has to be kept 'unborn'.]

15 June

B: How do *you* work? You're not only constructing my . . . our . . . analytic story, you're also doing something else of your own aren't you?

J: I too have an unconscious mind and hidden motives?

B: Yes . . . you hurt me yesterday when you put into words what I seemed to be expressing about being so stuck in my work: you said 'constipation'. That shocked me. But it was still harder to realize that I can't give. I particularly hated that because I cherish an image of myself as someone extremely generous whereas in fact it's quite untrue! I *can't* give; I'm *not* generous! But you aren't supposed to know that! [Long pause] I wonder how much this affects my work. With each piece of writing it's as though the first spurt is enough. I don't want to give any more of myself, or my story. The reader is supposed to *know* what the rest of the story is about.

J: You should be understood without having to use words?

B: Its not that I'm not saying anything—there is a public in my mind. But I think it's true that I'm holding back most of my 'contents'. My mother tried to get everything out of me as though all I had, all I was, belonged to her, not to me. So I'd die rather than give birth, or produce anything for her! [Long pause] I torture myself with the idea that the present novel, the constipated one, won't be up to everybody's expectations.

[We catch once again a glimpse of the immense importance of public recognition as a factor in convincing the creator that he or she is absolved for his or her fantasized transgressions.]

J: Still the shit fantasy?

B: Exactly! And then there's a difficulty with my characters. They have the same problems that I do . . . I've been going over this in my mind since yesterday . . . they can't do more than they're already doing, or they'd all fall off the page! If they try to reveal a little more of themselves, they become like my mother, lousy actors. It's all I can do to keep them on the page. I've only two alternatives: either I keep me together (that's to say my characters because they're part of me) or else we'll end up doing what my mother does—look real but in fact be completely phoney. So my book-child is a bit flattened out, two-dimensional.

J: To be or not to be—your mother? No third dimension?

B: That's right! In everything I've written my male characters all have to be killed. I guess they only come into existence to ressurect my father, and that done, they may just as well die. And there's always some shadowy plot underneath. It has to be shadowy because it must be expressed in a language different from my mother's. My language is either further ahead, or further behind (*en deça, ou en dessous*). It might be Martian language. Like my Martian body, ambiguous, with a shameful defect that always had to be hidden. I never had a normal body.

J: What's a 'normal' body?

B: It's the body of someone who *thinks* that the body he lives in is normal. You remember that years ago Marie Christine remarked on my public hair having a masculine distribution and I didn't look at myself in a glass nor even go in swimming for five years. I believed it had been a hormonal change after the death of Frédérique's husband. You allowed me to discover that it was a delusion on my part.[4] Meanwhile I looked desperately at other people's bodies and they seemed OK. Since then I've learned that most people are unhappy with their bodies. It helped a little to think others had some version of my suffering.

[Benedicte goes on to say that although she now knows she was not the only woman to feel such anguish nevertheless her childhood experiences had done nothing to help her construct a better body-image, and consequently, a better image of herself as an individual.

We catch a glimpse here of the link between the present-day trauma of the ovarectomy and the impact of the early psychic traumas that had given rise to her severely damaged, 'ambiguous' body-image. She now begins to link this new insight to her work inhibition.]

B: I wonder if this ambiguous feeling about my body and my sexuality affects my characters as well. Take the killer who's the central character—even his identity keeps changing. The reader will be constantly puzzled. Frédérique complained about that too.

J: The reader has to guess what the plot is? Like you had to do throughout your childhood about the mystery of your father's death? And the confusion over your own identity and sexuality?

B: Yes that's my problem . . . You must wipe out all trace of a body! Or at least it must pass unnoticed . . . just like I try to do in the street. It's my way of fooling everyone so they won't discover that I have a hideous ambiguous body. That's it, the reader has to guess, with no trace, nor clue to help him.

[We see that sexual differences and sexual identity have to be denied, but in addition separate identity, otherness itself, must become shrouded in mystery. The '*manque à être*' (in Lacan's terminology)—the 'something' that will always be missing in every terminology—the 'something' that will always be missing in every human being—must be denied. It is true that Benedicte's childhood experiences did not help her accomplish any of the mourning processes involved in the task of becoming an individual. She

---

[4] This incident, and its significant relationship to unconscious identification with her dead father, is recounted in McDougall (1989).

now tries to compensate for this through her writing—provided she can allow herself to work!]

16 June
B: From four pages its now become seven and a half. I'd love to bring both versions so you'd see what's missing in each. Of course I know what you'd say: 'You tell me what's missing; the missing part's inside you, obeying some unknown force'. Deep down I'm glad I can't and won't bring my work to you. the solution's inside me. You showed me that right from the beginning. [Long pause] You said yesterday I always sing in a low key. That's just the way I feel it. If I move into a higher key the terror of false notes will paralyze me . . . a voice inside me says: 'Christ! That's terrible!' . . . but it only speaks up when someone's going to *see* my work. Then I start to feel ghastly, terrified, and ashamed.
[We had worked for a long time on everything that Benedicte projects on to her public—and the parts of herself she gets rid of in this way. I begin to wonder which level of instinctual body-fantasy is coming to the surface now: the anal crime or the murderous one? . . . After a lengthy silence Benedicte continued:]

B: I suppose I'm my own mocking public much of the time—although there are days when my work isn't as good as it should be, so shame is sometimes justified too!
J: But we're trying to get to the destructive and shameful parts of yourself that you lend the public and with which your work then becomes identified. That's when you expect to be shamed and lend these attacking thoughts to your inner editor, and then pass them to the public.
B: It's this terror of producing something false—like my mother, with her tear-jerk artistry.
J: You're so often afraid of producing something false or shameful, something to be hidden . . . and these are the same terms you use whenever you speak of your mother. As though your mother were *your creation*, and a terrible one at that.
B: Oh! That's a new thought! It's true I was ashamed of her. Could I have done it to her?
[Benedicte has never accepted any interventions suggesting a period of her life when she might have felt dependent on her mother, loving her, needing her, wanting to cling to her. Possibly her need was so overwhelming after the death of her devoted father that the over-dependence may have fostered envious and detructive feelings toward her mother. Through the link with her work she is able, for the first time, to elaborate on possible guilt feelings toward her.)

J: Yesterday you saw me as broken up, alone, without a man.
B: Yes, I guess you were *her*. Perhaps I broke her up and made her into a reconstituted falsity? [Long pause] It's true I remember feeling that everything that was wrong with her was my fault. Because of me she had to move back to my grandmother's house where she was so unhappy. She hated her mother whereas I loved and needed her. If my mother hadn't had a child, if she'd just been a regular widow, her life would've been different. She wouldn't have had to go back. When she looked terrifying, or awful, I was sure I'd provoked that too. [Pause] You know, when one's mother can't answer a question eveything falls down. Up till then she's always been so intelligent.

Then one day you ask the question she can't answer—and suddenly, you've turned her into an ass! If I hadn't asked any questions . . . well what difference would it have made?

J: Ask me no questions I'll tell you no lies?

[I refer here to the fact that Benedicte's mother had lied for years about the father's death.]

B: That's it! If I hadn't asked the questions I wouldn't have got a pack of lies! Yes, I turned her into a liar. I did it to her. So what you're showing me is that this is the false note in my song . . . has this something to do with my blocked writing?

J: Maybe you're asking the wrong questions of your characters?

B: Yes! Before I trap them into words I've already locked them up—pushed them back into the house where they cannot breathe or live. Just like I pushed my mother back into her mother's house. And then after we left to live in the other house—I did feel ashamed of her most of the time. Especially with all her lovers—they were the punishment for my crimes, for not keeping my father alive, for what I'd done to her. I brought her nothing but harm. She made it very clear about her tragic situation—and of course I understood that *I* was the tragedy. I wasn't supposed to win after what I'd done. I had to be a loser. Maybe . . . I wonder, if that's what I'm still doing? When I write the way I do is it a way of repairing her? Or, when I'm blocked, of refusing to do so? You said yesterday that among the missing things in those inner voices was my father's voice. She had no answers—only false, secondhand ideas. I needed my father . . . I'm thinking of David . . .

[This was a man with whom Benedicte had had a lengthy love-relationship and with whom she has remained close friends. She refused to make her life with him—for many complicated reasons, some connected with her deep homosexual need to recover a feeling of bodily and narcissistic integrity by loving a woman. The normal integration of the primary homosexuality of childhood had gone awry, thus the missing identifications in her inner psychic world had to be sought in the external world. In other words, her love relations were intended, among other aims, to enable her to 'become a woman'.]

B: David's way of looking at things, of making me listen to another viewpoint, was a *man's* discourse. I felt his presence and the force of his difference. What he was telling me was important and I had to understand it. Maybe this is the missing element in my work? This is part of the low key of course, but something that has to remain so muted that I'm not actually listening to it fully.

J: As though you can't sing in different keys? Listen to both? Be both man and woman in your writing?

B: Yes, isn't that astonishing! I can't give my characters enough space . . . *because they're men* . . . and my terror of writing a soap opera is connected to this. If I turned my father or my grandfather into soap opera characters, without any reality, then I'd deserve to die.

J: So these male characters can't become fully alive? You might destroy them?

B: Oh, what a discovery! You know, all my male characters, though they're naturally good fathers—that's their vocation—in fact what they are, above all, is *good mothers*! [Long pause] Perhaps I believe that I'm unable to bring a man to life . . . maybe . . .

this is the secret of my loving? And of my blocked writing? Can I only recreate, only love a woman?

It is the end of the session. After Benedicte leaves I think to myself: how intricate and impalpable is the creative process . . . as intricate and mysterious as love!

REFERENCES

Freud, S. (1931/1961). Female sexuality. In *Complete psychological works of Sigmund Freud*, (standard edition, Vol. 21, pp. 225–43). Hogarth Press, London.

Freud, S. (1933/1964). Feminity. In *Complete psychological works of Sigmund Freud*, (standard edition, Vol. 22, p. 112–35). Hogarth Press, London.

Klein, M. (1945). the Oedipus complex in the light of early anxieties. *Int. J. Psycho-Anal.* **26**, 11–142.

Kestenberg, J. S. (1968). Outside and inside, male and female. *J. Am. Psychoanal. Assoc.* **16**, 457–520.

McDougall, J. (1970). Homosexuality in women. In *Female sexuality: new psychoanalytic views*, (ed. J. Chasseguet-Smiroel), pp. 171–212. University of Michigan Press, Ann Arbor.

McDougall, J. (1979). The homosexual dilemma: a clinical and theoretical study of female homosexuality. In *Sexual deviation*, (2nd edn), (ed. I. Rosen), pp. 206–242. Oxford University Press.

McDougall, J. (1989). The Dead Father: on early psychic trauma and its relation to disturbance in sexual identity and in creative activity. *Int. J. Psycho-Anal.* **70**, 205–20.

Panel Report. Renik, O. and Grossman, L. (1994). Contemporary theories of female sexuality: clinical applications. *J. Am. Psychoanal. Assn.*, **42**, 233–41.

11
Advances in the psychoanalytic theory and therapy of male homosexuality*

Charles W. Socarides

INTRODUCTION

In a new era of sexual permissiveness and intensive sociopolitical activism threatening to remove homosexuality as a psychopathological disorder and even proscribe its treatment, it is well to begin this chapter by a definition of homosexual and homosexuality, preceded by definitions of the words 'sexual', 'heterosexual', and 'heterosexuality'.

Sexual reproduction was antedated by asexual reproduction or fission, that is, one cell splitting into two identical cells. The word *sexual* is derived from biology and refers to a form of reproduction occurring between two cells which are different from each other. Their combined nuclear material resulted in completely new individual cells (germ cells differentiated as male and female). This event became the basis of the evolutionary differentiation of the sexes. Rado (1956, p. 187) notes: 'Taken in its entirety, the male–female reproductive pair is an emergent entity, a biological organization of a higher order. Produced by evolutionary differentiation, male and female germ cells, coital organs and *individuals* are but so many component parts of this new entity . . . The pattern of these early [alimentary] pairs is destined to exert a powerful influence on the individual's future sexual behaviour. Sexual activity began solely as reproductive activity. It was later enlarged to sexual pleasure activity, with or without reproduction.

Male–female sexual pairing is determined by two-and-a-half billion years of evolution, a product of sexual differentiation. Sexual activity was first based solely on reproduction and later widened to include sexual gratification; from one-celled non-sexual fission to the development of two-celled sexual reproduction, to organ differentiation, and finally, to the development of two separate individuals reciprocally adapted to each other anatomically, endocrinologically, psychologically, and in many other ways.

In man, heterosexual object choice is not innate or instinctual, nor is homosexual object choice; both are learned behaviours. The choice of sexual object is not predetermined by chromosomal tagging, but is outlined from birth by anatomy and then reinforced by cultural and environmental indoctrination. It is supported by

* Portions of this chapter, a revision and expansion of my chapter entitled 'The psychoanalytic theory of homosexuality with special reference to therapy' published in Ismond Rosen's (1964, 1979) books on sexual deviation, are adapted or replicated from my diverse writings on male homosexuality over a 35-year period (1968, 1974, 1978, 1988; Socarides *et al.* 1973).

universal human concepts of mating and the tradition of the family unit, together with the complementariness and contrast between the two sexes (Rado 1949, 1956).

Everything from birth to death is designed to perpetuate the male/female combination, a pattern not only anatomically outlined but culturally ingrained and fostered by all the institutions of marriage, society, and the deep roots of the family unit. The term 'anatomical outline' does not mean that it is instinctual to choose a person of the opposite sex (heterosexuality). The human being is a biological emergent entity derived from evolution, favouring survival.

In man, due to tremendous development of the cerebral cortex, motivation—both conscious and unconscious—plays a crucial role in the selection of individuals and/or objects that will produce sexual arousal and orgastic release. Massive childhood fears may produce a destruction of the standard male/female pattern. The roundabout method of achieving orgastic release is through instituting male/male or female/female pairs (homosexuality). Such unconscious fears are responsible not only for the later development of homosexuality but of all other modified sexual patterns of the obligatory type.

The term 'standard pattern' was originated by Rado (1956) to signify penetration of the male organ into the female at point before orgasm if possible and, of course, carries with it the potential for reproduction. Within the standard pattern, from which the foregoing characteristics are never absent, there are innumerable variations dependent on individual preference. Homosexuality is a modified pattern because it does not conform to the essential characteristics of the standard pattern. Other modified sexual patterns, also referred to as perversions or deviations, are fetishism, voyeurism, exhibitionism, paedophilia, etc. Individuals suffering from these conditions have in common the inability to perform in the standard male/female design, attempt to achieve orgastic release in a substitutive way. A homosexual, therefore, is an individual who engages repetitively or episodically in sexual relations with a partner of the same sex or experiences a recurrent desire to do so. If required to function sexually with a partner of the opposite sex, one can do so, if it all, with very little or no pleasure.

While Freud himself deplored the word 'perversion' because it carried a moralistic connotation, he continued to use it free from its pejorative meaning and in a scientific sense. He used it to denote sexual arousal patterns that are unconsciously motivated, stereotyped, and derived from early psychic conflict. Perversions, unlike neurotic symptoms, brought pleasure, not pain. In 1905, he coined the term 'inversion' for homosexuality and Ferenczi (1909) followed with his term 'paraphilia' to encompass all the perversions. The term 'sexual deviation' is a more acceptable one to many as it neither moralizes nor normalizes. Some behavioural scientists, especially those who believe that homosexuals can only achieve their proper civil rights through the normalization of this condition, insist that there are no sexual perversions and deviations, only alternative or different lifestyles, and that these conditions are merely a matter of social definition, some made permissible by society and others socially condemned. This is held to be especially true as regards homosexuality. It is my belief that the majority of psychoanalysts have no interest whatsoever in limiting the civil rights of obligatory homosexual men and women, especially since their disorder arises from unconscious conflict over which they have no control. Arlow (1986, p. 249) sums up as follows:

As scientists, our interest is in understanding the psychodynamics and the genesis of those patterns of sexual activity that deviate in a considerable degree from the more usual forms of gratification. While it is true that the term 'perversion' in current usage carries the connotation of adverse judgment, the essential meaning is a turning away from the ordinary course. As such, the term 'perverse' is an accurate one . . . The origin and meaning of unusual sexual behaviour is the subject matter of our scientific concern. The phenomenology of perversion should be approached from a natural science point of view, divorced from any judgmental implications.

We thoroughly deplore, therefore, those conclusions and interpretations as to the meaning, content, and origin of homosexuality which arise from political and social activists, psychiatrists, special advocates, and even some entrusted with the task of formulating and modifying recent psychiatric classification systems.

Psychoanalysts comprehend the meaning of a particular act of human behaviour by delving into the motivational state from which it issues. In their investigative and healing arms, psychoanalyst and psychodynamically oriented clinicians continually ask three questions: 'What is the meaning of an event or piece of behaviour or symptom?' (cause searching); 'Where did it come from?' (end-relating, means to ends); and 'What can be done to correct things?' (healing function). By studying individuals with similar behaviour we arrive at objective conclusions as to the meaning and significance of a particular phenomenon for that individual under investigation. Thus is insight achieved. To form conclusions as to the specific meaning of an event simply because of its frequency of occurrence is to the psychoanalyst scientific folly. Only in the consultation room, using the techniques of introspective reporting and free association, protected by professional ethics, will an individual, pressed by suffering and pain, reveal the hidden (even from oneself) meaning and reasons behind one's acts, and ascertain that obligatory homosexuality is a roundabout method for achieving orgastic release in the face of conscious and/or unconscious fears. The basic principle for understanding whether certain sexual activities can be considered deviations or not was supplied by Freud (1915–16, p. 40) when he stated: 'Let us once more reach an agreement upon what is to be understood by the "sense" of a psychical process. We mean nothing other by it than the intention it serves in its position in a psychical continuity'. Thus, whether or not homosexual acts can be termed sexual deviations or perversions can be justified by the study of the conscious and/or unconscious motivation from which they issue.

In considering the differences between normality and abnormality, Kubie's (1978) comments are invaluable. He concluded that stereotypy and automatic repetitiveness are signposts of the neurotic process. Therefore, when we describe homosexuality as not simply an alternative lifestyle or normal act, we are not issuing a judgment of value but rather a clinical description of attributes of behaviour common to neurotic action and absent from normal ones. The essence of normality is flexibility, in contrast to the

. . . freezing of behaviour into patterns of unalterability that characterizes every manifestation of the neurotic process, whether in impulses, purposes, acts, thoughts or feelings. Whether or not a behavioural event is free to change depends not upon the quality of the act itself, but upon the nature of the constellation of forces that has produced it. No moment of behaviour can be looked upon as neurotic unless the processes that have set it in motion predetermined its automatic repetition irrespective of the situation, the utility, or the consequences of the act. This may be the most basic lesson of human conduct that has been learned from psychoanalysis. Let me repeat: No single psychological act can be looked upon as neurotic unless it is the product of processes that predetermine a tendency to its automatic repetition. (Kubie 1978, p. 142).

Since the predominant forces in homosexual patients are unconscious, they will not respond to experiences of pleasure or pain, to rewards or punishments, 'neither to the logic of events nor to any appeals to mind or heart. The behaviour that results from a dominance of the unconscious system has the insatiability, the automaticity, and the endless repetitiveness that are the stamp of the neurotic process' (Kubie 1978, p. 143). Homosexual patients are unable to learn from experience, to change and to adapt to changing external circumstances. In the course of this chapter, the processes predetermining these tendencies will be explored and considered in detail.

The ego-syntonic nature of homosexuality requires clarification for it is often used to justify the view that obligatory homosexuality is a normal phenomenon and should not be subjected to psychoanalytic investigation and therapy. A number of ego-syntonic phenomena can be successfully analysed at the present state of our knowledge. These include neurotic character traits, addiction, psychopathy, borderline conditions, psychotic characterology, and perversions. When one speaks of the ego-syntonicity of homosexuality or any other deviant act, it is evident that we are dealing with two components: conscious acceptance and unconscious acceptance. The degree of conscious acceptance of a perverse act varies with a person's reactions to societal pressure and consciously desired goals and aspirations. The conscious part of ego-syntonicity can be more readily modified than its unconscious component. Analysis of perverse patients reveals that ego-syntonic formations accepted by the patients are already the end result of unconscious defence mechanisms in which the ego plays a decisive part. In contrast, where the super-ego or id plays a decisive role, the end result is often an ego-alien symptom. The splitting of the super-ego promotes ego-syntonicity. The super-ego is especially tolerant of this form of perversion as it may represent the unconscious acceptable aspects of sexuality derived from the parental super-ego. The split in the ego and the split in the object lead to an idealized object relatively free of anxiety and guilt. The split in the ego leads also to an ego, relatively free of anxiety, which is available for purposes of an incestuous relationship at the cost of renunciation of a normal one. A homosexual act differs from a neurotic symptom, first by the form of gratification of the impulse, that is, orgasm, and, second, by the fact that the ego's wishes for omnipotence are satisfied by the arbitrary ego-syntonic action. We may conclude that a homosexual act differs from a neurotic symptom in that the symptom is desexualized in the latter; discharge is painful in neurosis, but it brings genital orgasm in the homosexual enactment.

MAJOR PSYCHOANALYTIC FORMULATIONS

During the early years of psychoanalysis, the view of 'neurosis as the "negative" of perversion', as Freud put it (1905, p. 237) and of the pervert who accepted sexual impulses that the neurotic tried to repress, led to the general belief that homosexual patients could not be treated in analysis because they gratify their infantile wishes consciously, without interference from the ego or the super-ego. A successful analysis, it would seem, was only possible if the patient suffered from his symptoms, desired to eliminate them, and wished to co-operate in searching for the unconscious elements causing them. Since interpretation did not result in therapeutic change (i.e., the cessation of the homosexual act), the material elicited from the analysis of the homosexual patient was often considered by many to be of little or no value. If the patient repressed nothing, he had nothing for the analyst to uncover and decipher. As a result, many analysts were disinclined to treat homosexuality, or treated only the associated symptoms. Over time these obstacles were gradually overcome so that today they no longer pose serious problems. It became increasingly apparent that the homosexual had indeed repressed something: an unconscious conflict and aspects of his infantile sexuality. The part that was admitted to consciousness and was allowed gratification was connected to very strong pregenital fixation and helped eliminate the danger of castration. What was approved in the homosexual action was not identical with a component instinct and did not amount to a simple gratification of part of a polymorphous perverse activity of childhood. The component instinct had undergone extensive change and masking in order to be gratified by the homosexual action. This masking was conditioned by the defences of the homosexual ego. Thus the homosexual act, like the neurotic symptom, did result from a conflict among various agencies of the mind. It represented a compromise and contained elements of both instinctual gratification and frustration, all the while satisfying the demands of the super-ego. Similar to a symptom, this instinctual gratification could then be seen as taking place in a masked form, its real content remaining unconscious.

Comprehension of the psychopathology of the homosexual has been dependent upon the status of our theoretical and clinical knowledge of psychiatric disorders in general. Theoretical propositions have often preceded their clinical validation and, conversely, clear-cut and accurate distinctions have been made decades in advance of a theoretical understanding of the structure of the phenomena described. For example, Freud's (1905) observation that in homosexuals there is an early intense fixation to the mother were to be explored and documented by a number of investigators over a 75-year period (Fenichel 1945; Panel Report 1952; Klein 1946; Socarides 1974). The discovery of infantile sexuality and the view of 'neurosis as the "negative" of perversion' was of compelling significance in our approach to these patients during the early years of psychoanalysis, later giving way to newer information gained from advances in the formulation of ego psychology, improvements in analytic technique based on our understanding of the transference relationship and, more recently, research findings derived from psychoanalytic observational studies of the mother–infant relationship. Important contributions to this subject have been made by Stoller (1964, 1966, 1968, 1975); Roiphe (1968); Galenson and Roiphe (1973); Volkan (1979, 1982); and Mahler (1967, 1968); Mahler *et al.* (1969).

Freud (1905) clearly saw through the 'inverts' assertion that they could never remember any attachment to the opposite sex, realizing that in most instances they had only repressed their positive heterosexual feelings. He reviewed conceptions of homosexuality prevalent for centuries: it was innate, a form of degeneracy. Both he believed untrue and of no scientific value, since homosexuals appear otherwise unimpaired and may distinguish themselves by especially high intellectual and cultural development. Were homosexuality innate (hereditary or inborn), the 'contingent' homosexual (i.e., the non-obligatory homosexual), would be much more difficult to explain. Freud's assumption was that inversion is an acquired character of the sexual instinct, and he tested this hypothesis by removing inversion by hypnotic suggestion, an event he said would be 'astonishing' (1905, p. 140) if the condition were innate. He theorized that some experiences of early childhood had a determining effect upon the direction taken by the male invert's libido. In 'A child is being beaten' (1919), Freud stated that psychoanalysis had not yet produced a complete explanation of the origin of homosexuality. Nevertheless, it had discovered the psychic mechanism of its development and had made essential contributions to the statement of the problems involved. Foremost among these discoveries was his conclusion that in the earliest phase of childhood, future (male) inverts passed through a stage of very intense but short-lived fixation to a woman, usually their mothers, and, later, continued to identify themselves with a woman and took themselves as a sexual object. Proceeding from a 'narcissistic object choice' (1905, p. 146), they look for men resembling themselves and whom they may love as their mothers loved them. Freud (1905) underscored that the problem of inversion is highly complex in men. However, in the case of women it is 'less ambiguous' (p. 146) because active inverts exhibit masculine characteristics, both physical and mental, with peculiar frequency and look for femininity in their sexual object. He remarked, however, that a closer knowledge of the facts might reveal great variety in female inverts.

In 1905, Freud noted that psychoanalytic research decidedly opposes any attempt to segregate homosexuals from the rest of mankind as a group of special character, in that *all* human beings are capable of making a homosexual object-choice and that many have, in fact, made an unconscious one. Libidinal attachments to persons of the same sex play an important part in normal mental life and, as a motive force of illness, an even greater part than do similar attachments to the opposite sex. Freud believed that object-choice independent of sex—freedom to range equally among male and female objects (as is found in childhood and in primitive societies in the early phases of history)—is the basis for a subsequent restriction in one direction or the other, and from which both the normal and the homosexual types develop.

In the ensuing decade, Freud (1910, 1919, 1922), along with Ferenczi (1914, 1916, 1926, 1955), developed the formulation of the essential developmental factors in male homosexuality. (1) In the earliest stages of development, homosexuals experience a very strong mother-fixation. On leaving this attachment they continue to identify with the mother, taking themselves narcissistically as their sexual object. Consequently, they search for a person resembling themselves whom they may love as their mothers loved them. (2) The different types of narcissistic object-choice were outlined: one searched for a person one has loved; what one oneself is; what one oneself was; what one oneself would like to be; someone reminiscent of another who was once part of oneself (Freud 1914). A combination of these possibilities indicates the varieties of sexual object choice. (3) Clinical investigation of the genetic constellations responsible for this developmental inhibition—an over-strong mother-fixation with the resultant running away from the mother and a transfer of excitation from women to men in a narcissistic fashion—led to the discovery in these cases of an early positive Oedipus complex of great intensity.

Long before the advent of ego psychology, Freud remarked that ego-functions of identification and repression play an important part in homosexuality; and in homosexuals one finds a 'predominance of archaic constitutions and primitive psychical mechanisms' (Freud, 1905, p. 146, fn 1915). The lack then of a concept of ego psychology and development comparable to the already established phases of libidinal development presented difficulties for many years in the application of structural concepts to homosexuality.

Of considerable importance was Freud's (1920) comment that the late determinants of homosexuality come during adolescence when a 'revolution of the mental economy' (p. 231) takes place. The adolescent in exchanging his mother for some other sexual object may make a choice of an object of the same sex. In his (1910) work on Leonardo da Vinci, he pointed out that the absence of the father and growing up in a feminine environment or the presence of a weak father who was dominated by the mother furthers feminine identification and homosexuality. Similarly, the presence of a cruel father may lead to a disturbance in male identification.

The concept of bisexuality has erroneously been interpreted as a genetic (inborn) characteristic of attraction to persons of both sex. This was not Freud's meaning. He did not believe that any specific genetic (chromosomal) factor was capable of directing the sexual drive into overt homosexuality. He always believed that there are a number of factors which determine sexual integration: of these the psychodynamic ones were the most important. The constitutional factors determined only the strength of the drive.

There have been numerous and varied contributions to the theory, origin, and meaning of homosexuality over the decades since 1910. Ferenczi (1914) divided homosexuals into passive homosexual inverts and object homo-erotics; the latter remain masculine in their behaviour and may pursue another man as though he were a female. Thus, he differed from the observation that role reversal is more the rule than the exception. Fenichel (1945) maintained that homosexual love is mixed with characteristics of identification and generally agreed that there is an element of identification with the object in all homosexual love. Homosexuality, in his opinion, proved to be the product of specific defensive mechanisms that facilitate the repression of both Oedipus and castration complexes. He noted that a homosexual will reject a part of his or her personality, then externalize it on to someone else who becomes the sexual object. The homosexual is seeking an image of oneself in someone else. Anna Freud (1951) expounded the same views in considerable detail.

The idea that homosexuality was really a disguised form of psychosis was not borne out over the subsequent years. Homosexuality began to appear often during psychotic episodes where previously there had been no indication of its presence. In many others, however, homosexuality occurred without psychosis or disappeared during it.

Melanie Klein (1946) held that homosexuality was fundamentally concerned with the earliest phases of libidinal development. The chief factors, therefore, in the production of homosexuality are anxieties around the oral and anal phases. These anxieties produce insatiable needs that bind the libido to oral and anal forms. Such binding leads to profound disturbances of the genital function. The object-relationship of the genital phase became filled with the pattern acquired at the oral zone, including the unconscious phantasies and feelings of desire and fear. In many men this was interpreted as a fear of being devoured by the vagina. This is probably the most important factor responsible for psychosexual impotence in men. Similar unconscious phantasies may be responsible for the fear of the penis and for frigidity in women and therefore for the development of homosexuality. The Kleinian theoretical framework stressed the preoedipal, oral-cannibalistic phantasies as the basic psychological factor in the development of homosexuality. The Oedipus complex is a later development and the emotional patterns elaborated in object relations shifts during this period enter into the defences against both heterosexuality and homosexuality. The Kleinian school believed that the emotional nature and intensity of the oedipal phantasies are determined by the earlier repressed oral phantasies and their unconscious anxieties.

Sachs (1923) clearly demonstrated the 'mechanism' (p. 545) not the motive for perversion. He stated that we are not dealing simply with a fixation of the component sexual drive, as the dictum of the 'neurosis being the "negative" of perversion' (Freud 1905) would let us assume. Sachs' theory (which I paraphrase here) was of considerable importance in noting that in homosexuality one preserves a particularly suitable portion of infantile experience or phantasy in the conscious mind while the rest of the representatives of the instinctual drives have succumbed to repression, instigated by their all-too-strong need for gratification or stimulation. The pleasurable sensations of infantile sexuality in general are now displaced under the conscious 'suitable portion of infantile experience' (p. 540). This conscious suitable portion is now supported and endowed with a high pleasure reward—so high, indeed, that it 'competes successfully with the primacy of the genitals' (p. 540). Certain conditions make the fragment particularly suitable: the pregenital stage of development on which the homosexual is strongly fixated must be included in it. The extremely powerful partial drive must find its particular form of gratification and this particular fragment had to have some special relationship to the ego that allowed it to 'escape repression' (p. 540). In essence, there is a separation or split, in which the one piece (of infantile sexuality) enters into the service of repression and thus carries over into the ego the pleasure of a preoedipal stage of development, while the rest falls victim to repression; this appears to be the 'mechanism of perversions' (p. 542).

It could be seen, therefore, that in homosexuality the instinctual gratification takes places in a disguised form while its real content remains unconscious. The infantile expression of sexuality simultaneously serves to reassure the patient and to help him maintain a repression of his oedipal conflicts and other warded-off remnants of infantile sexuality. Repression is facilitated in homosexuality through the conscious stress of *some other aspect* of infantile sexuality. Therefore, it could be stated that homosexuality is a living relic of the past testifying to the fact that there was once a conflict involving an especially strongly developed component instinct in which complete victory was impossible for the ego and repression was only partially successful. The ego, therefore, had to be content with the compromise of repressing the greater part of infantile libidinal strivings (primary identification with the mother, intense unneutralized aggression towards her, dread of separation, and fear of fusion; at the expense of sanctioning and taking into oneself the smaller part). For example, the wish to penetrate the mother's body or the wish to suck and incorporate and injure the mother's breast undergoes repression. In these instances, a piece of the infantile libidinal strivings has entered the service of repression through displacement and substitution. Instead of the mother's body being penetrated, sucked, injured or incorporated, it is the partner's body which undergoes this fate; instead of the mother's breast, it is the penis with which the patient interacts. Homosexuality thus becomes the choice of the lesser evil. In this mechanism, two defence mechanisms—identification and substitution—play crucial roles. The male homosexual makes an identification with the masculinity of his partner in the sexual act. In order to defend himself against the positive Oedipus complex, that is, his love for his mother and hatred for his father and punitive, aggressive, destructive drives towards the body of his mother, the male homosexual substitutes the partner's body and penis for the mother's breast. Homosexuals desperately need and seek a sexual contact whenever they feel weakened, frightened, depleted, guilty, ashamed, or in any way helpless or powerless. In a patient's words, they want a 'shot of masculinity'. They then feel miraculously well and strengthened, thereby avoiding any tendency to disintegrative anxiety and enhancing their self-representation. They instantly feel reintegrated on achieving orgasm with a male partner. Their pain and fear and weakness disappear for the time being and they feel well and whole again. The male partners whom they pursue are representatives of their own selves in relation to an active phallic mother.

Other contributions were made by Bibring (1940); Bergler (1943, 1944, 1951, 1956, 1959); Weiss (1950); Greenacre (1953); Arlow (Panel Report 1952, 1954); Eidelberg (1954); and Litin *et al.* (1956).

In 1956, W. H. Gillespie presented his paper, 'The general theory of sexual perversion' at the International Psycho-Analytic Congress in Geneva. His formulations represented the status of our theory and understanding of sexual perversion as of 40 years ago. His paper was remarkably comprehensive, taking into account infantile sexuality and affirming that the problem of homosexuality, along with other sexual perversions, lies in the defence against oedipal difficulties. He underscored the concept that in sexual perversion there is a regression of libido and aggression to preoedipal levels rather than a primary fixation at those levels. He stressed the importance of ego-behaviour and ego-defence manoeuvres as well as the importance of the Sachs' mechanism. He delineated the characteristics of the ego that make it possible for the ego to adopt a certain aspect of infantile sexuality, thereby enabling it to ward off the rest. It was shown that the super-ego has a special relationship to the ego that makes the latter tolerant of this particular form of sexuality. A split in the ego often coexists with a split in the sexual object so that the object becomes idealized, 'relatively anxiety free and relatively guilt free in part' (Gillespie 1956, p. 402).

Over the years other analyst writers such as Fenichel (1945); Barahal (1953); Bychowski (1954); and Lorand (1956), began to show that there is a relationship of homosexuality to other perversions, especially fetishism. A review of these contributions is beyond the scope of this chapter.

In 1974, the Ostow Psychoanalytical Clinical Research Group, all experienced clinicians, reported an extensive study of over eight cases in detail and 35 vignettes of patients with perverse behaviour, including homosexuality, over a four-year period. They concluded that perversion and homosexuality were two aspects of the same disorder for the following reasons: (1) the developmental arrest required for one appeared to favour the other; (2) both phenomena represented infantile fixations with respect to the object in homosexuality and to the aim in other perversions; (3) narcissism, infantilism, and acting-out were common in both perversions and homosexuality; (4) homosexuality was sometimes used as a defence against other forms of sexual perversion predominant in heterosexual relations. This study adumbrated future developments in our psychoanalytic understanding by noting that there appeared to be gender disturbances, object-relations conflict, and severe disturbances in early ego-development in these individuals: this forecast was to be expressed with conviction, reinforced by further clinical experience 10 years later by one of the group (Arlow 1986) in his assertion that 'no matter what other factors pertain, perversions constitute problems of gender identity of male–female differentiation' (p. 248). The Ostow report (1974) made a great advance in theory and clinical study but did not suggest a comprehensive, integrated, and systematized theory of perverse development because theoretical constructs had not been made in the areas of the pathology of internalized object-relations, concepts of narcissism, and knowledge of the earliest primary psychic development derived from infant observational studies.

As noted over 40 years ago in *Psychoanalytic terms and concepts* of the American Psychoanalytic Association (Moore and Fine 1990), 'the outcome of the oedipal phase was considered the essential explanation for the origin of homosexuality and heterosexuality. More recent studies, however, of sexual orientation in early childhood development have emphasized preoedipal determinants that result in the failure to progress from the mother–child unity of earliest infancy to individuation. Although some cases may present a predominantly oedipal or preoedipal configuration, most involve mechanisms stemming from multiple levels of fixation or regression' (p. 86).

CLASSIFICATION

Over the last decade it became increasingly clear that one could not simply depend on dividing the homosexualities into reparative, situational, and variational types (Rado 1949) or Freud's (1905) subgroups of homosexuality into absolute, amphigenic, and contingent. As a result of extensive clinical experience, I noted that the deeper understanding of homosexuality could only be established by a psychoanalytic classification which embodied multiple frames of reference: we would be unable to comprehend this condition simply by a knowledge of the process of symptom formation or defences. Rather, as suggested by a panel (1960) on nosology, and Rangell (1965), we must adhere to a multi-dimensional approach, which should include data derived from a number of sources: (1) the level of libidinal fixation or regression (instinctual framework); (2) the stage of maturation, fixation, or regression of the ego (developmental framework); (3) the symptom itself as an 'end product'; (4) the processes of symptom formation; and (5) an inventory of ego-functions, including object-relations. Specific forms of homosexuality had to be seen in relation to other forms. A comprehensive classification had to correlate and integrate many factors in a logical fashion.

Three contributions aimed at describing the origins of homosexuality set the stage for attempting this comprehensive classification of homosexuality: the first by

Gillespie (1956), described above, the second by Greenacre (1968), and the third by this writer, Socarides (1968, 1974, 1978). Summing up extensive clinical research in 1968, Greenacre suggested that 'our most recent studies of early ego development would indicate that the fundamental disturbance is . . . that the defectively developed ego uses the pressure of the maturing libidinal phases for its own purposes in characteristic ways because of the extreme and persistent narcissistic needs . . . Probably in most perversions [including homosexuality] there is a prolongation of the introjective–projective stage in which there is an incomplete separation of the "I" from the "other" and an oscillation between the two. This is associated with a more than usually strong capacity for primary identification' (1968, p. 302).

In a 1967 paper (Socarides 1978) I suggested that the genesis of well-structured cases of homosexuality may well be the result of disturbances occurring earlier than had been generally assumed, namely in the preoedipal phase. I then divided the homosexualities into oedipal and preoedipal forms and described the characteristics of each (Socarides 1974). In 1978 I sorted the homosexualities into oedipal form, preoedipal Type I and preoedipal Type II, and schizohomosexuality. I considered these the clinical forms of homosexuality, and situational and variational forms not clinical. It appeared increasingly evident that the classification system I had suggested for the homosexualities (1978) could well be applied also to the various forms of other perversions. My classification demonstrated that the same phenomenology in homosexual men may have different structures in different individuals.

The essential ingredient of any homosexual act is the unconscious and imperative need to pursue and experience sexual pleasure and orgastic release in a particular manner and with a specific, particular object. This act expresses, in a distorted way, repressed, forbidden impulses, and usually brings temporary relief, either partial or complete, from warring intra-psychic forces. The homosexual mechanism for the relief of unconscious conflict exists at any level of libidinal fixation and ego-development, from the most primitive to the more highly developed levels of organization. The underlying unconscious motivational drives are distinctly different, depending on the level from which they arise. Oedipal homosexual activity arises from the phallic organization of development and must be differentiated from preoedipal homosexual behaviour, which arises from preoedipal levels of development. We associate narcissistic neuroses and impulse disorders with the latter. The homosexual symptom can operate at an anal level, especially when it represents a regression from a genital or oedipal phase conflict. In the schizophrenic, the symptom may represent an archaic and primitive level of functioning, a frantic and chaotic attempt to construct object-relations.

There is a wide range of clinical forms of homosexual behaviour, from those derived from the very archaic, primitive levels to products of more highly differentiated stages (Socarides 1978, 1988). Each case is hierarchically layered with dynamic mechanisms stemming from multiple points of fixation and regression. We can conclude that the clinical picture of the perverse homosexual activity itself does not necessarily correctly describe the origin of the particular mechanism responsible for it. This requires a study of the developmental stages through which the individual has passed, the level of fixation, the state of object-relations, and the status of ego-functions.

In 1974 and 1988 I described the general criteria for each form of homosexuality:

oedipal, preoedipal, latent, and schizohomosexuality. I detail the quality of object-relations and degree of pathology in each case, as well as describe pathological grandiosity, disturbances in super ego formation and freedom from internal conflict, defences in a primitive stage of development with splitting predominating over repression, degree of self-object differentiation, the nature and meaning of the sexually perverse activity, transference and therapeutic considerations, and criteria among perverse patients as regards the status of object-relations, prognosis for recovery, meaning of the perverse act, degree and level of fixation, class of conflict, the Sachs' mechanism and ego-syntonicity, tendency to regressive states, and degree of potential analysable transferences. I further clarify the capacity of the orgasm to restore the sense of having a bounded and cohesive self. The status of ego-functions other than object-relations is carefully differentiated among each type and I describe the defences present in each classification.

PSYCHOANALYTIC TECHNIQUE IN THE TREATMENT OF HOMOSEXUAL PATIENTS

Modifications

My technical procedures involve significant variations and departures from standard psychoanalytic technique and innovative procedures specifically designed for the alleviation of this disorder. As Anna Freud (1954, pp. 377–8) commented:

> Every discussion of therapeutic procedure in psychoanalysis derives added interest from the fact that it can never remain for long on purely practical grounds. In the history of psychoanalysis every advance and insight has been followed closely by an advance in technique; conversely, every technical rule has been considered valid only when rooted in a specific piece of analytic theory. Any doubt concerning the justification for a particular technique therefore, had to be dealt with by inquiry into the theoretical assumptions which had given rise to it . . . [One challenge to standard technique] is due to the widening of the field of application of the analytic therapy to patients with character structures different from those which the analytic technique was devised originally in this field. Eissler (1958a) has shown in a stimulating paper which deviations from our standard technique become necessary to meet deviations in the patient's ego structure and more than that—how technical experimentation in this respect may lead to new insight into abnormalities of structure. In this particular instance, theory profits from advances in technique.

Anna Freud expressed doubts as to whether 'our standard technique equips us for the undertaking of character analysis as adequately as it has equipped us for the analysis of the various forms of hysteria and the obsessional neuroses'. Perhaps the 'various forms of perversion, fetishism, homosexuality, etc. which we now consider accessible to treatment justify deviations of technique' (pp. 381–2).

In what follows I discuss my technical digressions against a backdrop of theoretical understanding, and justified on the basis of the deviations in the patient's ego-structure and the preoedipal origin for most types of homosexuality. It is my belief that, when homosexual patients are treated in the manner to be described, unconscious anxieties of the preoedipal period (as well as those anxieties of the oedipal period) become manifest and can be dealt with in a modified psychoanalytic therapy.

It is necessary that the analyst provide the patient from the outset with an opportunity to admit the extent of one's desolation to the paternal figure in the transference. Unconscious material revealing aspects of oneself which one abhors and wishes to change may not appear for a long time. Eventually, the patient realizes that he or she is the victim of childhood events and early intra-psychic conflicts that have produced an interference in normal sexual development and functioning. As a consequence, the patient is forced to utilize roundabout methods for sexual arousal and sexual gratification, both to provide orgastic pleasure and to defend against deeper anxieties. The pathological form of sexuality for which one seeks our help is, however, only one manifestation of a complex deeper disorder affecting all areas of development and functioning. The patient may fear the reawakening of hopes for heterosexuality, long suppressed, and express disbelief that anything can be done to remedy matters. Kohut's (1971) admonition to those who would treat narcissistic personality disorders should be well heeded in the treatment of homosexual individuals. He noted that therapists who do not enjoy putting a sympathetic and soothing tone in their voice will have a hard time treating preoedipal developmental arrests. One proceeds with correct empathy for the patient's feelings, ever mindful of his need for gratification through homosexual acts in order to ensure the development of both a relationship and a successful outcome. The patient's anxiety tolerance depends on his ability to identify with the therapist, who can both accept the patient's anxieties, his vulnerabilities and depressions, and pathological sexuality, as well as be a container for them.

Since the prognosis often depends on the patient's determination to change and the extent to which this determination can be awakened in analysis, it is important that no authoritative assertion of incurability be made regarding sexual practices. I make it clear from the outset that I view the obligatory performance of homosexual acts as a form of psychopathology, a disturbance in psychosexual functioning, a form of developmental pathology, and a consequence of preoedipal conflict. The essential task is the resolution of preoedipal conflicts in order to promote a process of developmental unfolding, in Spitz's (1959) words, 'free from the anxieties, perils, threats of the original situation' and through this 'transference relationship enable the patient to reestablish his object-relations or form new object-relations at the level at which this development was deficient' (pp. 100–1). The removal of these conflicts and obstacles makes it possible for the patient to progress along the road to heterosexual functioning as the need for perverse gratification becomes less obligatory. In time, it becomes neither tension-relieving, fear-reducing, nor a compensatory mechanism, and must then compete with newly established heterosexual functioning for pleasure and self-esteem. Thus, the treatment of all homosexual patients is the treatment of the preoedipal developmental arrest, which is the *fons et origo* from which the perverse activity emerged.

Obligatory homosexuals must be exposed to the information that neither homosexual *nor* heterosexual object choice is constitutionally determined, that is, hereditary in origin, biologically innate. Both are learned behaviours, the perverse act constituting 'abnormal learning' and the heterosexual act a normal form of sexual expression.

It is vitally important that when the patient asks the analyst if the analyst was somehow not 'born that way' (i.e., heterosexual), the analyst inform the patient that heterosexuals are not born that way either. It is well known that even when a patient announces at the beginning of therapy that one does not wish one's homosexual perversion to be changed and that one is undergoing analysis simply for the treatment of 'ancillary' symptomatology, psychoanalysis may well remove perverse activities (Anna Freud 1954).

In recent years, as mentioned earlier, the 'normalization' of exclusive homosexuality by non-analytic psychiatric establishments has led some well-intentioned but uninformed practitioners to express the view that the homosexuality of a patient be preserved and 'not tampered with' analytically because it is not a form of psychopathology. The extreme view held by some that the 'homosexual identity' of a patient should be 'preserved' (Isay 1985, 1986) destroys therapeutic effectiveness and eliminates the possibility of removal of symptomatology. Such a position may have various sources: sociopolitical activism in an era of sexual permissiveness and liberation, including genuine concern for but misguided efforts to remedy the plight of the homosexual who has suffered social disapproval for centuries for something over which he has no control; the ego-syntonic nature of homosexuality; and undue pessimism as to the value of psychoanalytic therapy for this disorder. To the clinician well versed in the treatment of homosexuality, however, unfavourable outcome in therapy should lead psychoanalysts to more rigorous pursuits of the theoretical and clinical understanding of this condition and the techniques most efficacious in its treatment and not to pronouncing it a 'non-disorder'. All homosexual patients wish *more* not less help from psychoanalysts. The growing tendency and even abhorrence in some quarters to view homosexuality as a clinical disorder and the criticism lain against those who treat such patients has been compared to the vilification heaped on Freud for his initial discovery of infantile sexuality and its consequences for normal and pathological development (Fine 1980). That sociopolitical activism, clinical naivety, personal bias, or therapeutic pessimism could be decisive in removing homosexuality from the realm of psychiatric inquiry represents a scientific travesty comparable to that which occurred in human genetics through the substitution of Lamarckian theory in place of Mendelian genetics for social/political purposes in the former Soviet Union. Those who take this position often rationalize it by the statement that homosexual individuals are thereby spared the pain of treatment and what they assume to be its inevitable failure. That political and social activist positions on a clinical disorder can lead to a compounding of ignorance is evident in the assertion by those who wish to 'normalize' homosexuality that analysts betray a basic principle of psychoanalytic therapy, namely the concept of neutrality, when they attempt to change one's 'homosexual identity' (Isay 1985). Espousers of this view unfortunately misunderstand the concept of neutrality as used in psychoanalysis. This concept does not mean that the analyst is 'neutral' as to whether the patient is helped in the removal of either phobia, obsession, or perversion; the analyst does care and the patient comes to the implicit understanding that the analyst wishes to help heal one's suffering through the analysis of preoedipal fixations and object-relations conflict, thereby eliminating perversion and opening the pathway to heterosexuality. Correctly used, the concept of neutrality means that the analyst must be neutral so that the patient's affects of the past can be projected; in other words, to promote the transference.

Exceptions to my position that homosexual patients may be treated successfully and much of their suffering alleviated are found in situations similar to those described by others, for example Kernberg (1985) in the treatment of severe personality disorders. A poor outcome may be predicted in those patients who exhibit severe antisocial personality structure; are unwilling or unable to attend sessions; show severe disturbances in verbal communication with an inability to make connections in the analysis; have a severely defective super-ego so that they are unable to profit either from the therapeutic alliance or the positive transference; engage in chronic lying and withholding of information; or are severely drug-dependent. The worst prognosis in my homosexual patients are those who are in the most severe range of narcissistic pathology (borderline cases who at times lose reality), who demonstrate severe splitting of the ego with projection more prominent than repression, and a tendency towards paranoid thinking of an insistent and intractable nature. They evidence psychosis-like transference reactions, such as chronic inclination to misunderstand others, and continually feel the analyst is letting them down. Under conditions of severe stress and environmental frustration of their unrealistic goals, they may retreat to a 'malignant part' of the pathological grandiose self (Rosenfeld 1949), a haven for revenge which is to be visited upon imagined depriving, powerful figures. These patients may remain in regression for extended periods of time, unaffected by interpretation and empathic responses.

Having defined the level of ego-developmental arrest, my overall strategy is to discover the location of the fixation point, to delineate ego-deficits in the type of object-relations dominating the patient's life. I make it possible for the patient to rediscover that part of development distorted by infantile or childhood traumas, conflicts, and deficiencies due to unmet needs and tensions. I eliminate compensatory reparative moves in the maladaptive process that have distorted and inhibited functioning, self-perpetuating defences. With their removal I encounter head-on preoedipal conflicts, especially re-enactments of rapprochement-subphase conflict, separation and fragmentation anxieties, disturbances in self-cohesion, and castration anxiety of both oedipal and preoedipal origin. No matter the form of homosexuality, I routinely find anxieties relating to separation from the mother which are then relived and abreacted to in the course of therapy. For all patients, the essential task is the elucidation of the three great anxieties of the rapprochement subphase (Mahler *et al.* 1975; Socarides 1980): fear of the loss of the object, fear of losing the object's love, and an undue sensitivity to approval and/or disapproval by the parents.

Any preoedipal developmental arrest must be treated with supportive measures until the patient can begin full analysis. A longer psychoanalytic treatment may be necessary in order to first break through the developmental arrest and the pathological character structure activated in the analysis. Defences in these patients may be immature, in a prestage of development, a pre-stage of defence (Stolorow and Lachmann 1978, 1980). In addition, there has been interference with appropriate self–object differentiation and integration. The need to engage in homosexual activity is a manifestation of this arrest in development: it is a developmental necessity, at least for the time being, and not a resistance. In such cases, special techniques are necessary to promote the maturation of arrested ego-functions. The aim of these techniques is to promote structuralization of ego-functions sufficient for later exploration of the defensive aspects of the patient's psychopathology in terms of the instinctual conflicts they serve to ward off. Developmental imbalances can be reconstructed from memories and dreams in the transference and can be placed correctly in the specific developmental stages to which they belong. This approach of permitting idealizing transferences with borderline patients is not, however, without its perils; for in a borderline preoedipal Type II narcissistic perverse patient there is a tendency to fusion with the object and confusion between self and object, between analyst and patient. The subsequent 'failure' of the object (analyst) to gratify the omnipotent and grandiose needs of the patient may be then responded to (if suitable interceptive interpretations are not made) with severe aggression, regressive paranoid feelings, and psychosis-like transference reaction.

In order to facilitate the structuralization of the psychic apparatus, the analyst must promote gradually differentiated and integrated self- and object-representations within the therapeutic relationship. During this period the analyst restricts interpretations to an empathic understanding of the patient's primitive arrested self- and object-representations which the patient attempts to restore. This ensures the continuation of the positive transference, whether or not these ego-deficiencies arise from the predominance of *aggressive* conflicts themselves in the earliest years of life (Kernberg 1975) or were due to a lack of empathic response from early caretakers (Kohut 1971). Neutrality and consistent understanding of archaic states promote differentiation and integration and contribute to the formation of the patient's new world of self- and object-representations. Once sufficient structuralization of the psychic apparatus has taken place, one may proceed with the analysis of transference manifestations of libidinal and aggressive conflicts as in any other psychoanalysis.

The bedrock of my therapeutic efforts rests on the establishment, consolidation, and maintenance of the therapeutic or working alliance (Greenson 1967; Greenacre 1971; Dickes 1975), the condition of 'basic trust' (Greenacre 1969) that allows the patient to follow the lead of the analyst in searching for the meaning, content, and genesis of one's condition.

These patients have failed to experience healthy ego-functioning, have not achieved object-constancy, and suffer from an inability to attain healthy object-relations. The analytic situation offers them the opportunity for experiencing in depth 'both the real and the unreal ways in which they deal with the world' (Greenson 1968). When I make interpretations to these patients, my aim is not only to remove their unconscious anachronistic anxieties but also to help them experience appropriate ego-functions and new object-relations. In this manner, structuralization of the mental apparatus takes place not only through interpretation and assimilation but by a positive recognition of the patient's effective level of performance. To achieve this there must be a 'real' non-transference relationship, all the while keeping an appropriate psychological and physical distance. Communication is designed to increase the development of object-relations and restore internal self-representations. In those patients with severe object-relations pathology (fusion between self and object) and in those with severe projective anxieties and tendencies or severe regressive episodes, the analysis proceeds for a long initial period in a face-to-face relationship. A unique indicator that a therapeutic alliance has been achieved is the patient's (especially the homosexual patient who has engaged in numerous face-saving rationalizations, including that of constitutional bisexuality to explain the need for same-sex partners) beginning awareness that one is not simply responding to an instinctual need in his perverse activities but is dominated by a tension which one can neither understand nor control.

Specific tasks

In what follows I describe four major tasks to be achieved for the successful psychoanalytic treatment of homosexual patients: (1) separating and disidentifying from the preoedipal mother; (2) decoding the manifest perversion; (3) providing insight into the function of erotic experience in homosexual acts; and (4) spoiling the perverse gratification. The delineation of these tasks fundamental for the treatment of all perversions in no way minimizes the importance of other tasks, either implicit with them or related to them: for example, promoting differentiation and integrating self- and object-representations; resolving castration anxiety of both preoedipal and oedipal phases; eliminating the 'narcissistic resistance' to change; diminishing unneutralized aggression, and so on.

1. Separating from the preoedipal mother

A primary task in the treatment of all male homosexuals is to disclose and define to the patient the primary feminine identification with the mother that has led to the disturbance in gender-defined self-identity, the core of the disorder. The ultimate purpose of this interpretation is to effect disidentifying (Greenson 1968/1978) from her (promote intra-psychic separation from her) so that a developmental step, previously blocked, a counteridentification with the father (analyst) may now begin to take place. (In the female homosexual, our aim is to allow the female to make her own unique feminine identification separate from a primary identification with the hated, feared, and malevolently perceived mother. The female does not have the double task of making a disindentification from the mother and also making a counteridentification with the opposite sex.) My aim is to aid the patient in successfully traversing separation–individuation phases and assume an appropriate gender-defined self-identity in accordance with anatomy. A consistent, disciplined, hopeful, and helpful attitude of the analyst towards the patient facilitates the identification with the analyst, a reopening of masculine identity in a new object relationship provided by the analysis, and extra-analytic experiences.

The patient is shown that the life-long persistence of the original primary feminine identification has resulted in conscious/unconscious pervasive feelings of femininity or a deficient sense of masculinity. The patient is symbiotically attached to the mother, has phantasies of fusing with her (as elicited in dreams, fantasies, and in actual interaction with her), but is also intensely ambivalent towards her. A severe degree of masochistic vulnerability is manifest, especially in relation to the mother, to whose attitudes and behaviour the patient is unduly sensitive. Early in therapy we encounter a deficit in body-ego boundaries accompanied by a fear of bodily disintegration, unusual sensitivity to threats of bodily damage by external objects explainable in part as a manifestation of castration anxiety, as well as threats of bodily damage involved with object-loss and inability to successfully differentiate oneself from the body of the mother. Aggressive impulses threatening to destroy both the self and the object are commonly found in this phase of treatment.

I demonstrate to the patient through interpretation of dreams, transference and extra-analytic events, and sexual enactments, that perverse practices preserve identification with the mother, albeit in a disguised form. The patient attempts to relieve anxiety, tension, depression, paranoidal feelings, and other intense archaic ego-states, including aggressive destructiveness, by pressing into service perverse enactments, making one feel secure because one has thereby reinstated the previously disturbed optimal distance from and/or closeness to the mother. (The term 'optimal distance and/or closeness' refers to a psychological state in which the patient feels secure against both the loss of the mother and the preoedipal need she supplies, and against the wish and/or dread of re-engulfment.) These interpretations occupy much of the course of the early and middle phases of the analysis, as the patient endlessly engages in an obsessive repetition of a pattern of perverse enactments in order to relieve oneself of intolerable anxieties, often made worse during this period of analytic investigation. While these acts represent flights from the mother, it is made clear that these perverse practices are simultaneously an attempt to maintain contact with her and constitute a reassurance against loss of self through merger in a somato-psychic fusion with her. They provide affirmation of one's individual existence through orgastic experience (Eissler 1958*b*; Lichtenstein 1983; Socarides 1978; Stolorow and Lachmann 1978, 1980).

To summarize what has already been stated: maturational achievements are unconsciously perceived and equated with intra-psychic separation and reacted to with anxiety and guilt of various degrees, which is then analysed in a manner similar to that used with neurotic conflict. These anxieties relate to actual or fantasized threats, intimidations by the mother, and are placed in a genetic restructuring of the patient's childhood. Archaic conflicts and rapprochement crises ultimately lose their strength and disappear. The patient, after the phobic avoidance is analysed and the genital schematization fortified through the patient's acknowledgment of the ownership of his own penis and elimination of castration anxieties of both preoedipal and oedipal periods, is then able to begin to function heterosexually, at first with and ultimately without perverse fantasies. Such therapeutic progress requires months of analytic work and mutual dedication to the task.

2. Decoding the manifest perversion

The perversion is an ego-syntonic formation, the end result of unconscious defence mechanisms accomplished with the Sachs' mechanism. The attachment to the mother, hatred towards the father, and punitive aggressive destructive drives towards the body of the mother have undergone disguise as the homosexual substitutes the partner's penis for the mother's breast. (The female homosexual substitutes the fictive penis of her female partner for the abhorrent maternal breast, resulting in a masculine attitude on the part of the female partner and/or herself.)

Through decoding, the patient can perceive the disorder in its original form: archaic longings and dreads, primitive needs and fears arising from the struggle to make a progression from mother–child unity to individuation. One can now perceive what one seeks to rediscover in one's object-choice and aims: the primary reality of narcissistic relations with different images of the mother and later with the father. The male homosexual perceives that his fear of engulfment due to a lack of separation from the mother and/or dread of fusing with her forces him to seek salvation from her by running towards men. Ironically, he does not seek femininity in approaching men but is attempting to regain lost masculinity so cruelly denied him in the earliest years of childhood. (The female homosexual is attempting to find her lost femininity in the body of the partner through resonance-identification.) Preoedipal Type II narcissistic homosexuals realize that they are in addition warding off threats to self-cohesion and fears of fragmentation and desperately need to experience emotions through the response of their self-objects, their sexual partners.

We should not overlook a unique function of all perversions including homosexuality: each dramatically restores the sense of having a bounded and cohesive self through the production of orgasm, which reinforces an 'incontrovertible truth' (Lichtenstein 1983) of the reality of personal existence separate from the mother. Therefore, orgasm in perversion has an 'affirmative function' (Eissler 1958b; Lichtenstein 1983).

3. Providing insight into the function of erotic experience

As the analysis progresses it becomes increasingly clear that it is not the fixated neurotic experience *per se* (the instinct derivation—its polymorphous perverse derivative) that is regressively reanimated in the patient's homosexuality, but rather it is the *early function* of the erotic experience that has been retained and regressively relied on (Socarides 1979; Stolorow and Lachmann 1978, 1980). In this way, through erotization, the patient attempts to maintain structural cohesion and implement the stability of threatened self- and object-representations.

The patient's erotic experiences are understood as providing two functions: a *warding-off function* to forestall the dangers of castration, fragmentation, separation anxieties, and other threats; and a *compensatory function* consisting of intra-psychic activities that help maintain and decrease threats to the self-representation and object-representations. Through erotization, anxiety and depressive affects are also eliminated (Socarides 1985). Depression is turned into its opposite through a 'manic defence' (Winnicott 1935), a flight to antidepressant activities, including sexuality.

4. Spoiling the perverse gratification

Perverse patients, unlike neurotic individuals, suffer from a widespread impairment of both libidinal- and ego-development throughout the major phases prior to the oedipal period. In these patients we are confronted at the outset with a seemingly insurmountable major task: stimulating sufficient neurotic conflict which can then be analysed. My intention is to bring about this conflictual situation. To this end I have adopted Kolansky and Eisner's (1974) phrase, 'spoiling the gratification of a preoedipal developmental arrest followed by analysis' (p. 24) to connote therapeutic activity which, although leading to discomfort and anxiety in relation to previously held ego-syntonic areas of immaturity, results in the conversion of an addiction or impulse neurosis or perversion into a condition similar to a neurosis. 'Spoiling' is accomplished through the analytic comprehension of the defined psychopathology resulting from the failure to make the intra-psychic separation from the mother, educating the patient as to the nature of specific vulnerabilities, and uncovering and decoding the hidden meaning and content of perverse acts and underlying fantasy system. This is accomplished with tact, without injury to pride, as traumas to these individuals are so early and severe that narcissistic defences are held on to tenaciously. It would be a narcissistic manifestation on the therapist's part to fail to acknowledge the difficulty or perhaps the impossibility in some instances of the patient ever giving up a specific need. On the other hand, we must keep in mind the *relativity* of the *need* for perverse gratifications. Such needs are determined by other needs, are not absolute or independent, but dependent for their existence, intensity, and significance on the total functioning of the individual. Kolansky and Eisner (1974), referring to such needs in impulse disorders and addictions, point out the distinctions between the phrases 'can not do' and 'will not do' and 'do not want to', and note that the analyst must question the 'can not' before the 'do not want to'. The same can be said for the phrase 'need for immediate gratification'. Is it a 'need' like breathing is a need or is it a 'wish' for gratification such as the wish for candy? There is a back-and-forth movement as to the relevant strength of 'need for gratification' at various points in treatment.

Lest I be misunderstood, I equal 'spoiling' to uncovering conflict and comprehending the meaning of symbols. For example, uncovering a homosexual's obligatory need to swallow another man's penis and semen is decreased when it is revealed to be a search for his own lost masculinity through the incorporation of the masculinity and body of another male, who also feels similarly deficient. It leads to relief rather than frustration as the patient is no longer a 'slave' to the imperativeness of a homosexual desire, nor driven by total reliance on a partner as a means of sexual arousal. It is an attempt to find lost masculinity rather than a desire for femininity. This interpretation has a profound effect on most homosexual patients, diminishing shame and guilt on an unconscious level, regular accompaniments, both conscious and unconscious, to homosexual practices. In such instances, 'spoiling' leads not to frustration but to an increase in self-esteem, a release from importunate tensions and obligatory performances, and sets the stage for previously blocked, new possibilities of sexual arousal and release.

'Spoiling' perverse gratifications in order to stimulate neurotic conflict that can then be analysed does not mean that a perverse patient remains without sexual pleasure during the analysis. Prohibitions against perverse activity should not be engaged in, as indicated by the rule of *non prohibere*. This rule, however, should not be misconstrued by the patient (and the analyst) as representing passive permission to persist in patterns of self-destructive, antisocial, perverse behaviour, or in inadvertent permissiveness which may precipitate acting out of perverse impulses. It is not a policy of indifference on the part of the therapist which would tend, according to Arlow, to perpetuate already established patterns of overt perverse behaviour (Panel Report 1954). The patient's increasing knowledge of the psychological conflicts responsible for the perversion and the analyst's position that the perversion is an end product of deep intra-psychic trauma/need, reinforced by continuous analysis of the motivational forces leading to each individual perverse act, militate against such misunderstanding. This therapeutic approach not only reduces the patient's feelings of failure when perverse practices continue for a lengthy period of time, but lessens countertransference reactions during periods of severe acting-out.

Once the perverse act is fully understood by the patient to be a symptom, that is, a compromise formation, a necessity in order to avoid more painful and damaging anxieties (a measure taken by the ego to ward off dangers and at the same time compensating for them), the patient may more actively join the analyst in seeking to modify the enactment of perverse needs. There may be a partial disbelief on the part of the patient that these activities may be modifiable; but ultimately the patient's belief in that possibility becomes as strong as that of the analyst. Modification of perverse practices should be first suggested by the patient, analysed fully before they are attempted, and undertaken only when a full knowledge of the underlying structure of the symptom is known and understood by both patient and analyst.

A survey of treatment results

In 1960, Edward Glover devoted considerable attention to the problem of therapy of male homosexuality. The Portman Clinic Survey in England reached the following conclusion: 'Psychotherapy appears to be unsuccessful in *only* a small number of patients of any age in whom a long habit is combined with psychopathic traits, heavy drinking, or lack of desire to change' (p. 236).

Glover divided the degrees of improvement into three categories: (1) cure, that is, abolition of conscious homosexual impulses and development of full extension of heterosexual impulse; (2) much improved, that is, the abolition of conscious homosexual impulse without development of full extension of heterosexual impulse; and (3) improved, that is, increased ego integration and capacity to control the homosexual impulse.

In conducting focal treatment (brief therapy aimed at the relief of the homosexual symptom), Glover commented on the significance of social anxiety present in these patients. This social anxiety, despite apparently rational justification, however, is based largely on a projected form of unconscious guilt. The unfortunate punitive attitude of society enables the patient to project concealed super ego conflicts on to society and the law.

Glover felt that almost from the outset the therapist must decide whether to conduct the treatment through the regular and prolonged course of analysis or through focal therapy of the symptom. In following the latter course, he would soon find that having uncovered some of the guilt, he would then strike against a core of sexual anxiety, and, in particular, the multifarious manifestations of the castration complex. At this point the history of the individual's familial relations, traumas, frustrations, disappointments, jealousies, and so on, would come to the surface or should be brought to the surface.

It is necessary to demonstrate the defensive aspects of the homosexual situation, for only by uncovering the positive aspects of his original relation to women (mother, sister) and by demonstrating the anxieties or guilts (real or fantasized) associated with a hostile aspect of these earlier relations can a path be cleared for the return of heterosexual libido.

An unpublished and informal report of the Central Fact-Gathering Committee of the American Psychoanalytic Association (1956) was one of the first surveys to compile results of treatment. It showed that of 56 cases of homosexuality undergoing psychoanalytic therapy by members of the Association, they describe 8 in the completed group (which totalled 32) as cured; 13 as improved, and 1 as unimproved. This constitutes one-third of all cases reported. Of the group which did not complete treatment (total of 34), they describe 16 as improved, 10 as unimproved; 3 as untreatable, and 5 as transferred. In all reported cures, follow-up communications indicated assumption of full heterosexual role and functioning.

A research team consisting of nine practising psychoanalysts and two psycho-analytically trained psychologists published the findings of a nine-year study of male homosexuals (Bieber *et al.* 1962). The team psychiatrist and 77 respondents to a 500-item questionnaire were members of the Society of Medical Psychoanalysts, whose roster consisted of faculty and graduates of the Psychoanalytic Division of the Department of Psychiatry of New York Medical College. The research sample consisted of 106 male homosexuals and a comparison group of 100 male heterosexuals, all in psychoanalytic treatment with members of the Society. The data obtained were analysed statistically in consultation with statistical experts and the clinical applications were carefully analysed and evaluated. The results of treatment were as follows:

> Of the 106 homosexuals who started psychoanalytic therapy, 29 were exclusively heterosexual at the time the volume was published. This represented 27% of the total sample. Fourteen of these 29 had been exclusively homosexual when they began treatment; 15 were bisexual. In 1965, in a follow-up study of the 29, I was able to reclaim the data on 15 of the 29. Of these 15 men, twelve had remained exclusively heterosexual; the other three were predominantly heterosexual, but had occasional episodes of homosexuality when under severe stress. Of the twelve who had remained consistently heterosexual, seven had been among the 14 who had been exclusively homosexual when they started treatment. Thus, seven men who started treatment as exclusively homosexual had been exclusively heterosexual for at least six or seven years. (Englehardt and Kaplan 1987, p. 424)

My own clinical experience with homosexual patients in private practice may well be, with the exception of Bergler, one of the most extensive. During a 10 year period from 1967 to 1977, I treated psychoanalytically 55 overt homosexuals: 34 of these patients were in long-term psychoanalytic therapy of over a year's duration (average 3.5 years). The number of sessions ranged from three to five per week. In this group there were only three females. The remainder (eleven) were in short-term analytic therapy (average six to seven months) at two to three sessions per week. Three were female.

In addition, full-scale analysis was performed on 18 latent homosexuals in which the symptoms never became overt, except in the most transitory form. Thus the total number treated in long-term analysis, whether overt or latent, was 63. In addition, over 350 overt homosexuals were seen in consultation (average one to three sessions) during this 10 year period.

I can report that of the 45 overt homosexuals who have undergone psychoanalytic therapy, 20 patients, nearly 50 per cent, developed full heterosexual functioning and were able to develop love feelings for their heterosexual partners. This includes one female patient. These patients of whom two-thirds were of the preoedipal type and one-third of the oedipal type, were all strongly motivated for therapy.

In addition, similar positive therapeutic results have occurred during the period from

1977 to 1988 in which I have treated over 50 more overt homosexuals in psychoanalytic therapy.

In answer to those who say a successful treatment has never been demonstrated in homosexual patients, I also report a seven-year follow-up of a patient who achieved full heterosexual function and the ability to love his opposite-sex partner (Socarides 1978, pp. 497–529).

Most recently, a report by MacIntosh (1994) reveals that in a response of a survey of 285 psychoanalysts who reported having analysed 1215 homosexual patients, 23 per cent changed to heterosexuality from homosexuality, and 84 per cent of the total group received significant therapeutic benefit.

During the early development of psychoanalysis reports of favourable outcome in the treatment of homosexuality rarely appeared; the outlook was pessimistic. Starting in 1944, Bergler published extensive studies confirming his finding that with suitable treatment, homosexuality could be reversed (1944, 1959). Bychowski (1945, 1954, 1956); Lorand (1956), and other workers including Gershman (1967); Ovesey (1969); Bieber (1967), and Socarides (1969) had also published significant material to this effect, including psychoanalytic, psychotherapeutic, and group therapy.

CONCLUDING REMARKS

In this chapter I have expanded and refined my earlier findings as regards the origins, symptoms, course, pathology, meaning, and function of obligatory male homosexuality. Despite the impediment of shrill sociopolitical activism surrounding psychoanalytic therapists who treat this disorder, and an attempt to declare it a non-disorder, significant progress has been made in two areas: a classification of the various types of homosexuality, as well as the general and specific techniques which should be employed in order to achieve a satisfactory result. The specific therapeutic tasks I describe should become a vital aspect in the treatment of any homosexual patient of the preoedipal type.

I wish to close this contribution by citing my comment in the earlier edition of Dr Rosen's work:

> One's compassion for the plight of the homosexual, his responsiveness as a patient, and his value as a human being in interaction with the scientific challenge and fulfilment posed by his intra-psychic conflicts, leads to a mutuality of gratitude and satisfaction between patient and psychoanalyst, which well justifies the commitment to the attempted alleviation of this important and serious disorder. (Rosen 1979, p. 275).

REFERENCES

American Psychoanalytic Association (1956). *Report of the central fact-gathering committee*. New York. (Unpublished.)

Arlow, J. A. (1986). Discussion of paper by J. McDougall and M. Glasser: Panel on identification in the perversions. *Int. J. Psycho-Anal.* **67**, 245–50.

Barahal, H. S. (1953). Female transvestitism and homosexuality. *Psychiat. Quarterly*, **27**, 390–438.

Bergler, E. (1943). The respective importance of reality and fantasy in the genesis of female homosexuality. *J. Crim. Psychopathol.* **5**, 27–48.

Bergler, E. (1944). Eight prerequisites for psychoanalytic treatment of homosexuality. *Psychoanal. Rev.* **31**, 253–86.

Bergler, E. (1951). *Counterfeit sex*. Grune & Stratton, New York.

Bergler, E. (1956). *Homosexuality: Disease or way of life?* Hill & Wang, New York.

Bergler, E. (1959). *1000 homosexuals: Conspiracy of silence on curing and deglamorizing homosexuality*. Pageant Books, Patterson, NJ.

Bibring, G. L. (1940). On an oral component in masculine inversion. *Int. Zeitschr. Psychoanal.* **25**, 124–30.

Bieber, T. (1967). On treating male homosexuals. *Arch. Gen. Psychiat.* **16**, 60–3.

Bieber, T., *et al.* (1962). *Homosexuality: A psychoanalytic study of male homosexuals*. Basic Books, New York.

Bychowski, G. (1945). The ego of homosexuals. *Int. J. Psycho-Anal.* **26**, 114–27.

Bychowski, G. (1954). The structure of homosexual acting out. *Psychoanal. Quarterly*, **23**, 48–61.

Bychowski, G. (1956). The ego and the introject. *Psychoanal. Quarterly*, **25**, 11–36.

Dickes, R. (1975). Technical considerations on the therapeutic and working alliances. *Int. J. Psycho-Anal. Psychother.* **4**, 1–24.

Eidelberg, L. (1954). *A comparative pathology of neurosis*. International Universities Press, New York.

Eissler, K. R. (1958a). Notes on problems of technique in the psychoanalytic treatment of adolescents: with some remarks on perversions. *Psychoanal. Study Child*, **13**, 223–54.

Eissler, K. R. (1958b). Remarks on some variations in psychoanalytic technique. *Int. J. Psycho-Anal.* **39**, 222–9.

Englehardt, H. T. Jr. and Kaplan, A. L. (ed.) (1987). *Scientific controversies: Case studies in the resolution and closure of disputes in science and technology*. Cambridge University Press.

Fenichel, O. (1945). *The psychoanalytic theory of neurosis*. Norton, New York.

Ferenczi, S. (1909/1955). More about homosexuality. In *Final contributions to the problems and Methods of Psycho-analysis*, pp. 168–74. Basic Books, New York.

Ferenczi, S. (1914/1950). The nosology of female homosexuality (homoerotism). In *Contributions to psychoanalysis*, pp. 296–318. Bruner, New York.

Ferenczi, S. (1916). *Contributions of psychoanalysis*. Badger, Boston.

Ferenczi, S. (1926/1950). *Further contributions to the theory and techniques of psychoanalysis*. Hogarth Press, London.

Ferenczi, S. (1955). *Final contributions to the theory and techniques of psychoanalysis*. Hogarth Press, London.

Fine, R. (1980). Presidential introduction to the first Sigmund Freud Memorial Lectureship Award, New York Center for Psychoanalytic Training. (Unpublished.)

Freud, A. (1951). Homosexuality. *Bull. Am. Psychoanal. Assoc.* **7**, 117–18.

Freud, A. (1954/1968). Problems of technique in adult analysis. In *The writings of Anna Freud*, Vol. 4, pp. 377–406. International Universities Press, New York.

Freud, S. (1905/1953). Three essays on the theory of sexuality. In *Complete psychological works of Sigmund Freud*, (standard Edition, Vol. 7, pp. 135–243). Hogarth Press, London.

Freud, S. (1910/1957). Leonardo da Vinci and a memory of his childhood. In *Complete psychological works of Sigmund Freud*, (standard edition, Vol. 11, pp. 59–137). Hogarth Press, London.

Freud, S. (1914/1957). On narcissism: An introduction. In *Complete psychological Works or Sigmund Freud*, (standard edition, Vol. 14, pp. 69–105). Hogarth Press, London.

Freud, S. (1915–16/1963). Introductory lectures on psychoanalysis. In *Complete psychological works of Sigmund Freud*, (standard edition, Vol. 15). Hogarth Press, London.

Freud, S. (1919/1955). A child is being beaten. In *Complete psychological works of Sigmund Freud*, (standard edition, Vol. 17, pp. 175–204). Hogarth Press, London.

Freud, S. (1920/1955). Psychogenesis of a case of homosexuality in a woman. In *Complete psychological works of Sigmund Freud*, (standard edition, Vol. 18, pp. 145–172). Hogarth Press, London.

Freud, S. (1922/1955). Some neurotic mechanisms in jealousy, paranoia and homosexuality. In *Complete psychological works of Sigmund Freud*, (standard edition, Vol. 18, pp. 221–32). Hogarth Press, London.

Galenson, E. and Roiphe, H. (1973). Object loss and early sexual development. *Psychoanal. Quarterly*, 42, 73–90.

Gershman, H. (1967). Psychopathology of compulsive homosexuality. *Am. J. Psychoanal.* 17, 58–77.

Gillespie, W. H. (1956). The general theory of sexual perversion. *Int. J. Psycho-Anal.* 37, 396–403.

Glover, E. (1960). *The roots of crime*. Selected Papers on psychoanalysis. Imago, London.

Greenacre, P. (1953). Certain relationships between fetishism and the faulty development of the body image. In Emotional growth: Psychoanalytic studies of the gifted and a great variety of other individuals, Vol. 1, pp. 9–31. International Universities Press, New York.

Greenacre, P. (1968/1971). Perversions: General considerations regarding their genetic and dynamic background. In *Emotional growth: Psychoanalytic studies of the gifted and a great variety of other individuals*, Vol. 1, pp. 300–14. International Universities Press, New York.

Greenacre, P. (1969/1971). The fetish and the transitional object. In *Emotional growth: Psychoanalytic studies of the gifted and a great variety of other individuals*, Vol. 1, pp. 315–34. International Universities Press, New York.

Greenacre, P. (1971). Notes on the influence and contribution of ego psychology to the practice of psychoanalysis. In *Separation-Individuation: Essays in honor of Margaret S. Mahler*, (ed. J. B. McDevitt and C. F. Settlage), pp. 171–200. International Universities Press, New York.

Greenson, R. R. (1967). *The technique and practice of psychoanalysis*, Vol. 1. International Universities Press, New York.

Greenson, R. R. (1968/1978). Disidentifying from the mother: Its special importance for the boy. In *Explorations in psychoanalysis*, pp. 305–12. International Universities Press, New York.

Isay, R. (1985). On the analytic therapy of homosexual men. *Psychoanal. Study Child*, 40, 235–54. International Universities Press, New York.

Isay, R. (1986). Homosexuality and homosexuals and heterosexuals. Some distinctions and implications for treatment. In *The psychology of men. New psychoanalytic perspectives*, (ed. G. I. Fogel, F. M. Lane, and R. S. Liebert), pp. 277–99. Basic Books, New York.

Kernberg, O. F. (1975). *Borderline conditions and pathological narcissism*. Jason Aronson, New York.

Kernberg, O. F. (1985). *Severe personality disorders: Psychotherapeutic strategies*. Yale University Press, New Haven, CT.

Klein, M. (1946). Notes on some schizoid mechanisms. *Int. J. Psycho-Anal.* **27**, 99–110.

Kohut, H. (1971). *The analysis of the self: A systematic approach to psychoanalytic treatment of narcissistic personality disorders*. International Universities Press, New York.

Kolansky, H. and Eisner, H. (1974). The psychoanalytic concept of the preoedipal developmental arrest. Paper presented at the American Psychoanalytic Association, December 1974. (Unpublished.)

Kubie, L. (1978). Distinction between normality and neurosis. In *Symbol and neurosis: Selected papers of L. S. Kubie*, (ed. H. J. Schlesinger), pp. 115–27. International Universities Press, New York.

Lichtenstein, H. (1983). *The dilemma of human identity*. Jason Aronson, New York.

Litin, E., Giffin, M., and Johnson, A. (1956). Parental influence in unusual sexual behaviour in children. *Psychoanal. Quarterly*, **25**, 37–55.

Lorand, S. (1956). The theory of perversions. In *Perversions: Psychodynamics and therapy*, (ed. S. Lorand and M. Balint), pp. 290–307. Random House, New York.

MacIntosh, H. (1994). Attitudes and experiences of psychoanalysts in analyzing homosexual patients. *J. Am. Psychoanal. Assoc.* 42, 1183–207.

Mahler, M. S. (1967). On human symbiosis and the vicissitudes of individuation. *J. Am. Psychoanal. Assoc.* **15**, 740–64.

Mahler, M. S. (1968). *On human symbiosis and the vicissitudes of individuation*, Vol. 1. International Universities Press, New York.

Mahler, M. S., Pine, F., and Bergman, A. (1975). *The psychological birth of the human infant: Symbiosis and individuation*. Basic Books, New York.

Moore, V. E., and Fine, B. D. (ed.) (1990). *Psychoanalytic terms and concepts*. American Psychoanalytic Association, New York.

Ostow, M., *et al.* (ed.) (1974). *Sexual deviations: Psychoanalytic insights*. Quadrangle/New York Times, New York.

Ovesey, L. (1969). *Homosexuality and pseudohomosexuality*. Science House, New York.

Panel Report (1952). Psychodynamics and treatment of perversions, J. A. Arlow, reporter. *Bull. Am. Psychoanal. Assoc.* **8**, 315–27.

Panel Report (1954). Perversions: Theoretical and therapeutic aspects, J. A. Arlow, reporter. *J. Am. Psychoanal. Assoc.* **2**, 336–45.

Panel Report (1960). An examination of nosology according to psychoanalytic concepts. N. Ross, reporter. *J. Am. Psychoanal. Assoc.* **8**, 535–51.

Rado, S. (1949/1956). An adaptational view of sexual behaviour. In *The psychoanalysis of behaviour: Collected papers of Sandor Rado*, Vol. 1, (rev. edn), pp. 186–213. Grune & Stratton, New York.

Rangell, L. (1965). Some comments on psychoanalytic nosology with recommendations for improvement. In *Drives, affects, behaviour*, Vol. 2, (ed. M. Schur), pp. 123–57. International Universities Press, New York.

Roiphe, H. (1968). On an early genital phase. *Psychoanal. Study Child*, **23**, 348–65.

Rosen, I. (ed.) (1964). *The pathology and treatment of sexual deviations*. Oxford University Press.

Rosen, I. (ed.) (1979). *Sexual deviation*, (2nd edn). Oxford Unversity Press.

Rosenfeld, H. A. (1949). Remarks on the relation of male homosexuality to paranoia, paranoid anxiety, and narcissism. *Int. J. Psycho-Anal.* **30**, 36–47.

Sachs, H. (1923). On the genesis of sexual perversion. *Int. Zeitschr. Psychoanal*, 172–82. [Trans H. F. Bernays (1964); New York Psychoanalytic Institute Library.] (Also in Socarides (1978). *Homosexuality*, pp. 531–46.)

Socarides, C. W. (1968). *The overt homosexual*. Grune & Stratton, New York.
Socarides, C. W. (1969). The psychoanalytic therapy of a male homosexual. *Psychoanal. Quarterly*, **38**, 173–90.
Socarides, C. W. (1974). Homosexuality. In *American handbook of psychiatry*, Vol. 3 (ed. S. Arieti), (2nd edn), pp. 291–315. Basic Books, New York.
Socarides, C. W. (1978). *Homosexuality*. Jason Aronson, New York.
Socarides, C. W. (1979). The psychoanalytic theory of homosexuality with special reference to therapy. In *Sexual Deviations*, (ed. I. Rosen), (2nd edn), pp. 243–77. Oxford University Press.
Socarides, C. W. (1980). Homosexuality and the rapprochement subphase crisis. In *Rapprochement: The critical subphase of separation-individuation*, (ed. R. F. Lax, S. Bach, and J. A. Burland), pp. 331–52. Jason Aronson. New York.
Socarides, C. W. (1985). Depression in perversion: With special reference to the function of erotic experience in sexual perversion. In *Depressive states and their treatment*, (ed. V. Volkan), pp. 317–37. Jason Aronson, New York.
Socarides, C. W. (1988). *The preoedipal origin and psychoanalytic therapy of sexual perversions*. International Universities Press, Madison, CT.
Socarides, C. W., *et al.* (1973). Report of the Task Force on Homosexuality of the New York County District Branch of the American Psychiatric Association. Homosexuality in the male: A report of a psychiatric study group. *Int. J. Psychiat.*, **11**, (4), 460–79.
Spitz, R. (1959). *A general field theory of ego formation*. International Universities Press, New York.
Stoller, R. (1964). A contribution to the study of gender identity. *Int. J. Psycho-Anal.* **45**, 220–6.
Stoller, R. (1966). The mother's contribution to infantile transvestic behaviour *Int. J. Psycho-Anal.* **47**, 384–95.
Stoller, R. (1968). A further contribution to the study of gender identity. *Int. J. Psycho-Anal.* **49**, 364–8.
Stoller, R. (1975). Healthy parental influence on the earliest development of masculinity in baby boys. *Psychoanal. Forum*, **5**, 234–40.
Stolorow, R. D. and Lachmann, F. (1980). *Psychoanalysis of developmental arrest: Theory and treatment*. International Universities Press, New York.
Stolorow, R. D. and Lachmann, F. (1978). The developmental prestages of defenses: Diagnostic and therapeutic implications. *Psychoanal. Quarterly*, **47**, 73–102.
Volkan, V. D. (1979). Transsexualism: As examined from the viewpoint of internalized object relations. In *On sexuality: Psychoanalytic observations*, (ed. T. B. Karasu and C. W. Socarides), pp. 189–222. Jason Aronson, New York.
Volkan, V. D. (1982). The transsexual search for perfection: Aggression reassignment surgery. Presented at Discussion Group on Psychoanalytic Considerations about Patients with Organic Illness or Major Physical Handicaps at the Annual Meeting of the American Psychoanalytic Association, New York City. (Unpublished.)
Weiss, E. (1950). *The principles of psychodynamics*. New York: Grune & Stratton.
Winnicott, D. W. (1935/1958). The manic defence. In *Collected papers: Through pediatrics to psychoanalysis*, pp. 129–44. Basic Books, New York.

12
Aggression and sadism in the perversions

Mervin Glasser

INTRODUCTION

Anyone considering sexual deviance should keep in mind the distinction between a true perversion and the deviant elements which may feature in the sexual life of normal people or people suffering from various forms of disturbance. The vast majority of people may, from time to time, indulge in sexual fantasies which deviate from the culturally accepted norms, and many people may even put such fantasies into occasional practice, particularly as foreplay. But when the sexual deviance is a persistent, constantly preferred form of sexual behaviour which reflects a global structure involving the individual's whole personality, I consider it appropriate to use the term 'perversion', despite its pejorative overtones, as a diagnostic designation like 'obsessional neurosis' or 'paranoid schizophrenia'.

The perversions should be identified by the specific nature of this global structure rather than by any manifest sexual activity. A deviant sexual act may be the expression of ego disintegration, such as an act of indecent exposure carried out by a person suffering from senile dementia, or we may learn that a man may carry out an act of apparently normal sexual intercourse only if he entertains, during the act, fantasies of being beaten by a big man.

Exploration of this global structure of the perversions shows it to be enormously complex, with numerous elements dynamically held together to form 'component complexes' which themselves are dynamically inter-related to each other. At the centre of this structure is such a component complex which we may refer to as the *core complex* because it is fundamental to the pervert's psychopathology and substantially influences all the other component complexes (see, for example, Glasser 1979*b*). When we have the opportunity to explore the components of the core complex through psychoanalysis we invariably find that an essential ingredient of the core complex is *aggression*; and it is to this aspect of the perversions that I shall be paying particular attention in this chapter.

ON THE NATURE OF AGGRESSION

I would like to clarify my understanding and usage of the term 'aggression'. In many psychoanalytic writings 'aggression' and 'sadism' have often been used interchangeably and this has led to confusion, both theoretically and clinically. It must be acknowledged that there is still no agreed conceptualization of 'aggression'. Unlike 'libido', which is a defined, theoretical concept, 'aggression' is a term taken from everyday language and this carries with it the ambiguities of everyday usage. Too often it is not clear in theoretical or clinical presentations whether what is being referred to is a primary instinctual drive (as discussed, for example, by Hartmann *et al.* 1949); or a behavioural response to, say, frustration; or an affect, such as hostility; or an attitude, such as antagonism. Even when it *is* established that 'aggression' is being regarded as an instinctual drive, there is the well-known uncertainty whether to consider it as a basic drive in its own right or an outwardly-turned expression of a more fundamental 'death instinct'.

Since 'aggression' is central to my discussion, I consider it unavoidable to lay down at least a working definition and set out the boundaries of my usage of this term. In approaching such a task I take up the same viewpoint as Brenner (1971) when he states: '[In psychoanalysis] an instinctual drive is a theoretical construct which serves the purpose of explaining the nature of basic motivation, of the prime impetus to mental activity', and later in the same paper: '. . . the evidence on which we base the concept of aggression as an instinctual drive is purely psychological'.

It is crucial to distinguish 'aggression' from 'sadism'. The easiest and most reliable way of making this distinction is not by trying to identify the nature of the drive involved, or even the developmental level on which the individual might be functioning, but rather the *attitude to the object* at the time at which the act is carried out. In the aggressive act, the elimination, exclusion, destruction—in essence, *negation*—of the object is the cardinal factor (as I shall elaborate at some length below); the object's emotional reaction, the meaning of the behaviour to the object, in a sense the object's fate in any other context, is irrelevant. In the sadistic act, on the contrary, the emotional reaction of the object is crucial: the specific aim is to cause the object to suffer, physically or mentally, crudely or subtly. Domination and control are obviously critical features common to both aggression and sadism and it will become clear later how they differ in this respect. Needless to say, the expression of both aggressive and sadistic motives may be achieved in the most covert and disguised ways as can be shown by the amount of psychotherapeutic work needed to identify and assess them when they are factors in a clinical condition.

The distinction I am making between aggression and sadism may be illustrated by some simple examples. The bank-robber who takes hostages and then proceeds to derive pleasure in frightening them or humiliating them while negotiating his escape is being sadistic; while the bank-robber who, in evading capture, shoots a guard dead, is being aggressive. An adolescent, who indulged in homosexual beating fantasies, spent a week having nothing to do with his parents, locking himself in his room and only opening it to receive trays of food and drink. Although emanating anger and hostility, he refused to talk to them, not even to explain why he was behaving in this way. His parents telephoned me to ask, in a troubled and exasperated way, what his behaviour was due to and what they should do about it. His behaviour was complexly motivated but it was clearly sadistic. In contrast, we can consider his behaviour after a homosexual man had made advances to him. He performed complicated stone-throwing rituals which expressed, among other things, his wish to eliminate the homosexual. This motive should be identified as aggressive. These examples bear out the clinical observation that anxiety is always absent in sadism whereas it is invariably present in aggression (although, through the operation of defence-processes, it may not be evident). These are critical considerations in the psychodynamics of the perversions as should become clear later when I elaborate how sadism is ultimately based on aggression.

Thus, crucial to the conception of aggression which I am proposing is that its aim is to remove or negate any element which stands between the individual and the meeting of his needs, or his survival. This conception agrees rather closely with that put forward by Gillespie (1971) where he regards aggression from the viewpoint that 'all instincts (Triebe) are essentially homeostatic' (see Cannon 1932). It is a fundamental task of the ego to guard the *psychic* homeostasis. The concept of psychic homeostasis is akin to, but not identical with, 'primary narcissism' which refers only to the disposition of libido. Taken from a physiological model, it implies a highly complex organization interrelating all psychological systems aimed at maintaining a *dynamic* balance, a steady state at optimum levels, rather than 'reducing [stimuli] to the lowest possible level; . . . [maintaining itself] in an altogether unstimulated condition' (Freud 1915), that is an inertia. I consider it is this way of thinking that led Freud to his formulation of the 'principle of constancy' and of the death instinct, concepts which my approach clearly rejects. The concept of 'psychic homeostasis' which I am putting forward is, perhaps, a more dynamic way of stating that the ego has to concern itself with demands and disturbances arising in the id, the super-ego, the external world, and within the ego itself. Maintaining a steady dynamic balance implies that over-gratification may be as disturbing as deprivation.

In considering aggression as an instinctual drive, we may follow the classical approach (Freud 1905, 1915) in regarding a drive as having a *source*, an *aim*, and an *object*. To this should be added that it also has a *stimulus*. In the context of psychic homeostasis, the stimulus of aggression would be any factor which threatens homeostasis; the aim of aggression is to eliminate the stimulus in one way or another; the object of aggression is the individual or thing responsible for the stimulus. I shall not attempt to identify the source of aggression but rather indicate its intrinsic nature by drawing attention to a quality of aggression which is not often appreciated, namely, how remorseless and single-minded it is—how, if its initial ideational and affective expression does not bring about appropriate adaptive moves by the ego it will proceed to its ultimate aim of destroying the threatening factor, even if this is at the expense of murdering the object, developing a psychosis or committing suicide. This illustrates the relationship between psychic homeostasis and aggression: that, ordinarily, increasing intensity of need, or put more generally, increasing disturbance of psychic homeostasis, is accompanied by increasing aggressiveness. This applies as much to purely psychological considerations, such as self-esteem, as to matters of life and death. It will be recognized that any stimulus of aggression could also be regarded as a stimulus of anxiety (Freud 1926). This indicates how intimate a relationship there is between anxiety and aggression and demonstrates the intrinsic relationship of this *psychological* response to the fundamental, *biological* 'fight-flight' response to danger (see Cannon 1929). This gives a basis for the usefulness of making a clear differentiation between the terms 'aggression' and 'violence' by limiting the usage of the former to the *psychological* and the latter to its counterpart in (observable) *behaviour*.

We may recognize how truly primitive a psychic phenomenon basic aggression is so that it may be regarded as an instinct in ethological terms (Lorenz 1966). This highlights at what primitive psychological levels certain violent individuals may be operating (Glasser 1983). Furthermore, it enables us to appreciate that anxiety may be the stimulus to aggression just as much as aggression may give rise to anxiety. This viewpoint differs from that of some schools of thought which consider aggression to be primary and basic anxieties a response to it (Klein 1948).

It is clear from the above that amongst the earliest capacities which the ego has to acquire is a refinement in its perceptual functioning so that it is able to identify the stimulus to aggression with precision, that is, to be able to distinguish between the object's stressful aspect and the object as a whole. Perhaps the Kleinian school has drawn attention more than any other to the crucial implications of this in the early object-relationships and this is complemented by the contributions of Anna Freud, Hartmann, and others in stressing the importance of the ego, its autonomous functioning, maturation and, in short, its guiding and controlling role in the individual's development. To give a simple example of how important it is for the ego to refine its perceptual functioning: a man who is furious with his car because it will not start on a cold morning needs to be able to know that he does not want to destroy the whole car but rather its 'not-starting-ness'. It is precisely this capacity which severely regressed patients, such as perverts, lose to a greater or lesser degree, so that they feel that their rage against a feature or piece of behaviour of the object threatens its total destruction.

The view of aggression which I have been proposing is, in fact, rather close to that expressed by Freud in his 'Instincts and their vicissitudes' (1915) where, in considering hate, *he* states:

> . . . the relation to *unpleasure* seems to be the sole decisive one. The ego hates, abhors and pursues with intent to destroy all objects which are the source of unpleasurable feelings for it, without taking into account whether they mean a frustration of sexual satisfaction or of the satisfaction of self-preservative needs. Indeed, it may be asserted that the true prototypes of the relation of hate are derived . . . from the ego's struggle to preserve and maintain itself.

Perhaps it is necessary to emphasize that the aim of the aggressive instinct is not the infliction of pain. Too often this is implicitly or explicitly thought to be so. for example, in an otherwise admirable paper, Brenner writes (1971):

> Aggressive aims vary with mental development and experience. They seem to be related to what hurts or frightens the child. Perhaps their close relationship to the aims of the libidinal component drives is due at least in part to the fact that the wishes connected with these sexual aims cause fear or pain, or both; the child hurts, or wants to hurt, someone else by doing to him what hurts or frightens the child himself.

I would say that Brenner is discussing sadism rather than aggression.

I have found the perspective given by regarding a threat to psychic homeostasis as the stimulus of aggression particularly useful clinically as the following example may illustrate:

At his initial interview a patient expressed great fear that his inability to control his temper would lead him to kill someone. He gave a number of illustrations of how he became 'fighting mad' and, making fists with both hands, said he would do anything I advised in order to overcome this threat to his future. The first illustration he gave was of how two men started teasing him in a public bar, commenting on the way he held his cigarette, the fact that he put his motorcar keys on the counter, the way he stood and so on. He replied in kind but kept quite calm. When he emerged a little later, he found the two of them waiting for him. They came at him and, feeling very frightened, he ran away. But after running about ten yards he had the thought 'Look what's happening to you!', whereupon he turned on his attackers in a wild rage and, in brief, assaulted them so fiercely that they both had to be taken to hospital. On another occasion, he was struck by the wing mirror of a careless driver. Before he knew what he was doing he was running after the car, calculating with a clear mind that he would reach it at the traffic lights. He did so and punched the driver in the face twice before the half-open window could be closed. He would have punched him through the window, heedless of any injury to himself, had he not calmed down. With great shame, he told me that on one recent occasion he had even punched his wife because of something she had said—something which he could not remember but which he thought implied humiliation. I shall not present any further clinical material except to mention that he was bullied by two older brothers in childhood and by older boys at school.

What stands out in this account is that it was of overriding importance to the patient that something must immediately be put right by the aggressive 'eliminating' of it and that his behaviour had a quality of panic to it. This 'something' may be considered to be any of a number of 'dangers': the blow to his self-esteem; the assault on his masculinity; his denigration to the same lowly position as he experienced with his brothers; an impulse to respond with a passive submission—no doubt further exploration in treatment would identify this; but the point relevant to the present discussion is that, whatever it might be, it constituted a serious threat to his psychic homeostasis and therefore provoked the extreme aggressive reaction he described. It is this which should initially guide the therapist in his management and approach to treatment, rather than a preoccupation with identifying the complex unconscious elements in the behaviour in question.

I would like to pursue this clarification further by distinguishing myself from those authors who consider aggression a special expression of the more fundamental instinctual drive of 'activity'; or, alternatively, those authors who consider 'activity' a derivation of the aggressive instinctual drive. For example, Spitz (1965) states:

> . . . it is rarely spelled out that the aggressive drive is not limited to hostility. Indeed, by far the largest and most important part of the aggressive drive serves as the motor of movement, of all activity, big and small, and ultimately of life itself.

Psychoanalysts like Spitz are no doubt influenced to such viewpoints by observing activities where aggression appears to be used constructively, for example, in chopping down trees to build a log-cabin or hammering away fragments of rock to form a piece of sculpture. From my theoretical position, the aggressive behaviour remains a destructive one: in the act of sculpting, the shapelessness, the irrelevant parts of the rock, the parts of the rock which stand between the sculptor and his expression of his deepest feelings, are removed, negated; in the example of the log-cabin, it is the 'homelessness' of the environment that is attacked, much like the 'not-starting-ness' of the car. Such an approach leads us to the seemingly paradoxical view that some of man's most creative activities make use of aggression; but we can recognize that this is because we almost automatically associate 'aggression' and 'destruction' with negativity and immorality.

It is these considerations which have led me to appreciate the clinical and theoretical usefulness of regarding aggression as essentially part of the ego's response to any dangers to psychic homeostasis. Amongst the most prominent of these encountered clinically are those which are ultimately experienced as threatening the survival of the Self.

Having elaborated my conception of the nature of aggression, I would now like to turn to a discussion of the core complex and the role aggression plays in it.

THE 'CORE COMPLEX'

When we treat perversions, we invariably come to recognize a particularly important complex of interrelated feelings, ideas, and attitudes. I refer to it as a *'core* complex' because the various elements that go to make it up are at the centre of the pervert's psychopathology and fundamental to it.

A major component of the core complex is a deep-seated and pervasive longing for an intense and most intimate closeness to another person, amounting to a 'merging', a 'state of oneness', a 'blissful union'. The specific versions of this longing are as varied as the individuals who express them. For example, a transvestite patient in the course of his treatment once spoke of imagining himself crawling up the birth passage and curling up snugly inside the womb; while on another occasion, when talking about the coldness and hardness of the city, he expressed his longing to be back in the country, 'at one with the earth and the grass and the trees, part of Mother Nature' (Glasser 1979b). This longed-for state implies complete gratification with absolute security against any dangers of deprivation or obliteration and, as will be seen later, a totally reliable containment of any destructive feelings towards the object.

Such longings are, of course, by no means indicative of psychopathology; on the contrary, they are a component of the most normal of loving desires. However, in the pervert it persists pervasively in this most primitive form even when later developmental stages modify its manifest appearance. Such 'merging' for him does not have the character of a temporary state from which he will emerge: he feels it carries with it a *permanent* loss of self, a disappearance of his existence as a separate, independent individual into the object, like being drawn into a 'black hole' of space. There are individual variations depending on the particular vicissitudes of the aggressive and libidinal elements involved: one patient may conceive of it as his passively merging into the object, another as being engulfed by the object, another as forcefully getting into the object or being intruded into by the object, and so on. But in one way or another the ultimate result is seen as his being taken over totally by the object so that his anxiety is of total annihilation. This wish to merge and the consequent 'annihilation anxiety' invariably comes into the transference—for example, as a fear of being 'brainwashed' by the analyst, or as intensely claustrophobic feelings in the consulting room.

Among the defensive reactions provoked by this 'annihilatory anxiety' is the obvious one of flight from the object, retreating emotionally to a 'safe distance' (i.e., essentially, a narcissistic withdrawal). This is expressed in such attitudes as placing a premium on independence and self-sufficiency. In therapy, it may be encountered as a wish to terminate treatment, as a constant argumentativeness or negativism, as the development of an intellectual detachment, and so on.

However, this 'flight to a safe distance' inevitably brings with it a situation of total emotional isolation with its attendant feelings of complete deprivation, abandonment, misery, and the low self-esteem consequent on the absence of narcissistic supplies. Furthermore, the only focus for the aggression initially directed towards the annihilating object is the self. These extremely painful affects (which in my experience are the commonest reasons for the pervert seeking treatment) prompt longings for a securely permanent, complete, indissoluble union with the object. We can thus observe that this aspect of the core complex has the quality of a vicious circle.

The emotional attitudes and fantasies I have described may well put one in mind of the 'symbiosis' and 'separation–individuation' stages of infant development (Mahler 1968) and since these stages are part of normal development it may be considered that I am not identifying anything specific to the pervert. I shal be taking up the discussion of the more specific factors later but at this juncture I would point out that the pervert differs from less severely disturbed individuals in that his core complex is fixated at these very early developmental stages. To envisage closeness and intimacy as annihilating, or separateness and independence as desolate isolation, indicates the persistence of a primitive level of functioning. What I have been referring to as the 'object' in my description of the core complex is thus ultimately the individual's mother (or the person who functioned in that capacity) during this early period of development.

Most workers in the field in recent times identify this early period as critical to the development of perversions, also laying stress on the impulses towards merging or primary identification with, and separation and individuation from, the mother, as well as the influence of introjective-projective mechanisms, (see, among others, Bak 1956, 1968; Chasseguet-Smirgel 1974; A. Freud 1968; Greenacre 1968; Khan 1962; Limentani 1989; McDougall 1970; Socarides 1973; Stoller 1976). There is less agreement over what particular factor or factors determine the establishment of a perversion rather than other equally disturbed forms of psychopathology. I believe important light is thrown on this problem by considering the role aggression plays in the core complex.

THE PART PLAYED BY AGGRESSION IN THE CORE COMPLEX

Aggression is an integral feature of the core complex. Earlier I described how the intense need for the mother mounts to a wish to merge with her and how this carries the implicit concomitant of a loss of a separate existence as an individual—'annihilation'. It will now be readily appreciated that this serious threat to psychic survival—ultimately psychic homeostasis—will provoke an intense aggressive reaction on the part of the ego aimed at the preservation of the self and the destruction of the mother. Such a destruction, however, would bring about complete negation of the mother and consequently all the gratification and stable security that would be achieved by merging with her.

With the limited resources the ego has at its disposal at this early stage of development, its efforts to deal with these conflicting considerations are inevitably crude and in the adult patient we can observe how inadequate these are. Thus, the ego may split its affective impulses towards the mother, attempting to deal with the aggressive component by denial. Often this aggressive component is then projected on to the mother so that *she* is experienced as threatening destruction.

Another way in which the ego attempts to deal with the aggression is to split the internal representation of the object, so that it retains the loving relationship with one part of the object and is aggressive to the other part. Again it requires later development to sustain this position—for example, by displacing the aggressive feelings on to another person, such as the father (see below; also see McDougall 1970 and Chapter 10). In this early period the only direction in which the ego can displace the split-off aggression is on to the self and frequently this is done onto the individual's own body: what may be termed 'somatic displacement'. There it is felt to be safely contained. It is because of this primitive vicissitude of aggression that the pervert is able to treat his bodily contents not only as vehicles for the expression of affects (most obviously in perversions involving urine and faeces) but also as objects. This basic mechanism of 'somatic displacement' is used in the establishment of hypochondria and psychosomatic conditions, so frequently found in the perversions.

The danger of 'abandonment' brought on by the need to destroy the engulfing, intrusive mother as much as by the wish to withdraw from her, will generally be dealt with by mechanisms which work towards enabling the re-establishment of contact with her; and the aggression will be focused on such factors as interfere with this aim. Some of the clinical features will be a result of these considerations. I have already discussed how the ego may seek to contain the aggresive intentions towards the mother by 'somatic displacement'. But it will also turn the aggression upon itself if other mechanisms seeking to re-establish contact with the mother are hampered by counter-considerations of the ego. For example, it may inhibit or negate its function of perceiving affects: the patient experiences a generalized 'numbness' so that there is no recognition of either missing the mother or wishing to destroy her. Such a 'numbness' is not the same as a developmentally later capacity to repress affects, being much more gross and generalized and amounting almost to a body-state. Suicide may be seen as an ultimate expression of such processes. If the internalized aggression is sufficiently intense it may run amok, so to speak, and be directed in crude, gross ways at the ego's basic functions—perception, synthesis, and so on—much as an animal bites at its painfully wounded leg. I am, of course, alluding to the development of a psychotic, disintegrative breakdown (see Glover 1964).

It should be appreciated that the dynamics I have been discussing are solely in terms of a two-person relationship. As I shall consider below (p. 291), the third person, ordinarily the father, is not involved. The vicissitudes of the core complex will naturally be influenced by the way the mother relates to her infant and I shall take this up more fully shortly. At this point I should simply like to put the reader in mind of the obvious ways in which the mother's attitudes and behaviour may disturb the psychic homeostasis of the infant and thus provoke further aggression, that is, by negligence or rejection on the one hand and by over-attentiveness and 'smothering' on the other (see Jacobson 1965).

The mental state of the infant in this core complex situation is far from placid and settled: it can be seen to be largely chaotic, fragmented, unintegrated, and threatening a profound disruption of psychic homeostasis. This state is not, however, unique to the perversions; in fact, I have come to consider it as a regular ingredient of normal infantile development. These features may thus be observed in the more severely disturbed conditions but what I am about to discuss *is* specific to the perversions and accounts, to an important extent, for the 'choice' of psychopathology—that is, why it is that the individual developed a perversion rather than some other form of disturbance.

THE ESTABLISHMENT OF THE SPECIFIC PREDISPOSITION TO PERVERSIONS

In the perversions, then, the ego attempts to resolve the vicious circle of the core complex and the attendant conflicts and dangers which I have indicated by the widespread use of *sexualization*. Crucially, aggression is converted into sadism. The immediate consequence of this is the preservation of the mother, who is no longer threatened by total destruction, and the ensuring of the viability of the relationship to her. The intention to destroy is converted into a wish to hurt and control. Henceforth, the (future) pervert is able to engage with the object to a varying degree of intensity but invariably in sadomasochistic terms. This keeps the object at a 'safe distance'—a distance which precludes trust and intimacy. Sexualization also acts as a binding, organizing force in the internal state of affairs, enabling defensive measures to be more effective and a certain stability to come about.

It is only when this process breaks down that sadism may revert to aggression. One can envisage a continuum starting at the one end with ordinary social teasing and moving via the cat-and-dog, sado-masochistic relationships which characterize some couples, to the perversion of frank sado-masochism; this in turn shades into sexual assault such as rape, moving through crimes of violence to homicide, which is the other extreme of the continuum. Quantitatively, sexuality is inversely present from one end of the continuum to the other with the appreciation of the object as a person decreasing in the process. When one works psychotherapeutically, as I do, with both delinquents and sexual deviants, one may, in some instances, actually observe the process of sexualization taking place before one's eyes, so to speak, in the course of the treatment. It was a characteristic of a burglar I treated that at certain times he would impulsively run amok in a house he was in the process of burgling: he would pull out all the contents of cupboards and drawers, rip clothing to pieces, slash cushions, hurl pieces of furniture about the room, and run through the rooms throwing flour, sugar, eggs, and other such things wherever he went. Finally he would leave the house without taking any of its valuables.

The analysis of his house-breaking revealed that the main motives involved were those of the core complex (illustrating, by the way, a development other than the creation of a perversion). We learnt through psychotherapeutic exploration that he would burgle at times when he felt particularly lonely. Entering the house represented entering his mother's body, and taking its valuables signified forcibly acquiring her precious love of which she had been so ungiving in his childhood. At the times he ran amok, some feature (such as an item of women's underwear) would have aroused his anger and his fear of being engulfed. His vandalizing behaviour was thus an expression of rage and panic in oral and anal terms, and his leaving the house reassured him he could escape being engulfed. At such times it was important not to take anything from the house since it would represent a claim of his mother on him. But what is of particular relevance to the present discussion is that, at the point in an extended treatment when he lost all desire to burgle, he started exposing himself indecently. This subsided with further therapeutic work when he established a satisfactory relationship with a woman whom he subsequently married.

With the contribution of other mental mechanisms, a more structured situation may be achieved, so that not only is there no evidence of aggression but even the sadism may not be immediately discernible. The favourite masturbation fantasy of a homosexual patient was to picture his lover sitting on a lavatory with himself astride his lap facing him and their both defecating and urinating. Bearing in mind the aggressive meanings which can be attributed by the ego to excretion, as well as the ejective significance such activities may have, it can be seen from this brief clinical example how sexualization protects the object from the aggression of the core complex and preserves the relationship. In this instance, the sadism is not evident—it is safely deposited in the lavatory bowl and flushed away.

It is important to recognize that very often a crucial component in sadistic pleasure is the implication that the object is experiencing what the individual wants him/her to experience. This is reassuring in a number of ways. It removes the sense of uncertainty as to what the object may be feeling: this uncertainty is a significant element in the relationship with the mother, as I shall discuss below. It also conveys the sense of both participants being absorbed in the same affective situation: this approaches the longed-for merging with the object but contains the safeguard against loss of self in the process. It is for these reasons that it is so often a condition of the sadist that the object does not wish to suffer—often a masochist is of no interest to the sadist. The sadist's fantasy often requires that the object does not wish to participate in the sexual experience and is actually antipathetic to it, but because of the overriding power or influence of the sadist, the object is carried away despite him- or herself and ultimately participates passionately in the experience. The exhibitionist, for example, prefers to observe an initial expression of shock or disgust on the face of the woman to whom he exposes himself, and he may even be aware of a vicious quality to his affects at the time, but then, in his fantasy, she is overcome by the sight of his penis and comes to give herself to him enthusiastically. A further illustration of this is the homosexual paedophile who preferred to carry out acts of anal intercourse on young adolescent boys who had not experienced this before. It was important to him that they should feel his penetration as painful and struggle to free themselves but then find themselves beginning to enjoy the experience sexually and eventually delight in it and want to repeat it. When he met mature homosexuals who would happily offer themselves for anal intercourse he was quite uninterested. An important element in this 'seduction' of the object is that it implies that there is no doubt that he is intensely wanted by the object but at the same time he controls the object's want and his own passions (as he often demonstrates to himself by 'coitus reservatus' and other such actions). Thus, through sexualization, all the disturbing components of the core complex are dealth with: the aggression no longer threatens destruction and loss and the dangers of both annihilation and abandonment are apparently averted. A further significance in the sadistic interplay with the object is that of revenge, basically on the mother. This is fully discussed by Stoller 1976 (see also Chapter 5).

I would like to make it clear that I do not consider that such sexualization of aggression results in the neutralization of the instinctual drives involved. I find myself unable to agree with those authors who seem to regard aggression and libido as 'equal but opposite', rather like acid and alkali, so that if they are mixed in suitable proportions they produce a 'neutral solution'. One can argue, for example, that the opposite of love is indifference rather than hate. This faulty approach is the result of allowing theoretical constructs to be applied too remotely from the clinical or behavioural phenomena they were set up to explain. It is also a clear implication of the viewpoint I have been elaborating that I do not regard sadism as part of the sexual drive, as Freud did and as many contemporary analysts still do (e.g. Gero 1962). Undoubtedly the anal-sadistic stage is an integral part of normal psychological development, but to deem that a different sort of libido is involved is as misleading as maintaining that a different sort of libido is involved in homosexuality as opposed to transvestitism, as opposed to fetishism, as opposed to heterosexuality.

In the perversions, no psychic institution or function is free from being libidinized. The functions of the ego may undergo this fate. This may be observed most frequently in those ego-functions which are employed to make the earliest contact with the object. I must make it clear that I am not here referring to how the ego-function may subserve a perverse sexual aim, such as the importance of smell in fetishism or looking in voyeurism; it is the actual ego-function itself that becomes sexualized. For example, a patient developed eye symptoms which eventually came to be understood as the result of the activity of looking being sexualized: it had the unconscious meanings of phallic intrusion into the object (as conveyed by such phrases as 'a penetrating gaze', 'a piercing look'), and of visual incorporation ('taking things in through one's eyes'). Needless to say, looking was a central feature of his perversion which, interestingly, was not voyeurism. Here the basic features of the core complex—being taken into the object, aggressive intrusion, and so on—found expression in an ego-function through its sexualization.

I would now like to indicate briefly what part the mother plays in the vicissitudes of aggression in the context of the core complex. Frequently, we have no objective information to corroborate the patients' depiction of their mothers, but one characteristic features so consistently in the accounts perverts give that one is safe to assume their veracity. This is that she has a markedly narcissistic character and relates to her child in narcissistic terms. To varying degrees with different patients, she is seen both to use her child as a means of gratification of her own needs and to fail to recognize the child's emotional needs. She is both over-attentive and neglectful and thus disturbs his psychic homeostasis in both ways. Her narcissistic over-attentiveness, in treating him as part of herself, reinforces his annihilatory anxieties and intensifies his aggression towards her and his need to get away from her. Her neglect, emotional self-absorption, and insensitivity to her child's needs will both frustrate him and arouse abandonment anxieties and again intensify his aggression towards her.

It may well be that the child's coming to deal with his aggression through sexualization is induced by his mother. There are many patients whose history contains accounts of manifest sexual stimulation of the child by his mother, this sometimes even extending into his adolescence: one patient will mention that his aunt told him how his mother used to play with his penis to stop him from crying; another will recall how, even at school-going age, he used to lie in bed with his mother fondling her bare breasts; another will mention in passing that his mother still bathes him at the age of 22. Even when the mother's sexual behaviour is less manifest, there is often the implication that the patient found his mother seductive. Many authors report such a finding. McDougall (1972) comments that 'complicity and seductiveness are attributed to the mother' and Bak (1968) describes the mother's seductiveness as being of a specific form: 'The boy is made to feel he is not only preferred, but closer to the mother through a bond of identity . . . In several instances the patients were close to the realization of incest'. Rosen (personal communication) stated that his clinical findings were similar and expressed his view that the crucial factor was that while the mother was particularly seductive, she never fulfilled her promise.

However, Limentani (1976) draws our attention to the fact that such findings are not invariable when he states: 'In my own experience the mothers of bisexuals who have come to my attention were not seductive mothers, as we often meet in the case of homosexuals'. Indeed, the whole matter is put in doubt by patients' accounts which present their mothers as emotionally remote and they state that they are unable to remember ever being cuddled or embraced or in any way experiencing a physical communication of warmth from their mothers. But such mothers are not physically inattentive; on the contrary, one invariably finds evidence of a definite involvement with their son's bodies so that one is led to consider whether a special bodily cathexis, or an unconscious communication of sexuality, does not pave the way to the utilization of sexuality even in such cases.

However attentive the mother is, she is inconsistent and, as mentioned above, often even 'teasing'. This in itself promotes both the anxiety of uncertainty and aggression and can be seen as an important determinant of the subsequent sadistic need to control the object and determine exactly how she feels and responds. In fact, in those patients with whom I have had the opportunity to study their early relationship to their mothers in detail, I have always found this to be predominantly sado-masochistic. Furthermore, I have not encountered clinically a true pervert who has not had a close relationship with his mother (or an adequate substitute). The more distant the relationship the more likely is the sadism to be predominantly physically aggressive. Those patients who have had a motherless childhood, having been brought up in institutions or passed from one foster-mother to another without the opportunity to form any relationships in depth, invariably have a markedly disturbed sexuality which is either severely inhibited or involves viciously sadistic fantasies or behaviour showing little or no concern for the object. In my opinion such patients are generally not perverts but borderline or psychotic individuals manifesting a deviant sexuality. This may be recognized in their lacking the cohesion and integration of the pervert's make up and in the impermanence of their form of sexual deviance, which now takes this form and now that.

I have elaborated on how the core complex occurs in the development of other conditions including, in fact, normality; and that what is specific to the perversions is the 'solution' found to the insoluble conflicting needs of the core complex, that is, the fundamental and widespread use of sexualization. In addition, a salient factor is the relative absence of the father, as mentioned above (see p. 286). At times, the pertaining circumstances lead him to be geographically absent but more often the history of the pervert includes the feature of the father being *emotionally* absent or peripheral. The father is thus not available to be utilized as an object with whom to identify or on to whom aggression and other feelings may be displaced. In the case of the future pervert, the core complex is thus essentially experienced and worked through in the dyadic context of mother and child.

Before concluding this section, I would like to discuss briefly the problem of masochism as a perversion. This may be discussed from many points of view (Freud 1924; Loewenstein 1957; Berliner 1958; Lihn 1971; de M'Uzan 1973); my comments are restricted to some aspects of the relation of masochism to the core complex. I think I can best convey my understanding of the role of masochism in this context by quoting a remark a female patient made when referring to the masochistic stories she read in her late teens, involving such events as a woman being raped by a group of conquering soldiers. 'Now I can only feel: Thank God she survived', she commented, 'but then I found it very exciting'. Sexualization preventing destruction again appears as the basic principle.

It will be remembered that one of the consequences of the withdrawal dynamic of the core complex is the turning on to the self of the aggression initially directed towards the annihilating object. This too is sexualized and thus converted into masochism. The object is retrieved and engaged with by what we may call a 'masochistic invitation' way of relating. Thus the 'seduction of the aggressor' (Loewenstein 1957) is based on the preliminary process of sexualization of the aggression directed towards the self.

It should be recognized that the masochist gives himself a sense of control of what transpires (as is most vividly illustrated in the 1973 paper by de M'Uzan). He is the master of operations, determining—often to the finest degree—in what way he will suffer in the role of the victim. A masochistic patient gave me an account of his encounters with a prostitute whom he would visit once every eight weeks. For the whole of the day he would play the role of the prostitute's servant, cleaning out her flat from top to bottom, cooking her food, running her bath, addressing her deferentially, and so on. At the end of the day, she would go on a walk of inspection of the flat and note any faults or oversights in his work—a trace of dust here, a fingermark there, an object not in place—and add these to the list of shortcomings he had displayed during the day. She would then make him stand submissively before her, reprimand him very sternly, and give him a cut on the hand with a cane for every fault found. Sometimes instead of this she would order him to stand in the corner with his trousers about his ankles and, after making him wait for some time, she would cane him on his bare bottom.

We can see that by-and-large he could determine what punishment he received. He could also be reassured that in this acted-out way his aggressive impulses were totally controlled, every fault being strictly noted and punished (thus, incidentally, giving externalized expression to his relationship to his super-ego, as discussed on p. 294).

At the same time, he could feel he could control when he came and went, that is the basic issue of moving towards or away from the object, in this way reassuring himself against both the annihilation and abandonment anxieties. It was relevant that while he was with the prostitute he would experience no sexual arousal whatsoever: only afterwards when he was at home would he masturbate with the memory of the day's events in mind—that is, when giving free expression to his passion did not carry the danger of his losing control of the situation in her presence and thus ensuring that he would not be engulfed by her. Studies of masochists bear out that they insist on laying down the conditions of their 'helpless suffering' most precisely. As Loewenstein states (1957): 'Masochists seek only certain specific and individually variable forms of suffering and humiliation. As soon as these reach greater intensity or take a different form, they are reacted to with the habitual fear and pain'.

Earlier (p. 291) I discussed how the pervert sexualizes the aggression which was turned inwards as a result of the narcissistic withdrawal from the object because of fear of annihilation and how this contributed to the individual's masochism. Now we can consider how the individual seeks to retain the object via masochism. At one and the same time, he makes the aggression in both himself and the object innocuous. By means of masochism it seems indisputably established that he is not attacking the object, which is therefore secured against destruction. At the same time, masochism prevents the danger of abandonment: 'it attenuates her anger into domination precluding desertion' (Loewenstein 1957). In addition, as I mentioned above in referring to the 'masochistic invitation', the masochist playing on the sadism of the object draws the object into an engagement with him/her. It should be added that in the actuality of such engagements the role of both participants should be characterized as sado-masochistic since they are invariably both sadistic and masochistic in relation to each other. These features are well-illustrated in the account of the masochist patient just described.

From the preceding discussion it can be seen that there is always an element of deception in masochism, always an arrogant contempt and assertion of control hidden behind the humiliation and submission. Extrapolating from this, one is led to recognize that there is always an element of deception in any perversion since, for the reasons I have elaborated, sado-masochism is so ubiquitous a feature in the perversions.

This is certainly substantiated by clinical experience and the therapist must be careful to watch out for it. One of the main areas in which such deception occurs is in relation to the super-ego and this is expressed in the transference. The fundamental motive for this deception is to ensure survival in terms of the core complex as the following section will elaborate.

AGGRESSION AND THE SUPER-EGO IN THE PERVERSIONS

In the perversions, the core complex dynamics are, of course, prominent in the *internal* object relations. This is particularly observable in the relationship of the pervert to his super-ego; and the part aggression plays in this is a crucial feature.

As do most psychoanalysts (see, for example, Goodman 1965), I would agree with Hartman and Loewenstein (1962) when they say that they consider the superego . . . as *one* system of personality . . . [and] . . . would not . . . consider the ego ideal as a separate system; that 'the connections between the ego ideal and the prohibitive aspects of the superego are so close that both should be considered as aspects of one and the same system.' Nevertheless, I have found that in practice, both clinically and conceptually it has been helpful to include in my considerations an approach advocated by authors like Lampl de Groot (1947), Novey (1955), and Piers and Singer (1953), that is, as I have stated elsewhere (Glasser 1978), I

> fairly firmly divide the super-ego functions into two sets. The first brings together those functions which are concerned with moral and ethical restrictions and prohibitions governing the individual's internal and external behaviour—the laying down of boundaries. Transgression of these boundaries is associated with a sense of guilt, wickedness, sin, feelings of remorse, and so on. This roughly corresponds to the superego-as-conscience and . . . [may be referred to] . . . as the *proscriptive superego*. The second set of functions are concerned with standards and goals of behaviour, the laying down of ideals and the making of demands of attainment for which the individual should strive. Failure in these respects is associated with such feelings as shame, inadequacy, low self-esteem, worthlessness and self-contempt, self-disdain or self-ridicule. This corresponds to the superego-as-ego-ideal . . . [and may be referred to] . . . as the *prescriptive* superego."

I consider it a quite inadequate account of the super-ego when authors such as Hartman and Loewenstein (1962) follow Freud (1923) and say 'it seems preferable to reserve the term superego . . . to that momentous step in structuralization which is linked with the resolution of the conflicts of the oedipal phase'. It simply does not comply with clinical experience (particularly in the transference) that the super-ego is: (a) solely the internalized father of the positive Oedipus complex and, rather as an afterthought, the internalized mother of the negative Oedipus complex; and (b) solely determined by castration anxiety. Rather, it must be regarded as the internalized aggregate of those aspects of relationships encountered in the individual's history which are to be characterized by the proscriptive and prescriptive constraints discussed above. The nature of these would of course change with the different developmental stages, as well as the individual's developing cognitive abilities, social interactions, and so on. The establishment of the super-ego is not complete until after the individual has passed through adolescence and I would maintain that the key feature of the mature super-ego is that it no longer exists as an internal object but is an integral part of the self which has become abstract and conceptual. Needless to say this is an end-point which none of us achieve entirely so that we share with those suffering from psychic pathology and therefore developmental fixations, relations with prohibitive and demanding internal objects.

If on no other grounds, these considerations point to how the perversions are psychopathological conditions. Their super-egos, to a substantial extent, do not achieve that abstract quality which is indicative of psychological maturity; that is to say, their super-egos feature predominantly as internal objects with whom they have an intense relationship. Furthermore, in examining the contributants to 'the internalized aggregate' of the super-ego of the pervert we find that these are preponderately the result of the introjection of the relevant *maternal* features with introjections of features of the father playing a much less influential role than is the case in the neurotic or normal individual.

A further indicator of the psychopathology of the perversions is that the relationship to the super-ego is conducted primarily in core complex terms. Thus, for example, harmony with the super-ego is regarded as an annihilatory merging, and must therefore be resisted. In pursuit of internal homeostasis, the pervert is constantly engaged in a sadomasochistic battle with his super-ego which leaves him with no peace.

He comes nearest to expressing frank aggression in his defiance of the proscriptive super-ego, often expressed towards external authority. Thus, a paedophilic patient, used to revel in detailed fantasies of carrying out acts of severe torture on his strict and rather sadistic manager at his place of work. These fantasies would sometimes involve open homicide—sanctioned by being in the service of justice: for example, transforming, in his fantasy, his manager into a dictator whom he would assassinate. This defiance of the proscriptive super-ego frequently takes a more hidden form expressed in subversive fantasies or activities aimed at undermining or destroying relevant figures in authority.

Such ingredients can often be seen to play a part in crimes, particularly sexual crimes. Careful exploration of the dynamics of the offence will reveal that the pleasure comes as much, if not more, from the excitement of defying the prohibitions as from the sexual acts themselves. Criminals know this 'dicing-with-death' thrill very well, even having a term for it, namely 'the adrenalin factor'. The excitement comes from the life-risking challenge to and imagined conquest of the omnipotent super-ego by demonstrating their own omnipotence (that is, essentially a manic denial). An exhibitionist patient, for example, said that, in his affair with a married woman, the greatest excitement he obtained was from the forbidden aspect of the sexual activity and the risk of being found out, rather than from the activity itself (Glasser 1978). A paedophile commented that what lent his activities a special kick was his knowledge that he was doing something so universally and intensely forbidden.

The opposition to the prescriptive demands of the super-ego characteristically takes the form of passive resistance with consequent feelings of inadequacy and low self-esteem. The characteristic under-functioning of the exhibitionist (Rooth 1971), for example, can be understood in this light. Thus, such a patient at the start of his psychotherapy had remained at the lowest position in the hierarchy of his place of work despite the fact that the work was well within his capabilities and his having an above-average intelligence (with a measured IQ of 120). He spoke shamefully of his lowly status and almost visibly squirmed at the contemptuous opinion he had of himself—and at what he believed others thought of him. (This well illustrates the sado-masochistic relationship between the pervert and his prescriptive super-ego.) It is relevant to note that he would report how irritated his senior would become with him over the mistakes he made. Needless to say this feature came into the transference and proved a most obdurate resistance. Nevertheless, he could gradually free himself of it so that at the time his treatment ended he was the head of his department.

We may now appreciate the importance to the pervert of his deceiving the super-ego: in both the proscriptive and prescriptive contexts deception is a covert way of attacking the super-ego. By protesting that it is regrettably beyond his capacities to carry out the demands of the prescriptive super-ego he 'innocently' forces it into a state of impotence. Similarly, his covert subversive acts defy the super-ego's prohibitions—a state of affairs which, expressed in the transference, may raise substantial therapeutic problems (particularly since the patient is mostly not conscious of these motives). The patient may say that he cannot report what he is thinking because there is nothing in his mind and as much as he tries he is simply unable to succeed. Or he may dutifully say whatever comes into his mind and report a series of incoherent thoughts and images of which the analyst cannot make head or tail. These deceptive engagements are clearly essentially sado-masochistic in nature, and one can identify their ultimately defensive function—a defence against the core complex danger of annihilation by the super-ego.

Perhaps the most vivid illustration of the sadomasochistic relationship of the pervert to his super-ego is seen in the child sexual abuser. As I stated elsewhere (Glasser 1988):

> It never fails to impress me how intense and desperate is the pervert's struggle with his superego. From the perspective of regarding his relationship with social morality as a reflection of his relationship to his internal morality, this is no more forcefully illustrated than by the paedophile who arouses the most extreme and universal condemnation, even to the extent of his needing to be isolated in prisons for his own safety.

This relationship to his super-ego may be illustrated in the following clinical material of a paedophile. In the session he referred to his strong attraction to two young boys he had seen at a swimming pool and went on to talk about how he despised this paedophilic part of himself. 'At the same time', he continued, 'it is a part of myself I am not prepared to hand over to you or anybody else. My attraction is very alive and a central part of my being: not to look [at the boys] is not to live'. I pointed out how he characterized me, the person he had come to for help, as seeking to induce him to hand himself over to me so that I could mould him to my moral requirements. He also experienced me as remote, hostile, and unable to understand his feelings. This led him to recall a dream he had had the previous night:

> He was driving his car to his execution—by hanging. There was nothing he could do about it, he just had to accept it. He thought of the pain of the rope and of his neck breaking. He was desperate to escape but knew he couldn't. He had a vague impression of the hangman coming from behind him to put the noose about his neck.

The only aspect of this dream that I would like to take up is the obvious way in which I, the analyst sitting behind him, had been constructed to be experienced as condemning of his paedophilia (which he regarded as an essential ingredient of his separate self) to the point of executing him—that is, the analyst is an externalized version of the remorseless, merciless and murderously aggressive authority that is his super-ego.

His relationship to his super-ego was generally and persistently sado-masochistic as was clearly reflected in his masturbation fantasies. These involved violent, ruthless spanking, and vicious anal intercourse, either with his being the passive recipient of these activities carried out by older men (that is, with him featuring essentially as 'the boy') or with him being the active perpetrator of these activities on young boys. In talking about these masturbation fantasies he mentioned that they *always* contained a component of corporal punishment. In fact, he said, this component was indispensible.

The men who featured as punishing him, the boy, always had the uniform of authority in a setting involving discipline such as the army or the navy or school. The spanking could often be provoked by a minor transgression—such as having a button of the army uniform undone, or coming back late from leave to the barracks or boarding school. In a number of sessions he recalled how it was his mother who administered punishment for his childhood transgressions, by slapping him on his bottom or spanking him with a wooden spoon.

Recognizing the role of aggression in the core complex helps us to understand more fully how it comes about that the development of the super-ego leads to the establishment of a channel whereby aggression can be directed against the self (Freud 1923, 1930, 1933; and others, such as Hartmann and Loewenstein 1962; Spitz 1953). The observed clinical facts are that patients can suffer greatly from the attack on themselves through feelings of guilt and shame (i.e., attacks from their super-egos). Freud understood this to come about through the internalization of the castrating, punitive oedipal father, as well as the instinctual defusion that occurs with identification (Freud 1923). But considering our clinical observations carefully we recognize that it is in the form of *sadism* that aggression is turned onto the self. In the pervert what is internalized is the sado-masochistic relationships to both the parental figures—predominantly the mother, as discussed above.

It should be recognized that it is generally rare to observe that aggressive (as opposed to sadistic) attacks on the self stem from the super-ego: rather they can be recognized to be the ego's responding to an aspect of the self which it considers to be a threat to its survival, this response thus being negating in intention. This dangerous aspect may be an internal object, including amongst others the super-ego (in which case the suicide is, psychologically, homicide) or an abhorrent quality. To be distinguished from this are the severe writhings of self-condemnation in the depressive, which can be seen to be essentially sadomasochistic, as careful study of 'Mourning and melancholia' (Freud 1917) bears out: the super-ego's criticism or condemnation is observably remorselessly cruel and with the masochistic co-operation of the self, causes extreme suffering. It is impressive to observe how the depressive, who is suffering so severely, resists any efforts to relieve him of his self-condemnatory suffering by reasoning, comforting, cajoling, or any other such attempts. And his covert sadism can be seen in how much the depressive makes those about him suffer. Thus it is doubtful that the suffering in itself leads to suicide. It is only when the sadism breaks down to release the underlying aggression that suicide takes place; the differentiation between attempted and successful suicide depends on whether aggression or sadism are the operative, driving forces.

This state of affairs is certainly characteristic of the perversions where feelings of guilt, self-condemnation, shame, self-contempt, and low self-esteem are intense.

Frequently this does not appear to be the case, so that, for example, the paedophile will show himself to be quite untroubled over the consequences of his abuse on his victims. Psychotherapeutic exploration reveals this to be the result of the intensive use of defence mechanisms, such as manic denial to cope with the extremely painful sadistic assaults of the characteristically severe, ruthless, and inflexible super-ego. These manoeuvres may be so extensive that he may even claim that his acts are benevolent and actually beneficial (see, for example, Brongersma 1984; Wilson and Cox 1983). It is only after substantial interpretive work that he will come to acknowledge and experience his intense guilt and shame.

It will thus be seen that, driven by the core complex dynamics, a consequence of the opposition to the super-ego is a much lowered sense of self-esteem and other evidence of narcissistic depletion. (For a fuller discussion of this aspect of the perversions, see Rosen, Chapter 3.)

CONCLUDING REMARKS

True perversions are complex mental structures involving the whole of the personality. As such, their ultimate form is shaped by the different stages of development that the individual must pass through, as well as by particular experiences. Consequently, individuals cannot be diagnosed as suffering from a true perversion until they have passed through adolescence, only after which the structure of their psychopathology is firmly established. In each of the stages, development will be influenced by the particular way the conflicting needs of the core complex are resolved (for an elaboration of this see Glasser 1979*a*).

I have made little mention of perversions in females because, although the early core complex development is the same for both sexes, the later developmental paths diverge. The whole question of perverse sexuality in females is an unclear one and is too extensive to be taken up here. (See Chapter 10.)

It is the nature of mental functioning that no element can be discussed in isolation without distorting it: it acquires a different character with different implications according to the context in which it is being considered. I have placed my discussion in the interrelated dimensions of the core complex and psychic homeostasis and proceeded to examine how aggression in these contexts make a fundamental contribution to the nature and structure of the perversions. Considered in this way, the perversions can be seen to serve the vital purpose of preventing the breakdown of the individual's object-relations and the psychic disintegration that would come about as a result of the unremitting demand of aggression to achieve its aim of negating the object which threatens psychic homeostasis.

REFERENCES

Bak, R. C. (1956). Aggression and perversion. In *Perversions: psychodynamics and therapy*, (ed. S. Lorand and M. Balint). Random House, New York.

Bak, R. C. (1968). The phallic woman. *Psychoanal. Study Child*, **23**, 15. International Universities Press, New York.

Berliner, B. (1958). The role of object relations in moral masochism. *Psychoanal. Quarterly*, **27**, 38.

Brongersma, E. (1984). Aggression against paedophile. *Int. J. Law Psychiat.* **7**, 79.

Brenner, C. (1971). The psychoanalytic concept of aggression. *Int. J. Psycho-Anal.* **52**, 137.

Cannon, W. B. (1929/1953). *Bodily changes in pain, hunger, fear and rage*. Charles T. Branford Company, Boston.

Cannon, W. B. (1932/1939). *The wisdom of the body*. Kegan Paul, Trench, Trubner & Co, Ltd. London.

Chasseguet-Smirgel, J. (1974). Perversion, idealization and sublimation. *Int. J. Psycho-Anal.* **55**, 349.

de M'Uzan, M. (1973). A case of masochistic perversion and an outline of a theory. *Int. J. Psycho-Anal.* **54**, 455.

Freud, A. (1968). Studies in passivity. In *Indications for child analysis*. International Universities Press [Vol IV], Aylesbury.

Freud, S. (1905/1953). Three essays on the theory of sexuality. In *Complete psychological works of Sigmund Freud*, (standard edition, Vol. 7, pp. 135–243). Hogarth Press, London.

Freud, S. (1915/1957). Instincts and their vicissitudes. In *Complete psychological works of Sigmund Freud*, (standard edition, Vol. 14, pp. 109–40). Hogarth Press, London.

Freud, S. (1917/1957). Mourning and melancholia. In *Complete psychological works of Sigmund Freud*, (standard edition, Vol. 14, pp. 239–60). Hogarth Press, London.

Freud, S. (1921/1955). Group psychology and the analysis of the ego. In *Complete psychological works of Sigmund Freud*, (standard edition, Vol. 18, pp. 67–143). Hogarth Press, London.

Freud, S. (1923/1961). The ego and the id. In *Complete psychological works of Sigmund Freud*, (standard edition, Vol. 19, pp. 12–66). Hogarth Press, London.

Freud, S. (1924/1961). The economic problem of masochism. In *Complete psychological works of Sigmund Freud*, (standard edition, Vol. 19, pp. 157–70). Hogarth Press, London.

Freud, S. (1926/1959). Inhibitions, symptoms and anxiety. In *Complete psychological works of Sigmund Freud*, (standard edition, Vol. 20, pp. 77–175). Hogarth Press, London.

Freud, S. (1930/1961). Civilization and its discontents. In *Complete psychological works of Sigmund Freud*, (standard edition, Vol. 21, pp. 59–145). Hogarth Press, London.

Freud, S. (1933/1964). New introductory lectures. In *Complete psychological works of Sigmund Freud*, (standard edition, Vol. 22, p. 5). Hogarth Press, London.

Gero, G. (1962). Sadism, masochism and aggression: their role in symptom-formation. *Psychoanal. Quarterly*, **31**, 31.

Gillespie, W. H. (1971). Aggression and instinct theory. *Int. J. Psycho-Anal.* **52**, 155.

Glasser, M. (1978). The role of the superego in exhibitionism. *Int. J. Psycho-Anal. Psychotherap.* **7**, 333. Jason Aronson, New York.

Glasser, M. (1979a). Some aspects of the role of aggression in the perversions. In *Sexual deviation*, (ed. I. Rosen) (2nd edn.), p. 278). Oxford University Press.

Glasser, M. (1979b). From the analysis of a transvestite. *Int. Rev. Psycho-Anal.*, **6**, 163.

Glasser, M. (1983). Some psychodynamic ingredients of violence. (Unpublished.) Opening paper, Portman Clinic Golden Jubilee Conference on 'Understanding Human Violence'. London, 1983.

Glasser, M. (1988). Psychodynamic aspects of paedophilia. Psychoanal. Psychother. **3**(2), 121.

Glover, E. (1964). Aggression and sado-masochism. In *The pathology and treatment of sexual deviation*, (ed. I. Rosen) Oxford University Press.

Goodman, S. (1965). Current status of the theory of the superego *J. Am. Psychoanal. Assoc.* **13**(1), 172.

Greenacre, P. (1968/1971). Perversions: considerations regarding their genetic and dynamic backgroud. In *Emotional growth*. International Universities Press, New York.

Hartmann, H. (1964). *Essays on ego psychology*. International Universities Press, New York.

Hartmann, H. and Loewenstein R. M. (1962). Notes on the superego. *Psychoanal. Study Child*, **17**, 42.

Hartmann, H., Kris E. and Loewenstein R. M. (1962). Notes on the superego. theory of aggression. *Psychoanal. Study Child*, **3**, 9.

Jacobson, E. (1964). *The self and the object world*. International Universities Press, New York.

Kahn, M. M. R. (1962). The role of polymorph-perverse body-experiences and object-relations in ego-integration. *Brit. J. Med. Psychol.* **35**, 245.

Klein, M. (1948). A contribution to the theory of anxiety and guilt. *Int. J. Psycho-Anal.* **29**, 114.

Lampl de Groot, J. (1947). On the development of the ego and the super-ego. *Int. J. Psycho-Anal.* **28**, 7.

Lihn, H. (1971). Sexual masochism: a case report. *Int. J. Psycho-Anal.* **52**, 469.

Limentani, A. (1976). Object choice and actual bisexuality. *Int. J. Psycho-Anal. Psychother.* **5**, 205.

Limentani, A. (1989). Clinical types of homosexuality. In *Between Freud and Klein*, p. 102. Free Association Books, London.

Loewenstein, R. M. (1957). A contribution to the psychoanalytic theory of masochism. *J. Am. Psychoanal. Assoc.* **5**, 197.

Lorenz, K. (1966). *On aggression*. Methuen, London.

Mahler, M. S. (1968). *On human symbiosis and the vicissitudes of individuation*. International Universities Press, New York.

McDougall, J. (1970). Homosexuality in women. In *Female sexuality: new psychoanalytic views*, (ed. J. Chasseguet-Smirgel). University of Michigan Press, Ann Arbor.

McDougall, J. (1972). Primal scene and sexual perversion. *Int. J. Psycho-Anal.* **53**, 371.

Novey, S. (1955). The role of the superego and ego-ideal in character formation. *Int. J. Psycho-Anal.* **36**, 254.

Piers, G. and Singer, M. B. (1953). *Shame and guilt*. Charles C. Thomas, Springfield, IL.

Rooth, F. G. (1971). Indecent exposure and exhibitionism. In *Contemporary psychiatry*, (ed. T. Silverstone and B. Barraclough), p. 212. Headley Brothers Limited, Ashford.

Socarides, C. W. (1973). Sexual perversion and the fear of engulfment. *Int. J. Psycho-Anal. Psychother.* **2**, 432.

Spitz, R. A. (1953). Aggression: its role in the establishment of object relations. In *Drives, affects, behaviour*, (ed. R. M. Loewenstein), p. 126. International Universities Press, New York.

Spitz, R. A. (1965). *The first year of life*. International Universities Press, New York.

Stoller, R. L. (1976). *Perversion: the erotic form of hatred*. Harvester Press, Hassocks, Sussex, UK.

Wilson, G. D. and Cox, D. N. (1983). *The child lovers*. Peter Owen, London.

13
Dynamic psychotherapy with sex-offenders

Murray Cox

INTRODUCTORY COMMENTS

Returning to a chapter written seventeen years ago is a salutary experience for an author. As it is reprinted *verbatim* in the present edition, certain introductory comments are called for. There are several matters of fact which are obviously now out of date. Since the 1979 edition the following changes have occurred. Broadmoor Hospital is now managed, not by the Department of Health and Social Security, but by the Special Hospitals Service Authority, which may become a 'purchaser' of that which a special hospital 'provides' if 'Trust status' is achieved. The Mental Health Act of 1983 has replaced that of 1959, so that restricted patients are now held under Sections 37/41, rather than 60/65, and the treatability issue with patients suffering from a psychopathic disorder has to be agreed at the point of admission. The hospital currently has approximately 500 patients, compared with the 700 of 1979.

However, these are all 'external' contextual facts. The inner world of the sex-offender patient has not changed. Neither has that of his psychotherapist, so that transference-countertransference issues are as alive as ever. King Lear's comments on 'thought-executing fires' (III, ii,4) are as relevant to sex-offenders, who are also arsonists, as they were hitherto or ever could be.

Re-engaging with his chapter, the author finds himself asking and trying to answer several challenging questions. Have recent advances in object-relations theory been matched by improvements in outcome studies of dynamic psychotherapy with sex-offenders? Where are dwindling resources best invested, when it comes to understanding and treating such patients? Knowing how difficult it is to treat sex-offenders 'successfully', is it possible to shift entrenched positions, so that both cognitive-behavioural and psychoanalytic approaches can admit that—rather than 'going it alone'—synergistic co-operation may be the way forward?

These are some of the questions posited by rereading my chapter for the third edition. Nevertheless, in addition to the fundamental challenge of endeavouring to distinguish that which has changed from that which has remained the same, there emerge three main areas which justify separate consideration in this brief introduction.

Note. The views expressed are those of the author and do not necessarily reflect those of the Special Hospitals Service Authority. Names, histories, settings, and other identifying features have been changed. Several incidents described are apocryphal, though they are based upon a corpus of experience. This camouflage does not diminish the human predicament of the disclosers and the clinical illustration they provide is not invalidated.

1. The impact of financial constraints on manpower resources

The prevailing presence of audit thrusts its interrogative impact on all workers in the field. Where are ever-diminishing resources best invested in research and clinical work for those undertaking dynamic psychotherapy with sex-offender patients? There are, and always will be, bright, politically prompted initiatives which usually receive brief headline status following 'sensitive' issues, such as re-offending, escapes, or 'high-profile' individuals. Even so, those in the know, are aware that long-term trends carry more weight that 'blips' on the screen or 'rogue' results in recidivism rates. Such insights are not new. Shakespeare, as always, is there before us:

> But shall we wear these glories for a day?
> *Or shall they last*, and we rejoice in them?
>
> (*Richard III*, iv, ii, 5. Emphasis added)

Economists, administrators, therapists, and patients are concerned to know whether rejoicing is permitted because 'these glories' last. Transient symptom relief, evanescent catharsis, and well-intentioned promises are unlikely to lead to enduring intra-psychic change and stable reciprocal object-relationships. Although money invested on sex-offender 'programmes' may have improved the quality of 'humane containment', it does not necessarily follow that such investment will have improved the capacity of the patient's psyche to contain explosive drives—particularly when they have once led to offences against the person and may well do so again if circumstances permit. The significance of the stated sequence of those who provide therapeutic facilities, or should benefit from them, is to be carefully noted. Each group has a vested interest in the 'success' of psychotherapy with sex-offenders, but it is their sequential ordering which is a certain indicator of changing times. We have just considered economists, administrators, therapists, and patients. Seventeen years ago reference would have been made to patients and therapists—in this order. Neither administrators nor economists (in that order) would have received mention, except in parenthesis or as a footnote. Except in exceptional circumstances (see below), forensic psychotherapy must not only be 'therapeutic' for patients, it must also manifestly prove its worth to those who pay the therapist. Those who sign the cheques call the tune. Paradoxically, audit is the one discipline which does not currently have to prove its worth. This attitude is likely to be reversed by our successors, who will be keen to audit audit. They will probably return to clinical priorities, where the current market-place therapeutic initiatives may engender a new and respected anti-symptom of 'therapeutic agoraphobia'. This implies cautionary doubt and even avoidance of the therapeutic market-place—which might not always be intrinsically 'therapeutic'.

Before we leave this theme, we need to explicate the inference of the sentence beginning 'except in exceptional circumstances . . .'. Reference was here being made to an unquantifiable, yet crucial, aspect of the consultant psychotherapist's work in a Special Hospital such as Broadmoor. Staff of all disciplines, at all levels, need a safe haven where nightmares, or other personal anxieties, can be safely ventilated; without receiving an indelible judgemental entry on a personal file.

> But I have words,
> That would be howl'd out in the desert air,
> Where hearing should not latch them.
>
> (*Macbeth*, iv, iii, 193)

At the other extreme of staff needs is the defensive anti-aggressive boredom, or the sheer *ennui* engendered by a case load which is far too large, intensified by the never-ending requests for more reports from those who have the authority to demand them. These comments apply just as much to senior managerial staff, who are themselves caught in the administrative web, as to those on whom the pressures are seen to focus. Society as a whole often seems particularly prone to be censorious of those who fail to treat sex-offenders 'successfully'. Public outcry against re-offending is understandably harsh and split projective identification, with both the offender and the victim, leads to the adoption of polarized, politicized positions.

It is entirely appropriate that the psychotherapist, like his professional peers, is also the subject of audit. Nevertheless, it is to be hoped that these strictures will be borne in mind. So that the time spent providing a place for the safe hearing of words that often need to be 'howl'd out . . . where hearing should not latch them' will be regarded as well spent.

2. The formal recognition of forensic psychotherapy as a discipline in its own right

It is probable that the majority of psychotherapeutic endeavours with sex-offenders now falls within the territorial preserve of the currently crystallizing discipline of forensic psychotherapy. The last few years have witnessed the establishment of the International Association for Forensic Psychotherapy (1991) which was inaugurated at a meeting in Leuven, Belgium. During the preceding year the first one-year day-release course in forensic psychotherapy was conducted at The Portman Clinic in London, under the direction of Estela Welldon. This is an emergent discipline which is just finding its feet. But, judging by the widespread interest shown by those representing several related disciplines, this confluence of interests brings Victor Hugo's words to mind: 'Mightier than an army is an idea whose time has come'. *Forensic psychotherapy* (ed. Cordess and Cox 1995) has since been published.

3. Aesthetic avenues of access to the hitherto inaccessible patient

Whereas the two preceding topics refer, for better or worse, to all those attempting to undertake dynamic psychotherapy with sex-offenders, the third reflects an increasing personal awareness of the significance of aesthetic avenues of access to the personality. It refers to a therapeutic emphasis known as the 'aeolian mode'. In collaboration with Professor Alice Theilgaard of the University of Copenhagen, I wrote *Mutative metaphors in psychotherapy: The aeolian mode* (1987). Its dynamic components are described as *poiesis*, aesthetic imperatives, and points of urgency, respectively. These ideas are further developed and applied to forensic psychotherapy in *Shakespeare as prompter: The amending imagination and the therapeutic process* (1994). Although it is of relevance to all psychotherapeutic endeavours, its strength is in establishing avenues of aesthetic access to the hitherto inaccessible patient through the use of mutative metaphors. It has a double forensic relevance. First, the very fact of *poiesis*—often defined as the calling into existence of that which was not there before—impinges directly upon therapeutic attempts with the sex-offender who presents clinically as a psychopath. Such narcissistic personalities tend to categorize stimuli into those which are ego-alien and others which are ego-syntonic. For obvious reasons, such a patient cannot habituate to that which is novel. This implies that the perennially unrehearsable response to the impingement of freshly culled mutative metaphors, which arise within the presented dynamic material, constantly keep the patient on his psychological 'toes'. The 'aeolian mode' rests on three theoretical foundations, namely, developmental psychology, neuropsychology, and phenomenological existential psychology. The presence of that which is new and remains so, through persistent *poiesis*, is in keeping with the neuropsychological work of Sokolov. In *Mutative metaphors* this process is illustrated by vignettes. They show how sex-offenders are confronted by the facilitated return of the repressed. Such an approach still falls within the wider framework of psychoanalytic psychotherapy. In other words, aesthetic access and mutative metaphors form a mode of presence intensification. This, in turn, facilitates the development of transference and its resolution.

In marked contrast to such a technique which allows contact to be made with psychopathic or personality-disordered patients, often regarded as inaccessible, the 'aeolian mode' also strengthens the possibility of empathic engagement with fragile, precarious psychotic patients who may also be sex-offenders. The mutative metaphor can be gentle, non-threatening, and enables the therapist to wait alongside the patient as presence intensification slowly augments the patient's resilience.

This is not the place to expand this approach which has proved to be of value when working with sex-offenders. It is clinically appropriate to a wide range of therapist/patient dynamic alignments and modes of clinical contact.

There is an ironic psychodynamic connotational relevance to the phrase 'achieving Trust status' which is the prevailing preoccupation of hospital managers and clinicians. Many of their sex-offender patients have attempted to achieve self-esteem regulation through sexual deviation. Psychoaetiologically, lack of basic trust was the prime pathology. Their primordial failure to 'achieve trust status', in relation to their primary object-relationships, led to their presence in this chapter. Paucity of early trustworthy experience, due to an imbalance between emotional 'providers' and 'purchasers', always leads to other avenues of self-esteem regulation. Sexual deviation is one of them and sex-offences may ensue (Rosen 1964; see Chapter 3.)—'The wheel is come full circle' (*King Lear*, v, iii, 175).

INTRODUCTION[1]

This chapter has a readily discernible, though heterodox, structure and its content is based on the clinical experience of working with a wide variety of sex-offenders in many settings. After defining 'dynamic psychotherapy' and 'sex-offender', there is an

---

[1] The remainder of this chapter is based on lectures given in Helsinki, 1974, at the invitation of the Finnish Psychiatric Association.

extended section on psychopathology. This is followed by a discussion of the setting and timing of the therapeutic alliance established between the sex-offender and the therapist. Setting and timing are inextricably involved with theoretical considerations which, in turn, underpin the indications for various therapeutic strategies. A rigorous structure is needed if a rambling, discursive approach is to be avoided in attempting to cover such a wide range of theoretical and practical considerations in the confines of one chapter. I hope the chapter will enable the reader to engage with its substance at the point of his need. For example, the following readers with widely differing needs may each justifiably hope to find relevant material in a chapter entitled 'Dynamic psychotherapy with sex-offenders'; the junior psychiatrist who is working for higher exams and yet has no personal forensic experience; the female probation officer counselling a rapist on parole; the psychoanalyst whose patient's sadistic fantasy is on the brink of erupting into reality, so that he fears his patient is about to become a 'sex-offender'; the experienced psychiatrist who, for the first time, is being called upon to undertake group therapy with sex-offenders either in a custodial or an outpatient setting; the general practitioner who finds that a patient, who ostensibly consulted him about organic illness, either discloses a fear of becoming a sex-offender or mentions that he has a record of such offences.

Any attempt to cover this field in one chapter necessitates the choice between a global, and inevitably superficial survey, and drastic selection with elaboration in depth of a few salient perspectives. I have chosen the second option, and hope that the discussion will act like a radiological tomogram, in which the subject is viewed from several angles, with varying degrees of penetration, so that contours and texture can be studied and a global appraisal attained.

DEFINITION

Dynamic psychotherapy

I regard dynamic psychotherapy as a process involving a professional relationship, in which the patient is enabled to do for himself what he cannot do on his own. The therapist does not do it for him, but he cannot do it without the therapist. Such therapy may be conducted on an individual or a group basis. When the group-as-a-whole forms the therapeutic unit, the group is enabled to do for itself what the group-as-a-whole could not do on its own. There is a perennial debate amongst therapists as to whether the individuals who constitute the group, or the group-as-a-whole as an irreducible entity, form the therapist's prime object of concern. This debate, although of academic interest, seems far removed from the practical world of therapeutic strategy. No therapeutic group is created *ex nihilo*, and each individual member of the group will have been referred to the psychotherapist by a general practitioner, a consultant psychiatrist, or other referral agency. Though the therapist may concentrate his attention on resistance, mobility, patterns of interaction, and corporate defensive strategies (such as scapegoating) adopted by the group-as-a-whole, he is nevertheless responsible for the individual patient who was referred to him for psychotherapy. The professional colleague who has referred a sex-offender for psychotherapy is concernred to know whether his patient is showing evidence of dynamic change, or whether his endopsychic patterning is becoming more firmly entrenched, with hardening of his defensive position. The vicissitudes of the cognitive-affective life of the group-as-a-whole is solely of peripheral interest to the 'referrer'. I cannot envisage the possibility of running a mixed group of sex-offenders (say, four rapists and four female patients) and disclaiming any concern for the progress (or regression) shown by the individual patient. If, however, the therapist ever loses sight of the group-as-a-whole, he or she runs the risk of missing phenomena which can only occur in a group matrix. These phenomena may be 'therapeutic', but can become catastrophically destructive, if they are not perceived and handled in the right way, in the right place, at the right time.

Dynamic psychotherapy can be conducted as 'pure', small-group psychotherapy on an outpatient basis. It may therefore take place within the community and be part of an interdisciplinary collaborative effort, involving the probation officer, the psychiatrist, the family doctor, the social services, and so on. It may also be part of the therapeutic programme within the confines of a total institution such as a prison, or a secure hospital, such as Broadmoor.[2] Some institutions are run solely on group lines, so that every patient is a member of a small group, a larger group (such as the ward meeting), and, frequently, a global group in which all members of the unit or the institution participate. Individual psychotherapy, group psychotherapy, mileu therapy, and the therapeutic community are all therapeutic settings in which a therapeutic alliance may be established between the psychotherapist and the patient who is a sex-offender.

The theoretical approach which I adopt rests upon both psychoanalytic and existential premises. Though this may appear to be Janusian, I find that it provides me with a coherent frame of reference affording both the rigours of psychic determinism and the flexible openness to the exigencies of the present moment, which the sex-offender demands from the therapist. In my experience, this approach is self-authenticating and is equally appropriate for the inadequate exposer on probation and for the sadistic homosexual patient, found guilty of dismembering his sexual partner.

I wish to dissociate myself from the claim that any single psychodynamic conceptual scheme can possibly have an exhaustive monopoly of clinical truth. Such complex phenomena as sex-offences are always over-determined, and personality characteristics, organic factors, modified inhibition due to drugs or fatigue, the detailed circumstances of the offence (including the specificity of the victim), together with the patient's previous life-experience, may all contribute to the patient's endopsychic patterning at the particular moment when he assaulted his victim. One brief example of an important variable in the pattern of relationships of the sex-offender is furnished by Hitchens (1972), who describes denial as 'a major theme' in the marital relationships of such patients. For this reason, it must never be assumed that dynamic psychotherapy is the only *via therapeutica* appropriate for the sex-offender. Each patient must be assessed *ab initio*, and only after the fullest possible

---

[2] The work described in this chapter would be impossible without the closest cooperation with staff colleagues at Broadmoor who refer patients, share in therapeutic work as co-therapists, assess patient's progress from many different perspectives, and, most important of all, spend long nursing hours in the life of the hospital when patients described in this chapter are *not* taking part in formal psychotherapy. Such work is possible only in a setting where the correct milieu is provided by a complex collaborative inter-disciplinary professional network. My gratitude to colleagues and patients is implicit on every page in this chapter, but it is made explicit here.

appraisal, from every conceivable angle, should a formal psychotherapeutic alliance be initiated. Physical treatments, medication, or behavioural modification (Bancroft 1976) may be appropriate, and frequently coexist alongside dynamic psychotherapy as part of a total therapeutic policy. The integration of all therpeutic energies within the life of a total institution or, in the case of the outpatient, the wider community, must not be forgotten in the subsequent discussion, which concentrates on one facet of offender-therapy. For example, the patient whose hypothyroid 'myxoedema madness' took the form of an escalating paranoid delusional system, in which a sexual assault was made on a stranger, although construed by the patient as an act of self-defence against 'the attack in his eyes', would need appropriate medical treatment to render the patient euthyroid, as well as appropriate psychotherapy. The schizophrenic may need medication, but this does not absolve the therapist from trying to understand what the patient understands and is endeavouring to express or conceal.

The sex-offender

McGrath (1976) has indicated the difficulty of defining a 'sex-offender'. The problem becomes even more complex when inner world phenomena, such as the patient's fantasy of a sexual offence which may accompany a sexually 'neutral' action, are to be encompassed in the discussion. We are here concerned with what the offence means to the patient rather than the legal definition. There is the '*overt*' sex-offence such as rape, in which the patient knew he was committing rape, his victim would be painfully aware that she was being raped, and bystanders would be fully prepared to witness on oath to what they had seen and heard. There is also the '*displaced*' sex-offence, in which the offence is correctly legally classified as, say, 'larceny of milk bottles'. However, during the course of subsequent psychotherapy, the patient eventually discloses that his prevailing fantasies at the time of the incident were of grabbing breasts, humiliating, and wounding women. Rubinstein (1965) has described sexual motivation in 'ordinary' offences. Thirdly, there is the sex-offence '*manque*' which *appears* to be identical to that described above as 'overt'. The difference is that the 'offender' is out of touch with reality, so that he is not aware that he was involved in a violent assault 'against the person'. In these circumstances psychotic ideation may protect the patient. His prevailing delusional system might include the girl he was seen to 'rape', but his social construction of reality, at the material time, was that he was an estate agent showing a prospective buyer round a new house. Finding the door a little tight, he had to force his way in and was surprised at the screams of delight with which his client enjoyed looking at the new premises.

Thus the term 'sex-offender' covers a wide range of human activity and motivation, ranging from an almost harmless and trivial deviation from a socially acceptable norm, such as the voyeur, to the extremely disturbed and disturbing homosexual killing, such as that described by Marlowe in *Edward II*.

> I know what I must do. Get you away:
> Yet be not far off; I shall need your help.
> See that in the next room I have a fire,
> And get me a spit, and let it be red-hot . . .
> (Need you anything besides?)

What else? a table and a feather-bed . . .
So now must I about this gear: ne'er was there any
So finely handled as this king shall be.
Foh, here's a place indeed with all my heart! . . .
If you mistrust me, I'll be gone, my lord.
(No, no, for if thou mean'st to murther me,
Thou wilt return again, and therefore stay.)
So, lay the table down, and stamp on it,
But not too hard, lest that you bruise his body.

(Edward II, 2480)

This detailed description so accurately conveys the jarring incompatibilities of the sadistic enjoyment of using a red-hot spit, and the bizarre gentleness of the injuction that the table should be stamped upon . . . 'But not too hard, lest that you bruise his body'. It was a body already bruised by penetration with a red-hot spit, yet it should be protected from bruising. Othello describes another killing, completely different from the homosexual sadistic murder just described, but the sexual provocation leading up to the act and Othello's comment '. . . I will kill thee, and love thee after' (*Othello*, v, ii, 28.) mean that, in the widest sense, this cannot be removed from the realm of the sex-offence. After smothering Desdemona, Othello stabs himself and falling upon her, cries 'I kiss'd thee ere I killed thee . . .' (v, ii, 358).

PSYCHOPATHOLOGY

There can be no unitary psychopathology underlying all sex-offences because of the over-determined, multicausal nature of the offence. There is no homogeneity of dynamic patterning behind the heterogenous offences 'against the person' known as sex-offences. The sex-offender is not confined to any single nosological classification. He (or she) may be appropriately diagnosed as neurotic, psychotic, psychopathic[3] or

---

[3] In this chapter, the term 'psychopath' is used to describe patients with a particular cluster of attributes, readily recognized by the clinician, although fashions in nomenclature change; for example, personality disorder, psychopath, sociopath, and sociopathic personality. However, narcissism and impoverished object-relations are core elements in the psychopathology of such patients. setting, where the safety mutual reciprocity with others, embarking upon the same risky business, can guarantee that the 'disclosure' is not 'solo'. This process is present in all group psychotherapy, wherever it is conducted, but when the patient is an offender-patient and, in particular, when he is a sex-offender, there is a snowball quality of escalation about disclosures. This means that a disclosure from one patient is frequently followed almost immediately by similar disclosures from other patients, 'I was waiting for you to start so that I could join in' . . . 'Funny, I was just going to say that'. In actual fact, the patient who was '*just* going to say that' was a reticent arsonist, terrified of making personal disclosures. But when, after 18 months in a group, another patient admitted that he was an arsonist, the certainty of not being the odd man out allowed him to say something that he had 'just' been going to say! Examples of this disclosure-fostering quality of shared group life could be extended almost indefinitely: thus, a patient discloses that his impotence *preceded* his excessive drinking, a dramatic reversal of his earlier statement that he was impotent *because* he has been drinking. This has a facilitating effect upon other patients, who find it easier to disclose homosexual orientation as the 'reason' for using a knife, because of doubts about the penetrating ability of 'anatomical weapons'. When such disclosures occur in mixed groups, the therapeutic effect can be profound. 'I never thought I could say this to anyone . . . let alone a woman.' 'We used to need to read the blanks between the lines . . . but now you are writing them in for us!' This comment indicates a marked progression in reciprocal disclosure from an earlier phase of cautious non-commitment, such as 'If you're always talking, how the hell do we know when you want to say something?'

subnormal and all possible organic causes must be considered. Within three minutes of raising this topic with a group of colleagues at Broadmoor Hospital, the following organic factors were mentioned as being part of a precipitating constellation which had led to the release phenomenon of violence; a ruptured cerebral aneurysm, acute porphyria, a pineal tumour, post-epileptic automatism, and many cases of disinhibition due to alcohol or other drugs.

Learning theory and psychoanalytic theory, sadly frequently presumed to be uneasy bedfellows, may each contribute understanding to this complex over-determined constellation of predisposing and precipitating factors. For example, one rapist may be patently 'modelling' himself on his father who was an infamous rapist, whereas object-relations theory may account for other rapists' offences where 'modelling' played no part.

Freud's famous essay 'Criminals from a sense of guilt' (1916) is usually regarded as the *fons et origo* of psychoanalytic criminology. The offence may be regarded as the offender's adaption to social stresses in the environment (Halleck 1967), whereas Tuovinen (1973) considers *Crime as an attempt at intrapsychic adaptation*. This excellent monograph discusses the work of Kernberg (1970) and the 'criminal' outlet of narcissistic personalities, and that of Kohut (1971, see also Kohut 1977), with special reference to the development of the grandoise self and of the idealized-parent-image out of the original primary narciss-ism. Tuovinen links this to deviant activity. Tuovinen (1972) has written a key paper on schizophrenia and the basic crimes (see pp. 69–73).

Once it is accepted that patients with a wide range of organic factors, personality characteristics, socially influenced motivation, and prevailing endopsychic pattern-ing may all commit sex-offences, then it clearly becomes impossible to do more than highlight certain features within the scope of one chapter. For example, the psychopathology of the psychopath who becomes a sex-offender is very different from that of the psychotic, who may commit an 'identical' offence. I am aware of the emotive quality of the word psychopath, but I use it as useful 'shorthand'; though, as I discuss further on, many 'psychopaths' subsequently prove to have borderline personality organization and may commit an offence during an ephemeral, micropsychotic episode.

A useful concept is that of the *offence as a defence*. Bernheim (1976, personal communication) has indicated that both acting-out and delusion may be a defence against anxiety for the psychopath who has relatively few inner conflicts. Primitive antisocial acting-out, involving assault, may be modified by psychotherapy into more acceptable styles of expression, and inner conflicts may be dealt with by increasingly differentiated and less antisocial defences.

The most ubiquitous and valuable concept in understanding the sex-offender is that of preservation of self. The *sense of self* of the sex-offender links so clearly with the work of Rosen (1968) on the self-esteem regulating quality of sexual deviation. In my experience, this profoundly influences the genre of appropriate psychotherapeutic management. Almost every mixed-group psychotherapy session in Broadmoor Hospital, where sex-offenders, say rapists, and female patients share in corporate group life, has moments of disclosure when a patient describes how his lost self-esteem was regained by committing the sex-offence or, for the first time, he experienced an enhanced sense of self—'I really became somebody'. This remark might refer to sexual potency, or it might refer to the stigmatizing negative labelling by society so that girls in the neighbourhood were warned, 'watch him, you know what he's like!' Part of the essence of dynamic psychotherapy with sex-offenders is to find alternative avenues of self-esteem regulation, which can provide more than an ephemeral, aggressive genital climax as the basis for enhancing self-esteem.

> The patient says that he feels there is a fault within him, a fault that must be put right. And it is felt to be a fault, not a complex, not a conflict, not a situation. Second, there is a feeling that the cause of this fault is that someone has either failed the patient or defaulted on him; and third, a great anxiety invariably surrounds this area, usually expressed as a desperate demand that this time the analyst should not—in fact must not—fail him. (Balint 1968)

The above quotation comes from *The basic fault*. There is a sense in which the sex-offender frequently suffers from an emotional deficiency disease, it is not so much a question of conflict as of primary deficiency. It is for this reason that third-level disclosures from sex-offenders are not always about psychosexual development, because sexual deviation itself may be a self-esteem regulator, and may cover a deeper pathology in which self-esteem is at risk, such as the threat of non-being. I have indicated (Cox 1973) the value of group psychotherapy as a milieu, in which fragile and negative self-definition can be 'redefined'. Such redefinition for the sex-offender lies in growing differentiation between who he is and what he does. 'I never thought anyone could love me. I couldn't believe I would get affection, so I took it'.' I wanted to live so that I had my life and she [mother] had hers . . . but it became her life. She pulled me back "with a rope" [an imperishable umbilical cord] . . . and this stopped heterosexual adventures and the rope, like a dog lead, only allowed "friendships with children"'. In this instance the psychopathology of paedophilia was as simple as the umbilical rope which 'stopped me becoming me'. The patient's self-esteem had been so low that he did not think that he was worth anything to another person, except a child. Psychotherapy and the unfolding of life events, which can never be dissociated, freed the patient from the restrictions imposed by low self-esteem and a dominating mother. 'I feel safer with kids under five or people over sixty-five . . . You really know that they want you'. 'Mum said she was going down the road for a loaf of bread and the bugger never came back . . . I'm less value than a loaf of bread . . . I hate women!' This disclosure speaks volumes and indicates key issues, such as low self-esteem and attitudes to women, which contributed to a violent assault.

A poignant aspect of precarious self-esteem is illustrated by the patient who said that no one had ever wanted a photograph of her and, in fact, she could never recall ever having her photograph taken. So that when her official photograph was taken for security purposes, she said to the photographer 'Can I have another copy please . . . to send to Dad?' (see Chapter 3).

Balint's 'basic fault' is an important primary deficiency which is intensified by, and declares itself within, an inability to love and trust. People with such a basic fault frequently become patients because they misinterpret social cues, so that their sexual advances will be doomed to failure. It is easy to see how stigmatization can lead to the experience of rejection which soon finds the patient living within a paranoid 'pseudo-community' (Cameron 1943).

In contradistinction to Balint's 'basic fault', repressed infantile sexuality and the failure to negotiate maturational phases appropriately, on account of defective capacities for relinquishment and/or attachment, underlie the specific psychopathology of the majority of sex-offenders. Nevertheless, however much castration anxiety, the inability to negotiate the depressive position or libidinal fixation, may describe inner world phenomena of the sex-offender, these factors never operate *in vacuo*. There is always a social setting in which the offence actually takes place, although it may have taken place in the patient's fantasy on many occasions in other settings. Exactly why the offence was committed *in this place, at this time, with this victim* requires the most detailed analysis involving sociological factors, a thorough assessment of possible organic precipitating events, and, indeed, access to all possible sources of information about the patient's inner and outer world. A psychoanalytic dynamic formulation alone does not account for the complex interaction which constitutes a sex-offence. There may be other people with identical inner world phenomena who 'behave' differently in a particular setting. It is not as naive and simplistic as it may first appear, if I underline the fact that *the sex-offence always involves action between two people*. The therapist is therefore not solely concerned with fantasy. Many sober citizens have fantasies of committing sexual offences, yet relatively few put them into practice. The psychopathology of the sex-offender is different from that of the law-abiding citizen whose 'sex-offences' remain safely within his fantasy world.

Sometimes the psychopathology of the sex-offender patient is crystal clear, and represents a fugue with various subjects which are interwoven, recapitulated and lead to an almost predictable conclusion. On other occasions psychopathology has the characteristics of a primitive, undifferentiated, chaotic affective surge . . . 'something came over me' . . . 'I had to do it' . . . 'I was powerless to resist'.

Victims may be 'killed again' if surrogates are sought and *it is therefore of cardinal importance that the therapist tries to reach the point of understanding what the offence means to the patient*. Only then is it possible for a realistic therapeutic policy to be formulated, because the goals of psychotherapy are inevitably influenced by the starting point of the patient's predicament which must include his way of viewing the world. The victim must have been a focal point in the patient's perception of reality, although defence mechanisms may have blurred awareness and/or tranposed location.

The sex-offender is frequently erroneously described as sadistic: this term should be restricted to the relatively small group of offenders in whom sexual arousal and orgasm only reach maximal proportions during the infliction of pain. Such a sadistic act may be homosexual or heterosexual and may be directed towards an adult or a child victim. True sadists should be distinguished from a different group of patients, frequently incorrectly called sadistic, whose expression of power and the assertion of dominance takes the form of humiliating and belittling another person. The first group only reach orgasm when inflicting pain (in fact or fantasy), whereas in the latter group the experience of sexual climax may not be associated with this personal statement of power, which may, however, lead to physical cruelty. The sex-offender may in fact occur in either category, though it should be noted that the sadistic sex-offender will have a different underlying psychopathology. In both categories the significance of emotional disclosure during the course of dynamic psychotherapy is central, although the content of the disclosure may vary. If the deviant behaviour is a self-esteem regulator, then it is likely that the deepest third-level disclosures (see below) will not be about the offence, but will refer to those other areas of experience where self-esteem was, at best, fragile and, at worst, shattered. This would clearly demonstrate that the offence had the function in the patient's psychic economy of recovering self-esteem.

The act designated as a sex-offence may be ego-syntonic or ego-dystonic for the offender. It may be prompted by conscious or unconscious factors. The latter may be exemplified by the patient who commits a sex-offence, ensures that he is detected, or actually gives himself up to the police. If such a patient subsequently enters psychotherapy, he may disclose the guilt which had previously been hidden. Such guilt is usually connected with forbidden acts, which led him to commit an offence which would be certain to attract a heavy sentence, and would thus give him the punishment which he felt he 'deserved', although never received. The exact nature of the early forbidden act will depend on his early experience of socialization and is therefore culturally determined, although at root it usually stems from sexual taboos. The unconscious motivation behind the sex-offence explains the panic which some patients experience, if they are 'reprieved', or merely receive a token sentence, after an act which they unconsciously expect will merit severe punishment to match their hitherto undisclosed guilt. It is, therefore, not surprising that third-level disclosures (see below) from sex-offenders frequently contain such material. Nevertheless, it cannot be repeated too often that it must not be presumed that, because a patient is talking about a sex-offence he is, *ipso facto*, disclosing the deepest recesses of his inner world.

When the therapist makes an intervention of the right texture and at the right time, he 'catches' the patient as he talks of two different worlds of discourse simultaneously, although prior to the intervention he is only aware of one. For example, the patient describing his feelings leading up to an incident involving multiple stabbing, because of his 'fascination with the blade', is suddenly (after the intervention) aware that a knife, unlike his anatomical 'weapon', would never lose its erection, would always elicit fear, and would never fail to penetrate. Such clinical experience is unforgettable for the therapist and dynamic theory comes to life in a self-authenticating way.

THERAPEUTIC ALLIANCE

Setting

Dynamic psychotherapy with the sex-offender may occur in several settings which inevitably have far-reaching consequences upon the patient's *modus vivendi* in general, and the nature of the psychotherapeutic alliance in particular. These vary from a custodial setting within a penal institution for a sentence of known duration (except for loss of remission or the granting of parole), to a time of unknown duration in the setting of a special hospital, such as Broadmoor. He may also be seen in an outpatient setting, which may involve psychotherapy in a hospital department or at a special unit, such as The Portman Clinic in London. Figure 13.1 illustrates at a glance the various settings in which patient and therapist may meet. The psychotherapy undertaken can range from 'pure' individual psychoanalysis to, say, group therapy sessions within Broadmoor. It should not be forgotten that, in Broadmoor, the psychotherapeutic group is a very small part of the 'treatment' the patient receives; because such therapy takes place within the intense microcosm of life in the hospital, with its complex matrix of staff–patient, staff–staff, and patient–patient interactions which all form part of the ongoing community life. Nevertheless, in whatever setting the patient and therapist meet, it is the patient's response as a whole person to the totality of therapeutic influences bearing upon him that guides prognosis. Psychotherapy may help him to understand and modify his inner world of fantasy and his idiosyncratic construction of reality, which led to an incident in his outer world of action and designated him as a sex-offender.

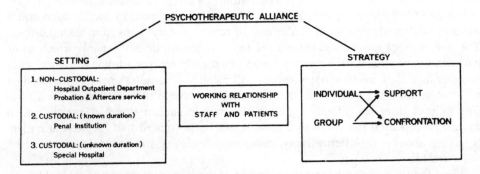

Fig. 13.1 Settings in which a patient and therapist may meet. Reproduced by kind permission from *Brit. J. Crim.* (Cox 1974).

Timing

> Look to the lady:
> (*Lady Macbeth is carried out*).
> And when we have our naked frailties hid,
> That suffer in exposure, let us meet,
> And question this most bloody piece of work,
> To know it further.

(Macbeth, ɪɪ, iii, 126)

Figure 13.2 graphically portrays the chronological sequence of events from the pre-offence phase A to the post-trial phase C, where a patient may be, say, in Broadmoor 'without limit of time'. This brings a new set of variables into the discussion about dynamic psychotherapy with the sex-offender. For example, in phase A the patient is not, strictly speaking, an offender-patient because he has not yet committed an offence. Nevertheless, he may present to his general practitioner or the social services department, saying that he feels he is going to stab someone 'if something is not done', or that he has read about 'baby batterers' and thinks that he may become one, if he is not rehoused. This frontline clinical situation, which the general practitioner or the social worker may have to face single-handed, demands almost impossible wisdom in differentiating the manipulative threat, from a genuine fear that 'if something is not done I will stab, rape, kill'. Some patients who ultimately commit sex-offences may give warnings of their intent, but there are vastly greater numbers whose thoughts of giving such warnings are not put into effect, and are subsequently dismissed by the comment 'I never really thought I'd do it'.

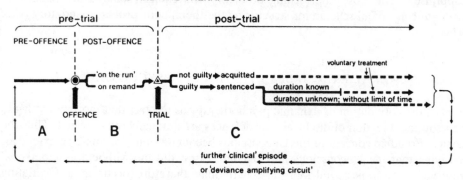

TIME AND THE THERAPEUTIC ENCOUNTER

Fig. 13.2 A deliberately simplified flow chart. Higher and Lower Courts, etc., are not distinguished.

There is no easy rule of thumb to guide the general practitioner or the social worker in such situations, but an increased level of awareness grows from the assurance gained from inter-disciplinary staff support groups with experienced colleagues. These act as emotional resource points for the worker who battles with the need to 'worry along with each one'.

The timing of the first encounter between patient and therapist can have a critical effect on the subsequent course of the therapeutic alliance. It can be seen in Fig. 13.2, phase B, that the patient 'on the run' may have very different disclosures to make from the patient who is on remand and being interviewed by a psychiatrist preparing a report for the court. The patient 'on the run' may have returned to his old, trusted family doctor and confessed 'I'm in dead trouble'.

Phase C, shows the circumscribed or extended duration of the therapeutic encounter upon which the therapist and patient may embark. Therapeutic space takes on entirely different qualities in the various post-trial patient–therapist alignments. The diagram speaks for itself, but it must be added that when a patient is resident without limit of time, both patient and therapist have long enough to share therapeutic space until it is no longer necessary. However, the bottom line in Fig.13.2 indicates that one post-trial phase *may* usher in a future pre-trial phase. Recidivism is always an over-determined phenomenon. I have discussed group psychotherapy in a secure setting (Cox 1976), where this aspect of the work is amplified. There is a unique quality of relationship which can pervade therapeutic space and permeate the life of the group when therapist and patient are together 'without limit of time'.

The physical setting and timing of initiating the therapeutic alliance, shown in Figs 13.1 and 13.2, respectively, are important in all psychotherapeutic work, although they have an added significance in psychotherapy undertaken with offender-patients including the sex-offender. For example, an entire chapter could be written on the dynamics underlying the optimal handling of the difficult therapeutic alliance in which a rapist on parole finds he is attracted towards his female probation officer. Both the setting and the timing of the encounter are of cardinal importance and, as with all supervision groups for, say, general practitioners or probation officer, the structuring of time, depth, and mutuality need to be rigorously scrutinized and constantly reappraised. The close interlocking of theory and clinical management makes an adequate conceptual scheme for structuring the therapeutic process mandatory (Cox 1978a).

GENERAL PRINCIPLES OF DYNAMIC PSYCHOTHERAPY

I regard the core datum of dynamic psychotherapy as the fact that movement always occurs in the direction of disclosure, as defences are gradually relinquished. Thus the classical Freudian concept of the Unconscious becoming Conscious may be extended, by saying that the Unconscious may become Conscious-but-withheld as a personal preserve of awareness. Further disclosure may therefore occur in a facilitating environment, when the patient is enabled to disclose, to others, material which he has hitherto kept as a 'secret'; although it may be a secret of which he is painfully conscious. The total process can therefore be stated as follows: Unconscious Conscious-withheld Conscious disclosed. The final step is greatly facilitated in a group

Dynamic psychotherapy with sex-offenders frequently confronts not only the patients, but also the co-therapists, with facts about the pervasive influence of unconscious mental processes which may have been previously dogmatically denied! For example, the cynical psychopathic rapist who may join a group because it will give the impression that he is cooperative, with the barely disguised determination to disclose nothing whatever about his personal world, is shattered when such events as a shared group-dream occur. He is immediately aware that 'something is going-on'. Another patient in the group describes, in considerable detail, a dream which she had during the previous night, and he, almost too shaken to hold a lighted match in one place long enough to ignite his cigarette, says 'Good God, that was my dream too!' In the same way, the junior therapist, who may be well-trained academically but has comparatively little clinical experience, is startled when a patient who had certainly never read Freud says 'Hey, wait a minute, I know it sounds crazy, but could there be any connection between the feelings I had when I first broke into a house and when I first had sex with a girl? I know they are so different and yet in a funny way I had the same kind of feeling'. This is likely to be followed by disclosures from other patients in which 'forcible entry into forbidden territory', and the knowledge that the patient always chose to break into a locked house and had no interest whatsoever in entering an invitingly open door, plays a major part. Raping a prostitute might be equally uninviting. The trainee therapist is here confronted by clinical reality. Either this is a genuine third-level disclosure or the patient has 'read the right books and knows the right noises to make!'

Levels of disclosure

During the course of psychotherapy the words spoken by the patient, and the affective penumbra in which they are uttered, fluctuate across the boundaries between three levels of disclosure. The first is trivial, bus-stop 'chat': 'I thought I saw frost this morning'; the second is personal, but emotionally neutral: 'I am breeding budgies' (parakeets in the USA); the third is both personal and emotional: 'I never had a childhood'.

By definition, a third-level disclosure is difficult to make; it is either painful, shame-inducing and embarrassing, or 'precious' and not for public scrutiny. Thus, sadistic fantasies or the intimate information that 'I can never listen to Mahler without crying' could be third-level disclosures; although disclosures of sadistic fantasies are not *necessarily* third-level, a patient might enjoy recounting them.

The ability to distinguish between these levels depends upon the therapist's capacity to perceive what the disclosure means to the patient. It depends upon the clinical skill of experiencing 'vicarious introspection', which was Kohut's (1959) brilliant definition of empathy. For example, the disclosure 'I was born in Birmingham' is, for me, a second-level disclosure. I am neither particularly proud and want to publish the fact, nor anxious to conceal such information. Nevertheless, it is possible that the statement 'I was born in Birmingham' might be a third-level disclosure for someone other than myself, if, say, a strong Birmingham accent had blocked a life-long ambition to be a newsreader on television. The therapist learns to gauge what the disclosure means to the patient on the basis of the cognitive-affective qualities of the disclosure. It is the physiological concomitants of changing levels of anxiety, such as posture, gesture, rate of respiration, vocal rhythm and pitch, whether the direction and intensity of the gaze-pattern changes (either in the direction of becoming fixed or floating), which furnish evidence to confirm or contradict the overt affective 'statement' of feeling.

One of the axiomatic facets of psychotherapy training is to enable the trainee to be relatively 'uncluttered' by himself so that he has sufficient available energy, and the affective freedom, to recognize a patient's third-level disclosure and to distinguish it from what would be a third-level disclosure if he (the therapist) had said it.

The concept of disclosure levels is pertinent to all dynamic psycho-therapy, but it is particularly relevant in offender-therapy. The fact that a sex-offender may be discussing rape does not, *ipso facto*, mean that he is making a third-level disclosure. A psychopath may discuss the incident with bland detachment or undisguised relish. The trainee therapist may be understandably impressed that the patient has been able to disclose such intimate phenomena, although, in fact, he or she needs to remember the caveat that such a disclosure may not be a genuine third-level disclosure for the patient. It is not infrequent for a third-level disclosure for such a patient to relate to various facets of an adolescent identity crisis; for example, he was teased at school because he had no public hair; he was the only boy in Borstal whose 'beard' did not register the fact that the daily distribution of razor blades had been withheld, because of a rumour that one had been stolen. Female sex-offenders often give overwhelming evidence that their third-level disclosures are concerned with the uncertainty of their sexual identity ('I didn't know if I was a man or a woman'), presenting as an adolescent identity crisis. For example, when a girl of 12 says 'I set fire to a convent', it is not unlikely that the most painful sense of emotional vulnerability and defencelessness might occur when she said 'The little girl in me still wanted to be cuddled but I felt torn apart because I hated the feeling that mum was superior and controlling . . . when I heard about *The* Mother Superior it was more than I could bear . . .' Another patient indicated that he could never share his life with another person, 'I could *never* share what I think of myself'.

Third-level disclosures of sex-offenders may be inextricably involved with self-esteem enhancement, and the offences often carry the secondary benefit of regaining peer group esteem or, if it has never been experienced previously, of establishing it for the first time.

It will be seen that levels of disclosure are intimately related to the psychoanalytic concept of the unconscious becoming conscious. Indeed, a third-level disclosure often occurs as the patient 'receives' into consciousness aspects of himself of which he was previously unaware. This has the effect of the disclosure having a novel 'startling' quality, not only for the other members of the therapeutic group, but for the disclosure himself. 'Blimey, I never knew I felt like that before.' A third-level disclosure is rarely accessible to introspection, except in retrospect. (The hypothetical constructs of disclosure levels as elaborated in Cox 1976, and various visual display systems of disclosure phenomena are described in Cox 1978*a*,*b*).

The phenomenon of the pseudo-disclosure merits a separate paragraph. In conventional psychotherapy it is important, although subsidiary, to the three levels already discussed; whereas in offender-therapy in general, and in sex-offender therapy in particular, it assumes major significance.

The psychopath and pseudo-disclosure

A third level disclosure is always a cognitive-affective phenomenon, and the non-verbal facets of communication, together with the physiological concomitants of change in the level of anxiety (either reduced or increased) are hallmarks of the affective components which accompany the cognitive 'statement'. Indeed, without such ancillary evidence, it is unlikely that third-level disclosure is occurring.

When the patient *seems* to be talking about disturbing, intimate, affect-laden material with simulated anxiety which does not 'ring true', then it is probable that the therapist is receiving a pseudo-disclosure. I regard the task of distinguishing pseudo-disclosure, beloved by the psychopath, as one of the most important skills in offender-therapy. Ultimately, the psychopath hopes to find that he cannot 'con' the therapist, though he may have an escalating life-long 'conning' pattern which enhances his defences, so that he may need fiercely incursive confrontation if his jealously guarded preserves of feeling are to be tapped. It must not be forgotten that 'confrontational therapy' is *confrontation with self*, facilitated by the therapist, not confrontation with the therapist.

The pseudo-disclosure of the psychopath is not a lie

Although this sounds a truism, it needs to be stressed, because it is so frequently presumed that because a particular patient is in the habit of lying, therefore whatever he may disclose about his inner world is, *ipso facto*, a lie. He may have lied about his involvement in a 'gang-bang' (a multiple rape), or about the number of robberies he has committed. Put bluntly, these are lies and not pseudo-disclosures. The essence of the pseudo-disclosure is that it is genuine in the sense that it describes certain facets of experience which are true, but which, nevertheless, are not related to the prevailing core psychopathology. The pseudo-disclosure is not a lie, but neither is it a third-level disclosure, although it may seem so to the therapist inexperienced in treating sex-offenders and, in particular, psychopaths who are sex-offenders. In my experience, it is possible to fail the patient precisely at the point where he is most vulnerable and indeed welcomes further confrontation with himself. For example, if the therapist diverts the attention of the group immediately a patient has described the incidents which led up to an incident of rape, there may be an implicit assumption that 'John has got it off his chest at last . . . he's been in the hot seat long enough . . . this is what we've been working towards for months'. He may have failed to discern that this was in fact a pseudo-disclosure. It may have been difficult for John to describe the incident of rape, and this pseudo-disclosure was most certainly not a lie, but an accurate account of what happened. Nevertheless, the crucial concept is that for John the genuine third-level disclosure, which lay behind the events which culminated in rape, would have related to impotence and homosexuality. 'I *know* I'm queer . . . I've known it for ages . . . it's a relief not to need to hide it any more . . .' this could easily be a rapist's third-level disclosure. The therapist can put the clock back almost indefinitely, if he misinterprets a pseudo-disclosure as a genuine third-level disclosure. What may be regarded as having 'struck oil' may in fact be nothing more than the removal of top soil.

The sex-offender frequently adopts the defensive manoeuvre of saying that he is now concerned to look ahead and 'face life' and it is not healthy to 'go back over the past and dig it all up'. The therapist's task is always that of facilitating disclosure, and I would never regard psychotherapy with a sex-offender as satisfactory if he discussed, with appropriate affect, everything *except* his offence. *Per contra*, it is equally unsatisfactory if he *only* discusses his offence. This always suggests that he is in fact making pseudo-disclosures because genuine third-level disclosures about a sex-offence always lead back to earlier relationships (in fact or fantasy) which were unsatisfactory. And, as in conventional psychotherapy, again and again the patient retraces his emotional footsteps to early life-experience. If he remains fixated at the point of discussing his offence it is either an indication of an unsuccessful attempt to 'con' the therapist, or it indicates that there are more painful earlier experiences which he is not yet able to tolerate so that he is therefore relatively more at ease 'living with' his offence.

> . . . where the crime's committed, the crime can be forgot.
> (*A woman young and old*: W. B. Yeats)

However, as far as psychotherapy with the sex-offender is concerned it is fallacious to assume that the crime can be, or should be, 'forgot'. In clinical practice the crime often needs to be renegotiated, almost to the point of tedium, until the patient not only understands what happened, but has been able to incorporate hitherto intolerable parts of himself which, prior to psychotherapy, may have been consciously denied and were often totally repressed.

Once the therapeutic alliance is firmly established, the patient no longer regards the therapist's incursive activity as an attack. It is gradually reconstrued as the necessary, although painful, cooperation of an 'ally'. When this stage is reached, the patient, himself, will be aware whether the 'crime can be forgot . . . [yet]'. '*I don't linger long* [in the traumatic past] *but the feeling comes back with me and lasts quite a long time*. It's very strong and tails off'. There is an entirely different ethos about the patient who is aware that he can safely turn to the future because 'the crime can be forgot' in the sense that, following in the wake of insight, endopsychic patterning has been changed. For example, when the rapist who had built-up an infamous local reputation for being a 'lad with the girls' has become conscious of, and able to tolerate, his homosexuality, he can experience an emotional relief after years of emotional smoke-screens and pretending to be what he was not. Such a patient is in marked contrast to a fellow member of a therapeutic group, who still avoids the past at all costs, denies that he has any problems and is anxious to convince staff and fellow patients alike that 'all is well'. Such a patient may eventually begin to discover things about himself when, as a member of a mixed therapeutic group (four male and four female patients), he learns through the third-level disclosure of the most attractive girl in the group, that she has an exclusively lesbian orientation and is therefore impervious to his desire to impress her. An interesting question was raised in such a group: 'Is this really a mixed group if we are either male homosexuals or lesbians?'

Nuclear disclosures

A nuclear disclosure is a third-level disclosure which so captures both core psycho-pathology and the process pattern of life predicaments that the therapist senses that what 'surfaced' during a transient, almost casual, disclosure, would furnish the 'skeleton' which extended interviewing or numerous therapeutic sessions would invest with detail. When a nuclear disclosure occurs, it makes such a vivid impact on the therapist that it is like reading a page of English literature, where five words 'stand out' because they are in another language. It is difficult to give examples of nuclear disclosures, because what would be a nuclear disclosure for one patient would not necessarily be so for another. Furthermore, sex-offenders are no more likely to make nuclear disclosures than any other patients in psychotherapy; although when they do, like all other nuclear disclosures, it is unforgettable. However, for three patients with different realms of experience, different psychopathology, and different clinical presentations, the following disclosures are examples of nuclear disclosures: 'we were her [mother's] life, so when we went there was nothing left'; '. . . the more things that are hurled at you, the less painful it becomes . . . It's like scar tissue'; 'when I lost my temper, I seemed to *lose myself* in my temper'.

Disclosures such as these occur as individual patients and the group-as-a-whole free-associate. The way in which this process was described by a member of a group of sex-offenders to a new member, who had just joined a long-established group, exemplifies his awareness of psychic determinism and the existential exigency of the present moment. Although his description is in basic English, it is infinitely more articulate than any technical words used in this sentence. When he was asked what happened in the group, how did people know what to say, and so on, he replied '. . . in the group we do what happens'.

Probably the most frequent topic for discussion in the post-therapeutic session between co-therapists, revolves around the differential diagnosis of a genuine third-level disclosure and a psychopathic pseudo-disclosure, so eloquently described by a patient as 'a sub-scription to rent-a-mouth'! The problem is compounded by the psychotic whose disclosure may, paradoxically, appear to be 'too good to be true', that is a pseudo-disclosure, and yet, when perceived as part of a delusional system, may be a psychotic third-level disclosure.

The psychotic and the group-as-a-whole

Fascinating though the psychotherapy of the psychoses is as a topic in its own right, and particularly as many sex-offenders have psychotic phases, it can receive no more than a passing reference here. However, supportive psychotherapy with the psychotic sex-offender (alongside appropriate medication) must take the form of conveying to the patient by posture, gesture, and word that he is taken seriously as a person. 'I'm blind because I see too much, so I study by a dark lamp' comes from a psychotic[4] arsonist with archetypal primitive disclosures and too little ego to defend. The therapist's role with such a patient is therefore that of acting as guardian for a man who cannot guard himself. I have frequently found that one such patient in a group confers a reciprocal benefit on both the psychotic and the non-psychotic. In an almost inexplicable way, the psychotic himself finds that the group is supportive, and this may be because of such 'trivial-significant' events as the sharing of sweets or cigarettes, and possibly because the psychotic's loose hold on reality protects him from the overt confrontation which may occur in such a group between, say, the sadistic paedophiliac and the psychopathic murderer. The non-psychotic patients gain, although painfully, by the blunt emotional broadside from the psychotic who has no customary defences of tact and caution which protect most of us in social situations, and therefore the question 'Why don't you talk about why you killed your mother?' takes on a strangely penetrating quality. The psychopath, who could bounce such a question back from a patient with similar psychopathology, does not know how to cope with a patient who is, in one sense, out of touch with reality, and, in another, able to penetrate defences with unerring accuracy.

When conducting small group psychotherapy with sex-offenders, there are advantages in making the group mixed, as far as the sex of the patients is concerned, and also in achieving the optimal, although heterodox, amalgam of having one psychotic in a group of psychopaths: however, for obvious reasons, the psychotic must be sufficiently stable and in touch with reality to be able to make the journey to the group room and to be aware of what is going on. The inherent buoyancy of a group constituted in this way offers both the psychotherapist and his colleague, the responsible medical officer, many advantages. First, it fosters more accurate diagnostic appraisal than is possible in the early stages of assessment. However appropriate the nosological classification 'psychopathic' may be, it frequently becomes clear that the patient exhibits borderline personality organization (Wolberg 1973; Kernberg 1975) see also Hartocollis (1977). Such patients have capricious, mercurial, rapidly fluctuating defence organization, so that the sex-offence may have been committed during a transient psychotic

---

[4] I know of no textbook which has so accurately captured the ethos of the psychotic's changing perception of the world as Hannah Green's novel, *I never promised you a rose garden* (1964).

micro-episode which, though catastrophic, was only a fragment of the patient's history which otherwise has the classical stamp of the psychopath. The presence of an overtly psychotic patient in the presence of a group of 'psychopaths' can evoke painful memories of the occasion when the 'cool, calculating' psychopath lost his 'cool' and was temporarily disorganized and chaotic.

Secondly, a group constituted in this way has an idiosyncratic orchestration so that the following vignettes are possible: 'I remember raping the girl next door', a pseudo-disclosure from a psychopath intent on impressing the group, and possibly succeeding, with all except the psychotic, whose reply follows: 'was she in a bungalow or a house?' The recipient of the disclosure is totally unimpressed, and this may push the discloser in the direction of genuine third-level disclosures. There is an infectious, escalating quality about genuine third-level disclosures, whether they come from the psychopath or the psychotic. Indeed, the following disclosure was from a psychotic patient, but it 'rang true' for almost every member of the group, although it was embedded in a jungle of disordered thoughts: 'the weakness I have in myself is what is in you . . . it's loneliness and desertion'.

No one in the group could deny that this, in part, had been their experience too, and a genuine sense of corporate solidarity was achieved in the group by the disclosure from the psychotic, which had acted as a Trojan Horse and taken the psychopaths from within.

Another example is furnished where a psychotic girl breaks into a psychopath's pseudo-disclosure and asks whether it matters if she has a spot on her dress. The ensuing free-association about blemishes; going through bad patches; having faults that people see; those that are hidden; having a 'stained soul' as being more disturbing than a stained dress; once again led the group to a disclosure level where the psychopaths were able to risk the vulnerability of disclosure. Such examples could be continued 'without limit of time', but I hope the few instances cited have indicated the vital fact that in conducting group psychotherapy with sex-offenders (as with all patients in group psychotherapy), the members of the group ultimately form their own best facilitators and become co-therapists for each other, although, for many technical reasons, there must always be professional co-therapists.

Ideally, there should be a therapist of each sex. Whenever possible members of the nursing staff should be fully integrated into a group therapy programme as co-therapists. The contribution of the nursing staff, who see the patient in formal 'small-group psychotherapy' as well as being intimately involved in the day-to-day events of his life within the total institution, is invaluable, and can never be exaggerated.

Brancale *et al.* (1971) describe a special treatment unit which is part of the New Jersey Program for sex offenders. The seven principles and guidelines they suggest are as follows:

1. Group therapy is more successful and longer lasting than individual therapy.
2. Sex offenders are generally too passive and inadequate for standard group therapy techniques and need more directive treatment, even to the point of re-educational methods.
3. Group therapy has to be supplemented by sex education sessions, since sex offenders are most often grossly misinformed or sexually naive or both.

4. Homogeneity of grouping by offence has been found to be useless and even potentially detrimental to successful treatment.
5. The sex offence itself must be understood by patient and therapist to be a symptom only and not the problem itself. It then follows that:
6. The 'whole man' treatment philosophy should be employed.
7. Emotional release is an essential element in the treatment process.

Each one of these 'guidelines' is debatable, although they all raise issues which every therapist experienced in working with sex-offenders would acknowledge. Although I agree in general terms, my reservations are as follows (I use the same numbered paragraphs as Brancale).

1. A small minority of offender-patients, who have been exposed to the emotional pressures in a group and yet remain impervious, are referred to my colleagues who conduct individual psychotherapy. Occasionally individual psychotherapy 'strikes oil' where group therapy fails. Not surprisingly, there is also a reciprocal flow of patients in the opposite direction!

2 and 3. Not all sex-offenders are 'too passive and inadequate for standard group therapy techniques'. The great advantage of mixed group psychotherapy, with male sex-offenders and female patients, is that it not only demonstrates the way in which the offender relates (or fails to relate) to the opposite sex, but it also provides 'education' in addition to the dynamic aspects of psychotherapy.

4. I entirely disagree with guideline 4 as a general statement. Group psychotherapy where the group is homogeneous as far as the offence of 'killing' (whether legally defined as murder or manslaughter) is concerned, can facilitate third-level disclosures at a rate rarely attained in heterogenous groups. (There are, of course, other advantages in heterogeneous groups, but that is not being debated.)

5, 6, and 7. I agree with these guidelines, although methods of facilitation, participation and 'regulation' of 'emotional release' depend on a complex network of 'domestic' relationships within the total institution.

Dynamic psychotherapy with sex-offenders brings into sharp focus two of the ubiquitous and perennial questions facing all psychotherapists. The first relates to the techniques of facilitating psychodynamic change so that movement in the direction of disclosure takes the following course: Unconscious . . . Conscious-withheld . . . Conscious-disclosed. The questions confronting the therapist are 'How can I facilitate disclosure in this individual or group setting?', and what are the risks for the patient and/or the community in which he lives, if the sex-offender is enabled to make such disclosures, which frequently relate to his offence, or, *per contra*, if he remains unable to do so?' The second question is an inevitable consequence of the first. 'Having at last [in Broadmoor, we might substitute 'at long last'] enabled the patient to make third-level disclosures, what does the therapist do, that is, how does he respond to these disclosures from his patient?' This not a textbook on general psychotherapeutic theory or strategy, but once again the sex-offender patient presents, in an inescapable way, topics which arise with every patient in psychotherapy. How do I facilitate disclosure? How do I respond to the disclosures once they have occurred, and, even more important, how does the patient 'respond' to his own disclosures?

SPECIAL ASPECTS OF THE THERAPEUTIC RELATIONSHIP
WITH SEX-OFFENDERS

I have discussed elsewhere (Cox 1974) the psychotherapist's anxiety with special reference to the offender-patient. Change in established defence patterns takes place in all dynamic psychotherapy, and that undertaken with the sex-offender is no exception. During individual psychotherapy, as transference is established and develops, the therapist is invested with feelings which the patient had previously invested in 'significant others'. The victim of his sex-offence may have been a specific 'target' whom the patient had been pursuing for many months; on the other hand, the victim might have been an unfortunate casualty who 'happened' to be present. During the course of dynamic psychotherapy, the therapist may have invested in him feelings transferred from this particularly significant 'significant other' in the life of the sex-offender—the victim. The therapist will be aware that, say, a victim has been killed, and there is no theoretical reason why this attack should not be repeated.

Arnold and Stiles (1972) write: 'Group methods have become one of the most widely used therapeutic techniques in our correctional institutions'. This, like conventional group psychotherapy, may have come about initially on economic grounds or because of the scarcity of trained personnel, although there is currently a striking shift in emphasis towards an appreciation of the intrinsic value of the group process itself. This applies both in terms of the facilities for enhanced dynamic understanding of the patient, and also as a therapeutic milieu. It may be that it was in a group setting that the patient originally established a deviant identity and, *ipso facto*, a group setting may also provide the redefining process in which the patient's self-definition may be changed, in the direction of greater personal fulfilment in socially acceptable patterns. Group therapy therefore has an important redefining function. Tuovinen (1973) writes: 'The only opportunity to study these problems is via individual psychotherapeutic work', which supports Ormrod (1975): 'Unless the study of offenders is undertaken on an individual basis, little progress will be made'. I disagree with these statements if they are taken to imply that it is *only* on an individual basis that the study of the individual can be furthered. In my experience, the greatest study of the individual is facilitated when he takes part in mixed group therapy and collateral individual appraisal is possible. It is in such settings that the rapist's relationship with women can be studied in great detail over a prolonged period of time. I am aware that this privileged therapeutic opportunity is only likely to occur in hospitals such as Broadmoor, where mixed dynamic group therapy is an established part of the total therapeutic thrust of the hospital.

One special aspect of working with the sex-offender is the demand made on the therapist to understand both the inner world of the patient, and the exact way in which the patient construed the context in which the offence was committed. To neglect either the inner world or the context betrays the patient. To concentrate solely on the ambient circumstances of the offence and to rely on objective, external sources of information about the offence fails the patient at his point of greatest need. It is one of the advantages of group psychotherapy with sex-offenders that the patient is constantly finding his/her own inner world confronted by the external world of fellow-patients. They, better than any therapist, know the importance of the need to bring together their early blurred conception of 'how it was' with the undeniable facts, perhaps seen in legal depositions or even photographs, of how 'it really was'. The therapist needs both a macrocosmic and a microcosmic approach to the assessment of the significance of a sex-offence for a particular patient. The former is like a panoramic view, the latter like a zoom lens which closes-in. Thus, for one patient a long-perspective macrocosmic view is necessary if sense is to be made of his offence. His arson was no substitute sexual activity, but rather a way of getting his family, highly respectable and respected in the local Cornish village, into the headlines of the local paper, by ensuring that the reporters knew of his activity: 'Fancy one of them doing that. They were always such a good family!' In such an event, the patient's comment that he set out to 'blacken the family name' by this form of indirect attack had succeeded. The microcosmic perspective may be needed for another patient, where the prevailing endo-psychic patterning of the sadistic homosexual killing, such as that described in such lurid detail by Marlowe (pp. 306–7), may be infinitely more important than the wider perspective of killing the king. The microcosmic perspective demands a close-up, detailed analysis of the context of the offence, and careful scrutiny of its relevance to the inner world of the patient; whereas the macrocosmic perspective involves standing back and seeing what the offence meant in its totality, such as 'blackening the family name'. Appropriate psychotherapy therefore depends on the global appraisal of endopsychic patterning and its relation to *contextual analysis* which may need to be micro- or macrocosmic.

In addition to such indubitably important topics as the relationship between transference phenomena developing during psychotherapy with the sex-offender and the possibility that the therapist may be perceived as a victim-surrogate, and the perennial debate between the value of individual and group methods of offender-therapy, there are other aspects of the therapeutic relationship with the sex-offender which must be discussed. I am referring to three phenomena which are of importance in all dynamic psychotherapy, but assume even greater significance when the patient is a sex-offender. These are the existential concept of *fragestellung*, the concept of 'therapeutic space', and the '*Weltanschauung* of the therapist'. These will now be considered in turn.

Fragestellung[5]

There appears to be no English equivalent to this German term, which I am therefore retaining. It means literally 'the putting of the question', and refers to the totality of ideas which lead to the question being put in the first place. It implies that the answer to a question may be influenced by the way in which the question is asked, and can be demonstrated in the following example. The question, 'Why *did* you kill your mother?' may be asked forcefully in an early interrogation, or it may be asked with the greatest possible tact and diplomacy in a pre-trial psychiatric interview while the 'patient' is on remand. The question may be answered in several ways. The patient may be suffering from global or focal amnesia which may be organically or psychodynamically determined. He may be only too well aware of the event, but deny that he did it, or say that she was unduly provocative or that he was drunk and did

---

[5] Part of this and the subsequent section are taken from Cox (1978*a*)

not intend to do it. The same question, 'Why did *you* kill your mother?', asked by a fellow patient in the context of group psychotherapy at Broadmoor, where perhaps everyone else in the group was aware that it was a group of killers, might facilitate an entirely different answer. An identical question, but in a different setting, and with a totally different *fragestellung*. The first had the implication 'Come on, tell us . . . we know you did it'; the latter was, in effect, asking the question 'Why did *you* kill your mother? . . . I know why *I* killed mine!', and this obviously alters the ethos pervading therapeutic space. It is this facilitating process which allows third-level disclosures to occur. It must be remembered that the physiological concomitants of third-level disclosures usually enable the therapist to recognize them without difficulty, although the perennial trap for the therapist unaccustomed to working with offender-patients is to presume that, because a patient is talking about his offence, he is *ipso facto* making a third-level disclosure. For example, the patient who describes how he fatally stabbed a white-haired parish priest may be making a third-level disclosure, but on the other hand it may be a psychopathic pseudo-disclosure. Thus, the patient might describe with disinterested, trivializing, detachment how he stabbed the priest, whereas he might find it almost overwhelmingly embarrassing, on a subsequent occassion, to disclose the fact that he was the only boy in his year at school whose voice had not broken. The trainee therapist might think that it was much easier to admit to a voice sounding feminine than to stabbing a priest, but he is not his patient. It is this ability to enter the inner world of the patient, and yet remain sufficiently detached to be objective, which is the hallmark of making progress in the growth of psychotherapeutic experience. Siirala has so admirably described psychotherapy training as a 'suffering-maturation process' (1974, personal communication).

The concept of *fragestellung* is relevant to many aspects of psychotherapy with the sex-offender. It refers not only to the 'putting of the question' by the therapist to the patient but, to a much greater extent, to the putting of the question by one patient to another within the shared group. The therapist's task is to so modify disclosure depth that it is balanced between the invitational edge of the intolerable and the easily tolerable safety of inactivity. The poignant fact is that each patient in the group knows that, at some stage, he has to face the intolerable parts of himself. 'I have the burden of having no burden.' The *fragestellung* is a conceptual device which aids the therapist in monitoring disclosure potential, not only for the individual patient but for the group-as-a-whole.

Therapeutic space

This term is used in several ways by different authorities: Moreno uses it to describe the 'stage' upon which psychodrama in enacted; whereas others use it to describe intra-psychic space, that is that realm within the personality in which there is room for manoeuvre and growth.

There has recently been a growing interest in the concept of therapeutic space. Khan (1974) in a chapter entitled 'The role of illusion in the analytic space and process' writes:

Clinically the unique achievement of Freud is that he invented and established a
therapeutic space and distance for the patient and the analyst. In this space and distance
the relating becomes feasible only through the capacity in each of sustain illusion and to
work with it . . . It is my contention here that Freud created a space, time and process
which potentialize that area of *illusion* where symbolic disclosure can actualize.

The clincial experience of working with many patients whose lives have included
incidents involving the 'basic' crimes, such as murder and incest, has convinced me
that therapeutic space, although symbolic, is much 'firmer' and part of a joint reality
than can be conveyed by the word 'illusion'. Khan writes 'the relational process
through which the illusion operates is the transference'. The transference may be an
illusion but it is not the whole content of dynamic psychotherapy, though its inherent
dynamic pervades it.

Psychotherapeutic work with the offender-patient can provide a corrective emotional experience for the therapist! By this I mean that it reminds him or her that
the ubiquitous and timeless fantasies of murder, and other destructive activity, may
erupt into reality in a catastrophic manner. Much literature on psychotherapy often
states explicitly, or conveys by an implicit *timbre*, that destructiveness is confined
to intra-psychic fantasy or attenuated in the clinical presentation of verbal abuse
or hostile silence. When the patient has actually killed someone, the conceptual
boundaries between 'that area of *illusion* where symbolic discourse can actualize',
and that area of *reality* where the 'hard' non-symbolic facts are disclosed, is of
paramount importance. It is the merging of the *fact* that Donald killed his father with
the *transference 'illusion'* (when the therapist may transiently vicariously represent
the un-killed father, or whoever Donald's father stood for in his social construction
of reality), which sharpens the significance of reality testing. Such dynamic events are
part of an established therapeutic alliance (whether on an individual or group basis)
within therapeutic space. In my view, there is a danger of simplistic reductionism if
the concept of therapeutic space is restricted to an illusion, on the one hand, or 'these
four walls', on the other. In the same way that a patient who has actually killed his
father reminds me that fantasy may become fact, so therapeutic space which may be
an illusion can become 'factual' if enclosed within concrete boundaries.

The setting in which much offender-therapy takes place may be 'secure' so that
therapeutic space takes on a literal 'concrete' quality, readily discernible in the form
of bars at the windows and locks on the doors. These are constant reminders to both
patient and therapist that therapeutic space has undeniable boundaries. Such therapy
may be conducted in the 'group room' set aside for this purpose in a hospital, or
prison, or a probation officer's office. In this sense, therapeutic space is the exact
opposite of an illusion. My experience is that such custodial emblems as bars and
keys intensify, rather than diminish, the affective flow of the therapeutic encounter.
'We are in this together' has a double meaning. There is the symbolic illusion of
therapeutic space but this 'takes place' in a physical space (confined by a secure
perimeter) which is also therapeutic. This existential blending, of the symbolic and
the literal, intensifies transference phenomena and therefore facilitates individual and
group dynamic psychotherapy when conducted within a secure setting.

In view of the many connotations of the term 'therapeutic space', it is essential that
I clarify my own perspective. I regard it as a term which can be used metaphorically

to describe an invisible boundary to the 'space' within which the therapist and patient meet, and where the phenomena of transference and countertransference are 'housed'. It may therefore embrace both an individual therapeutic encounter or a total group matrix, involving eight patients and two co-therapists. In a more global sense it could include all the space within a hospital. Who would not regard the hospital football pitch, on which a patient might learn to improve physical co-ordination and at the same time learn the values of team-work and personal sacrifice, as therapeutic? However, the term usually refers to that space within the between those who share in a formal psychotherapeutic alliance. In other words, it includes the intra-psychic space of both patient and therapist and the inter-personal space between them. It is the shared air they breathe.

Even without bars and keys, I could not work if I felt that the therapeutic space which I shared with a patient was ever *solely* an illusion. I regard it as a 'concrete' existential fact that the patient and I are 'in this together'. Winnicott (1945) describing the feeding of the infant writes: 'I think of the process as if two lives came from opposite directions, liable to come near each other. If they overlap there is a moment of *illusion*—a bit of experience which the infant can take as *either* his hallucination *or* a thing belonging to external reality'.

Dynamic psychotherapy with sex-offenders frequently needs to get back to this early nurturing situation, and this implies that the therapist may become a transitional object. This links closely with Balint's concept of the 'basic fault'. When the therapist is working at such a primitive level with his patients, he may be perceived as a transitional object, but this is only while his patients need to perceive him in this way. It is of the essence of psychotherapy training that the patient's prevailing needs determine the therapist's response. In this instance it would be disastrous if the therapist's personal 'need' to be seen as a transitional object, 'overruled' the fact that his patient had now reached a stage where he could safely relinquish such transitional maturation facilitation. It is logically impossible to be a permanent transitional object, and therapy has ceased to be dynamic if the patient's emotional needs and perceptions of the therapist do not change. Winnicott's comment about infant feeding is also exactly on target at the deepest level of dynamic psychotherapy with the sex-offender: the nourishing experience may be taken 'as *either* his hallucination *or* a thing belonging to external reality'.

Barker and Mason (1968) have taken Buber's theme *Between man and man* (1947) and look at the implications for treating patients 'confined by law, against their will, until they change' in '*Buber behind bars*'. The probation officer is literally in the same prison cell as his client, and the psychiatric nurse in a secure hospital shares therapeutic space in a more than symbolic sense. It is true that one member of the alliance has a key and the other does not, but both are locked in together, and it is in the intensity of this 'locked in-ness' that many of the dynamics I have already discussed take place. From my office at Broadmoor I have a panoramic view covering three countries, with the horizon eighteen miles away. From my desk I can only see the view, but when work is over I can, if I wish, enter and enjoy what I have previously only seen. My patient has the same view, he has no keys and the countryside can be nothing other than a view for him. In spite of the patient's knowledge that I alone have a key, he and I together share therapeutic space.

Hitherto the patient has been stigmatized as 'that bloody rapist', or 'that monster'. The judge, vicariously representing society, has pronounced him guilty of rape and he may, for example, have been admitted to Broadmoor under Sections 37/41 of the Mental Health Act (1983) 'without limit of time'. He and I know the terms of reference within which we meet to share therapeutic space. It is no facile evasion or mere playing with words to state that, by his therapeutic presence, which may be conveyed by gesture, posture, and expression long before words have been necessary (and possibly also when they have ceased to be necessary), the therapist conveys to the patient with whom he shares therapeutic space the realization that *'one of us* has done this'. This is not to condone or in any sense approve of the offence, but there is a profound difference in therapeutic perspective when the patient senses that he is able to say 'I have done this', because the therapist is aware that 'one of us has done this'. This is in marked contrast to conditions previously obtaining when he was being confronted and challenged by 'you have done this', which may have made him retreat into the defensive position of rationalizing the particular episode of his history, deliberately denying it, or even being focally amnesic due to repression.

Within the context of a hospital such as Broadmoor, the fostering of the sense of therapeutic space occurs focally in the particularly intense cosmos of what would be formally known as 'small-group psychotherapy', and in wider life of the institution as a whole. This permeates the many-faceted staff–patient interactions, ranging from that with the football coach and the conductor of the choir, via that with staff undertaking more conventional nursing activities, to that with staff using specialized techniques, such as dream interpretation, or appropriately dealing with other 'pure' psychotherapeutic topics, such as group transference.

The concept of therapeutic space serves to counteract the previous stigmatizing experiences described by sociologists such as Goffman (1963), Chapman (1968), and Matza (1969). Merton (1949) warns us against the dangers of the 'self-fulfilling prophecy', and this is closely linked to the idea of 'controlling identity' elaborated by Matza. Attention is drawn to the risks inherent in limiting the patient's possible future by extrapolating from his past, though the clinician is always aware of the 'natural history' of disease processes. This applies, *a fortiori*, to the profound clinical and moral implications of decisions, relating to the release of dangerous offenders such as the sex-offender, in whom there might be an 'outcropping' of violence after a five-year gap of impeccable social behaviour. The therapist is therefore warned against therapeutic nihilism implicit in the statement 'because the patient has behaved like this in the past, he will therefore continue to do so in the future', and the therapeutic naiveté implicit in the remark 'the patient now has insight into what he has done and therefore he will not do it again'! However, Matza's concept of the controlling identity, implicit in the stigmatization 'the patient is a thief', merits serious consideration. In fact, this may only apply to one brief incident in the life of the patient, who may otherwise be a bank clerk, a psychotherapist, an out-of-work labourer, or a retired general! Matza develops the argument that this indulgence in deviant activity incurs running the risk of intervention, apprehension, and signification. This leads to the enhancement of the identity in terms of the characteristics signified: that is to say, 'to be signified a thief is to lose the blissful identity of one who among other things happens to have committed a theft. It is a movement, however gradual, toward being a thief and representing theft'.

It need scarcely be added that if the word 'arsonist', 'rapist', or 'murderer' replaces the word 'thief' in the preceding sentence, then an entirely different dimension of significance applies, not only to the individual concerned but to society as a whole.

Sociologists quite correctly point to the risks of labelling, although the clinician is aware that a firm diagnosis of schizophrenia has many more prognostic and therapeutic implications than the mere attachment of an appropriate 'label'. However, in day-to-day professional work a label such as 'psychopathic' is useful shorthand because it conveys 'infinite [diagnostic] riches in a little room'. By describing a patient as a psychopath, it is implied that there has been escalating antisocial behaviour, that he has low impulse control, and that he is not psychotic, but we must be careful that such a label does not lead to the implication that the patient will never improve, that he is always lying and therefore everything he tells you is untrue, and so on. In this way it is easy for a self-fulfilling prophecy to emerge which takes the following form: 'This patient is a psychopath. He will not respond to treatment. Therefore we will not offer him treatment'.

Many psychopaths do mature, and one of the functions of psychotherapy with such patients is to hasten the maturational process, and to monitor and reappraise it as the patient encounters opposition and provocation, when he confronts 'himself' in other members of the group. Bolingbroke was describing the maturation of the psychopath with prophetic insight, although it was in the days before formal group psychotherapy could claim any share in the maturational process!

> As dissolute as desperate, yet thro' both I see some
> Sparkles of a better hope, which elder days may happily bring forth.
>
> (*Richard II*, v, iii, 20)

In spite of Matza's strictures about the dangers of a controlling identity, it is perfectly true that if any staff member working in an institution concerned with treating the mentally abnormal offender-patient asks 'What did he do?' with reference to a particular patient, the answer is likely to be 'He shot his boss', 'He raped an usherette', or 'He set fire to a hotel'. This answer is, of course, only describing a fragment of the patient's history, but anyone who regards homicide, rape, or arson as a fragment and unimportant for the patient or society, must be out of touch with reality.

Weltanschauung of the therapist

The psychotherapist sharing therapeutic space with the sex-offender comes closer to the inner life of the patient than the psychiatrist whose work is predominantly involved with overall treatment strategies and administration. If an effective global therapeutic strategy is to be able to 'hold' a patient, the psychotherapist needs to work in a particularly close relationship with his colleague, the responsible medical officer. This has been discussed elsewhere (Macphail and Cox 1975). The responsible medical officer has to make many executive clinical decisions about his patient (Loucas and Udwin 1974), whereas the psychotherapist spends the majority of his time 'being with' the patient rather than 'doing to' the patient. When the patient is invited to 'say anything', then the therapist has, by implication, made the far-reaching claim that he can 'hear everything'. This may therefore stretch his personal emotional resources to the limit, and will inevitably call his *Weltanschauung* into play. The therapist never fully knows what content his patient's disclosures may carry. 'Looking back on it all now, do you see it very clearly or is part of it baffling and confusing?' Such an invitation to disclosure may yield material which is painful, though in a different way, to both therapist and patient. Yet he remains a human being, and there is no doubt whatever that his inner world may be invaded by that of his patients, and his own smouldering doubts and anxieties may be re-ignited by those with whom he shares therapeutic space. He is exposed to the awareness that his patients may be vicariously carrying his murderousness. He is not 'wholly other'. His patients therefore confront him with part of himself which is usually hidden. In the words of Prospero: 'This thing of darkness I acknowledge mine' (*Tempest*, v, i, 275). If he does not bring the sense of being a person and therefore partially vulnerable to the group, he will be construed as being 'remote and clinical'. If, on the other hand, he appears too soft and fragile, then the patients may feel either that he is unable to take their violence or aggression or, *per contra*, that if they 'go to pieces' the therapist will follow suit. This stretching of the therapist's personal *weltanschauung* underlines the following paradox: he needs to be ruthlessly rigorous in diagnostic appraisal, alert for any disclosures, and aware of the risks of acting-out (particularly by patients who have known histories of violent offences against the person); yet, at the same, he needs to retain warmth and a sense of being at ease with himself. This is an ideal which no individual can ever achieve completely by either personal endowment or technical mastery. The longer I spend in therapeutic space with such patients, the more I feel that I am growing in two directions at once; namely by becoming more rigorous in my objective dynamic formulation of events and, *pari passu*, of accepting my patients as people who are in so many ways just like me. This links closely with the existential approach. It provides the therapist with an awareness of the dangers of foreclosing and pre-empting any fresh disclosures from a patient, if he has already made a cast-iron dynamic formulation based upon rigid psychic determinism. He may in fact run the risk of not hearing what does not fit into his presumed formulation of the patterning of the patient's endo-psychic life. If the therapist is to be able to retain this Janusian quality of adopting both a deterministic and existential outlook, he will discover many surprising things. For example, he will learn that many psychopaths, far from being affectless people, have previously often been particularly vulnerable and formed strong emotional bonds on at least one occasion, but, having been betrayed, they have withdrawn from any further deep relationships. Third-level disclosures from psychopaths often take the form of personal reminiscence about tenderness, beauty, or the betrayal by a trusted ally, which frequently justifies the comments 'Never again, mister'; 'I can't get what I love, so I hate it'. I recall such a disclosure from a man with many violent offences 'against the person', who yet just withheld tears as he described scenes of fantasy from his childhood, which were not only Calibanesque but almost an exact paraphrase of '. . . the isle is full of noises,/Sounds and sweet airs, that give delight, and hurt not . . ./ . . . that, when I waked,/I cried to dream again' (*Tempest*, iii, ii, 144). This patient, 'classified' correctly as an aggressive psychopath, showed a degree of tenderness which many would find it hard to believe, yet it was quite different from the incongruous tenderness of the sadistic homosexual killer, so vividly portrayed in the quotation from *Edward II*.

Bush (1975) in 'Sex offenders are people!' describes her involvement as a volunteer therapist in a group of sex-offenders. (There is a poverty of publications concerning the role of the psychiatric nurse in forensic psychiatry, although in a hospital such as Broadmoor the weight of therapeutic initiative rests on the relationship between the nursing staff and the patients. Consultants come and go. The nursing staff are involved 24 hours per day 'without limit of time'.)

CAVEAT

No single theoretical approach holds a monopoly of truth in determining the predisposing and precipitating factors leading to a sex-offence. Therefore, there cannot logically be a single therapeutic modality which is universally indicated.

It is for this reason that psychotherapy with the sex-offender is such an excellent *métier* for teaching both theory and clinical strategy. The trainee may indulge in elaborate psychodynamic hypotheses to account for his patient's behaviour, but he is brought down to earth by the personal confrontation with the question posed by the patient's legal representative, and society as a whole, 'Is John Smith "ready" to go yet?' There is a paradigmatic quality about mixed-group psychotherapy when, say, rapists and female patients share therapeutic space. This makes the therapist tighten up his dynamic formulations with the utmost rigour, and yet, simultaneously, demands that he remains open towards the patients' unfolding disclosures. Dynamic psychotherapy with sex-offenders therefore makes particular emotional demands on the therapist which, although present in every therapeutic alliance, here assume heightened significance. There is a need for constant reappraisal of endo-psychic patterning, and the monitoring of changes in defence organization which must occur within an emotional climate that facilitates disclosure and provides a therapeutic presence.

The 500 (in 1996) patients in Broadmoor form a highly selected population and provide a unique opportunity for the psychotherapist. He is able to share therapeutic space with patients 'without limit of time', and at a depth of facilitated vulnerability impossible in any other setting. He is cautiously allowed to enter the outer world of his patients, and gradually, but only after repeated testing-out, is he accepted in their inner world. A therapeutic group slowly achieves an autonomous life of its own, and the paradoxical status of the therapist takes on its characteristically chameleon-like quality . . . 'He is one of us but he is not one of us . . . the group goes on without him, but not if he is not there . . . He is there at the beginning and the end, but seems to go away in the middle'. The long temporal perspective allows the 'trust-testing' see-saw to oscillate until it finally rests on trust, and the consequent disclosure of hitherto unconscious or 'conscious-withheld' material gives the therapist in Broadmoor unrivalled access to inner world phenomena of the sex-offender. It is from life within the intense arena of group psychotherapy, with male and female patients, when therapeutic space has been shared for literally thousands of hours, that the following dogmatically antidogmatic reflections come. Prolonged exposure to the inner and outer world of the rapist, the arsonist, or the killer convinces me that any statement about 'The' psychopathology of such offences inevitably implies that the author must have limited personal experience and be basing such remarks upon the comparatively few such cases he has seen. There is a great danger in extrapolating from a few cases to assume that there is a universally applicable psychopathology of a particular offence. Nevertheless, there is clinical validation and an authenticating experience for the therapist, when disclosure at depth and of prolonged duration has occurred from hundreds of sex-offenders: A member of one such group, seeking reassurance, asked anxiously in a pre-therapy assessment interview 'It will be a group of killers, won't it?' and his question implied not only that there is 'safety in numbers', but also that group cohesion is fostered and disclosure facilitated if the murderer is exposed to the 'benevolent ordeal' (Haley 1963) of psychotherapy in a murderer's peer group.

ARSON: A PARADIGM OF OVER-DETERMINISM

I shall love you horribly because you let me unlove you so soon . . .

I want horribly to burn a house, Alyosha, our house. You don't believe it, do you? . . . Why not? There are even children about twelve years old who want very much to burn things, and they do. (*The brothers Karamazov*, Dostoevsky)

It is in the nature of extreme self-lovers, as they will set a house on fire, and it were but to roast their eggs. (*Of age and youth*, Bacon)

. . . thought-executing fires . . . (*King Lear*, iii, ii, 4)

The arsonist may be diagnosed as subnormal, neurotic, psychotic, or psychopathic. The act may be of profound symbolic importance to the patient or almost incidental. It may be of overt sexual significance, and the patient will claim that he has his best ever orgasm as he watched the flames leaping up, or that his greatest moment of sexual excitement was when he was helping the fire service unsuccessfully to put out the fire which he had started. ('I started something which was so out of control that even I and the fire service could not deal with it.') In this instance the act is overtly and expressly sexual. On other occasions the act may be symbolically associated with love or hate ('My best flame, you set me on fire, burning anger' . . .). The arsonist may show psychotic concrete thinking so that self-immolation occurred when Charles Wesley's hymn, 'Kindle a flame of sacred love on the mean altar of my heart', was taken literally. The act may be the quickest way of damaging the property of an enemy. It may be part of a deliberate sexual assault, either in fact or fantasy. One arsonist said that radiotherapy worked by the burning out of cancer, and therefore a really big blaze would destroy all the cancer cells in the vicinity and thus protect his children.

Thus, the almost limitless range of clinical presentations means there is no neat unitary hypothesis which can underlie the behaviour of all patients convicted of arson, which may or may not be part of a sexual offence.

The endo-psychic patterning and defence organization of patients committing arson recall us to the importance of studying the individual. However valuable statistical surveys may be, work at Broadmoor constantly reminds us that although we may have seen a hundred arsonists, we must remain open to what *this* patient is telling us about himself. Hurley and Monahan (1969) were unable to demonstrate any psychopathology specific to arsonists, which reinforces an editorial comment in the *British Journal of Delinquency* (1957) 'the dynamic approach to the individual aspects of crime is not yet exhausted', and Ormrod (1975), already quoted, 'unless the study of offenders is undertaken on an individual basis, little progress will be made'. The therapist working with such patients must welcome any possible exploratory avenue of research which might conceivably go some way towards answering the many unanswered questions.

OFFENDER–VICTIM ALIGNMENTS

Classical quotations can serve as a backcloth to various sexual offences: the deliberately fostered morbid jealousy of Othello, or the 'textbook' homosexual sadistic murder of Edward II. The porter in *Macbeth* made comments about the effect of alcohol on sexual performance which have never been bettered:

> . . . much drink may be said to be an equivocator with lechery; it makes him, and it mars him; it sets him on, and it takes him off; it persuades him, and disheartens him; it makes him stand to, and not stand to . . . (*Macbeth*, ii, iii, 31).

Many sex-offences are precipitated by alcohol or other drugs.

The following is a brief list of the range of clinical presentations: the psychotic killer who rapes and strangles a girl, he 'takes a life' because he needs a life; the woman who castrates her lover and then enucleates her own eye, because she sees what she has done and obeys the injunction 'If thine eye offend thee, pluck it out'; the anxious 'blameless' schoolmaster who confesses to the police that he has exposed himself to a 'sober-suited matron all in black' in the local park and admits that although he was not seen, let alone caught, he feels he ought to have been and has therefore given himself up; the ferocious homosexual dismemberment of a faithless partner; the man convicted of house-breaking who experiences the same excitement of forceful entry into forbidden territory as on his first illicit sexual adventure; the arsonist who burned her lesbian friend's flat, who now presents as psychotically deluded, claiming that her clitoris is protruding from her ear; the rapist whose victim had to be 'a stranger but look like Mum'; the unmarried man with a shoe fetish who can only masturbate when wearing stolen high-heeled shoes and who is charged with 'larceny of a pair of shoes'; the phobic housewife who stabbed a postman because the tubular parcel he handed in was 'too big to squeeze through your letter-box'. Some are 'overt', some are 'displaced', and some sexual offences '*manqué*.' One of the least understood, but most pressing, problems is the relationship between the offender and his victim. This highlights the immense complexity of the subject and rules any simplistic interpretations out of court. Howells (1977), using a standard form of repertory grid, studied the way in which mentally abnormally aggressive offenders perceive their victims subsequent to the actual offence. He uses a grid in which eighteen representative persons from the patient's life (including victim, mother, father, self, ideal self) are used to elicit fifteen constructs from the patient, so that it is possible to identify whom the victim resembles, and which constructs differentiate the victim from other people. Such information will be useful diagnostically and prognostically when used in conjunction with data from many other sources, not forgetting the primacy of the clinical presentation of the patient and the relationship he has with all members of the staff involved in his 'treatment'.

Whether or not the offence is victim-'specific', transference phenomena can induce the therapist, his colleagues, or other patients to be perceived as victim surrogates. Unremitting vigilance is therefore an inextricable facet of the therapist's use of self as he engages with a mentally abnormal sex-offender in therapeutic space. An additional complication is that of the masochistic victim who provokes assault.

'DISPOSAL OPTIONS'

These have been briefly indicated in Figs 13.1 and 13.2. In the interests of protecting society and the offender-patient himself, we are forced into making legal judgements and therefore deciding the appropriate 'disposal' of the offender-patient, while still very much in the dark as far as the individual patient's inner world is concerned. To describe him as being psychotic or psychopathic may have certain administrative and custodial implications, but it is often only after prolonged psychotherapy that we begin to understand what 'makes him tick'. Such executive decisions inevitably have to be made in the presence of incomplete knowledge. However, it is important to remember that such executive action must not be taken to imply that we know more about the patient than we do. Nosology may be administratively essential and yet be dynamically barren. We may have done what is right for society and for the patient at a particular time in his history, but this may mark the beginning of a psychotherapeutic encounter (Fig. 13.2) rather than the end of 'appropriate disposal'. Nevertheless, there is sometimes a marked contrast between the cautious, provisional statements of psychiatrists in executive positions of authority and the dogmatic certainty about inner world dynamics suggested by psychotherapists—which cannot be proved and is not put to the test! Scott (1964, 1969, 1970, 1974), Tennent (1971), Gunn (1976, 1977), together with editorials in professional journals, e.g. *British Medical Journal* 1975), 'Patients or criminals'), and the national press (e.g. *The Times* 2 October 1973, 'Therapy for criminals' all draw attention to the dilemma with which the offender-patient confronts society. To punish or to treat? Scott (1977) underlines the crucial fact of 'involvement on a long-term basis' in 'Assessing dangerousness in criminals'.

It is undeniable that phenomenological identification and the gradual differentiation of syndromes, such as those demarcated by forensic psychiatrists, are of help in terms of assessing the outcome and the likely recrudescence of violence. I refer to the work of Mowat (1966) and Brittain (1968, 1970) who described morbid jealousy and sadistic murderers, respectively.

The studies of Williams (1964) draw attention to a small group of sexual murderers who have similar psychopathology (although many do not). 'The idea of a focalized lesion breaking loose and taking over the whole personality in certain circumstances for a brief but crucial period would correspond to Wertham's catathymic crisis (1949)'. Working with such patients can be one of the most testing experiences for those who share therapeutic space. The encapsulated enclave may be touched upon in a mixed group and, when the 'flash' occurs, the therapist tries to hold the group at a disclosure level where such primitive sequestrated energy can be discharged in safety. Other group members frequently act as 'hosts' for the temporary investment of the energy which streams out like volcanic lava. It is after such experiences that patients and therapists alike are aware that dynamic psychotherapy can be hard work!

'Listen to the patient, he is telling you the diagnosis' was William Osler's advice to clinical students, and it is equally applicable to those undertaking psychotherapy with the sex-offender patient. If we listen to the patient long enough, he may tell us not only the diagnosis but also disclose the dynamics of his inner world. Once the dynamics underlying a sex-offence are understood, an appropriate therapeutic policy can be initiated, although two caveats must be made. First, one of the paradoxes of psychotherapy is that disclosure proceeds as the therapeutic alliance matures; that is, 'diagnosis' becomes more sharply delineated as 'treatment' progresses. Second, the mentally abnormal sex-offender may need psychotherapy for many reasons, such as coming to terms with his past, understanding himself, facing a prolonged period in a secure hospital, among others. Therapy may be 'effective' for such matters but this is *not* equivalent to stating that the patient is now 'safe' and will not rape again. *The reduction of re-offence potentiality is an extremely important parameter, but it is not the only reason why a sex-offender may need psychotherapy*. Dynamic psychotherapy with sex-offenders is likely to be a long and arduous process with many turbulent phases, although it is possible to reach a stage when therapeutic work is complete. Global generalizations about 'the' psychopathology of sex-offenders are doomed to failure; but the detailed 'close-up' of inner world phenomena disclosed in therapeutic space can furnish vital material which is impossible to glean in any other way. Tuovinen (1973) has drawn attention to *Crime as an attempt at intrapsychic adaptation* and psychotherapy may therefore be 'disturbing' to a balanced endopsychic system, with the result that the patient experiences new needs. In the long run, the patient may become 'safer'—but, during those unavoidable phases of the therapeutic process in which defence patterns are changing, he may become temporarily less stable and more dependent on therapeutic proximity.

It is for this reason that the psychotherapist and the psychiatrist (responsible medical officer), who has overall clinical and legal responsibility, work in a particularly close double-harness. Yet each operates within a preserve of autonomy, so that the patient's response to the responsible medical officer provides dynamic material for the psychotherapist and, *ipso facto*, the responsible medical officer can monitor the patient's adaptive response to a formal therapeutic 'session' and compare it with his response to other less-structured encounters.

The implications of this chapter may only be fully understood when considered within the special milieu constituted by Broadmoor Hospital which, as a 'Special Hospital', provides the conditions for dynamic psychotherapy with serious sex-offenders.

REFERENCES

Arnold, W. R. and Stiles, B. (1972). A summary of increasing use of group methods in correctional institutions. *Int. J. Group. Psychother.* **xxii**, 77.

Balint, M. (1968). *The basic fault: therapeutic aspects of regression.* Tavistock, London.

Bancroft, J. (1976). The behavioural approach to sexual disorders. In *Psycho-sexual problems*, (ed. H. Milne and S. J. Hardy). Bradford University Press, Bradford.

Barker, E. T. and Mason, M. H. (1968). Buber behind bars. *Can. Psychiat. Assoc. J.* **13**, 61.

Brancale, R., Vuocolo, A., and Prendergast, W. E., Jun. (1971). The New Jersey program for sex offenders. *Int. Psychiat. Clin.* **8**, 145.

British Journal of Delinquency (1957). **8**, 82.

British Medical Journal (1975). **ii**, 70.

Brittain, R. P. (1968). In *Gradwohl's legal medicine*, (2nd edn), (ed. F. E. Camps). Bristol.

Brittain, R. P. (1970). The sadistic murderer. *Med. Sci. Law*, **10**, 198. Wright.

Buber, M. (1947). *Between man and man*, (trans. R. Gregor Smith). Routledge & Kegan Paul, Trench Trubner, London.

Bush, M. (1975). Sex offenders are people! *J. Psychiat. Nurse Ment. Hlth Serv.* **13**, 38.

Cameron, N. (1943). The paranoid pseudo-community. *Am. J. Sociol.* **46**, 32.

Chapman, D. (1968). *Sociology and the stereotype of the criminal.* Tavistock, London.

Cordess, C. and Cox, M. (ed. 1995). *Forensic psychotherapy: crime, psychodynamics and the offender patient.* Jessica Kingsley, London.

Cox, M. (1973). Group psychotherapy as a redefining process. *Int. J. Group Psychother.* **xxiii**, 465.

Cox, M. (1974). The psychotherapist's anxiety: liability or asset? With special reference to the offender-patient. *Brit. J. Crim.* **14**, 1.

Cox, M. (1976). Group psychotherapy in a secure setting. *Proc. Roy. Soc. Med.* **69**, 215.

Cox, M. (1978a). *Structuring the therapeutic process: compromise with chaos.* Oxford. Reprinted 1995. Jessica Kingsley, London.

Cox, M. (1978b). *Coding the therapeutic process: emblems of encounter.* Oxford. Reprinted 1988. Jessica Kingsley, London.

Cox, M. and Theilgaard, A. (1987). *Mutative metaphors in psychotherapy. The Aeolian mode.* Tavistock, London.

Cox, M. and Theilgaard, A. (1994). *Shakespeare as prompter: The amending imagination and the therapeutic process.* Jessica Kingsley, London.

Freud, S. (1916/1957). Some character types met with in psychoanalytic work. III. Criminals from a sense of guilt. In *Complete psychological works of Sigmund Freud*, (standard edition, Vol. 14). Hogarth Press, London.

Goffman, E. (1963). *Stigma: notes on the management of spoiled identity.* Jason Aronson, New Jersey.

Green, H. (1964). *I never promised you a rose garden.* Holt, Rinehart & Winston, New York.

Gunn, J. (1976). Sexual offenders. *Brit. J. Hosp. Med.* **15**, 57.

Gunn, J. (1977). Criminal behaviour and mental disorder. *Brit. J. Psychiat.* **130**, 317.

Gunn, J. (ed.) (1978). Sex offenders: a symposium. *Special Hospitals Research Report*, No. 14.[1]

Haley, J. (1963). *Strategies of psychotherapy.* Grune & Stratton, New York.

---

[1] Although not directly focused on dynamic psychotherapy with sex offenders, this is an important source of collateral and complementary material.

Halleck, S. L. (1967). *Psychiatry and the dilemmas of crime*. New York.
Hartocollis, P. (1977). *Borderline personality disorders: the concept, the syndrome, the patient*. International Universities Press, New York.
Hitchens, E. W. (1972). Denial: an identified theme in marital relationships of sex offenders. *Perspect. Psychiat. Care*, x, 152.
Howells, K. (1977). Social perception in 'abnormal' aggressive offenders. PhD thesis, University of Birmingham.
Hurley, W. and Monahan, T. M. (1969). Arson: the criminal and the crime. *Brit. J. Crim.* 9, 4.
Kernberg, O. (1970). Factors in the psychoanalytic treatment of narcissistic personalities. *J. Am. Psychoanal. Assoc.* 18, 51.
Kernberg, O. (1975). *Borderline conditions and pathological narcissism*. Jason Aronson, New York.
Khan, M. M. R. (1974). The role of illusion in the analytic space and process. In *The privacy of the self*. Hogarth Press, London.
Kohut, H. (1959). Introspection, empathy and psychoanalysis. *J. Am. Psychoanal. Assoc.* 7, 459.
Kohut, H. (1971). *The analysis of the self*. International Universities Press, New York.
Kohut, H. (1977). *The restoration of the self*. International Universities Press, New York.
Loucas, K. and Udwin, E. L. (1974). The management of the mentally abnormal offender. *Brit. J. Hosp. Med.* 12, 285.
Macphail, D. S. and Cox, M. (1975). Dynamic psychotherapy with dangerous patients, Proc. 9th Int. Congress Psychother., Oslo 1973. *Psychother. Psychosom.* 25, 13.
McGrath, P. G. (1976). Sexual offenders. In *Psycho-sexual problems*, (ed. H. Milne and S. J. Hardy). Bradford University Press, Bradford.
Matza, D. (1969). *Becoming deviant*. Prentice Hall, New Jersey.
Merton, R. K. (1949). *Social theory and social structure*. The Free Press, Chicago.
Mowat, R. R. (1966). *Morbid jealousy and murder*. Tavistock, London.
Ormrod, R. (1975). The debate between psychiatry and the law. *Brit. J. Psychiat.* 127, 193.
Rosen, I. (1968). The basis of psychotherapeutic treatment of sexual deviation. *Proc. Royal Soc. Med.* 61, 793.
Rubinstein, L. H. (1965). Sexual motivations in 'ordinary' offenses. In Sexual behaviour and the law, (ed. R. Slovenko). Charles C. Thomas, Springfield, IL.
Scott, P. D. (1964). Definition, classification, prognosis and treatment. In *The pathology and treatment of sexual deviation*, (ed. I. Rosen). Oxford University Press.
Scott, P. D. (1969). Crime and delinquency. *Brit. Med. J.* (i), 424.
Scott, P. D. (1970). Punishment or treatment: prison or hospital? *Brit. Med. J.* ii, 167.
Scott, P. D. (1974). Solutions to the problem of the dangerous offender. *Brit. Med. J.* iv, 640.
Scott, P. D. (1977). Assessing dangerousness in criminals. *Brit. J. Psychiat.* 131, 127.
Tennent, T. G. (1971). The dangerous offender. *Brit. J. Hosp. Med.* 6, 269.
The Times (1973). 2 October.
Tuovinen, M. (1972). Schizophrenia and the basic crimes. In *Psychotherapy of schizophrenia*, (ed. D. Rubenstein and Y. O. Alanen). Excerpta Medica, Amsterdam.
Tuovinen, M. (1973). *Crime as an attempt at intrapsychic adaptation*. University of Oulu, Finland.
Wertham, F. (1949). *The show of violence*. Doubleday, New York.
Williams, A. H. (1964). The psychopathology and treatment of sexual murderers. In *The pathology and treatment of sexual deviation*, (ed. I. Rosen). Oxford University Press.
Winnicott, D. W. (1945). Primitive emotional development. *Int. J. Psycho-Anal.* 26, 137.
Wolberg, A. R. (1973). *The borderline patient*. Thieme-Stratton, New York.

14
Child sexual abuse

Israel Kolvin and Judith Trowell

INTRODUCTION

Over the two last decades sexual abuse of children has now come to be seen as one of the new 'epidemics' of childhood and yet previously it must have been present in communities; the question arises, why was it not viewed as pathological behaviour and a serious problem affecting children's physical and psychological health. It would seem that multiple factors must have contributed to what appears to be a suppression of the facts, or perhaps it was a reluctance to acknowledge the presence of sexual abuse. For instance, it might have been seen as having little to do with the wider community, but rather attributable to social or psychiatric deviance (R. S. Kempe and C. H. Kempe 1978). Recent reviews suggest a multiplicity of factors as contributing to the apparent increase of prevalence—a greater ease of disclosure, a greater sensitivity by professionals to the possibility of abuse, more knowledge about the relevant suspicious signs and symptoms, and the greater openness about sexuality (Smith and Bentovim 1994).

DEFINITION

The definition of what constitutes child sexual abuse varies widely according to the discipline of the defining professional. However, definitional differences reflect conceptual differences (Haugaard and Reppucci 1988). An older general definition which still has wide currency is that of Schechter and Roberge (1976); 'the involvement of dependent developmentally immature children and adolescents in sexual activities that they do not fully comprehend, are unable to give informed consent to and that violate the social taboos of family roles'. A tighter pragmatic descriptive definition was provided by D. Mrazek and P. Mrazek (1985) who suggested that sexual abuse could be conceptualized as one of four types: (1) exposure (viewing of sexual acts, pornography, and exhibitionism); (2) molestation (fondling of either the child's or adult's genitals); (3) sexual intercourse (oral, vaginal, or anal on a non-assaultive and chronic basis); and (4) rape (acute assaultive forced intercourse). Such a typology has high credibility in forensic situations.

Another useful typology is that developed by Jones and colleagues in Oxfordshire (OACPC 1992). They maintain that the key issue in assessing whether sexual abuse has occurred is that of exploitation. They classify sexual acts *first* as *direct*, for instance, where there is genital, or anal sexual contact between a child and adult; penetration—anal, vaginal, or oral; or other acts where the child is the object of the adult's sexual gratification (e.g., bondage, ejaculation on the child, etc). *Second*, as *indirect*, which includes genital exposure and exposure to pornographic materials. *Third*, there is *exploitation*, this refers to the balance of power between the child and other person at the time the sexual activity first occurred. Thus, exploitation is considered to have occurred if the activity was unwanted when it first began, and/or involved a misuse of conventional age, authority, or gender differential. In the above definitions the key considerations concern questions of consent and the issue of exploitation. The last definition takes into consideration abuse by adolescents or peers and this is particularly important as recent work has demonstrated that a substantial minority of abuse is perpetrated by adolescents. Yet others, Finkelhor and Hotaling (1984), chose to emphasize a definition that includes any sexual contact that occurs as a result of force, threat, or deceit, etc., or through exploitation of an authority relationship, irrespective of the age of the partner.

PREVALENCE

Estimates of prevalence are bedevilled by differences of definition and methods of study, and are closely tied to the population source of the information. In his original study, Finkelhor (1979) reported rates of 19 per cent of female and 9 per cent of male college students who had been sexually abused as children. In the United Kingdom, Baker and Duncan (1985), using a MORI poll of those aged 15 years and older, calculated that 12 per cent of women and 8 per cent of men had abusive experiences in childhood. Unfortunately, even these population surveys are open to criticism of either flawed method, and/or not being representative of the general population (Markowe 1988). For example, few of the earlier studies distinguished between the four types of abuse, described by D. Mrazek and P. Mrazek (1985). In a review of four studies, Wyatt and Peters (1986) investigating methodological differences, demonstrate that the lower rates tended to be based on questionnaire surveys using broad questions. Higher rates were obtained from direct interview techniques. Other studies have demonstrated that where less restrictive definitions are used, mainly referring to exhibitionism and/or touching, very high rates of abuse were reported in women (59 per cent) and less than half of this in men (27 per cent). However, when more restrictive definitions are used these rates fall dramatically (Kelly *et al.* 1991). Rates of abuse also differ according to whether the information concerning biological father or step-father is explored—only 2 per cent of women raised by biological fathers report sexual abuse, as against 17 per cent raised by step-fathers. Higher rates are reported by younger respondents (Russell 1984). However, even when such studies have no such methodological flaws, it is not easy to identify those children who have been abused, as often there is no witness and no clear-cut physical evidence. Sexual abuse only emerges in about 15 per cent of girls at any point in time (Kerns 1981). Finally, it is accepted that official statistics will always underestimate the size of the problem as there is an unwillingness by victims to report abuse (Markowe 1988).

PRESENTATION

Information about sexual abuse can present in different ways—the various forms of presentation can be summarized as follows: based on *accounts* by the *child*; based on *disturbed behaviour* or *changes* in behaviour; with *physical symptoms* or *signs* associated with *other forms of maltreatment*; with *allegations by parents, relatives* or other adults (Jones and McQuiston 1986; Kolvin *et al.* 1988). Some presentations have an established association with child sexual abuse whilst others are more tentatively linked in terms of having a low or only possible association (Kolvin *et al.* 1988). Irrespective of the source of information, it is evident that the most common form of presentation is through *accounts* by the child (Conte and Berliner 1988). Nevertheless, subjects who have been sexually abused often delay reporting what has transpired (Meiselman 1978, Conte *et al.* 1989). However, there is apparently less delay in reporting incidents by a stranger (Jones 1992). Accounts by children may be given to friends and less often to parents. Telephone help-lines are currently a common form of anonymous presentation (Smith and Bentovim 1994). Jones (1992) points out that disclosure happens at a variable time after the abuse has been initiated; and there are differing patterns according to the age and stage of development at which abuse occurs. For instance, some begin in infancy, whereas for others the start is in the teenage years.

From a comprehensive review of the literature, it has been reported that few presentations are likely to be conclusively diagnostic of a child's sexual abuse (Browne and Finkelhor 1986). Some cases have multiple modes of presentation, such as behaviour and physical signs or symptoms, as well as accounts by the child. Often, accounts by the child are not welcomed by caretakers. There is continuing evidence that some children report being disbelieved when they make their first disclosure (Burgess and Holmstrom 1975; Jones 1992). Furthermore, children, especially younger children, may disclose only a part of what has occurred, perhaps waiting to see the caretaker's response and if they receive a (an accepting or supportive) response they may feel secure enough to give more (Jones 1992).

Some children may present with a change in behaviour and this will be discussed later. Changes in behaviour, or other behavioural or psychological warnings may constitute crucial evidence as only a minority of children (under 14 per cent) who have been abused show physical signs (Royal College of Physicians 1991).

Behavioural associations of child sexual abuse

Children can respond with a wide variety of symptoms to specific forms of sexual abuse. These can be viewed as signs or symptoms which alert professionals to the possibility that the child may have been sexually abused. Whilst this is a useful exercise such patterns are not necessarily specific and only a minority of children who have shown these behaviours will actually have been abused. Some of these symptoms have an established association with sexual abuse, whilst others only have low or possible associations.

CLASSIFICATION OF BEHAVIOURAL FEATURES

Behavioural features associated with abuse may be categorized under a number of headings (Jones and McQuiston 1986).

1. Early warnings

Jones (1992) developed a concept of early warnings which occur in the field of physical abuse (Ounsted and Lynch 1976). In sexual abuse some behaviours are tantamount to early warnings in which the child tries to alert the world to his or her plight. For instance, the child may make an ambiguous statement ascribing his or her own experience to another mythical child or else, the child may simulate sexual behaviour, or even intercourse, with a friend in order to alert parents or professionals. In a similar vein Jones points out that older more verbal children may offer hints about their unwanted sexual experiences to either peers, or significant others in their family or social environment.

2. Social relationships

These may consist of a disturbance in relationships and attachments. There may be phobic avoidance of males (Sgroi 1982), the child may show mistrust of adults in general (Herman *et al.* 1986), or show impaired peer relationship (Adams-Tucker 1982). Some children may also not trust their mothers, presumably because of their failure to protect them. Some children may become over and inappropriately friendly with adults seeking close physical contact indiscriminately, some may seek and touch body parts or expose themselves as a means of initiating a relationship.

3. Disturbed behaviour

Post-traumatic stress disorder syndromes

Many children may develop post-traumatic stress disorder (Conte and Berliner 1988). This disorder consists of a sense of unexplained arousal or distress, often with numbed emotional affect, anticipation of future attacks, fears of helplessness, and re-experiencing of the traumatic events which may be 'flashbacks'. There are also memory problems (psychogenic amnesia) and some children may show a degree of hyper-awareness, sleep problems, night terrors, nightmares, and dissociative episodes.

Other behaviours

Regressive behaviour has been reported and features representative of neurotic disorder have been found, such as anxiety and agitation, and again, nightmares and night terrors. Some children may develop phobias, or a sense of general fearfulness. In others, features representative of antisocial behaviour may be found. Somatic symptoms and eating problems, or even anorexia, have been reported (Browning and Boatman 1977; Oppenheimer *et al.* 1985). Symptoms of depression and parasuicidal behaviour are common.

Self-harming behaviour and drug and alcohol abuse are not uncommon. (James and

Meyerding 1977; Conte 1985). School and academic problems consisting of deterioration in behaviour in school and with school work has been reported (Goodwin 1982). This may be because the children's anxiety and distress impedes their concentration and, hence, their ability to achieve.

Some of the above occur more frequently in younger children, whilst others more frequently in older children, and some are found across the age range. When they occur after the abuse may be significant but the picture is not a simple or clear one. For instance, some behavioural features may reflect recent abuse, whereas others may be seen as longer-term affects (Green 1986). However, these behavioural features are often similar to those occurring in children attending child guidance, or child psychiatry clinics, and cover almost the total spectrum of child psychiatric disorders. Thus, the presence of disturbed behaviour is not diagnostic of sexual abuse (Jones and McQuiston 1986). Looked at from the other end of the telescope it is estimated that a minority of disturbed children attending child psychiatric clinics have been sexually abused (Kolvin *et al.* 1988). There is evidence that whilst many behaviours may be commonplace in sexually abused children, they are not specific; that is, only a minority of children with such behaviours would have been abused (Kolvin *et al.* 1988). Finally, a minority of sexually abused children do not show behavioural features, at least in the short term (Jones 1992), whilst others may present with behaviours and other responses which constitute 'accommodations to sexual abuse' (Summit 1983)—the latter constitutes a syndrome which is described more fully in a later section.

4. Attitudinal problems

Some sexually abused children may report feelings of worthlessness and poor self-esteem (Sgroi 1982), which may become enduring personality traits. They may blame themselves or feel irrevocably damaged by their experiences. Some may also experience shame and self-disgust if their bodies responded to the sexual excitement.

5. Psychosexual disturbances and allied problems

Some younger children may present with what can be described as sexualized behaviour in which they are precociously preoccupied with adult types of sexual behaviour (Mian *et al.* 1986; Friedrich *et al.* 1986). Some older children may show disturbances of sexual behaviour—becoming sexually disinhibited, or may behave provocatively, or occasionally turn to prostitution. Some young people become sexually inhibited, avoiding peer sexual contact, and others are confused about their sexual orientation.

Presentations in adulthood

Not all sexually abused children present with disturbed behaviour in childhood and many do not do so until adulthood. Those behavioural symptoms presenting in adulthood have been summarized by Cotgrove and Kolvin (1994) who conclude that there are four main long-term associations with child sexual abuse.

1. Psychological symptoms consisting of depression, anxiety, low self-esteem, guilt, sleep disturbance, and dissociative phenomena.

2. Problem behaviours including self-harm, drug use, prostitution, and running away.
3. Relationship and sexual abuse problems: social withdrawal, sexual promiscuity, and victimization.
4. Psychiatric disorders, particularly eating disorders, sexualization, post-traumatic stress disorders, and borderline personality disorders. (See Chapter 15.)

MULTI-FACTORIAL ORIGINS OF DISTURBED BEHAVIOUR IN SEXUALLY ABUSED CHILDREN

It is commonplace to assert that all disturbed behaviour with which sexually abused children present is a consequence of the abuse. It is very important that this assumption is *not* made—due weight must be given to the effect of the level of dysfunction in the family and the environmental pathology. It is essential that the literature on child sexual abuse is studied with care and rigour. The data on which the main body of knowledge derives is often rather flawed, this is because of the nature of the study and sample and, generally, the absence of comparison groups. Perhaps the most cogent criticism of the search for behavioural association of child sexual abuse is provided by Jones (1992). He concludes that child sexual abuse is not a unitary phenomenon, but covers a wide variety of activities and situations. For instance, children may have been assaulted by strangers, or have been the victims of incest for many years. Furthermore, there are a diversity of environmental factors; such as accompanying neglect, emotional abuse, deprivation, or physical abuse. Available research does not necessarily specify whether there has been any pre-existing maladjustment. Other workers have sought evidence of a relationship between age of the child when first abused and evidence of disturbed behaviour as an indicator of more serious disturbance in younger children, but the evidence is contradictory. However, there does seem to be positive evidence of more serious disturbance when the abuse is coercive, or when it includes the use of physical force or violence (Finkelhor 1979; Fromuth 1986). In a similar vein, abuse which includes penetration appears to be associated with greater degrees of disturbance (Russell 1984; Mannarino *et al.* 1992). The nature of the relationship with the abuser seems significant—abuse by biological parents and step-parents, is associated with the greater severity of disturbance occurring where the abuser is a step-parent (Gomes-Schwartz *et al.* 1990). These authors also demonstrated that when mother showed negative responses to the disclosure of abuse, this was associated with an increased severity of disturbance in the child.

Psychology of child sexual abuse

A number of different theories have been advanced in an attempt to explain the psychology of sexually abuse: factors in the perpetrator; factors within the child; and family factors.

Factors promoting abuse

Finkelhor (1984) has conceptualized four basic 'preconditions' which may promote abuse. First, an adult who is sexually aroused by children, together with the ability to fantasize a sexual interaction with the child. There may also be an impaired capacity to have normal and sexual relationships with adults and the potential abuser may have been sexually abused as a child. Not all these features necessarily coexist in the one individual. Second, there may be a relative lack of internal restraints, determined by inadequate acquisition of socially appropriate norms, compounded by poor personal controls or other personality problems. In addition, alcohol and/or drugs may reduce normal inhibitions. Third, there may be inadequate external inhibitions in the shape of social and family forces which constrain the predisposition to sexual abuse, particularly the protection afforded to the child by the mother. Fourth, the ability of the child to resist abuse, which is enhanced by parental teachings and educational programmes; in addition, some children have a poor sense of danger perhaps linked to vulnerability factors. While the above stereotypes allow a better understanding of factors which have the potential for promoting or preventing sexual abuse, it can give rise to a too high expectation of the prevalence of child sexual abuse which can seriously mislead the inexperienced.

Adaptation to abuse

A number of authors (e.g., Summit 1983; Jones and McQuiston 1986) provide convincing accounts of the psychological processes by which the child and family may adapt to abuse. Often, the potential abuser has become the most available care giver some time before the abuse occurs, so the child and the care giver become mutually absorbed and closer together. The non-involved spouse becomes aloof and excluded. The relationship between the abuser and the victim gradually becomes sexualized by what appears to be a growing process, starting with closer physical contact and culminating in inappropriate sexual contact. In the process, children become very confused and while they may suspect that such behaviour is wrong, they do not wish to lose the close emotional ties and younger children may even begin to wonder if this is a normal process which happens to all children. The abuser abuses the care giving relationship with the child and asks the child to keep their 'special secret', misusing adult or parental authority to maintain control. Alternatively, gifts or threats of break-up of the family or threats to a beloved relative (Lister 1982) are used to ensure secrecy.

In this way the child's feelings are harnessed and exploited by the abuser. In the course of time the child develops a sense of fear and guilt (Conte *et al.* 1989), compounded by a desire to be loved and for some children some sexual pleasure. A child whose personal security and that of their family is threatened by the abuser, may find it hard to escape from this situation or to prevent a recurrence of the abuse. A child thus trapped is under a great deal of stress and develops a sense of helplessness, indeed a sense of learned helplessness (Seligman and Peterson 1986) as any action he or she may take may be seen as having dreadful personal and family repercussions.

Perpetrator and victim

Intra-familial abuse is common in clinical studies and stranger abuse is relatively common in non-clinical studies (Finkelhor *et al.* 1986; Baker and Duncan 1985). Furthermore, abuse by siblings occurs relatively frequently in population studies, perhaps even as common as abuse by fathers (Finkelhor 1979; Anderson *et al.* 1993). There are a number of other important patterns reported in the literature. For instance, girls with step-fathers are at much higher risk of being abused than those with biological fathers. And abuse by step-fathers tends to be associated with more serious disturbance (Russell 1984). Another pattern is that girls are more likely to be abused within the family and boys more so by strangers (Kelly *et al.* 1991; Haugaard and Reppucci 1988). Finally, a minority of the abuse occurring while still inside the home, is by caretakers who are not related to the family, mainly by female perpetrators who are mostly in their teenage years. Much of this abuse had taken place whilst the caretaker was functioning in a baby-sitting capacity (Margolin 1991).

Reliability and validity of alerting symptoms

Although the above-mentioned alerting or warning symptoms and behaviour patterns may be common in abused children, they are not specific (i.e., only a minority of children with such behaviours will be found to have been abused). Thus, these features should be seen as screening measures, always bearing in mind that such measures are of limited diagnostic utility and the data must be interpreted cautiously. A single feature must be seen as an indicator, and not necessarily as definitive evidence of sexual abuse. The validity of these screening measures increases according to the number that coexist, the sources of information, and where this is supplemented by corroborative evidence from further careful assessment.

Two concepts derived from epidemiology—sensitivity and specificity—are particularly useful in validation of screening criteria. In this respect, sensitivity can be defined as the capacity of a measure to select a child who has been abused; it represents the proportion of true cases out of all possible cases selected by that particular screening measure. In contrast, specificity is the capacity of a screen measure to identify children who are truly free of sexual abuse by keeping the number of false negatives to a minimum. Such validation exercises need to be complemented by reliability checks.

It is crucial that the judicial system, the professions, and society must give attention to the twin issues of which is worse or which is better—more false positives, and to have an excess of families under question; or more false negatives and to have more missed cases of child sexual abuse. How much uncertainty we are willing to accept as a society and which way we prefer to err currently fluctuates.

The basis of suspicion

Professional suspicion may be justified but professional opinion about probability must be based on appropriate assessment. Jones (1992) clearly points out that when approaching assessment the over riding general principle is that the interview is not of a sexually abused child, but rather a child who may have been abused. The clinician has to consider a number of factors, including the source of the suspicion and the quality and objectivity of the information that is offered (Kolvin *et al.* 1988). It is essential that pre-judgement of issues is avoided. It should be emphasized that the basis of suspicion is a step which enables the professional to proceed to the next stage of evaluation but is not tantamount to confirmation of that suspicion (Kolvin *et al.* 1988). If clinicians are overly suspicious they are likely to identify an excess of false positive cases; in contrast, if the threshold of suspicion is too low, there will not only be a reduction in true positive cases but a simultaneous excess of false negatives.

Consent to assessment

In the wake of the Cleveland inquiry (Butler-Sloss 1988), a sensible policy of seeking parental consent for assessment of the child, and the consent of the older child, must be established. It is suggested that parental consent is implicit for standard clinical assessments which include routine physical inspection of the child and screening questions. However, for more detailed assessment, parental consent should be obtained and, when appropriate, agreement of the child as well. It is thought that such consent should apply as well to special methods of recording. It is also wise to obtain written consent if the assessment is going to be beyond the routine. Complementary to consent is the necessity for openness and honesty and the avoidance of misguided attempts at reassurance that 'all will be well'. Both child and parents should be kept informed about the possible consequences of the assessment (Jones 1992). Just occasionally, where suspicion is high that the parent is the abuser, after debate at a case conference, it may be decided that for the child's safety consent should not be sought and the parent be informed after an investigative interview.

Tailoring the assessment

It has been suggested that it is necessary to adjust the intrusiveness and breadth of the professional evaluation according to the level of suspicion that exists in the individual case (Kolvin *et al.* 1988). It is not possible to provide a rigid description of this tailoring: broadly, the stronger the basis of suspicion the fuller the paediatric/psychiatric/social investigation. When the basis of suspicion is weaker, a further filtering/screening exercise would help to gauge the appropriate depth of the investigation. The response to such screening measures can then indicate whether further psychological evaluation should be considered. The extent of assessment will also be guided by careful scrutiny and evaluation of the prior history and any social, psychological, school, and medical records (Jones 1992).

Principles in relation to evaluation and examination

The professional should avoid bias, pre-judgement, emotional overtones, and an accusatory stance, and should display an open-minded reaction to their accounts (Goodwin 1982). The clinician must provide a comprehensive, sensitive, and multi-disciplinary approach. The findings should be communicated to the parents and the need for further investigations explained.

In the examination of the child a number of principles or practices appear to be sensible: children should not be subjected unnecessarily to repeated examinations or disclosure interviews; the examiner must be cautious about the use of facilitatory questions and leading questions; it is helpful to interview the child in a sensitive atmosphere, always ensuring that the child is as comfortable as possible; finally, investigations need to be child-focused rather than attempting to fit the child into the system. The child needs to be allowed to proceed at his or her own pace.

Psychiatric assessment

There are a number of potential pitfalls in psychiatric assessment and the following approach will help the clinician to avoid them. In all cases, a carefully taken history is essential to understand the child's past history, developmental level, and family context. An abuse history is then needed to allow information about the psychological background of sexual abuse to emerge, together with the gathering of information about immediate and long-term possible sequelae and any changes in the child after the alleged experience. In addition, the history may provide clues regarding the reliability of the accounts by the child and the parents. The child's psychiatric examination must, first and foremost, address itself to the child's psychiatric status, including mood, capacity for relationships, personal strengths, defence mechanisms, extent of fantasizing, and any evidence of disorders of behaviour, including sexual behaviour (Kolvin and Kaplan 1988).

In the above, a distinction should be drawn between the standard clinical psychiatric assessment and the disclosure interview. An investigative interview may occur within the psychiatric assessment but may well be a separate interview arranged in the light of the information discovered during the initial interview. The basis of the investigative interview is that skilled, sensitive interviewing will allow children to confide (disclose) their secrets. Unfortunately, this has become questionable as it incorporates the preconception that non-disclosure is tantamount to denial. This can preclude the possibility that sexual abuse has not occurred (Kolvin *et al.* 1988; Jones and McQuiston 1986).

Disclosure techniques include the use of drawings and play, the validity and utility of which may be hampered by suggestions, leading questions, and the possibility that the investigative procedure itself, when unwisely conducted or prolonged, may become sexualizing and abusive.

Many authorities take the view that evaluative assessment is preferable to an investigative interview. Evaluative assessment follows the same principles as a general psychiatric examination, while bearing in mind the following points. Interviewers or assessors need to be knowledgeable and experienced, as there are potential civil and criminal implications; they require traditional interviewing skills and a background knowledge of the child's play, language, and memory, as well as knowledge of normal and abnormal sexual development and the psychology of child sexual abuse (Kolvin and Kaplan 1988). The interviewer needs to build a supportive and honest relationship with the child, while recognizing that no guarantees can be offered about confidentiality. The initial questioning should be flexibly open-ended, with little or no leading questions or suggestions. The child should be encouraged to talk spontaneously. The pace of the interview is also a factor, with some authorities recommending a slower pace and frequent contact, whereas others are concerned that the interview process, when prolonged and focusing on 'disclosure', may become abusive in itself, it is certainly important to ensure the investigative process is time-limited. Other facilitating techniques, such as the use of hypothetical questions, have been seriously questioned by some authorities. There is general agreement that facilitative techniques should not be used in the first stage of interviewing. When these techniques are used, great skill is required to avoid the extreme of being overtly leading during questioning, or insufficiently enabling. The use of different degrees of facilitation in questioning has been outlined by Jones and McQuiston (1986). As part of this facilitating exercise, an anatomically correct doll may be used in the assessment of suspected sexual abuse. Unfortunately, such dolls are often used by those who are not trained to use them: they should not be used without an understanding of child development, play, fantasizing, and psychopathology. However, they are thought to be particularly useful when a younger child has indicated sexual abuse at some level but then has become stuck, or wishes to describe a particular detail about sexual abuse but does not have the words or concepts to do this (Jones and McQuiston 1986). The dolls can also be useful when interviewing children with learning difficulties who may lack the language and, rarely, some very shy inhibited children and young people. Any interviewer using anatomically correct dolls needs to bear in mind that many questions remain concerning their validity and reliability.

The stages of interviewing with a younger child consist of an introductory free period with open-ended questioning: seeking of evidence of traumatization; attachment problems; behaviour and social relational problems; unusual attitudes; sexualized behaviour; and possibilities of fabrication. A second stage of facilitative interviewing requires experience and skilled interviewing.

FAMILIES AS VICTIMS OF PROCEDURES

Children as procedural victims

When there is a presumption of abuse without adequate attempts at comprehensive assessment and validation, it becomes apparent that children may be exposed to traumatic procedures by professionals which may be extremely distressing and anxiety-provoking. For instance, children may be exposed to multiple coercive questioning and unnecesarily be removed from their families and familiar environments. Another aspect of this is the induction of an expectation whereby children obtain the impression that they have to give the 'right response' to be allowed to go home. Children may be treated with inadequate sensitivity; there may be lengthy delays in the assessment and other procedures; there may be forceful separation of children from parents. Hence, foremost in the expert's mind must be the question what is in the child's best interest and whether the needs and rights of children are being respected. Many questions remain as to how the experiences and views of the children can best be ascertained, and how investigative procedures can be controlled so that they are not misapplied. This is currently an area of considerable debate (Kolvin 1992).

Assessors or experts need to be supportive and honest in their approach and should avoid collusion and promises or guarantees which cannot be kept. They also have to exercise maximum discretion in using 'encouraging' or 'facilitating' interviewing techniques. In the interview, they need to be guided by the level of suspicion, the level of the child's distress, and the possible value of, and objectives met by, this information. However, they must also respect the child's persistent refusal to talk about their experiences. They have to ask themselves whether the investigatory processes are in the best interests of the child's psychosocial needs and whether the child's welfare is totally dependent on obtaining the 'truth'.

MEMORY

It is only possible to touch on some salient aspects of the psychology of memory. This will be supplemented by sections covering psychodynamic understanding of memory, post-traumatic stress disorder, and the so-called 'false memory syndrome'.

Psychology of children's memory

Fundudis (1989) notes that a child who is alleged to have been sexually abused is likely to be interviewed by several professional including the police. Hence, the reliability of the child's memory has a central role in the credibility of the evidence. Further, there has been a tendency of some experts to doubt the ability of younger children to 'observe and recall events reliably' (Goodman *et al.* 1984), but later research has shown such doubts to be unfounded (Ceci *et al.* 1987). Jones (1992) concludes that the poorer ability of children than adults to remember events in detail is because of children's lesser experience, poorer grasp of language, conceptual level of development, and the inadequate assessment skills of professionals in assessing this memory (Loftus and Davies 1984). However, what children remember does not differ substantially from what adults remember—and in children it depends on language, conceptual level of development, and the style and manner in which their memory is assessed (Fundudis 1989). Furthermore, although children may have better recall in relation to certain aspects of memory, the development of memory is not linear, with some components becoming more reliable and others less reliable with age. An important theme is that some children may even be able to recall memorable events which occurred prior to them being able to speak (Todd and Perlmutter 1980). Children's *recognition memory*, for example, where a physical stimulus is present (e.g. a face in a picture, and the child must decide whether it is familiar or not) is better than in *free recall*, which involves recollection of past information or events and includes recounting rather than merely recognizing information or events from the past (Fundudis 1989). There are two other important factors: first, as in adults, memory does decay over time and, second, as the child grows older, the memories may be influenced by suggestion (Goodman and Clarke-Stewart 1990). It is important to note that salient events are often remembered well by children, and they also place them in an appropriate sequence (Gelman 1978). The salient events need to be emphasized as both children and adults are less likely to remember accurately events with less in the way of personal poignancy for the subject (Jones 1992). In addition, young children are particularly influenced by the authority of the interviewer, misleading questions, and suggestibility (Jones and Krugman 1986; Goodman and Clarke-Stewart 1990).

It also needs to be remembered that interviewer techniques can seriously distort children's memories—in particular, leading questions combined with relentless probing for detail (Moston 1990), with a particular influence on the younger child (Jones 1992). Fundudis (1989) recommends that younger children need to be given opportunities to provide their accounts in their own way. For instance, allowing the child the freedom to report on personally relevant details (this constitutes script memory), rather than according to the expectations or demands of the interviewer. This can be followed by simple, unambiguous questions both as an aid to the child and to clarify any inconsistencies. Another factor in apparent forgetting is that the children may be exposed to circumstances where they are told not to tell or reveal information and thereby conceal information, fearing repercussions (Jones 1992). Much can be done to help the child to remember events by gentle open-ended questioning and the availability of appropriate historical props reminiscent of their everyday experiences, such as a dolls house, toy motor cars, etc. (Jones 1992).

A psychodynamic understanding of memory

In childhood sexual abuse, many processes are at work to try and enable the child to survive. These coping strategies are the usually intra-psychic mechanisms, but in addition the trauma provokes the use of other mechanisms. Normal events that cause anxiety or conflicts may be repressed, that is, removed from the conscious into the unconscious. The memory may at some later date re-emerge in the consciousness of the individual directly, or may emerge indirectly linked to some other event or stimuli. This process does not seem to be a mechanism that is capable of helping a child 'forget' sexual abuse, where the violation of the body produces very powerful emotions. Similarly, displacement cannot really help the child: this is where the affect and the surrounding conflicts are transferred from one event, or individual, on to another. Disavowal may be helpful—Freud defined it as 'a specific sense of a mode of defence which consists of the subject's refusing to recognize the reality of a traumatic perception'. It is seen as enabling the individual to deal with external reality by holding two incompatible ideas at the same time. In childhood sexual abuse, the child can simultaneously believe 'this is a kind caring father', 'this is a bad frightening person who hurts me'. Disavowal may sometimes enable a child to survive, but frequently it is not sufficiently robust to keep the terror from consciousness.

If the emotions are too painful the individual can resort to using earlier or infantile mechanisms: splitting-off and denial, or projection. An overwhelming or unbearable experience may be denied and split-off: this is not in the conscious mind but in the deep unconscious, the event having been such as to pass through the conscious and preconscious into the unconscious. The split-off and denied piece of experience remains encapsulated, unintegrated into the rest of the internal world. However, it has consequences for the individual, entrapping with it other areas of functioning, such as cognitive capacity or the capacity to distinguish fantasy from reality or the capacity to relate, empathize, be sensitive, and responsive. In some individuals this split-off and denied experience does not remain encapsulated but is projected outwards on to other individuals who are then seen as threatening and dangerous or very vulnerable. Mothers who may themselves have been abused but do not recall it, can present their daughters as sexual abuse victims and the child shows some symptoms. This can be understood as the mother 'communicating' the abusive experince to the child, probably via projective identification. This process occurs at an unconscious level and needs to be distinguished from 'coaching' the child as happens in some divorce allegations.

These split-off experiences can re-emerge in consciousness and frequently this is very distressing. It can happen spontaneously, or during some form of therapy, perhaps for altogether other reasons. However, these memories once recalled do usually have some associated material detailing the abuse, or the environment. The memories can also re-emerge at specific points in the individual's lifecycle when married or pregnant or when their child reaches the age when they were abused.

Recently, there has been interesting corroboration of this hypothesis that certain very emotionally charged traumatic experiences can be split-off and denied. New psychological research has indicated that such experiences produced neurological responses that cannot be registered in the normal memory bank. They remain unprocessed, that is, they do not enter explicit memory but are presumed to be located in implicit memory. In addition, there is often a failure of development of normal object-relationships: each individual, as they develop, builds up an internal world, which contains, at an unconscious level, representations of themselves and significant others. In the unconscious this is thought to start as 'part objects', eyes, hands, body, etc., and then these come together as 'whole objects'. The child who is treated as a sexual object develops a model of themselves as 'part object', not a whole person, and this can give rise to difficulties in thinking, in remembering and making sense of experiences.

Post-traumatic stress disorder

This provides another conceptual framework to try and understand the response to a traumatic event or events. Where the individual experiences a stress outside the range of usual human experience, there can be re-experiencing of traumatic experiences shown by recurrent and intrusive recollections, recurrent distressing dreams, sudden feelings as though the event is recurring ('flashback'). In these manifestations the memory could be viewed as stuck, repetitive, and out of control. Or individuals may show persistent avoidance of thoughts and feelings of situations or activities that might provoke memories, or 'forgetting' of important aspects of the trauma (psychogenic amnesia). They may also show diminished interest in activities, feel detached, and have a restricted range of affect. In these manifestations memory is limited or lost and this mechanism is labelled dissociation.

Dissociation describes how memories are pushed away, out of consciousness but, as indicated, they can break through as flashbacks or re-experiencing. Where the trauma has been extensive and prolonged the dissociation can appear as lapses which may be mistaken for *petit mal*. The child briefly appears to be detached and unavailable. More frequently, this manifests as a flatness, an absence of liveliness, warmth, and spontaneity; this is because with the avoided memories go feelings and thoughts. Dissociation does not include a description of where the memories go other than out of awareness. Dissociation is described as a numbing process or distancing strategy (B. Justice and R. Justice 1979; Sgroi 1989). Dissociation can become a life-long coping mechanism that the survivor repeatedly invokes when triggered by minimal cues—perhaps a means of autohypnosis (Sgroi 1989).

False memory syndrome

In the 1990s a new syndrome has emerged—false memory syndrome—largely identified by parents who have been the subjects of allegations of sexual abuse. They maintain that in some cases where sexual abuse is alleged, particularly where the 'survivor' is in therapy, the allegations arise through the over-zealous attitude of the therapist in searching for repressed memories of sexual abuse in childhood. The therapist is believed to have suggested to their patient, with great conviction, their understanding that their patient's problems and difficulties arise because he or she must have been sexually abused. The therapist and patient then explore together the abusive experience the patient must have had. The patient becomes convinced of the reality of the abuse and blames the alleged abuser. This has occurred most frequently where the patients are young women and where they 'recall' sexual abuse in their early childhood. The parents argue that the young women are suggestible and vulnerable and easily believe what therapists tell them, particularly if this is conveyed with insistence. They claim these memories are not corroborated by independent evidence nor supported by other members of the family.

The question arises of whether this syndrome exists or whether it is a defensive manoeuvre developed by alleged abusers joining together. The nature and basis of the syndrome and of limited concepts are being debated strongly in the literature (Mersky 1995). The validity of the syndrome is dependent on three main factors: first, whether there is scientific evidence that memories can be repressed; second, whether earlier life forgotten memories can be recovered; third, whether there is independent corroborative evidence of sexual abuse. So far, research by academic psychologists has failed to support the notion of widespread repression of early life memories (Holmes 1990). As to clinical research, Loftus *et al.* (1994) revealed that one in five sexually abused women had had episodes of forgetfulness but, unfortunately, the nature of the amnesia was not clarified at interview. However, such findings cannot be discounted totally because of lack of clarification.

An important study by Femina *et al.* (1990) throws new light on relevant processes. They studied some 70 adults whose serious abusive experiences had been recorded during adolescence. However, only about 60 per cent reported this abuse at subsequent interview. About half of those who did not report abuse were re-interviewed and all revealed that they remembered abuse but *consciously* wanted to *forget* the painful experience or wanted it *to be private*, or wanted *to minimize it*. A worrying development in some recent reviews is a tendency by 'purist' researchers to want to underplay the fear and terror in sexually abused children that causes them to suppress their memories (Russell 1986). Nevertheless, so far there is neither definitive evidence that early-life forgotten memories cannot be recovered, nor definitive evidence that painful memories cannot be repressed. However, it is clear that any *demonstrated repression* will not prove to be a widespread phenomenon. But in one case study where a woman in her early thirties was in therapy for relationship problems, the patient and her therapist insisted she had been sexually abused but there was no confirmatory details of any abusive incident. There was only a conviction that the patient and her therapist believed it had happened and the traumatic experience explained her problems. A second-opinion interviewer found it impossible to discover any more information to question or doubt the above conviction. Perhaps the main support for repressed memory phenomena derive from clinical anecdotes. And it is these case anecdotes, where forgotten memories appear to have re-arisen spontaneously, which cannot be discounted.

SOME DYNAMICS SURROUNDING THE MANAGEMENT OF SEXUAL ABUSE

Once sexual abuse has been suspected or disclosed powerful feelings may arise in carers or attendants such as shock, horror, fear, anxiety, rage, revulsion, distress, and sadness. But at the same time there may be both a denial—it cannot be true, these things do not happen, and not in this family that I know quite well. Or a wish not to know, a desire to walk away and not become involved. At every stage with cases of child sexual abuse, there may be the same conflict, the wish to rescue and protect and the wish to ignore in the hope it will go away. Child sexual abuse can be understood as the abuser psychically 'raping' the child's mind, that is, a piece of madness is forced into the child's mind so that the child can no longer make sense of their experiences, thoughts, and feelings. This same process can happen to those who then become involved.

The consequences of suspecting abuse or hearing a child disclose inevitably means there needs to be action. The person told must inform the responsible statutory agencies (e.g., the social services). It will also be necessary to have strategy meetings, investigative interviews, and case conferences. The child and his or her family are likely to be split up one way or another; the alleged abuser may leave, or the child may be removed, with consequent further emotions of shame, confusion, guilt, doubts, and disbelief.

If the abuser is the father, or step-father, the mother is precipitously placed in a conflict of loyalty situation between her partner—her emotional support and bread-winner, or her vulnerable child who is in need of protection. If the mother's relationship with her child has previously been poor, the decision to believe and support the child may be difficult or impossible. If the child has a disability or exhibits antisocial behaviour the mother may find it very hard to decide between her partner and her child, particularly if the child reminds her of someone in her own background. Extended families usually become drawn in, in one way or other way—taking sides with 'their daughter', or 'their son', or the grand-child. Ripples spread into the community, the school is likely to be involved, also neighbours, the family doctor, the community, and the legal system. Inevitably, child sexual abuse, especially associated with obvious uncontrolled sexuality and probably aggression, and also the abuse of power, provoke very powerful feelings (Furniss 1991; Glaser and Frosh 1991; King and Trowell 1992).

The inter-agency professional network that must assess the case and then carry through any legal action is always subjected to this emotional barrage—their capacity to hold on to clear rational objective thinking is imperative, but is all too frequently lost. Often, there may be revulsion, disgust, and outrage. Different agencies and different professionals easily become identified with different members of the family (Hay *et al.* 1991). This process is known as mirroring, and if not expected and anticipated can lead to inter-professional and inter-agency conflict. Police are likely to want evidence for a criminal prosecution, social workers will want to protect the child and to keep the child's world child-centred and not cause too much disruption, and health workers will want to care and treat the child. All too frequently, these different professional aims can lead to conflict and fragmentation of the network. Often, professionals will not want to work with or have dealings with the alleged abuser, except to convict. All the professionals ostensibly want to 'help' the child but may compete for this role. However, the social worker may become very involved in supporting the mother and may lose sight of her parenting inadequacies. It is frequently the case that mothers have been physically and/or sexually abused themselves and need much help and support (the abusers have also, many of them, been physically or sexually abused). The child's needs, once the abuse has stopped and the child is safe, can be lost sight of because of the greater needs of the mother. It may well be that the health visitor, the family doctor, or the school are the professionals that are in touch with the child's pain and distress after the initial tasks of child protection have been implemented.

In case discussions and conferences these divergent views about needs can lead to rather heated, and at times, acrimonious discussions. The professionals speaking for the child may feel ignored, put down, or attacked; the professionals speaking for the mother may feel misunderstood; any thought or plan for the abuser may be lost other than punishment. With good professional skills based on appropriate training, many of these difficulties can be anticipated and dealt with so that the decisions made are not too biased or distorted by these identifications. If the decision is to go for Court action, civil and/or criminal, sadly all too often the conscious conflicts and unconscious dynamics can be reactivated and dominate the legal process unless this phase is handled with awareness, sensitivity, and care. Once decisions in Court are made, the dynamics can again be acted out. Where is the emphasis to be—the need for help, treatment, or the need for punishment? Whose need in a time of limited resources? Moreover, agreeing a treatment plan for parents, abuser, abused child, and siblings can be skewed unless there is constant vigilance and a monitoring of the process of decision-making because, again, the identifications with the different family members and their needs is so powerful.

Therapy

All members of the family system are likely to need treatment from the following menu:

Adults
Abuser

- individual psychotherapy (focused or long-term); group therapy; cognitive-behavioural therapy.

Non-abusing parents

- help with parenting issues; individual psychotherapy; group therapy; marital therapy; parent/child work.

  Foster/substitute carers

- support and management help.

Children

Abuse survivor (victim)

- individual psychotherapy (focused or open-ended); group therapy (to reduce isolation); cognitive-behavioural (to enhance self-esteem); group psychotherapy (psychodynamic, psycho educational); parent/child work; educational therapy.

Siblings

- individual psychotherapy; group psychotherapy.

Family

Family work

- re-establishing family structuring.

Family therapy

- rehabilitation of abuser, or rehabilitation of child survivor.

In addition, there may be a need for work with the school and the community. As all the work is likely to be very stressful and demanding, therapists need regular supervision if they are to retain their capacity to function effectively. It bears remembering that all the dynamics present within the family may be repeated in the treatment.

The child

The child may have difficulty in talking about the abuse, or may talk of nothing else. It is important to work with the whole child—not to see the child only as a victim of abuse. However, the child by oscillating between projection, projective identification, introjection, and introjective identification can from moment to moment change from, for example, an abused victim, being rather vulnerable and distressed, to an excited sexualized being, to an autocratic sadistic abuser, or to a depressed or ignoring preoccupied indifferent carer. The therapist has to deal simultaneously with all these different experiences, in addition to helping the child make sense of his or her life experiences as well as the other traumatic or depressing experiences he or she may have had. This requires considerable skill and sensitivity. Part of the initial assessment is to decide whether the child would be more likely to benefit, from group or individual therapy as well as all the support and management work listed above.

The parents and school

Parents may need help in their own right. The abuse of their child may have stirred up memories of their own childhood difficulties and they may need help to work through these, so as not to repeat earlier experiences with their children. Parents may need to be seen individually or as a couple if there are parenting or marital difficulties. Many of the mothers are vulnerable, traumatized, and depressed individuals. The guilt for them is very painful. Helping mothers to see that the abuser must take responsibility for his or her own actions is very important. It is a delicate exercise because many mothers are aware, with hindsight, of noticing something different, but at the time they did not realize they should be suspecting abuse. The mother must believe she is not responsible for the abuse, and yet she also has to think about how to protect her child in the future.

Whilst this emotional maelstrom is being worked through with the child in therapy, there are practical management and educational issues. Many of the children are depressed and under-functioning academically. Many of them will be presenting behavioural problems. Hence, teachers are likely to need support and help in order to educate and manage the child. In addition, carers may need support as they attempt to provide for these children's physical, emotional, and psychological needs.

The abuser

Abusers need advice and help from highly skilled and very dedicated professionals. The work is difficult and demanding and keeping hope alive is particularly difficult. We now know that abusers have often been having sexual fantasies about children for long periods and that it is very difficult to change these. What can be done – it is hoped – is to reduce their intensity and help the abuser find coping strategies.

Rehabilitation

The child

A crucial question is whether a child, who has been removed from his or her family, can ever return? Equally, if an abuser has been excluded from the home can he or she ever return? Most sexually abused children remain in their families and there are very few criminal prosecutions (30 per cent of cases), and very few of these result in convictions. Thus, in reality most children remain in their families or return to them. Court proceedings to protect the child are becoming more common and the child may be received into the care of the local Authority. Most of such children eventually re-establish contact with their families or at least by the age of 16 or 18 years when they leave care. In some families, where the abuse is completely denied but the child has clearly been abused, the child may be permanently removed and freed for adoption. However, in most cases where the child has been sexually abused, they remain or return to their home with at least one natural parent.

The abuser

There are differing views on rehabilitation of abusers. One set of experts considers it imperative that the abuser admit their guilt and take full responsibility. Another view is that if the alleged abuser and the non-abusing parent can agree that the child has been abused, and what needs to be in place to protect the child, and they take responsibility for the protection, then it may be possible to consider rehabilitating the child.

If the abuser has been excluded it is not easy to judge when, or if, they may return. Many abusers move away and find new families, and only a few are willing to undertake the long-term commitment to treatment that is required. However, even at the end of treatment professional anxieties remain.

Racial, cultural, and gender issues

In order to understand the significance of the abuse to the child and family there must be adequate knowledge of the child's heritage and culture. If therapists are of the same heritage and culture this is ideal, but usually these are not available. Access to suitable consultation and advice then becomes important. It is also sensible to talk to the child and family about cultural issues and to be honest about the limits of one's knowledge.

Some experts advise that male and female children require male and female therapists, respectively. However, a child or young person may have a very strong preferences and this should be respected. In reality, because there are many more female therapists and as most children prefer a woman there is no problem. A small number of girls ask for a male therapist and if this can be provided, then it makes sense to do so. There is, however, an issue about male therapists and many experts question whether men should undertake this work at all. Another view is that it is important that men are involved, in order to provide a good male role model. However, perhaps much more important are the qualities of the therapist rather than their gender as the outcome of therapy is likely to depend on whether the therapist is skilled, competent, sensitive, and thoughtful. In long-term work it appears doubtful that the gender of the therapist determines the outcome. It is definitely not the same experience with a man or a woman—it is different, but, it is hoped equal.

Disabilities

Disproportionately more disabled children are abused than the able-bodied. Seriously disabled children, particularly deaf children are a high-risk group; children with learning difficulties who may have speech and language problems, or may be viewed as too cognitively impaired to be believed (Sinason 1992) and children with physical disabilities or those that are temporarily or permanently immobilized, are the most vulnerable groups. Offering treatment to these children and young people requires special communication skills and awareness (Sinason 1992) and ideally some professionals will require training such as *Signing* or *Maketon*. But in reality such skills will only occasionally be available.

Many sexually abused children have been unable to concentrate, learn, and think, and so present as learning disabled. Thus, assessment of these individuals is important so as to be sure about the basis or extent of their disability. Other disabilities may have been exacerbated by the abuse or threats of violence. Again, it is important to ascertain what is due to the disability and what is the secondary disability due to the trauma, shock, and disassociation of the abuse.

CONCLUSION

Child sexual abuse is a complex and distressing issue for society and professionals. We do not fully understand the impact on the children, but we do know it is a major mental health problem in countries where basic physical needs—food, warmth, and clothing are not met. Inter-generational abuse is a frequent occurrence alongside inadequate parenting. Considerable resources have now been used and abused children are being identified. The pressing need now is to have treatment available when the child is ready to work through any of their worries or distress. The children need to be allowed to remember in their own time so that they can forget in a healthy way, letting go, so that they can rediscover their humanity and get on with their lives.

REFERENCES

Adams-Tucker, C. (1982) Proximate effects of sexual abuse in childhood: a report on 28 children. *Am. J. Psychiat.* **139**, 1252–6.

Anderson J. C., Martin, J. L., Mullen, P. E., Romans, S. E., and Herbison, P. (1993). The prevalence of childhood sexual abuse experiences in a community sample of women. *J. Am. Acad. Child Adol. Psychiat.* **32(5)**, 911–19.

Baker, A. W. and Duncan, S. P. (1985). Child sexual abuse—a study of prevalence in Great Britain. *Child Abuse Negl.* **9**, 457–67.

Browne A. and Finkelhor, D. (1986). Initial and long-term effects: a review of the research. In *A sourcebook on child sexual abuse*, (ed. D. Finkelhor). Sage, Beverley Hills.

Browning, D. H. and Boatman, B. (1977). Incest: children at risk. *Am. J. Psychiat.* **134**, 69–72.

Burgess, A. and Holmstrom, L. L. (1975). Sexual trauma of children and adolescents: sex, pressure and secrecy. *Nurs. Clin. N. Am.* **101**, 551–63.

Butler-Sloss, Lord Justice, E. (1988). *Report of the inquiry into child abuse in Cleveland (1987)*. HMSO, London.

Ceci, S. J., Toglia, M. P., and Ross, D. F. (1987). *Children's eyewitness memory*. Springer, New York.

Conte, J. R. (1985). The effects of sexual abuse in children and suggestions for future research. *Victimology*, **10**, 110–30.

Conte, J. and Berliner, L. (1988). The impact of sexual abuse on children: the empirical findings. In *Handbook on sexual abuse of children: Assessment and treatment issues*, (ed. L. Walter), pp. 72–93. Springer, New York.

Conte, J. R. and Schuerman, J. R. (1987). Factors associated with an increased impact of child sexual abuse. *Child Abuse Negl.* **11**, 201–11.

Conte, J. R., Wolfe, S., and Smith, T. (1989). What sexual offenders tell us about prevention strategies. *Child Abuse Negl.* **13**, 293–301.

Cotgrove, A. J. and Kolvin, I. (1994). The long-term effects of child sexual abuse. In *Basic child psychiatry*, Vol. 1 *(Research and clinical)* (ed J. Tsiantis), pp. 85–102. Kastaniotis, Athens.

Femina, D. D., Yeager, C. A., and Lewis, D. O. (1990). Child abuse: adolescent records vs. adult recall. *Child Abuse Negl.* **14**, 227–31.

Finkelhor, D. *et al.* (1979). *Sexually victimised children*. Free Press, New York.

Finkelhor, D. (1984). *Child sexual abuse. New theory and research*. Macmillan, London.

Finkelhor, D. and Hotaling, G. T. (1984). Sexual abuse in the National Incidence Study of Child Abuse and Neglect: an appraisal. *Child Abuse Negl.* **8**, 23–33.

Finkelhor, D. *et al.* (1986). *A sourcebook on child sexual abuse*. Sage, Beverly Hills.

Friedrich, W., Urguizon A., and Berlke, R. (1986). Behaviour problems in sexually abused young children. *J. Paediat. Psychol.* **11**, 47–57.

Fromuth, M. E. (1986). The relationship of childhood sexual abuse with later psychological and sexual adjustment in a sample of college women. *Child Abuse Negl.* **10**, 5–15.

Fundudis, T. (1989). Children's memory and the assessment of possible sexual abuse. *J. Psychol. Psychiat.* **30(3)**, 337–46.

Furniss, T. (1991). *The multiprofessional handbook of child and sexual abuse*. Routledge, London.

Glaser, D. and Frosh, S. (1991). *Child sexual abuse*. Macmillan, Basingstoke.

Gomes-Schwartz, B., Horowitz, J. M., and Cardarelli, A. (1990). *Child sexual abuse: The initial effects*. Sage, Beverly Hills.

Gelman, R. (1978). Cognitive development. *Ann. Rev. Psychol.* **29**, 297–332.

Goodman, G. S. and Clarke-Stewart, A. (1990). Suggestibility in children's testimoney: Implications for sexual abuse investigations. In *The suggestibility of children's recollections*, (ed. J. Doris). American Psychological Association, Washington, DC.

Goodman, G. S., Golding, J. M., and Health, N. (1984). Jurors' reactions to child witnesses. *J. Soc. Iss.* **40**, 139–53.

Goodwin, J. (ed.) (1982). *Sexual abuse: Incest victims and their families*. John Wright, Boston.

Goodwin, J. and Owen, J. (1982). Incest from infancy to adulthood. A developmental approach to victim and families. In *Sexual abuse: Incest victims and their families*, (ed. J. Goodwin). John Wright, Boston.

Green, A. H. (1986). True and false allegations of sexual abuse in child custody disputes. *J. Am. Acad. Child Psychiat.* **25**, 449–56.

Haugaard, J. and Reppucci, N. D. (1988). *The sexual abuse of children*. Jossey-Bass, London.

Hey, A., Minty, B., and Trowell, J. (1991). Interprofessional and interagency work; Theory practice strategy in the nineties. In *Right or privilege?* (ed. M. Pietroni). CCETSW, London.

Herman, J., Russell, D. E. H., and Trocki, K. (1986). Long term effects of incestuous abuse in childhood. *Am. J. Psychiat.* **143**, 1293–6.

Holmes, D. (1990). The evidence for repression: an examination of sixty years of research. In *Repression and dissociation: Implications for personality, theory, psychopathology and health*, (ed. J. Singer), pp. 85–102. University of Chicago Press.

James, J. and Meyerding, J. (1977). Early sexual experience as a factor in prostitution. *Arch. Sex. Behav.* **7**, 31–42.

Jones, D. P. H. (1992). *Interviewing the sexually abused child*. Royal College of Psychiatrists. Gaskell., London

Jones, D. P. H. and Krugman, R. (1986). Can a three year old child bear witness to her sexual assault and attempted murder? *Child Abuse Negl.* **10**, 253–8.

Jones, D. P. H. and McQuistion, M. (1986). The process of validation. In *Interviewing the sexually abused child*, Vol. 6, Ch. 5, (2nd edn). The C. Henry Kempe National Center for the Prevention and Treatment of Child Abuse and Neglect, Denver, Colorado.

Justice, B. and Justice, R. (1979). *The broken taboo*. Human Sciences Press, New York.

Kelly, L., Regan, L., and Burton S. (1991). An exploratory study of the prevalence of sexual abuse in a sample of 16–21-year-olds. Polytechnic of North London.

Kempe, R. S. and Kempe, C. H. (1978). *Child abuse*. Fontana/Open Books, London.

Kerns, D. L. (1981). Medical assessment of child sexual abuse. In *Sexually abused children and their families*, (ed. P. B. Mrazek and C. H. Kempe). Pergamon, Oxford.

King, M. and Trowell, J. (1992). *Children's welfare and the law. The limits of legal intervention*. Sage, London.

Kolvin I. and Kaplan C. (1988) Sex abuse in childhood. In *Recent advances in clinical psychiatry*, (ed. K. Granville-Grossman). Churchill Livingstone, Edinburgh.

Kolvin, I., *et al.* (1988). Child sexual abuse—principles of good practice. *Brit. J. Hos. Med.* **39**, 54–62.

Kolvin, I. (1992). Diagnostic thresholds in child sexual abuse. In *Mental health in the family*. World Health Organization, Geneva.

Lister, E. D. (1982). Forced silence: a neglected dimension of trauma. *Am. J. Psychiat.* **139**, 872–5.

Loftus E. F. and Davies, G. M. (1984). Distortions in the memory of children. *J. Soc. Iss.* **40**, 51–67.

Loftus, E. F., Polonsky, S., and Fullilove, M. T. (1994). Memories of childhood sexual abuse: Remembering and repressing. *Psychol. Women Quarterly*, **18**, 67–84.

Mannarino, A. P., Cohen, J. A., Smith, J. A., and Moore-Motily, S. (1992). Six and twelve month follow-up of sexually abused girls. *J. Interpers. Viol.* **6**, 494–511.

Margolin, L. (1991). Child sexual abuse by non-related caregivers. *Child Abuse Negl.* **15**, 213–21.

Markowe, H. (1988). The frequency of child sexual abuse in the UK. *Hlth Trends*, **20**, 2–6.

Meiselman, K. C. (1978). *Incest: A psychological study of causes and effects with treatment recommendations*. Jossey Bass, San Francisco.

Mersky, H. (1995). Multiple personality disorder and false memory syndrome. *Brit. J. Psychiat.* **166**, 281–3.

Mian, M., Wehrspann, W., Klajner-Diamond H., Le Baron, D., and Winder, C. (1986). Review of 125 children 6 years of age and under who were sexually abused. *Child Abuse Negl.* **10**, 223–9.

Moston, S. (1990). How children interpret and respond to questions: situational sources of suggestibility in eyewitness interviews. *Soc. Behav.* **5**, 155–67.

Mrazek, D. and Marazek, P. (1985). Child maltreatment. In *Child and adolescent psychiatry. Modern approaches*, (ed. N. Rutter, L. Hersov, and E. Taylor). Blackwell, Oxford.

Oppenheimer, R., Howells, K., Palmer M. L. and Challoner, D. A. (1985). Adverse sexual experience and clinical eating disorders. University of Leicester.

Ounsted, C. and Lynch, M. (1976). Family pathology as seen in England. In *Child Abuse and neglect: The family and the community*, (ed. R. E. Helfer and C. H. Hempe), pp. 75–86. Ballinger, Cambridge, MA.

OACPC (Oxfordshire Area Child Protection Committee) (1992). *Child protection procedures*. Oxfordshire Social Services Department, Oxford.

Royal College of Physicians (1991). *Physical signs of sexual abuse in children*. Royal College of Physicians, London.

Russell, D. E. H. (1984). The prevalence and seriousness of incestuous abuse: stepfathers vs. biological fathers. *Child Abuse Negl.* **8**, 15–22.

Russell, D. E. H. (1986). *The secret trauma: Incest in the lives of girls and women*. Basic Books, New York.

Schechter, M. D. and Roberge L. (1976). Sexual exploitation. In *Child abuse and neglect: The family and the community*, (ed. R. E. Helfer and C. H. Kempe). Ballinger, Cambridge, MA.

Seligman, M. E. P. and Peterson, C. (1986). A learned helplessness perspective on childhood depression: theory and research. In *Depression in young people: Developmental and clinical perspectives*, (ed. M. Rubler, C. E. Izard, and P. B. Read) pp. 223–50, Guilford Press, New York.

Sgroi, S. M. (1982). *Handbook of clinical intervention in child sexual abuse*. Heath, Lexington, MA.

Sgroi, S. M. (1989). Vulnerable populations. In *Sexual abuse treatment for children, adult survivors, offenders, and persons with mental retardation*, Vol. 2. Heath, Lexington, MA.

Sinason, V. (1992). *Mental handicap and the human condition*. Free Association Books, London.

Smith, M. and Bentovim A. (1994). Sexual abuse. In *Child and adolescent psychiatry*, (ed. M. Rutter, E. Taylor, and L. Hersov), pp. 230–51. Blackwell, Oxford.

Summit, R. C. (1983). The child sexual abuse accommodation syndrome. *Child Abuse Negl.* **7**, 177–93.

Todd C. and Perlmutter, M. (1980). Reality recalled by preschool children. In *New directions for child development*, (ed. M. Perlmutter), No. 10, pp. 69–85. Jossey-Bass, San Francisco

Trowell, J. (1991). Teaching about child sexual abuse. In *Right or privilege?* (ed. M. Pietroni), pp. 85–93. CCETSW, London.

Wyatt, G. E. and Peters, S. D. (1986). Issues in the definition of child sexual abuse in prevalence research. *Child Abuse Negl.* **10**, 231–40.

15
The adult sequelae
of childhood sexual abuse

Ismond Rosen

INTRODUCTION

This chapter briefly reviews the clinical consequences and psychodynamic treatment in adults who have experienced sexual abuse in childhood. (See also the recent review by Green 1993.)

No specific syndrome exists for the adult consequences of child sexual abuse, the contributory factors and responses being so varied. Psychiatric symptoms may occur such as anxiety, phobias, depression, and low self-esteem, together with physical manifestations of a psychosomatic kind.

Because the effects of child sexual abuse are understood dynamically as the reaction to trauma, these experiences are being placed on a par with other traumas, such as physical abuse and severe emotional deprivation, and discussed as such. Anna Freud (1982) regarded the intensity of the harm done by childhood sexual abuse as higher in degree than abandonment or neglect, physical maltreatment, or any other form of abuse. From a psychoanalytical point of view the after-effect of serious abuse is of several kinds. Conflicts engendered by the abuse unconsciously motivate a repetition of the experience, either directly in the role of the seducer or the seduced, or symbolically in the events of everyday life. Unconscious ego defence mechanisms usually associated with psychic trauma, such as avoidance, inhibition, repression and denial, are stimulated to help the individual deal with the abuse. These are directed against sexuality as such. These psychic effects may lead in later adolescent or adult life to a lack of sexual satisfaction or to psychiatric symptomatology, particularly in women where actual incest has occurred. Abused men may suffer compulsive repetitions or problems of potency. More specific unconscious defences have been reported in sexually abused persons such as 'somatization' (Buriss (1994); Kramer 1994); symbolization of everyday life events in terms of seduction or its avoidance; and the unconscious organization of mental life around the abuse.

For the immediate effects in childhood of sexual abuse, see Chapter 14. Some authors regard the effect of severe childhood sexual abuse as compatible with post-traumatic stress disorder. (Goodwin 1985; Kiser et al. 1988; McLeer et al. 1988; Green 1993). In stressed child victims, symptoms may occur immediately with anxiety manifesting as avoidances, phobic reactions, sleep disturbances, aggression, and depression. Later there may be disturbed sexual behaviour and a disordered gender identity. Learning difficulties may be a feature due to the inhibition of perception and an unwillingness to engage with external objects. Sinason (1992) has reported cases where learning difficulties can be caused by abuse. Also, that where learning difficulties are organic in origin, such as in the mentally handicapped, sexual abuse can produce a lowered level of functioning and exacerbate their problems.

Cotgrove and Kolvin (1994) state that some sexually abused children may not produce symptoms until adulthood. Terr (1990) has discussed the literary descriptions of childhood abuse experiences by Virginia Woolf and their effects in her life. She 'suffered the special signs and symptoms of long-standing childhood psychic trauma—sexual numbing, emotional distancing, self-hypnosis, splitting, and dissociation. She also suffered some of the more ordinary signs and symptoms common to most sexual traumas—fears, perceptual repetitions, and repetitions in behaviour'. Terr points out that Woolf's fictional characters suffer similar symptoms which often evoke in the reader a response similar to that evoked by sexual abuse victims—boredom, disbelief, and failure to respond.

A dynamic definition of child sexual abuse is by Brandt Steele (1990) in Howard Levine's (1990) book describing the work of the study group at the Boston Psychoanalytic Association (see also Steele 1991, 1994).

> Childhood sexual abuse is the involvement of dependent developmentally immature children in sexual activity that they do not fully comprehend, which takes place without consideration for their stage of psychosexual development, something done for the adult, or the seducer, rather than for the child.

Sexual abuse of children occurs in many varieties and can happen at any age from infancy through adolescence, with various family members, relatives, or strangers. It can be a single isolated incident, or repeated frequently over many years. It may be homosexual or heterosexual with either girls or boys and involve anything from fondling to full genital intercourse or variations of oral and anal contact. It may be done with some degree of love and gentleness or involve various threats and actual physical violence. In addition to this wide degree of aetiological factors, the effects of childhood sexual abuse must also be assessed within the context of the family relationships and the developmental phase of the child victim.

In the family, dominant–submission patterns are usually found. Much of male–daughter incest takes place against a background of maternal rejection and emotional deprivation. The deprived child may a willing partner to apparently affectionate overtures. Where these go too far, the result is that dependency needs are short-circuited and unconscious sexual fantasy or genital development are disastrously advanced. From the child's point of view, sexual abuse is a breach of dependency, of trust, and a breaking of taboos. Loving and caring are interfered with by the substitution of a sexual experience. The psychological accompaniments of conflict and guilt may then undergo repression, leading to a devalued self and an inhibited personality. There may be no complaints by the child. Subsequently, adult symptoms are regarded as unrelated to the childhood experiences.

PREVALENCE OF CHILDHOOD SEXUAL ABUSE IN ADULTS

Incest and the taboos against it are age-old and universal. From being a phenomenon comparatively ignored clinically, sexual abuse in the last decade has become the focus of growing professional, public, and media interest. There is current alarm over its prevalence and the implications attendant on its discovery and treatment.

Community surveys in the United States of adult females with a history of child abuse varied from 6 to 62 per cent (Siegel *et al.* 1987). This wide statistical divergence was attributed to the difference in definition of sexual abuse used by the investigators. Definitions ranged from witnessing male genital exposure, to being fondled, or actual bodily penetration. The statistics being as discrepant as the definitions, they were regarded with reserve.

A more accurate study based on national rather then community surveys was made by Finkelhor *et al.* (1990). He surveyed all residential-phone users in the United States, Alaska, and Hawaii. In the sample of 2626 men and women over 18 years of age, sexual victimization was reported by 27 per cent of the women and 16 per cent of the men. These were unknown people contacted randomly at home by telephone. They were not complaining of anything. The author felt that this first US national study was an important confirmation of compatible community researches into the nature and impact of child abuse.

Finkelhor examined the risk factors as to whether sexual abuse resulted in an adverse or not-so-bad experience for the child. He concluded that growing up in an unhappy family appeared to be the most powerful risk factor for abuse. Further, in both women and men who described their families as unhappy, they were more than twice as likely to have been abused. A child growing up in an unhappy family might be more vulnerable to the manipulations of an abuser offering affection or companionship. Such children might also receive less supervision when away from home.

Growing up without a natural parent was another significant factor. Girls were particularly at risk when living alone with the father or with two non-natural parents. Boys were primarily at risk in two family constellations: when they lived with their mothers alone or with two non-natural parents. It would seem that almost any long-term disruption of the natural parent situation was risky for girls but not for boys. The transition from a single mother alone to a single mother with step-father increased the risk for girls but not for boys.

Finkelhor's study confirmed that most of the abusing experiences were at the hands of a person known to the child. Many of the victims never disclosed to anyone what had happened. The average age at which the abuse took place was 9 years.

Female sexual abuse of children is currently emerging as an area of research which has been under a cloud of prejudice that such abuse should occur. The literature has been summarized by Jennings (1993) in a book by Michele Elliott startlingly entitled, *Female sexual abuse of children: the ultimate taboo*. Elliott (1994) described how difficult it is for child victims of female sexual abuse to be believed, even in adulthood. A television hotline produced a flood of calls by adult victims abused in childhood of whom approximately two-thirds were female. Those 'sexually abused by their mothers seemed to have an overpowerig need to find bonding mother-love'. Although they hated their mothers for what they did, they still wanted to be loved by them and would never confront them. Some of the men felt a hatred of and sense of violence towards women and girls. Ninety-six per cent of the 95 female and 32 male victims in her study said that the abuse they had suffered dramatically affected their lives adversely. Twelve per cent of the male victims said that the effect had been beneficial and that some continued into adult life.

Wilkins, in Craig (1994) divided female sexual abusers into two groups, co-perpetrators and independent perpetrators: 'Those acting independently are frequently divorcees; have been themselves abused as children; and have been married as teenagers but are now living independently from their partner. Emotional disturbance, alcohol and drugs are other factors. The co-offenders are often bored young couples living in a polyincestuous situation. Again alcohol and drugs and a history of abuse themselves as children were factors'.

Further research is necessary to determine the prevalence of female abusers and the best way to treat their victims.

THE IMPACT OF CHILDHOOD SEXUAL ABUSE ON ADULT HEALTH

Surveys of the literature emphasize the widely varying differences in the late effects of childhood sexual abuse (Bachmann *et al.* 1988; Kinzl and Bield 1991). These range from severe behavioural and character disorders to having very little effect. It is difficult to assess the truth of claims that childhood sexual abuse produces very little after-effect. Further research is needed to distinguish between an actual minimal effect and the inhibitions produced by unconscious defence mechanisms. In the psychotherapeutic and psychoanalytical treatment of adults, sexual abuse may be reported in the history without complaint thereof. When the repression of affect and denial is lifted by analysis, intense pain, anxiety, and anger may emerge.

Psychiatrists treating adults sexually abused in childhood have reported symptomatology of frigidity, difficult sexual relationships, anxiety, phobias, and depression (see Palmer 1992). Research has been conducted on the relationship between child abuse and specific conditions such as mental health (Mullen *et al.* 1993); patients in general practice (Palmer *et al.* 1993); the effect on social, interpersonal, and sexual function (Mullen *et al.* 1994); community studies (Walch and Broadhead 1992; Anderson *et al.* 1993); the relationship with borderline personality structure (Salzman *et al.* 1993); and with anorexia nervosa and bulimia (Herzog *et al.* 1993).

Mullen *et al.* (1988) studied the 'Impact of sexual and physical abuse on women's mental health'. They randomly selected 2000 women living at home in five parliamentary constituencies in New Zealand. Women with a history of being abused were more significantly likely to have raised scores on two tests for disordered psychopathology and to be identified as psychiatric cases. Twenty per cent of the women who had been sexually abused as a child were identified as having psychiatric disorders, predominantly depressive in type, compared with 6.35 per cent of the non-abused population. Similar increases in psychopathology were found in women who had been physically or sexually assaulted in adult life. Most of the women reported their child abuse to have been of a gross genital experience. They were conservative in their personal assessments of any link between their experience of childhood abuse and their current mental states. The authors found depression, anxiety, and phobias, which had continued for many years, to be the predominating symptoms in this sample of women who had not presented themselves for help, but were cooperating in a general health survey. See also Mullen (1990,1991).

Arnold *et al.* (1990) in Bristol, England, examined the medical problems of adults sexually abused in childhood. They focused on a small group of difficult psychiatric patients who had made the rounds of various departments of medicine and surgery, complaining of pelvic and abdominal pain for which no physical cause was found despite many investigations and operations. Only later was the factor of childhood sexual abuse discovered in these patients. I am reminded of group of women patients seen during my early psychiatric training at Tara Hospital in Johannesburg (around 1950), whom we referred to as 'Railway Tummies'. The name referred to the many parallel abdominal laparotomy scars from repeated operations. Investigative medicine and surgery had failed to discover the cause of their abdominal pains which were then referred as being of psychological origin. No links were considered at that time between the women's abdominal pain and any childhood sexual abuse, even as a possibility, by the psychiatrists who were unsuccessful in relieving the psychosomatic condition. The surgeons had succeeded in the production of ice-cold abdominal walls.

Dubowitz (1991) and Green (1993) complained of the lack of longitudinal studies on the effect on physical health outcomes in childhood sexual abuse. Zimrin (1986) used longitudinal studies to investigate the factors inaugurating successful psychological defences which acted as a buffer against the stress of childhood sexual abuse. Of 28 abused children followed-up for 14 years, 19 exhibited significant pathology, but 9 did not. Of special interest were those survivors who had experienced no harmful effects. They were found to be optimistic with high self-esteem, were in charge of their lives, and had no self-destructive behaviour. Their cognitive ability was higher, they had hopeful fantasies, tended to be belligerent, had a supportive adult in their lives, or were responsible for caring for someone else. The significant differences between the two groups were the quality of their coping skills and having a relationship with supportive adult. The best buffer against the long-term effects of childhood abuse and neglect was having a confident mother.

West (1988) quotes Kilpatrick concerning retrospective surveys of population samples of adult women where no detectable long-term effects were found in the majority of those who recalled childhood sexual contacts with older persons. The most common complaint was of frigidity or unease in heterosexual relationships. In contrast to the above, a high rate of incidence of sexual abuse was found in samples of adults in penal settings or undergoing treatment for various disorders. The belief that incest was liable to provoke disturbances in later years led to the association between child abuse and a host of conditions. These included personality disorders, prostitution, alcoholism, drug abuse, promiscuity, lesbianism, eating disorders, suicidal attempts in the case of females, and in the case of male victims, aggressive sex crime and homosexual prostitution. West pointed to the fact that not all surveys of deviant groups, such as prostitutes and addicts, show an aetiological link with sexual abuse in childhood. In other words, one cannot base the psychopathology of any of the above conditions on some single or multiple event of childhood sexual abuse. Profound illnesses or character disorders result from cumulative traumas or a summation of aetiological influences, of which sexual abuse is but one factor.

The adult consequences of child abuse are the result of an interaction of three dimensions:

1. Family and social effects as discussed in Chapter 14.
2. The individual's inner psychological responses: especially the debilitating effect of shame and guilt; increased unconscious defence mechanisms; a distorted self-esteem regulatory system and a devalued self.
3. The presence of additional traumas and deprivations; the predisposition to psychiatric illness or psychosomatic ill-health.

Some authors go so far as to say that in sexual abuse, the physical act has little or no intrinsic meaning apart from its social and psychological connotations. While there are obvious exceptions to this view, the resulting psychological accompaniments in the abused child stem from the victim's distorted perception of themselves, consciously and unconsciously. Psychological abuse always accompanies sexual or physical child abuse. Lowered self-regard is particularly induced where victims experienced ambivalence about the sexual abuse. Due to the physical pleasure or fulfilment of unconscious sexual fantasies in the abuse, they see themselves in a bad light, may feel guilty and ultimately responsible, with a sense of worthlessness and disordered self-esteem regulation. The resultant effects are influenced by the developmental phase in which the relevant traumas occurred, especially during the oedipal phase or if there are unresolved oedipal conflicts. In therapy, such patients require special attention to relieve their guilt and elevate their sense of worth.

The discrepancies of incidence and effects reported in the literature may therefore be partly determined by the varying presence and strength of family factors, object-loss, unconscious defensive processes, such as denial, and the repression or somatization of affects. The need for substantial unconscious defensive processes occurs where the child has experienced the triad of sexual experience of an intense bodily kind, unconscious conflicts of desire and guilt, and the self-doubts and diminution in self-esteem that come from imposed secrecy and a betrayed trust. The loss of external objects, personal integrity, and lowered self-regard predisposes to depression. Unconscious defence mechanisms which may be found in sexually abused patients are manifold. They include inhibition, the compulsion to repeat, turning passive into active, identification with the aggressor, disavowal, somatization, and in severe cases, denial, projection, and splitting of the ego, the object and the super-ego.

THE UNCONSCIOUS COMPULSION TO REPEAT THE ACT

A high incidence of re-victimization occurs in child abuse victims: 65 percent of the victims of incest and 36 per cent of those with a history of sexual abuse by a non-family member, were subjected to rape or attempted rape after the age of 14 (Russell 1986). Sexual abuse within the family increases the compulsion to repeat, probably because of the unconscious oedipal conflicts which are aroused and intensified. Some authors believe that the repetition of victimization is due to the victim's changed notion of themselves following the initial abuse. Their assumptions about themselves and their world appear to have been shattered, they no longer feel emotionally invulnerable or physically intact. Normal self-regard presupposes 'I am all right . . . nothing is going to happen . . . one can walk about freely . . . nothing adverse will occur'. Sexually abused people may expect things to happen, and may also allow themselves to be victimized, even if only symbolically. At times they may provoke such occurrences. Their perceptions of themselves and the world as meaningful may be impaired. Wilkins, in a symposium on women and crime (Craig 1994), reported that when women became the criminal abusers of their own children, they were usually found to have been abused themselves in childhood. These mothers tended to be placed on probation, whereas for a similar offence, a father would be sent to prison.

Snow and Sorensen (1990), who reported on ritual child abuse in a neighbourhood setting, found two significant points of interest. One was that the perpetrators and seducers were themselves often the victims of incest. The other was the need to maintain secrecy by the adult perpetrators. They used powerful threats against their child victims which led to defences of splitting, denial, and psychological layering, or contributed to multiple personality development. The need to hide unpalatable facts is put forward by Sinason (1994). Discussing the treatment of survivors of Satanist abuse, she describes the conflict of opinion among experts and officials over the very existence of ritual abuse.

In sexually abused adolescents or young adults, resulting negative emotions such as revulsion, fear, anger, and a sense of powerlessness may be activated during their first dating or sexual experiences. It is nowadays fashionable to talk about 'date rape' on college campuses. Young students out on a date may be unsure of what to expect or allow sexually. If either or both persons has previously been abused, their ambivalent attitudes may contribute to a sexual misunderstanding. The problem may then go beyond an immature social or sexual attitude, based on inexperience, and be compounded by a disordered sense of reality in the sexual situation. Instead of thought, they may proceed directly into action.

THERAPIST–PATIENT ABUSE

Female incest victims appear to produce an arousing effect on males when it is revealed that they have been sexually abused. They appear to be particularly at risk of re-victimization by professional advisers. These include doctors, dentists, and lawyers. In particular, general practitioners, gynaecologists, psychiatrists, and psychotherapists are cited. Therapist–patient seduction, as it is now termed, includes female as well as male therapists, is becoming a focus of attention for authorities responsible for medical ethics as well as in the literature. New terms for the sexual abuse of patients by therapists have been proposed: 'therapist–patient abuse'; 'therapist–patient sex syndrome' (Gutheil 1992), and 'sexual boundary violations in psychotherapy' (Lymberis 1994). Boundary violations may also be non-sexual. See also 'Incest, erotic countertransference, an analyst–analysand boundary violations', an editorial by Margolis (1994).

Patients who were sexually abused in childhood and then seduced by their therapists pose particular problems which are dealt with in detail below. Not only does a subsequent therapist require particular skill and sensitivity in the therapeutic relationship so that trust may be built-up, but the problem also arises of what ethical attitude the new therapist should adopt towards the previous abusing therapist. It is argued and rationalized that because such patients may be attractive and seductive, the abusing therapist has little hope of resisting, especially if the therapist falls in love, or fantasizes that they are acting in the patient's best interests by providing an emotional need. The onus rests on all professional advisers and carers not to violate the patient's real needs, which are for understanding, security, and emotional growth. See Kernberg (1994) p. 441.

Kluft (1989), by analysing the literature, reported that of psychiatrists and clinical psychologists studied, between 5 and 7 per cent had sexual involvement or intercourse with their patients. The seduced patients were graded into three levels of risk. The majority of these patients came from the high-risk group which was categorized as having a history of hospitalization, suicidal attempts, major psychiatric illnesses, and drug or alcohol addiction problems. Exploitation by a therapist resulted in some patients becoming transiently overwhelmed or mildly disturbed, but the majority had become severely symptomatic and were the victims of incest or other severe abuse.

Experience in the United Kingdom would suggest that the incidence of therapist–patient abuse is somewhat lower because of the stringent General Medical Council regulations. However, it is not unusual to have to treat patients seduced by a previous therapist. In my experience of a few cases the patients were physically and sexually attractive. In spite of traumatic experiences resulting from the therapist seduction they unconsciously repeated being seductive during treatment. It was as if they had turned their childhood experience of being passively seduced into an active but ambivalent conquest of the previous therapist as proof of being lovable. Therapists who seduce a patient are either unscrupulous, inexperienced, or act from false motives of providing warmth, satisfaction, or love to the emotionally deprived. The seduction is consciously or unconsciously enacted more for the satisfaction of the therapist's emotional needs than that of the patient, for whom it provides a spurious sexual comfort. At the point where sexual intimacy occurred with the therapist in the patients cited, the notion of therapy came to an end, because the patient felt once more let down, abused, and unprotected by a carer. Some patients protect their therapists from disclosure similarly to the way child incest victims will not inform about a relative. Therapist–patient seduction always transcends the therapeutic task which is that of understanding and interpretation. Garrett and Davis (1994) profiled abusing therapists in a UK clinical psychology survey. They found that the vast majority of abusers were older men and the patient-victims were young women. The abusing therapists were found to suffer from stress, broken marriages, mid-life crises, and narcissistic personality disorders. The prognosis did not appear to be good for the treatment of abusing therpists, especially where they were serial offenders. Women abusers of patients formed a very small minority, and in one study reported, these women therapists were themselves involved sexually with their teachers, supervisors, or therapists.

The therapeutic relationship between patient and therapist develops and continues to exist on a basis of trust. Breaching this trust is particularly traumatizing to the patient as well as constituting a grave professional risk for the practitioner. These dangers and pitfalls exist where inadequately trained or insufficiently analysed therapists fail to comprehend or respect the patient's transference needs. These are for verbalization instead of re-enactment of the experiences of sexual abuse within the therapeutic relationship. This does not mean that the therapist must not be warm and compassionate towards the patient. Gabbard (1994) discussed sexual excitement in the analyst. He recommended greater openness by analysts in this area. Where the analyst experiences loving or sexual feelings towards a patient, these should be contained and constructively processed within the analyst. This would provide creative understanding, helpful for the patient's progress in therapy, instead of a destructive acting-out of such impulses. Kernberg (1994) described the technical management of an erotic countertransference, and stressed the need for the analyst to able to explore his/her own feelings without constraint. 'Powerful sexual feelings towards patients can compel us into action and bring us perilously close to the abyss of sexual transgressions. However, only by tiptoeing on the edge of that abyss can we fully appreciate the internal world of the patient and its impacts on us. The value of consultation with a colleague cannot be overemphasized.' Psychoanalysts burdened by an erotic countertransference may find it easier to find and approach a helpful colleague. This may be more difficult for psychotherapists, doctors and others, who have looser professional affiliations. Health care professionals require education and available help in the form of supervision in this area. Kluft (1989) regards the following issues as being central to the subsequent treatment of patients seduced by a previous therapist:

> . . . addressing their helplessness, their ambivalence about the exploitive therapist, their difficulties with trust, their guilt, their depression and pressures toward self-harm, their confusion over sexuality, their post-traumatic and dissociative features, their severe symptoms, and the diagnostic confusion this involves, and the counter-transference pressures upon the therapist.

The abused patient's fantasies are of being seductive as a means of being desirable and therefore being valued and acceptable—basically because they feel worthless. These women during therapy are only partially emotionally or sexually adult, they are also children reliving their traumatic early experiences. Any therapist's notions of providing regressed or immature patients with adult love and sex as a corrective emotional experience are totally erroneous. They indicate the need for therapy or further analysis of the therapist. The counter-argument in favour of the doctor's becoming intimate with the patient is that some doctors have a restricted social life and turn to their patients whom they often marry.

Conflicting attitudes exist towards sexual misdemeanours by doctors between medical and legal authorities in different countries, as well as in different states such as in the United States. The Australian Medical Association were of the opinion that doctors struck off for sexual misconduct by medical tribunals should not have their sentences reversed on appeal by the common law courts, which were regarded as too lenient (Zinn 1994). Lymberis (1994) discusses the recent developments of legislation by individual US states and national professional organizations against professional abuse and sexual boundary violations in psychotherapy. Medical ethics are accepted as the basis for medical practice, with the basis of the doctor–patient relationship being that of informed consent. Dryer (1988) describes the revisions of medical ethics made by the American Medical Association in line with modern practice. The American Psychiatric Association, through its Ethics Committee, has developed two educational videotapes on the problem of sexual involvement with patients (1986, 1990). Borruso (1991) formulated a model Uniform Criminal Statute applicable in every US state to deal with the alarming rate of sexual exploitation of patients by psychotherapists. At the state level, he regarded the licensing boards, whose duty it was to enforce codes prohibiting sexual contact between therapist and patient, as possessing inadequate powers to deter. These boards had no jurisdiction over unlicensed therapists, or licensed therapist-exploiters who on discovery switched residence to new states.

Currently, legislation in different countries on the need for doctors to disclose information on the sexual abuse of their patients, is transcending the hitherto sacrosanct area of doctor–patient confidentiality. In Wisconsin and California it is the duty of therapists to inform authorities of previous sexual abuse of patients. In Britain, the General Medical Council (GMC) has ruled separately in terms of the doctor's duty to patients and to other doctors. But these rules apply with regard to the welfare of patients. Para 83 of the *Professional conduct and discipline: Fitness to practice* (December 1993) states 'where a doctor believes that a patient may be the victim of abuse or neglect the patient's interest are paramount and will usually require a doctor to disclose information to an appropriate, responsible person or officer of a statutory agency'. This section, while not specifying the age of the patient, has been quoted with regard to children in an Addendum (DOH 1994) to *Child protection: Medical responsibilities*, issued by the Department of Health, the British Medical Association, and the Conference of Medical Royal Colleges.

The GMC rules govern the duty of doctors to inform on the fitness of colleagues to practice. Where previous doctor–patient sexual abuse is revealed, the treating doctor would be required to obtain the consent of the patient to disclose this to information to any appropriate authority. If, however, in the considered opinion of the doctor, there was a danger to other patients of continued abuse by the previous doctor, it would be the duty of the doctor to report without necessarily obtaining the patient's consent. Para 81 states 'Doctors who are faced with the difficult decision whether to disclose information without a patient's consent must weigh carefully the arguments for and against the disclosure. If in doubt, they would be wise to discuss the matter with an experienced colleague or seek advice from a medical defence society or professional association'.

THE QUESTION OF THE REALITY OF CHILDHOOD SEXUAL ABUSE EXPERIENCES

For clarification of the relationship between fantasy and actual seduction we must examine the history of psychoanalytical ideas in this area. Freud (1896*a, b*) proposed that sexual seduction was the origin of neurosis. On the basis that so many people could not all have been sexually abused in childhood, Freud made the creative jump to the idea that the patient's accounts of sexual abuse were due to their unconscious sexual fantasies. Masson (1984) denied the pathogenicity of fantasies, and falsely claimed that Freud had abandoned the reality of sexual abuse and trauma in childhood, ascribing it instead to fantasy. Freud however continued to accept the reality that childhood seduction occurred and was traumatic. This did not contradict his view that unconscious sexual fantasy and conflict were pathogenic for personality development. See Levine (1990) where this is discussed in detail.

Patients in therapy at times question themselves and the therapist as to whether the apparent memories of sexual abuse actually happened as recalled, or are due to fantasy. This may occasionally be extremely difficult to determine. Depending on the child's age when it occurred, there may be a mixture of memories of the event and fantasies consistent with the phase of development. One may be helped by the sequential logic of the recall or reconstruction of the events may be corroborated by other psychic material. Difficulties arise in assessing descriptions of early sexual seductions because reality events commingle with the current sexual fantasy-life of the child. This is intensified where there are unconscious conflicts of an oedipal and preoedipal nature. A more accurate picture may be constructed from the variable versions of the event as they are worked through in psychotherapy and repeated in the transference. With this process, clarity and cohesion occurs between the inner and outer perceptions, between past reality and fantasy which fosters personality integration. This dilemma of the truth of a person's recall of earlier sexual abuse is but one aspect of current controversy. The other is the 'false memory syndrome', where notions of having been sexually abused in childhood are foisted upon adult patients by therapists or counsellors with preconceived ideas (see below and pp. 348–52).

Self-doubt and the questioning by the patient of whether some event really occurred should make the therapist seriously assess the reality dimension of inferred sexual abuse. Especially in today's climate of sexual abuse as a weapon between divorcing parents, or children and parents, which may be the basis for litigation, (see the case report by Good 1994: 'The reconstruction of early childhood trauma; fantasy, reality, and verification'). Raphling (1994) described the psychodynamic factors in a patient who claimed she had been sexually abused. The patient used the alleged sexual abuse trauma to account for her misery and to assign blame, to expect compensation and enjoy vengeful fantasies. The abuse was never substantiated.

Brenneis (1994) contrasted two paradigms using reconstruction in the recovery of fully repressed memories from childhood. One is the belief that such early traumatic experiences can be reconstructed in the absence of memories as proof. Many analysts regard this with scepticism as it provides a fertile ground for overt and covert suggestion. Where an anxious or unconsciously motivated patient complies with such constructions, false memories may be produced. The other paradigm is where the analyst uses reconstructions as a holding environment in ongoing therapy, while repressed memories may be uncovered. There is a fine distinction between these two paradigms, which run in a complementary series. Analytic opinion, however, sees the suggestion hypothesis as the likely outcome. Whichever paradigm is chosen, the clinical implications are enormous. See also Shevrin (1994) and Person and Klar (1994).

During or after therapy, the return from repression of hostile feelings towards the abuser from childhood, may give rise to direct confrontation with the abuser, leading to rifts even with family members. In well-analysed cases, a reassessment of the relationships may occur, where understanding may lead to forgiveness. International press publicity was recently aroused by a lawsuit in the United States, where 'abuse memories' interpreted by a therapist were used by a daughter to confront her father. The father denied the allegation and successfully sued the therapist for the defendant's use of 'drugs and quackery' in 'helping' his daughter to 'recover' lost memories. These were regarded as unsubstantiated. Following this trial, Purves (1994) in a press report, pointed out that 400 in Britain were now claiming that their children's sudden accusations of child abuse were false ones implanted by their therapists. She warned all so-called 'recovered memories' therapists that they were now not only answerable to their own patients, but also to others affected by their 'airy diagnoses'. The suggestion was made by Macintyre (1994) that some therapists are under-trained and 'too eager to leap to the conclusion that an individual is repressing a memory that may not exist'. The danger now arises, because of these legal implications, that truly abused victims will not get a proper hearing, and that false allegations may be made against innocent persons. Walter Reich writing in the *New York Times* (1994), summed up the position as follows: 'Not all recovered memories are true, though many surely are, and not all accused abusers are guilty, though many surely are'.

FURTHER PSYCHOLOGICAL ASPECTS

Understanding the patient's relationship with their mother is crucial in therapy. Evidence of maternal deprivation is significant and the consequences may take many forms. In cases where incest between father and daughter has occurred, the mother may have suffered from depression or a personality disorder, resulting in the emotional deprivation of both father and child. This may have thrown the latter two together emotionally, leading to a sexual relationship, at times extending into latency or the early adolescent phases. Where the girl is deprived by her mother and feels close to her father, his breaching her trust by sexually abusing her means she stands to lose both parents and become emotionally abandoned. She not only has to cope with a damaged and devalued self, but may feel forced not to divulge in order to protect the only significant parental relationship she has.

The line between good bodily parental care of the child and actual sexual abuse is usually clearly drawn, based on the carer's knowledge, experience, and emotional attitude. Depressed mothers may interfere with the child's early development by paying too much or too little attention to the child's bodily needs. The mother's attitude to cleaning rituals may colour the child's attitudes to his or her body and subsequent sexuality. One patient reported how her mother took her as an infant into the bathroom in order to clean her vagina. She did not mind being cleaned but was affected thereafter by her mother's surreptitious attitude and her insistence on closing the bathroom door, which was usually left open. The event was thus turned into a secret activity for which she felt guilty and which became linked retrospectively with a phobia of lesbianism.

The question arises as to how adults, prevously sexually abused in childhood, regulate their self-esteem. One mechanism is through the unconscious repetition-compulsions of the abuse. This has parallels with self-esteem regulation in the perversions (see Chapter 3), and in social and domestic violence (Rosen 1991). Adolescents who have been abused then or in childhood often feel worthless, which increases their exposure to repeated sexual traumas, homelessness, and drug addiction. They are often impulsive, with poor controls. Their cognitive abilities and capacity for symbolization may be affected, interfering with their learning processes. In some cases the whole psyche appears disorganized. Compliance is another mechanism of self-esteem regulation which is also employed in the successful avoidance of rejection. But this results in the formation of a false or social self and the denial of personal identity, which is simultaneously self-devaluing. Abstinence, denial of desire, and masochistic relationships may also be unconsciously elevating of self-esteem.

Childhood sexual traumata stimulate precocious personality organization in the form of fixation, which may manifest as obedient compliance. Loss of parental protection, with intense conflicts over abandonment and separation, reinforces the struggle to hang on to a primary object, such as the mother, even if she is rejecting, making for a rigidity in the organization of the abused person's inner object- and self-representations. Reaction formations of shame, disgust, and guilt, further strengthen the defensive personality organization. In therapy, the growth of personal desires, identity, and free choice in the adult patient creates anxiety on an infantile level, due to the unconscious risk of separation, object-loss, and abandonment. These issues have to be very carefully balanced and handled in therapy as they are being worked through in the transference.

THERAPY WITH ADULTS SEXUALLY ABUSED IN CHILDHOOD

Some abused patients attending for assessment or treatment give no history of abuse, and are diagnosed as suffering from depression, phobias, anxiety, or psychosomatic complaints. Others may readily give full accounts of their childhood or earlier abuse, but do so without any show of feelings or sense of relevance for their present condition. Under the surface, these patients may gradually reveal a common scenario of an impaired ability to relate sexually; secretiveness, preferring to keep their experience of abuse to themselves; a history and ongoing compulsions to repeat their victimization in actual or symbolic ways; relationships and events in their daily lives unconsciously repeat symbolically their victimization in the previous abuse. This repetition-compulsion of the trauma and the defences maintained against it to avoid the pain of recall, is repeated within the treatment situation.

Treatment selection for these patients depends on two main factors. The strength of the patient's ego to face the traumata and their accompanying affects, and the availability of skilled therapy or supervision. Psychoanalysis may be the preferred choice, requires considerable ego-strength, but is not realistically available to the majority of patients outside major centres in the Western world. Analytical principles, as applied in psychotherapy, are extremely helpful for all concerned in the treatment of this world-wide condition. Some patients may need supportive therapy over a long period of time as they slowly come to terms with their traumatized feelings. Others may benefit in the short-term from focal therapy which allows them to analyse their depession in terms of their guilt over the pleasure in either being an abuser or being abused. One young woman, pregnant with her first child, was depressed with the phobia that the child would be born deformed. The fears and depression disappeared prior to the birth, with weekly psychotherapy, in which the links were made with her guilt and repressed fantasies of destruction and the pleasure in examining the genitals of the baby boy in her care as a child-minder.

The therapist may therefore be kept unaware of any abuse due to the patient's unconscious repression, denial or dissociation, or a conscious need for secrecy. This information may only be divulged when the patient feels a sufficient sense of trust. Even then, when the facts are shared, the patient may still feel too ashamed or defended to be able to reveal the full extent of their feelings. The patient should be allowed to explore these feelings in their own time, consistent with their sense of comfort and increasing trust in the therapeutic relationship.

The initial task in therapy is the establishment of a working alliance, leading to the development of a sense of trust. Without this trust and a positive transference, no progress can take place and the patient may leave. With trust, the therapist becomes the longed-for, caring parent, which can become internalized and therefore a stable influence in life. Patients may be resistant to the development of a therapeutic alliance due to their powerful erotic or negative reactions when in a relationship. Hostile defences, calculated to prevent emotional involvement because of the fear of rejection must be analysed. Some patients cannot bear separations during therapy, such as over the therapist's holidays, and may act-out accordingly (see the case of the female exhibitionist sexually abused by being looked at, p. 174). When necessary during such breaks, arrangements should be made for another therapist to be available for the patient.

It may take some time before the patient feels secure enough to explore the sexual trauma. The fact of their being able to do so is indicative of sufficient trust having been built up. The relationship with the therapist may be described as a mixture of defensive dependency and manifest self-sufficiency. From a diagnostic point of view, these patients may be thought of as having a split-ego organization in which a healthier or neurotic aspect of personality alternates with a more primitive impulsivity.

Trust is accumulated through the careful analysis of the actual or symbolic victimization the patient experiences in the minor but meaningful events of therapy or daily life. This allows for the working through of affects and defences stemming from the original traumatic experiences, in ways which are acceptable and valuable to the patient. Progress becomes manifest when, with understanding, they are able to alter the circumstances of their real everyday existence, and gain enhanced self-esteem. Such gains allow the patient to reveal more of their inner selves in the therapy.

The therapist has to be particularly careful as to how they relate to the patient, because the patients unconsciously transfer on to the therapist the expectation of seduction or their exploitation. If the therapist is too nice, they may be suspicious of the intention; if the therapist is not nice enough, may feel unconsciously rejected or abandoned. A very fine balance of attitude has to be maintained by the therapist of interest in and acceptance of the patient. Because sexual abuse is usually associated with unhappy or disrupted family life, both these aspects enter inextricably into the treatment. Child psychiatrists specializing in child abuse may deal with the whole family in therapy. Adults are usually treated in individual therapy. Preparatory group therapy in adults has been recommended where the sense of self is so weak that they require the support of the group in order to able to talk about themselves at all. Having had the benefit of the group they may proceed to individual therapy.

Abused patients pose much difficulty for the therapist who has to accomplish two main tasks:

1. The maintenance of the patient's good sense of self which they have been able to build-up by experience, despite the devaluations occasioned by the abuse and deprivations in childhood.
2. Facilitating the patient's recall of the repressed memories of the sexual abuse, and encouraging expression of the associated repressed affects. From a psychoanalytical point of view, these should be worked through in the transference. The therapist should treat the patient as a whole person. Focusing exclusively on the sexual abuse may reinforce the patient's view of their themselves and their identity as a victim of abuse.

Phyllis Greenacre (1956) observed that the fantasies required to be worked through were rarely typical. Rather, they were characteristic childhood sexual fantasies which had been given a special strength, form and pressure for repetition, through having been confirmed by external events. The childhood fantasies which are aroused by the actual experience colour the child's response to the abusing event. The mixture of inner and outer psychic reality will be co-determined by the quality and nature of the event and the intra-psychic state of the child's frame of mind.

Traumatized feelings emerge during treatment when the details of the experiences of abuse are re-lived. Beneficial effects may arise from such explorations provided that certain technical transference problems are handled correctly. In my experience of treating patients with less than severe symptoms of guilt and depression, who were abusers or had been abused, of both sexes, alleviation of symptoms and guilt occurred when the unconscious pleasure in the act was worked through. Sexual activity has a pleasure element inherent in it, even though it was originally or repeatedly stimulated inappropriately. Any pleasure in the act of abuse is usually overshadowed by the anger and rage that are aroused at the time of the trauma and subsequently augmented by growing awareness of the narcissistic hurt and the fantasies of revenge. These feelings may be augmented in later life by the narcissistic interplay between the victim and the original abuser. Child abuse is not purely a sexual act, it is also a statement of omnipotence and narcissistic power on the part of the abuser towards the victim. Intra-familial abuse or its effects, tends to be denied by the abusers, who may arrogantly retain their abusing attitudes towards the victim in a narcissistic demeaning way. When the narcissistic compliance towards the person in question is analysed in therapy, a good deal of anger towards the abuser and those who failed to protect is released. This rage underlies the psychosomatic symptoms such as headaches, abdominal pain, cramps, and fears of death or illness. These symptoms, though multi-determined, are alleviated or removed when the anger is worked through, which is usually a lengthy process. Patients in treatment should ideally be able to accept their affects of anger and pleasure in past sexual experiences and be free to experience desire and satisfaction in the present relationships. Price (1994) describes how chronically abusive child–parent interactions often become the blueprints for later interpersonal interactions: 'Reenactments of abusive relationships are frequent in the lives of adults with a history of incest. They represent attempts to enact a relationship with a powerful person in which both members are merged and idealised'.

TRANSFERENCE AND COUNTERTRANSFERENCE

Transference is the reproduction by the patient in therapy of their inner psyche, their experiences, relationships, fantasies, and feelings, which are projected on to the therapist, who comes to represent any or all of the figures and meaningfulness of their past or present life. The transference may vary from a re-living to the most subtle symbolic manifestation. The timing and sequence of transference revelations is determined by the unconscious, which, thereby reveals the developmental patterning of infantile relationships, traumas, conflicts, and defences. Understanding the patient's material must be understood in relation to their inner and external reality, in a process called working through. The most efficacious therapy is achieved when the transference is worked through. An ideal interpretation helps the patient to understand material that relates simultaneously to infantile experience, present reality in their everyday lives, and in the transference. In cases of abuse, a great deal of working through has to be accomplished, with much pain, against strong resistances, which accounts for the lengthy treatment. In time, patients develop a style of working through affects in sequences in the transference. When painful experiences and affects arise in the transference, it is comforting for both therapist and patient to share that they will be successfully worked through and diminished or eliminated on the basis of an established style and capacity.

The modern meaning of countertransference is the therapist's awareness within themself of all their reactions and feelings during therapy. This is a broadening of Freud's original description of countertransference as the therapist's response to the patient's transference. The simplest way to understand this phenomenon is to regard the therapist's awareness as the repository into which the patient unconsciously projects their psyche. The therapist may feel emotions akin to those experienced by the patient, or the emotional tone of the person who produced past affects in the patient. The therapist may feel themselves to be blank, affecting the tone of an emotionally empty, depriving mother. Such otherwise inexplicable responses in the therapist are invaluable in understanding the patient's past object-relationships and what they are experiencing in the transference. Countertransference awareness is especially valuable where repression and inhibition limit conscious recall.

Patients who have been seriously sexually abused also have a history of emotional deprivation. In the transference they display subtle mixtures of emotional withdrawal, painful recall of abuse, and defences against eroticism. They fear a repetition of physical or emotional abuse or abandonment in the transference, in ways which may threaten their psychic integrity. One abused and deprived patient entering analysis firmly declared that she knew patients always fell in love with their analyst. This was never going to happen with her. When she eventually fell in love, it was in an immature, demanding way, with an unsuitable man who rejected her, causing an immense trauma, which took an age to work through. I felt one had to allow her the experience of falling in love and not interfere by interpreting her love as the displacement of an infantile transference reaction which it undoubtedly was. Erotization of the therapeutic relationship may function defensively in some patients, because it protects against any emotional involvement with its subsequent danger of loss, rejection, and abandonment. The erotized transference, which unconsciously serves to keep the therapist interested and at bay, is preferable to experiencing what is underneath, an empty, worthless self, fixated on internalized, emotionally depriving, parental figures.

The situation of re-living deprivation is very testing of both patient and therapist. One particular patient suffered enormously in the phase of re-living the maternal deprivation, which went on for some years. When I felt uncomfortable with the mutual strain of her suffering her emptiness, I tried to reassure her by saying,'You are not nothing, not worthless, but of value'. She became enraged and rebuked me with 'Why can't you accept me as I am? Aren't I good enough as I am?' . . . 'If I was good enough, why did my mother ignore me and leave me unprotected to become sexually abused'. She was quite correct in her remarks to me, and I learned the hard way to respect and accept my patient's emotional reality without interference on my account. I had felt alienated and unsympathetic to the patient's unending rages, but admiring of her courage and determination in working through them. The reward for both of us was the discovery of early good relationships away from her mother, which had been totally repressed. These were hypothesized and interpreted on the basis of her positive attitude to working through in the transference. Regular late night childhood incest was experienced as a show of kindness and interest, which was rendered mortifying by day, as she was ignored and terrified of discovery. From such patients one learns to appreciate the significance of countertransference phenomena, the foremost principle of which is the accepting of the patient's reality in the transference. The therapist may be tested emotionally in the countertransference in varying ways, being made to experience boredom, deadness, or inadequacy of understanding the complex projections of their abused inner selves and psychic reality. Any experience which may drive the therapist to break the ordinary bounds of therapeutic neutrality, by offering more positive help may be more than the patient can deal with and be experienced as a rejection or seduction.

Working with seriously abused patients some analysts have reported feelings of confusion, helplessness, and being made to feel outraged like an abused child. In severely deprived and abused cases, the therapist must be prepared to be immersed in an ungratifying situation of rages, seductions, or emotional deadness for long periods until the massive withdrawal of affect is understood, recovered, and worked through. These treatments may be long and stormy, with periods of distrust and intense negative and erotic transferences. In the opening phases there may be impulsive tendencies with primitive dissociative reactions, in which there is a blurring of the boundaries between fantasy and reality, with recourse to archaic defence mechanisms such as projection, splitting, and denial. The therapist may be subjected to being the witness in a voyeuristic fashion of sexual acting-out in real life, unable to control it. This may occur where patients were subjected to intense bodily stimulation very early in life, including repeated primal scene experiences. They use the defence of turning passive into active, so that the therapist is controlled, rendered passive and impotent, and abused in the way they were themselves.

The transference becomes very intense due to the unconscious pressure to repeat, so that the patient relives in the therapeutic situation, the trauma of seduction or failure to be protected. The therapist is experienced by the patient as rejecting, devaluing or not protecting; taking advantage, or using the patient for the therapist's own selfish, unconsciously narcissistic or erotized needs, everyday decisions and experiences take on a symbolic meaning of abuse and victimization. The recognition of this symbolism and its unconscious re-enactment in the transference, allows for an acceptable working through in minute ways of the much more intense underlying affects. The patient's view of themselves as a victim has to be dealt with. A basic aim of treatment is to view the patient as a whole person who has access to normal desire and pleasure which had become distorted and unavailable due to the act of abuse. Modification must be made of the ensuing guilt and inhibition and a sense of equality established in personal relationships, stemming from the shared understanding in therapy.

The therapist may have to depart from a standard technique to suit each patient, but basically the therapist must patiently present a balanced understanding of the patient's needs while remaining emotionally neutral. That is the core of the therapeutic problem. See the chapter by Levine (1994) and the section on 'Treatment challenges with the traumatised patient' in Sugarman (1994), a Ralph Greenson Monograph by the San Diego Psychoanalytic Institute. Clinical experience shows that it is possible to help such patients, even with less than perfect technical expertise, provided the caveats and guidelines described above are observed. The pressing problem is the lack of skilled personnel to provide proper training and therapy. Macpherson and Babiker (1994) found that over half the mental health professionals in a Bristol, England, NHS Trust Hospital were working with abused patients. They complained of the lack of training and lack of skilled supervision and called for an 'agreed strategy involving training, supervision and inter-cooperation to deal with this increasingly common problem'.

REFERENCES

American Psychiatric Association (1986). Videotape. *Ethical concerns about sexual involvement between psychiatrists and patients.* American Psychiatric Press, Washington, DC.

American Psychiatric Association (1990). Videotape. *Reporting ethical concerns.* American Psychiatric Press, Washington DC.

Anderson J., Martin, J., Mullen, P. E., Romans, S., and Herbison, P. (1993). Prevalence of childhood sexual abuse experiences in a community sample of women. *J. Am. Acad. Child. Adol. Psychiat.* **32**, 911.

Arnold, R. P., Rogers, D., and Cook, D. A. G. (1990). Medical problems of adults who were sexually abused in childhood. *Brit. Med. J.* **300**, 705.

Bachman, G. A., Moeller, T. P., and Benett, J. (1988). Childhood sexual abuse and the consequences in adult women. (Review with 94 references). *Obstet. Gynae. Col.* **71**, 631.

Borruso, M. T. (1991). Sexual abuse by psychotherapists: the call for a uniform criminal statute. *Am. J. Law Med.* **3**, 289.

Brenneis, C. B. (1994). Belief and suggestion in the recovery of memories of childhood sexual abuse. *J. Am Psychoanal. Assn.* 42, 1027–53.

Burris, A. M. (1994). Somatisation as a response to trauma. pp. 131–140. In *Victims of abuse*. (ed. A. Sugarman). International Universities Press. Madison, CT.

DOH (Department of Health) (1994). *Child protection: Medical responsibilities. Addendum to: working together—under The Children Act 1989*. HMSO, London.

Cotgrove, A. J. and Kolvin, I. (1994). The long-term effects of child sexual abuse. In *Basic child psychiatry*, Vol. 1: *Research and clinical*, (ed. J. Tsiantis), pp. 85–102. Kastaniotis, Athens.

Craig, I. (1994). Women who sexually abuse children: the psyciatric perspective. In 'Women and crime', symposium contribution. *J. Roy. Soc. Med.* **87**, 174.

Dryer, A. R. (1988). *Ethics and psychiatry*. American Psychiatric Press, Washington DC.

Dubowitz, H. (1991). The impact of child maltreatment on health. In *The effects of child abuse and neglect. Issues and research*, (ed. R. H. Starr and D. H. Wolfe), p. 278. Guilford Press, New York.

Elliott, M. (ed.) (1993). *Female sexual abuse of children: the ultimate taboo*. Longman, Harlow.

Elliott, M. (1994). Female sexual abuse of children: the ultimate taboo. *J. Roy. Soc. Med.* **87**, 691.

Finkelhor, D., Hotaling, G., Lewis, I. A., and Smith, C. (1990). Sexual abuse in a national survey of adult men and women; prevalence, characteristics, and risk factors. *Child Abuse Negl.* **14**, 19.

Freud, A. (1982). A psychoanalyst's view of sexual abuse by parents. In *Sexually abused children and their families*, (ed. P. B. Mrazek and C. H. Kempe), p. 33. Pergamon, Oxford.

Freud, S. (1896a/1962). Further remarks on the neuropsychoses of defence. In *Complete psychological works of Sigmund Freud*, (standard edition, Vol. 3, p. 157). Hogarth Press, London.

Freud, S. (1886b/1962). The aetiology of hysteria. In *Complete psychological works of Sigmund Freud*, (standard edition, Vol. 3, p. 191). Hogarth Press, London.

Gabbard, G. G. (1994). Sexual excitement and countertransference love in the analyst. J. Am. Psychoanal. Assn. **42**, 1083–1107.

Garrett, T. and Davis, J. (1994). Epidemiology in the U.K. In *Patients as victims: Sexual abuse in psychotherapy and counselling*. (ed. D. Jehu). John Wiley, Leicester.

General Medical Council. *Professional conduct and discipline: fitness to practice*. December 1993, para 83.

Good, M. I. (1994). The reconstruction of early childhood trauma: fantasy, reality and verification. *J. Am. Psychoanal. Assoc.* **42**, 79.

Goodwin, J. M. (1985). Post-traumatic symptoms in incest victims. In *Post-traumatic stress disorder in children*, (ed. S. Eth and R. Pynoos). American Psychiatric Press, Washington, DC.

Green, A. H. (1993). Child sexual abuse: Immediate and long-term effects and intervention. *J. Am. Acad. Child Adol. Psychiat.* **32**, 890.

Greenacre, P. (1956). Re-evaluation of the process of working through. in *Emotional growth*, (ed. P. Greenacre), p. 641. International Universities Press, New York.

Gutheil, T. G. (1992). "Therapist-patient sex syndrome": the perils of nomenclature for the forensic psychiatrist. *Bull. Am. Acad. Psychiat. Law*, **20**, 185.

Herzog, D. B., Staley, J. E., Carmody, S., Robbins, W. M., and van der Kolk, B. A. (1993). Childhood sexual abuse in anorexia nervosa and bulimia nervosa: a pilot study. *J. Am. Acad. Child Adol. Psychiat.* **32**, 962.

Jennings, K. (1993) Female child molestation: a review of the literature. In *Female sexual abuse of children: the ultimate taboo*, (ed. M. Elliott). Longman, Harlow.

Kernberg, G. T. (1994). Love in the analytic setting. *J. Am. Psychoanal. Assoc.* **42**, 1137–57.

Kinzl, J. and Biebl, W. (1991). Sexual abuse of girls: aspects of the genesis of mental disorders and therapeutic implications. *Acta Psychiat. Scand.* **83**, 427.

Kiser, L. J., *et al.* (1988). Post-traumatic stress disorder in young children: a reaction to purported sexual abuse. *J. Am. Acad. Child Adol. Psychiat.* **27**, 645.

Kluft, R. P. (1989). Treating the patient who has been sexually exploited by a previous therapist. *Psychiat. Clin. N. A. M.* **12**, 483.

Kramer, S. (1994). Further considerations of somatic and cognitive residues of incest. pp. 69–96. In *Victims of abuse* (ed. A. Sugarman). International Universities Press, Madison, CT.

Levine, H. B. (ed.) (1990). Introduction and overview. In *Adult analysis and childhood sexual abuse*, (ed. H. B. Levine). Analytic Press, New Jersey and London.

Levine, H. B. (1994). Repetition, reenactment and trauma: Clinical issues in the analytic therapy of adults who were sexually abused as children. pp. 141–164. In *Victims of abuse*, (ed. A. Sugarman). International Universities Press, Madison, CT.

Lymberis, M. T. (1994). Boundary violations in psychotherapy: sexual and nonsexual pp. 165–186. In *Victims of abuse*, (ed. A. Sugarman). International Universities Press, Madison, CT.

Margolis, M. (1994). Incest, erotic countertransference, and analyst–analysand boundary violations. Editorial. *J. Am. Psychoanal. Assn.*, **42**, 985–9.

Macintyre, B. (1994). Man gets damages over daughter's 'abuse memories'. *The Times*, 16 May.

Macpherson, R. and Babiker, I. (1994). Who works with adult victims of childhood sexual abuse? *Psychiat. Bull.* **18**, 70.

McLeer S. V., Deblinger, E., Atkind, M. S., Foa, E. B., and Ralphe, D. L. (1988). Post-traumatic stress disorder in sexually abused children. *J. Am. Acad. Child Adol. Psychiat.* **27**, 650.

Masson, J. M. (1984). *The assault on truth. Freud's suppression of the seduction theory*. Farrer, Strauss, Giroux, New York.

Mullen, P. E. (1990). The long-term influence of sexual assault on the mental health of victims. *J. Forensic Psychiat.* **1**, 13.

Mullen, P. E. (1991). The consequences of child sexual abuse. *Brit. Med. J.* **303**, 144.

Mullen, P. E., *et al.* (1988). Impact of sexual and physical abuse on women's mental health. *Lancet*, **1**, 841.

Mullen, P. E., Martin, J. L., Anderson, J. C., Romans, S. E., and Herbison, G. P. (1993). Childhood sexual abuse and mental health in later adult life. *Brit. J. Psychiat.* **163**, 721.

Mullen, P. E., Martin, J. L., Anderson, J. C., Romans, S. E., and Herbison, G. P. (1994). The effect of child sexual abuse on social, interpersonal and sexual function in adult life. *Brit. J. Psychiat.* **165**, 35.

Palmer, R. L. (1992). Effects of childhood sexual abuse on adult mental health. *Brit. J. Hosp. Med.* **48**, 9.

Palmer, R. L., Coleman, L., Chaloner, D., Oppenheimer, R., and Smith, J. (1993). Childhood sexual experiences with adults. *Brit. J. Psychiat.* **163**, 499.

Person, E. S., and Klar, H. (1994). Establishing trauma: the difficulty distinguishing between memories and fantasies. *J. Am. Psychoanal. Assn.* **42**, 1055–1081.

Price, M. (1994) Incest and the idealized self: Adaptations to childhood sexual abuse. *Am. J. Psychoanal.* **54**, 21.

Purves, L. (1994). When therapy rapes the mind. *The Times*. 16 May.

Raphling, D. L. (1994) A patient who was not sexually abused. *J. Am. Psychoanal. Assoc.* **42**, 65.

Reich, W. (1994). *New York Times*. 16 May.

Rosen, I. (1991), Self-esteem as a factor in social and domestic violence. *Brit. J. Psychiat.* **158**, 18.

Russell, D. E. (1986). *The secret trauma: Incest in the lives of girls and women*. Basic Books, New York.

Salzman J. P., *et al.* (1993). Association between borderline personality structure and history of childhood abuse in adult volunteers. *Comp. Psychiat.* **34**, 254.

Shevrin, H. (1994) The uses and abuses of memory. Editorial. *J. Am. Psychoanal. Assn.* **42**, 991–6.

Siegel, J. M., Sorenson, S. B., Golding, J. M., Bumam, M. A., and Stein, J. A. (1987). The prevalence of childhood sexual assault. The Los Angeles Epidemiologic Catchment Area Project. *Am. J. Epidemiol.* **120**, 1141–53.

Sinason, V. (1992). *Mental handicap and the human condition*. Free Association Books, London.

Sinason, V. (ed.) (1994). *Treating survivors of Satanist abuse*. Routledge, London and New York.

Snow, B. and Sorensen, T. (1990). Ritualistic child abuse in a neighborhood setting. *J. Interpers. Viol.*. **5**, 474.

Steele, B. (1990). Some sequelae of the sexual maltreatment of children. pp. 21–34. In *Adult analysis and childhood sexual abuse*, (ed., H. B. Levine). Analytic Press, New Jersey and London.

Steele, B. F. (1991). The psychopathology of incest participants. In *The trauma of transgression*. (ed. S. Kramer and S. Akhtar). Aronson, Northvale, NJ.

Steele, B. F. (1994). Psychoanalysis and the maltreatment of children. *J. Am. Psychoanal. Assn* **42**, 1001–26.

Sugarman, A. (1994). *Victims of abuse*. International Universities Press, Madison, CT.

Terr, L. C. (1990) Who's afraid in Virginia Woolf? Clues to early sexual abuse in literature. *Psychoanal. Study Child.* **45**, 533–46.

Walch, A. G. and Broadhead, W. E. (1992). Prevalence of lifetime sexual victimization among female patients. *J. Fam. Pract.* **35**, 511.

West, D. J. (1988). Incest in childhood and adolescence: long-term effects and therapy. *Brit. J. Hosp. Med.* **40**, 352.

Zimrin, H. (1986). A profile of survival. *Child Abuse Negl.* **10(3)**, 339–49.

Zinn C. (1994) Editorial. Australian doctors get tough on sexual misconduct. *Brit. Med. J.* **308**, 1185.

16
Behavioural therapy treatment for sex-offenders

Gene G. Abel and Candice A. Osborn

INTRODUCTION

Behavioural therapy evolved out of learning theory and is used to evaluate and treat psychiatric and psychological symptoms by directly decreasing the frequency of pathological behaviours and increasing the frequency of appropriate behaviours. Behavioural therapy for sex-offenders initially focused on single treatment interventions, such as aversion therapy, to change the paraphiliac's deviant behaviour.

Behavioural therapy for offenders has changed profoundly in the last 20 years due to three primary factors. First, the public has become sensitized to sexual crimes as a result of the rape crisis movement's public awareness campaigns and increasing research documenting the frequency of sex-crimes. Large numbers of sex-offenders have subsequently come forward or have been forced forward into treatment, inundating treatment programmes. Second, cost containment has permeated all categories of health care, including evaluation and treatment programmes for sex-offenders. Modern treatment must not only be effective, but also must be cost-effective. Finally, there has been an integration of various forms of behavioural therapy with other systems of intervention to stop sex-crimes. Each of these factors has changed behavioural therapy for sex-offenders, and has rushed behavioural therapy forward on a wave of political, economic, and therapy changes.

INTEGRATION OF MULTIPLE BEHAVIOURAL THERAPIES

Behavioural therapy initially involved aversion therapy as the treatment for sex-offending under the premise that the control of deviant arousal would stop the paraphiliac's offending. Electrical aversion and emetic aversion therapies based on animal learning studies were the source of clinical treatment for paraphiliacs. As behavioural therapists expanded their experience, they first added other forms of aversion therapy, and then extended treatment to correct the offender's social and assertive skills deficits, lack of victim empathy, cognitive distortions that justified committing paraphilic acts, frequent correlates of sex-offending, such as alcohol and drug abuse, victimization issues, lack of the offender structuring his time with prosocial behaviours, deficits of sexual education and knowledge, sexual dysfunctions, and organic illnesses that increased the risk of paraphilic behaviour. Currently no behavioural treatment programmes exist which treat paraphiliacs with behavioural therapy for only one of these problem areas.

Behavioural therapy programmes now combine a variety of behavioural therapies into a unified, integrated treatment plan called cognitive-behavioural treatment. Table 16.1 identifies the most effective or most commonly used components of integrated cognitive-behavioural treatment programmes for paraphiliacs. Each therapy component has been identified by whether it is implemented by the patient (P) or requires implementation by the therapist (T); whether it can be implemented in an individual (I) or group (G) setting; its level of cost-effectiveness, high (H), medium (M), or low (L); and its level of intrusiveness, high (H), medium (M), or low (L). References are also provided for the details of each treatment.

How cognitive-behavioural therapies have been combined and integrated is best exemplified in the work of Pithers (Pithers 1990; Pithers *et al.* 1983, 1988, 1989; Marques (Marques and Nelson 1989; Marques *et al.* 1989), and others on relapse prevention.

Three types of behavioural therapy for sex-offenders warrant further description because they provide innovative approaches: imaginal desensitization, relapse prevention, and modified aversive rehearsal. Imaginal desensitization is based on the premise that a behavioural completion mechanism is established in the central nervous system when a behaviour becomes habitual. When an offender is in the presence of stimuli that, in the past, have been associated with offending, or when the offender fantasizes or has urges to carry out deviant sexual behaviour but does not complete that behaviour, the behavioural completion mechanism is activated causing the perpetrator to feel tense and anxious. This increased emotional response is believed to increase the probability that the perpetrator will carry out his paraphilic behaviour in order to alleviate his discomfort.

Imaginal desensitization involves the offender developing a few imaginal scenes that typify his usual paraphilic behaviour, but rather than the scenes ending with completion of the act, the imaginal scenes end with the paraphiliac overcoming his urges to offend. The paraphiliac is then taught progressive muscle relaxation and imagines the various components of each scene, periodically pausing to practise relaxing when elements of the deviant scene cause him emotional discomfort. McConaghy (1985) and McConaghy *et al.* (1990) have demonstrated that imaginal desensitization is equally, if not more, effective than covert sensitization when applied to a variety of paraphilias. In contrast to aversion therapies, this therapy decreases the emotional discomfort the paraphiliac experiences when he tries to avoid giving in to deviant urges rather than specifically decresing his deviant interest. The importance of this treatment intervention is that it is a non-invasive procedure that effectively reduces re-offence rates without the potential ethical problems of implementing aversion therapy which can reduce the perpetrator's self-esteem and potentially be misused.

Relapse Prevention (RP) is a treatment model initially developed as a maintenance programme for use in the treatment of compulsive behaviours such as alcohol and drug abuse, cigarette smoking, gambling, and over-eating (George and Marlatt 1989). RP is psychoeducationally based and combines behavioural skill-training procedures with

Table 16.1 Behavioural therapy techniques: decreasing deviant arousal

Therapy	Character-istics	Cost-effectiveness	Intrusive-ness	Procedure	References
Olfactory aversion	P	H	M	Patient pairs anteecendents to deviant behaviour with noxious odour, e.g., ammonia	Laws *et al.* 1978 Laws & Osborn 1983
Covert sensitization	P,T	H	M	Patient pairs anteecendents to deviant behaviour with aversive consequences	Abel & Rouleau 1990 Abel *et al.* 1984
Imaginal desensitization	T	L	L	Patient verbalizes antecendents to deviant behaviour using relaxation techniques to reduce negative feelings usually associated with deviant urges	McConaghy 1990 McConaghy *et al.* 1985
Masturbatory satiation	P	H	H	Patient masturbates to ejaculation to non-deviant fantasy, then masturbates to boredom with deviant fantasy	Abel *et al.* 1984 Laws *et al.* 1987
Verbal satiation	P	H	M	Patient verbalizes deviant fantasy to boredom	Laws & Osborn 1983
Assisted covert sensitization	P,T	M	M	Patient pairs deviant scene with aversive imaginal consequence combined with noxious odour	Maletzky 1980
Aversive behavioural rehearsal	T	L	H	Patient carries out deviant behaviour in front of audience who provide feedback	Wickramsekera 1976 Wickramsekera 1980 Serber 1970 Smith & Wolfe 1988
Modified aversive behavioural rehearsal	T	M	M	Patient carries out simulated deviant behaviour with a mannequin while being videotaped. Videotape played to audience for feedback to patient	
Electrical aversion	T	L	H	Patient receives electrical shock when responding to deviant stimuli	Rice *et al.* 1991a
Fading	T	L	M	Patient presented deviant stimuli, gradually faded to non-deviant stimuli as patient can tolerate	Barlow *et al.* 1975

Technique					Description	References
Thematic shift	P	I	H	H	Patient masturbates to point of orgasm to deviant fantasy, then shifts to non-deviant fantasy. Patient learns to shift earlier and earlier in the sequence	Conrad & Wincze 1976; Marques 1970
Fantasy alternation	P	I	H	H	Patient masturbates to orgasm, alternating between deviant and non-deviant fantasies. Patient gradually drops out deviant fantasies	Abel et al. 1975; Leonard & Hayes 1983
Directed masturbation	P	I	H	H	Patient masturbates exclusively to non-deviant fantasy, and stops masturbating to deviant fantasy	Kremsdorf et al. 1985; Maletzky 1985
Exposure	T	I	H	M	Patient views erotic, non-deviant sexual movies to increase non-deviant sexual fantasies	Barlow et al. 1975
Social skills training	T	G,I	H	L	Patient learns how to initiate and maintain conversation through role-playing exercises	Abel et al. 1984; Marshall 1971; Whitman & Quinsey 1981
Assertiveness training	T	G,I	H	L	Patient learns how to appropriately express his thoughts, feelings and wants through role-playing	Abel et al. 1984
Sex education Sex dysfunction training	T	G,I	H	L	Didactic training focused on basic anatomy and elements of healthy sexual communication and relationships	Abel et al. 1984; Quinsey et al. 1987
Cognitive restructuring	T	G,I	HL	M	Didactic therapy to challenge cognitive distortions which support inappropriate sexual behaviour	Abel et al. 1985; Lange 1986; Murphy 1990
Victim awareness	T	G,I	HL	HM	Patients are presented written and videotaped vignettes of sexual abuse victims to enhance their awareness of the consequences of molestation	Knopp 1984; Hildebran & Pithers 1989

P, patient-implemented; T, therapist-implemented; G, group format; I, individual format; H, high; M, medium; L, low.

cognitive intervention techniques. Pithers *et al.* (1983) modified the self-management model of RP for application with sex offenders. The RP self-control programme is designed to teach the paraphiliac how to anticipate and cope with the problem of potential relapse of paraphilic behaviour. It conceptualizes behaviour change as a multi-stage process, minimally a treatment stage (stopping the behaviour), and a maintenance stage (preventing relapse).

Relapse Prevention was not designed to be used as an isolated treatment, but as 'a maintenance strategy intended to preserve gains made in whatever treatment preceded it' (Laws 1989, p. viii). Some treatment programmes employ RP as a sort of umbrella concept, under which a variety of activities are conducted (Marques *et al.* 1989; Pithers *et al.* 1989), while other programmes employ RP as one of a variety of treatment components, and then as a maintenance procedure (Jenkins-Hall *et al.* 1989).

The patient first learns to identify the factors which contribute to or trigger paraphilic urges and learns how to cope effectively with these situations. These coping strategies include avoidance of risky situations, reduction of deviant interest, and control of deviant urges with behaviour therapy techniques, reduction of anxiety with relaxation techniques, skills training, self-efficacy enhancement, etc. The patient then develops methods to monitor accurately his therapy progress including tracking the frequency of deviant sexual urges, tracking and monitoring motivation, etc. The patient also develops social support networks to assist him through his transition from a paraphilic to a non-paraphilic lifestyle through emotional support, external monitoring of the patient's behaviour, social contact to appropriately cope with loneliness, etc.

Overriding all these components, the patient learns that his deviant lifestyle is learned and thus can be unlearned or modified. This requires that the patient accepts that, in order to maintain a non-deviant lifestyle, he cannot conduct his life in the same manner he did prior to treatment. The patient learns to develop and maintain a balanced lifestyle that will 'inoculate' him against the covert antecedents to relapse and will promote mental and physical well-being, incorporating appropriate methods to reduce stress, reducing his sense of deprivation by participating in enjoyable activities, avoiding situations which increase the likelihood of relapse, and practising urge-control techniques.

Relapse Prevention, therefore, provides a framework within which various behavioral and cognitive interventions can be integrated to provide treatment for paraphiliacs. Additionally, it provides a long-term maintenance strategy previously missing in comprehensive treatment programmes.

Modified aversive behavioural rehearsal is a final form of behaviour therapy showing considerable promise. This treatment is a modification of the work of Serber (1970) and Wickramsekera (1976, 1980), who describe a type of aversion therapy in which tranvestitic fetishists and exhibitionists carry out their deviant behaviour in front of a small audience who in turn give feedback to the perpetrator regarding his deviant behaviour. Smith and Wolfe (1988) have modified this earlier therapy so it is applicable in the treatment of paedophiles (or rapists) by having the paedophile carry out paedophilic behaviour with a child mannequin while being videotaped. This videotape is then played back to the perpetrator in the presence of the therapist, other paraphiliacs, or the paraphiliac's significant others. Although not articulated in the literature, the direct observation of the paraphiliac carrying out his deviant behaviour with a mannequin affords an opportunity to identify and correct the paraphiliac's cognitive distortions that he has used to justify and rationalize his paraphilic behaviour. This modification of aversive behavioural rehearsal, although containing elements that can be interpreted as an aversion therapy, is better seen as a therapy designed to deal with the paraphiliac's cognitive distortions.

Therapy begins with an extensive discussion of the anticipated treatment, its effects, and potential side-effects, and an opportunity for the perpetrator to sign a statement of informed consent. A paedophile, for example, is asked to carry out his typical acts of child molestation on a child mannequin (of the preferred gender). The molestation is videotaped with major emphasis on asking the paedophile to externalize his usual self-statements before, during, and after the actual molestation (e.g., how he feels touching the child). He is also queried regarding his perception of the victim's experience during the molestation as well as being asked to imagine possible sequelae for the child.

The presence of the child mannequin, contrary to what one might expect, allows most paedophiles to carry out their typical molestation behaviour, since the mannequin's small size and appearance provoke the typical kind of feelings, emotions, and fantasies that paedophiles have during the actual commission of child molestation. The videotaped molestation captures not only the physical aspects of the molestation, but also the perpetrator's inner self-statements.

In two, and sometimes three, subsequent replays of the videotaped molestation of the mannequin, the videotape is reviewed with the perpetrator, the therapist, and two or three individuals who provide a critique of the perpetrator's self-statements, based on their own experience or their knowledge of what child victims have typically reported regarding the impact of victimization. The immediacy of viewing the molestation of the mannequin, concomitant with the paedophile's verbalization of his rationalizations and justifications to neutralize the consequences of the experience for the victim, coupled with the immediate feedback from the audience, has a profound influence on the perpetrator's belief system. Most perpetrators find it untenable to maintain their cognitive distortions in the midst of repeated feedback. Other methods directed at normalizing the paedophile's false beliefs about paedophilic behaviour can be problematic since investigation of these beliefs leads the paedophile to retreat from verbalizing his cognitive distortions. The capturing of the molestation of the mannequin and the perpetrator's self-statements on videotape allows the subsequent sessions to hone in on these cognitive distortions. This procedure shows great potential for dealing with the cognitive distortions of any category of paraphilia where cognitive distortions occur and perpetration of the simulated act can be captured on videotape.

INTEGRATION OF COGNITIVE-BEHAVIOURAL THERAPY WITH OTHER THERAPIES

As cognitive-behavioural therapy has matured and expanded its treatment components, the behavioural therapist has become more acquainted with other categories of therapy and has incorporated these into programmes that focus on the total needs of sex-offenders. Drug intervention involving oral or intramuscular cyproterone acetate, medroxyprogesterone acetate, and leuprolid acetate are the more commonly used hormonal agents to rapidly reduce sexual drive and thereby reduce the risk of relapse while waiting for the effects of cognitive-behavioural therapy to impact on the paraphiliac. These hormonal interventions do not detract from cognitive-behavioural treatment, but instead complement it. More recently, serotonin reuptake inhibitors, such as sertraline, fluoxetine, and paroxetine, have been added as a first step in drug intervention, to be followed by hormonal intervention if the serotonin reuptake inhibitors are ineffective at rapidly reducing sexual drive and providing the paraphiliac better control (Abel and Osborn 1995).

A number of other treatment interventions have also been incorporated with behavioural therapy. The Sexual Addiction Model, relying heavily on a 12-Step Alcoholics Anonymous theoretical background, has been included, especially the incorporation of the sexual addiction, self-help groups. Such self-help programmes are cost-effective and expand the network available to the perpetrator to assist in monitoring and supervising his maintenance therapy (Carnes 1990).

The Sexual Trauma Model is predicated on the assumption that a frequent initiator of sex-offending is the perpetrator's own victimization when he or she was a child (Schwartz and Brasted 1985). This model is particularly helpful in understanding the adolescent sex-offender who will frequently begin to offend shortly after he or she is offended upon. The feelings and emotions of the adolescent victim/offender are frequently detailed to help the adolescent perpetrator understand his or her feelings about having been victimized and are also used in aversive and/or empathy training material to help the adolescent perpetrator appreciate the negative consequences of his or her offending on others.

Research data indicate that approximately 30 per cent of those who molest girls, exclusively molest children in their own home (Abel *et al.* 1989). The perpetrators of such crimes have the lowest recidivism rate of any category of paraphilia, irrespective of the theoretical orientation or the specific type of therapy provided, with most recidivism rates running at less than 5 per cent (Marshall and Barbaree 1990). The complexities of the family interaction and the apparent role reversals resulting before or during incestuous involvement emphasize the need for a family systems intervention with this category of sex-offence, especially when reunification of the perpetrator with the family is to be considered. For this reason, a Family Systems intervention has been incorporated into many integrated programmes.

As a result of the integration of the various theoretical treatment models for paraphiliacs, standards of care for treating sex-offenders have been set forward so as to improve the quality of treatment for sex offenders (ATSA 1993; Dwyer and Coleman 1990). In the United States, this has extended to state law determining the specialized training and experience needed by therapists providing treatment for adjudicated offenders or those under supervision by state child protection agencies (SOTP 1991).

The impact of the integration of cognitive-behavioural therapy with other therapies for the treatment of sex-offenders can be appreciated by a survey completed in 1992 (Knopp *et al.* 1992) that reviewed 1461 programmes in the United States which specialize in the treatment of sex offenders. The majority of treatment

Table 16.2 Treatment modalities used by sex-offender treatment programmes

Treatment modalities	Cognitive-behavioural programmes (%)	All treatment programmes (%)
Victim empathy	97	96
Cognitive distortions	95	91
Anger/Aggression management	91	90
Sex education	90	88
Relapse prevention	89	86
Communications	89	89
Assertiveness training	87	87
Relapse cycle	87	84
Personal victimization trauma	80	80
Pre-assault/Assault cycle	78	74
Thinking errors (same now)	78	77
Conflict resolution	76	77
Victim apology	74	74
Frustration tolerance/Impulse control	74	76
Relaxation techniques/Stress management	74	70
Journal-keeping	73	70
Positive/Prosocial sexuality	68	65
Values clarification	67	70
Aftercare planning	67	66
Fantasy work	66	64
Covert sensitization	65	43
Sex-role stereotyping	63	67
Waiving of confidentiality	59	58
Homosexuality/Homophobia	57	56
Employment/Vocational issues	54	54
Sexually transmitted disease	54	51
Sexual arousal measures (plethysmography)	46	28
Addictive cycle	44	49
Masturbatory satiation	43	29
Alcoholics Anonymous	42	43
Polygraph	35	24
Masturbatory conditioning	35	23
Modified aversive behaviour rehearsal	31	24
Aversive conditioning (olfactory)	31	19
Masturbatory training	30	23
Narcotics anonymous	27	28
Adult children of alcoholics	27	28
Sexual arousal card sorts	26	15
Minimal arousal therapy	26	17
Sexual attitudes reassessment	20	20
Medroxyprogesterone acetate (depo form)	19	14
Hypnosis	12	14
Dissociative state therapy	11	14
Shame aversion	9	8
Bio-feedback	7	8
Aversive conditioning (faradic)	3	2
Bodywork/Massage therapy	3	3
Fluoxetine	24	21
Minor or major tranquillizers	22	20
Antipsychotic medication	22	20
Lithium carbonate	19	19
Clomipramine	15	13
Buspirone	13	12

programmes reported their treatment orientation as cognitive-behavioural, 41 per cent; followed by psychosocioeducational, 25 per cent; relapse prevention, 16 per cent; psychotherapeutic, 11 per cent; family systems, 2 per cent; sexual addictive, 2 per cent; behavioural only, 1 per cent; psychoanalytic, 0 per cent; biomedical only, 0 per cent; and other, 2 per cent.

Table 16.2 shows the treatment modalities employed by these programmes and a subgroup of 597 programmes that defined themselves as cognitive-behavioural in their orientation. An examination of Table 16.2 indicates that treatment components normally associated with the cognitive-behavioural model are commonly seen at a high percentage in all treatment programmes. Those programmes that identify themselves as cognitive-behavioural also use a wide variety of treatment components that fall outside of the cognitive-behavioural label. Plethysmography is used in 32 per cent of all programmes and polygraphy in 24 per cent; electrical aversion is virtually unused, 2 per cent, and only 3 per cent use faradic aversion.

INTEGRATION OF MULTIPLE SYSTEMS PROVIDING INTERVENTION FOR SEX-OFFENDERS

The magnitude of the efforts taken to stop sex offences is currently reflected in a variety of different systems that are combined into a unified effort to treat the public health problem of sex-offences. Treatment programmes for paraphiliacs began as isolated programmes in the provinces of Canada and in a few states in the United States. Government funds channelled through federal research grants eventually allowed the bringing together of representatives from these isolated programmes to compare evaluation and treatment strategies.

These isolated programmes were further stymied because the professional literature lagged sorely behind clinical treatments. This has changed as articles on the evaluation and treatment of sex-offenders have increasingly appeared in such journals as *Annals of Sex Research, Journal of Interpersonal Violence, Child Abuse and Neglect, Criminal Justice and Behaviour, Violence Update, Journal of Sex Research, Annual Review of Sex Research*, and *Archives of Sexual Behaviour*. The primary organization for researchers and clinicians in the area of evaluation and treatment of sex-offenders, the Association for the Behavioural Treatment of Sexual Aggressives, changed as a result of the movement from exclusively behavioural treatment to integrated treatment programmes and is now the Association for the Treatment of Sexual Abusers.[1]

It is now possible to attend international meetings encompassing systems of intervention for sex-offenders, including cognitive-behavioural treatment, drug intervention, sexual addiction, family systems, and the sexual trauma model. In the United States, the Association for the Treatment of Sexual Abusers and the Safer Society Program provide information on the availability of programmes throughout North America, their treatment components, and their theoretical orientation.

Victim organizations, probation and parole officers, the criminal justice system,

---

[1] Association for the Treatment of Sexual Abusers, P.O. Box 866, Lake Oswego, Oregon 97034–0140, USA.

treatment programmes for sex-offenders, and the legal sector are now attempting to come together to ensure a unified effort to stop sex-offending.

INTEGRATION OF ASSESSMENT SURVEILLANCE SYSTEMS

Plethysmography

Penile plethysmography with sex-offenders involves direct measurement of the perpetrator's erection size while concomitantly presenting him with slides, audiotaped descriptions, or videotapes of paraphilic and non-paraphilic sexual stimuli. Based on early volumetric plethysmography studies by Freund and his associates (1967, 1979, 1981) and the development of the circumferential penile transducer (Bancroft *et al.* 1966), penile plethysmography has played a critical role in the behavioural assessment and treatment of sex-offenders. Because some paraphiliacs cannot or will not identify the full extent of their paraphilic interest, plethysmography has been successfully used to help break through the paraphiliac's denial by identifying his sexual interests (Abel 1989).

Penile plethysmography has been exceedingly helpful but it has a number of limitations. It is relatively invasive in that it requires the perpetrator to place a penile transducer around his penis and necessitates presenting stimuli depicting paraphilic themes. Some paraphiliacs can suppress deviant, or augment non-deviant, arousal by voluntary means, and some paraphiliacs 'flatline' (fail to have any arousal during such an assessment, Murphy and Barbaree 1988). Plethysmography has not passed the Frye test for admissibility in court.[2] Objection has also been made that depictions of children during plethysmography is a victimization of children. In spite of the limitations of plethysmography, it has brought some degree of objectivity to the assessment of the potential paraphiliac and contributes to the prediction of post-treatment relapse (Barbaree 1990). Evidence of its general acceptance is demonstrated by numerous scientific articles regarding its use and the existence of standards for plethysmographic measurement of sex-offenders (ATSA 1993).

Polygraphy

Polygraphs are another physiological assessment methodology employed during assessment, treatment, and/or post-treatment follow-up. Twenty per cent of treatment providers use polygraphy to assist in identifying the types and numbers of sex-offences an individual has been involved in before treatment begins, or more importantly, as a periodic means of identifying subsequent relapses post-treatment (see Table 16.2). Polygraphs, like plethysmographs, do not meet the Frye standard of admissibility in court, but serve as a useful adjunct to the clinical interview for gathering information regarding the perpetrator's behaviour outside the treatment setting (S. Abrams and J. B. Abrams 1993).

---

[2] The Frye test is based upon *Frye v. United States* (1923) which determined that polygraph evidence was not admissible because the theory on which it is based had not crossed the 'line between the experimental and the demonstrable stages', and 'such evidence should not be admitted until the underlying scientific principles have become sufficiently established to have gained general acceptance in the particular field in which it belongs'.

Surveillance systems

One reason professionals are reluctant to treat sex-offenders is that, when relapse occurs, not only is there a sense of failure for the perpetrator's relapse, but more importantly, others are victimized. A major change in cognitive-behavioural therapy for sex-offenders has been the development of systems of surveillance for closer supervision during the maintenance portion of treatment. Such surveillance systems involve participation of the offender, the offender's therapist, and individuals from his family, work and social environment, to identify observable behaviours and personality characteristics or stressors that have been antecedent to the sex-offender's prior relapses. These relapse characteristics are incorporated into report forms that are completed by those in the perpetrator's environment and which are advanced to the therapist twice per month (Abel and Rouleau 1990).

When the sex-offender is a professional whose inappropriate sexual behaviour extends into his professional activities (professional sexual misconduct), this reporting system incorporates staff and other professionals working with the impaired professional. It can also include feedback from the offender's patients, clients, or parishioners to further enlarge the sources of feedback regarding possible prerelapse behaviours (Abel *et al.* 1992; Abel and Osborn in press).

When the perpetrator is on probation or parole, surveillance has been expanded to incorporate probation and parole officers. These criminal justice officers are important contributors to the surveillance system since adherence to treatment guidelines can be incorporated into the legal requirements of probation and parole (Pithers *et al.* 1989).

The purpose of treatment of sex-offenders is to stop sexual violence and victimization. No system of treatment or theoretical orientation has achieved 100 per cent success in the treatment of sex-offenders. The use of plethysmography, polygraphy, and surveillance systems provide useful extensions so that the therapist can more accurately monitor potential relapse.

TREATMENT OUTCOME

Treatment outcome studies are nearly impossible to attempt with sex-offenders. These studies have been hindered by the following factors:

1. Outcome is usually measured by recidivism. Most paraphilic acts are considered felonies. Sex-crimes such as paedophilia revealed to therapists must, by law, be reported to state child protection agencies or the criminal justice system. The sex-offender runs the high probability of felony charges and/or incarceration if he accurately reports his recidivism, thus inhibiting his willingness to do so. Should the therapist develop a system to obviate reporting, the therapist will be criticized by victim advocates as being unethical and supportive of child molestation. Also, arrest records are a very inaccurate measure of recidivism since perpetrators often carry out many offences for which they are not caught. Thus, while recidivism is the primary measure of outcome, it is extremely difficult to determine accurately.

2. Baseline rates for various paraphilias are dramatically different (Abel *et al.* 1987). If outcome studies include heterogeneous groups of paraphiliacs, recidivism rates can be significantly influenced by the unequal numbers of various paraphiliacs in either the control or experimental groups. Attempts to control the heterogeneity of paraphiliacs leads to treatment of a single category of paraphilia, thereby diluting the number of subjects available for outcome research.

3. Virtually all large treatment programmes involve multiple-treatment components which are then difficult to separate for analysis.

4. The establishment of a control group is virtually ethically impossible since it would require not treating potentially dangerous paraphiliacs.

5. Lawsuits are becoming increasingly common. Programmes treating paraphiliacs are at risk for such lawsuits; those with controlled studies are at increased risk.

6. The cost of evaluating treatment outcome has continued to spiral upward along with all medical care costs. Burdened by the rapidly increasing numbers of paraphiliacs needing treatment, treatment needs have been given priority over evaluating treatment, at most treatment centres.

7. Academic settings have avoided training clinical staff in the assessment and treatment of paraphiliacs but have focused instead on less controversial psychiatric problems. As a result, those having contact with the largest numbers of paraphiliacs with which to conduct outcome studies tend to have better clinical than research skills.

8. Political and legal sources have impacted on the classification nomenclature to such an extent that the definitions of various categories of paraphiliacs have been blurred by legal, political, and scientific jargon making outcome studies more difficult to compare due to the resultant confusion in diagnostic labels (Okami and Goldberg 1992).

9. Finally, our culture is so incensed with outrage at the occurrence of violence, and specifically sexual violence, that it is unsuportive of scientific studies that seek to measure treatment outcome with offenders and is more supportive of a 'lock them up and get them away from us' approach.

Relapse rates

Reviews of behavioural treatment with sex-offenders have generally involved comparison of relapse rates from treated versus untreated sex offenders. Treatment outcome from programmes with only a marginal emphasis on maintenance, surveillance, and relapse prevention indicates that recidivism is decreased by approximately 20 per cent from untreated control groups (Marshall and Barbaree 1990). Such untreated groups, however, are generally composed of individuals who have been offered therapy but who have refused for geographical, financial, or time restraints. These controls, therefore, are not perfectly matched with the experimental group.

When analysis of treatment outcome has been attempted (Furby *et al.* 1989), the studies reviewed for meta-analysis have usually been from programmes initiated from 15 to 20 years ago using therapies no longer in practice (Pithers 1993). When emphasis is placed on behavioural treatments including victim empathy training and a relapse prevention model that incorporates close supervision by therapists and parole or probation officers, recidivism rates fall to less than 10 per cent (Pithers 1993).

Current research on treatment effectiveness has investigated multi-component treatment to identify which factors best predict success. These factors include the paraphiliac having a single paraphilia (as opposed to a variety of different paraphilias); a history of successful adult attachment and support for a non-paraphilic lifestyle; an IQ above 70; the absence of antisocial personality traits (as measured by the Hare Scale of Psychopathy, Hare 1991); the absence of non-sexual, antisocial behaviours; low paraphilic arousal prior to the initiation of treatment; the absence of concomitant alcohol and drug problems; if involved in incestuous child molestation, not to have had intercourse with one's own child; the absence of cognitive distortions supportive of paraphilic acts; and evidence of behavioural change toward normative patterns during the implementation of cognitive-behavioural treatment (Abel *et al.* 1988; Harris *et al.* 1993; Quinsey *et al.*. in press; Rice *et al.* 1991*b*).

CONCLUSIONS

The belief that behavioural therapy would emanate from animal laboratory studies to lead to specific treatments testable in a human paraphiliac population has not come to fruition. Well-controlled studies of narrow behavioural treatments have been pushed aside by economic considerations requiring cost-effectiveness, a burgeoning number of sex-offenders needing treatment, and the clinical realities that effective treatment demands an integration of multiple cognitive-behavioural therapies, other therapies, and multiple systems dealing with sexual violence. The integration of efforts to stop sexual violence has been at the expense of completing controlled outcome studies. The temporary winners in this sea of change are potential victims, sex-offenders, and society in general, since more forces are at work to stop sexual violence. The scientific issue, however, remains. Can we devise controlled outcome studies that can meet the necessary scientific, ethical, and safety standards needed to demonstrate which therapies are effective with which categories of paraphiliacs?

REFERENCES

Abel, G. G. (1989). Paraphilias. In *Comprehensive textbook of psychiatry*, Vol. 3, (ed. H. I. Kaplan, B. J. Sadock, and J. Benjamin), pp. 1069–85. Williams & Wilkins, Baltimore, MD.

Abel, G. G. and Osborn, C. (1995). Treatment for pedophilia. In *Treatment of psychiatric disorders: The DSM-IV edition*, (ed. G. O. Gabbard). American Psychiatric Press, Washington, DC.

Abel, G. G. and Osborn, C. (in press). Cognitive-behavioural treatment of professional sexual misconduct. In *Current dilemmas in the approach to sexual misconduct among physicians*, (ed. J. Bloom, C. Nadelson, and M. Notman). American Psychiatric Press, Washington DC.

Abel, G. G. and Rouleau, J.-L. (1990). Male sex offenders. In *Handbook of outpatient treatment of adults*, (ed. M. E. Thase, B. A. Edelstein, and M. Hersen), pp. 271–90. Plenum, New York.

Abel, G. G., Blanchard, E. B., Barlow, D. H., and Flanagan, B. (1975, December). *A case report of the behavioural treatment of a sadistic rapist*. Paper presented at the 9th Annual Convention of the Association for the Advancement of Behaviour Therapy, San Francisco, California.

Abel, G. G., Becker, J. V., Cunningham-Rathner, J., Rouleau, J. L., Kaplan, M., and Reich, J. (1984). *The treatment of child molesters*. Behavioral Medicine Institute of Atlanta, Atlanta, GA.

Abel, G. G., Mittelman, M. S., and Becker, J. V. (1985). Sex offenders: Results of assessment and recommendations for treatment. In *Clinical criminology: The assessment and treatment of criminal behavior*, (ed. M. H. Ben-Aron, S. J. Hucker, and C. D. Webster), pp. 191–205. M & M Graphics, Toronto, Canada.

Abel, G. G., *et al.* (1987). Self-reported sex crimes of nonincarcerated paraphiliacs. *J. Interper. Viol.* 2, 3–25.

Abel, G. G., Mittelman, M. S., Becker, J. V., Rathner, J., and Rouleau, J.-L. (1988). Predicting child molesters' response to treatment. *Ann. N.Y. Acad. Sci.* 528, 223–34.

Abel, G. G., Becker, J. V., Cunningham-Rathner, J., Mittelman, M. S., and Rouleau, J.-L. (1989). Multiple paraphilic diagnoses among sex offenders. *Bull. Am. Acad. Psychiat. Law*, 16, 153–68.

Abel, G. G., Barrett, D. H., and Gardos, P. S. (1992). Sexual misconduct by physicians. *J. Georgia Med. Assoc.* 81, 237–46.

Abrams, S. and Abrams, J. B. (1993). *Polygraph testing of the pedophile*. Ryan Gwinner Press, Portland, OR.

ATSA (Association for the Treatment of Sexual Abusers) (1993). *The ATSA practitioner's handbook*. ATSA Lake Oswego, OR.

Bancroft, J. H. J., Gaynne Jones, H., and Pullan, B. R. (1966). A simple transducer for measuring penile erection, with comments on its use in the treatment of sexual disorders. *Behav. Res. Ther.* 4, 239–41.

Barbaree, H. E. (1990). Stimulus control of sexual arousal: Its role in sexual assault. In *Handbook of sexual assault: Issues, theories, and treatment of the offender*, (ed. W. L. Marshall, D. R. Laws, and H. E. Barbaree), pp. 115–42. Plenum, New York.

Barlow, D. H., Agras, W. S., Abel, G. G., Blanchard, E. B., and Young, L. D. (1975). Biofeedback and reinforcement to increase heterosexual arousal in homosexuals. *Behav. Res. Ther.* 13, 45–50.

Carnes, P. (1990). Sexual addiction: Progress, criticism, challenges. *Prev. Psychiat. Neurol.* 2, 1–8.

Conrad, S. R. and Wincze, J. P. (1976). Orgasmic reconditioning: A controlled study of its effects upon the sexual arousal and behavior of adult male homosexuals. *Behav. Ther.* 7, 155–66.

Dwyer, M. and Coleman, E. (1990). Proposed standards of care for the treatment of adult sex offenders. *J. Offender Rehabil.* 16, 93–106.

Freund, K. (1967). Erotic preference in pedophilia. *Behav. Res. Ther.* 5, 339–48.

Freund, K. (1981). Assessment of pedophilia. In *Adult sexual interest in children*, (ed. M. Cook and S. K, Howell), pp. 139–79. Academic Press, London.

Freund, K., Chan, S., and Coulthard, R., (1979). Phallometric diagnosis with "non-admitters". *Behav. Res. Ther.* 17, 451–7.

Frye v. *United States*, 293 F. 1013 (D. C. Cir. 1923).

Furby, L., Weinrott, M. R., and Blackshaw, L. (1989). Sex offender recidivism: A review. *Psychol. Bull.* 105, 3–30.

George, W. H. and Marlatt, G. (1989). Introduction. In *Relapse prevention with sex offenders*, (ed. D. R. Laws), pp. 1–31. Guilford Press, New York.

Hare, R. D. (1991). *Manual for the revised Psychopathy Checklist*. Multi-Health Systems, Toronto, Canada.

Harris, G. T., Rice, M. E., and Quinsey, V. L. (1993). Violent recidivism of mentally disordered offenders: The development of a statistical prediction instrument. *Crim. Just. Behav.* **20**, 315–35.

Hildebran, D. and Pithers, W. D. (1989). Enhancing offender empathy for sexual-abuse victims. In *Relapse prevention with sex offenders*, (ed. D. R. Laws), pp. 236–44. Guilford Press, New York.

Jenkins-Hall, K. D., Osborn, C. A., Anderson, C. S., Anderson, K. A., and Shockley-Smith, C. (1989). The center for the prevention of child molestation. In *Relapse prevention with sex offenders*, (ed. D. R. Laws), pp. 268–91. Guilford Press, New York.

Knopp, F. H. (1984). *Retraining adult sex offenders: Methods and models*. Safer Society Press, Syracuse, NY.

Knopp, F. H., Freeman-Longo, R., and Stevenson, W. F. (1992). *Nationwide survey of juvenile and adult sex-offender treatment programs and models*. The Safer Society Program, Orwell, VT.

Kremsdorf, R. B., Holmen, M. L., and Laws, D. R. (1980). Orgasmic reconditioning without deviant imagery: A case report with a pedophile. *Behav. Res. Ther.* **18**, 203–7.

Lange, A. (1986). *Rational-emotive therapy: A treatment manual*. Florida Mental Health Institute, Tampa, FL.

Laws, D. R. (1989). Preface. In *Relapse prevention with sex offenders*, (ed. D. R. Laws), pp. vii–ix. Guilford Press, New York.

Laws, D. R. and Osborn, C. A. (1983). How to build and operate a behavioral laboratory to evaluate and treat sexual deviance. In *The sexual aggressor: Current perspectives on treatment*, (ed. J. G. Greer and I. R Stuart), pp. 293–335. Van Nostrand Reinhold, New York.

Laws, D. R., Meyer, J., and Holmen, M. L. (1978). Reduction of sadistic sexual arousal by olfactory aversion: A case study. *Behav. Res. Ther.* **16**, 281–5.

Laws, D. R, Osborn, C. A., Avery-Clark, C., O'Neill, J. A., and Crawford, D. A. (1987). Masturbatory satiation with sexual deviates. Unpublished manuscript. University of South Florida, Florida Mental Health Institute, Tampa, FL.

Leonard, S. R. and Hayes, S. C. (1983). Sexual fantasy alternation. *J. Behav. Ther. Exp. Psychiat.* **14**(3), 241–9.

Maletzky, B. M. (1980). Self-referred versus court-referred sexually deviant patients: Success with assisted covert sensitization. *Behav. Ther.* **11**, 306–14.

Maletzky, B. M. (1985). Orgasmic reconditioning. In *Dictionary of behavior therapy techniques*, (ed. A. S. Bellack and M. Hersen), pp. 157–8. Pergamon, New York.

Marques, J. (1970). Orgasmic reconditioning: Changing sexual object choice through controlling masturbation fantasies. *J. Behav. Ther. Exp. Psychiat.* **1**, 263–71.

Marques, J. K. and Nelson, C. (1989). Elements of high risk situations for sex offenders. In *Relapse prevention with sex offenders*, (ed. D. R. Laws), pp. 247–67. Guilford Press, New York.

Marques, J. K., Day, D. M., Nelson, C., and Miner, M. H. (1989). The sex offender treatment and evaluation project: California's relapse prevention program. In *Relapse prevention with sex offenders*, (ed. D. R. Laws), pp. 247–67. Guilford Press, New York.

Marshall, W. L. (1971). A combined treatment method for certain sexual deviations. *Behav. Res. Ther.* **9**, 293–4.

Marshall, W. L. and Barbaree, H. E. (1990). Outcome of comprehensive cognitive-behavioral treatment programs. In *Handbook of sexual assault: Issues, theories, and treatment of the offender*, (ed. W. L. Marshall, D. R. Laws, and H. E. Barbaree), pp. 363–85. Plenum, New York.

McConaghy, N. (1990). Assessment and treatment of sex offenders: The Prince of Wales programme. *Austral. N. Zealand J. Psychiat.* **24**, 175–81.

McConaghy, N., Armstrong, M. S., and Blaszczynski, A. (1985). Expectancy, covert sensitization and imaginal desensitization in compulsive sexuality. *Acta Psychiat. Scand.* **72**, 176–87.

Murphy, W. D. (1990). Assessment and modification of cognitive distortions in sex offenders. In *Handbook of sexual assault: Issues, theories, and treatment of the offender*, (ed. W. L. Marshall, D. R. Laws, and H. E. Barbaree), pp. 331–42. Plenum, New York.

Murphy, W. D. and Barbaree, H. E. (1988). *Assessments of sexual offenders by measures of erectile response: Psychometric properties and decision making*. National Institutes of Mental Health, Washington, DC.

Okami, P. and Goldberg, A. (1992). Personality correlates of pedophilia: Are they reliable indicators? *J. Sex Res.* **29**, 297–328.

Pithers, W. D. (1990). Relapse prevention with sexual aggressors. In *Handbook of sexual assault: Issues, theories, and treatment of the offender*, (ed. W. L. Marshall, D. R. Laws, and H. E. Barbaree), pp. 343–61. Plenum, New York.

Pithers, W. D. (1993). Treatment of rapists: Reinterpretation of early outcome data and exploratory constructs to enhance therapeutic efficacy. In *Sexual aggression: Issues in etiology, assessment, and treatment*, (ed. G. C. Nagayama Hall, R. Hirschman, J. R. Graham, and M. S. Zaragoza), pp. 167–96. Taylor & Francis, Washington, DC.

Pithers, W. D., Marques, J. K., Gibat, C. C., and Marlatt, G. A. (1983). Relapse prevention with sexual aggressives: A self-control model of treatment and maintenance of change. In *The sexual aggressor: Current perspectives on treatment*, (ed. J. G. Greer and I. R. Stuart), pp. 214–39. Van Nostrand Reinhart, New York.

Pithers, W. D., Kashima, K. M., Cumming, G. F., Beal, L. S., and Buell, M. (1988). Relapse prevention of sexual aggression. In *Human sexual aggression: Current perspectives*, (ed. R. Prentky and V. Quinsey), pp. 244–60. *Ann. Acad. Sci.*, New York.

Pithers, W. D., Martin, G. R., and Cumming, G. F. (1989). Vermont treatment program for sexual aggressors. In *Relapse prevention with sex offenders*, (ed. D. R. Laws), pp. 292–310. Guilford Press, New York.

Quinsey, V. L., Chaplin, T. C., Maguire, A. M., and Upfold, D. (1987). The behavioral treatment of rapists and child molesters. In *Behavioral approaches to crime and delinquency: Application, research, and theory*, (ed. E. K. Morris and C. J. Braukmann), pp. 363–82. Plenum, New York.

Quinsey, V. L., Rice, M. E., and Harris, G. T. (in press). Actuarial prediction of sexual recidivism. *J. Interper. Viol.*

Rice, M. E., Harris, G. T. and Quinsey, V. L. (1991a). Evaluation of an institution-based treatment program for child molesters. *Can. J. Prog. Eval.* **6**, 11–129.

Rice, M. E., Quinsey, V. L., and Harris, G. T. (1991b). Sexual recidivism among child molesters released from a maximum security psychiatric institution. *J. Consult. Clini. Psychol.* **59**, 381–6.

Schwartz, M. and Brasted, W. (1985). Sexual addiction. *Med. Asp. Hum. Sexual.* **19**, 103–7.

Serber, M. (1970). Shame aversion therapy. *J. Behav. Ther. Exp. Psychiat.* **1**, 213–5.

SOTP (Sex Offender Treatment Providers) (1991, May). 18.155.010–.902 RCW.

Smith, T. A. and Wolfe, R. W. (1988). A treatment model for sexual aggression. *J. Soc. W. Hum. Sexual.* **7**, 149–64.

Whitman, W. P. and Quinsey, V. L. (1981). Heterosocial skill training for institutionalized rapists and child molesters. *Can. J. Behav. Sci.* **13**, 105–14.

Wickramsekera, I. (1976). Aversive behavioral rehearsal for sexual exhibitionism. *Behav. Ther.* **7**, 167–76.

Wickramsekera, I. (1980). Aversive behavioral rehearsal: A cognitive behavioral procedure. In *Exhibitionism: Description, assessment and treatment*, (ed. D. J. Cox and R. J. Daitzman). Appleton-Croft, New York.

17
Sexual deviance and the law

Michael Freeman

INTRODUCTION

Sexual mores vary from culture to culture, and there is an approximate correspondence between the law and the pattern of accepted behaviour. A survey of the world's legislation on sexual deviance and methods of treating it would thus present a variegated picture. The United States of America, according to Slovenko (1965), has more laws on the subject than all of the European countries combined. The world-wide trend is towards liberalization, 'decriminalization' as it is often called, and this is also the tendency in the United States, although hiccups such as *Bowers* v. *Hardwick* (1986) and *R.* v. *Brown* (1993) show the trend is not all one way. No purpose can be served by cataloguing the world's laws. This chapter, accordingly, concentrates on the law of England and Wales, although references are made where appropriate to other systems. Indeed, some of the discussions of the effects of legal intervention, while theoretically sound wherever the locale, are particularly apposite to the American situation.

The need for law

Every society must set up norms for the regulation of sexual conduct (Davis 1976). In contemporary societies, the law is the principal vehicle of standard-setting. But such regulations must not be looked upon as altogether restrictive. In a broader sense, law is a programme for living together (Fuller 1969; Unger 1976): society is not a suicide club (Hart 1961), and much can be gained even from restrictions. Without limits on sexual expression, there could be no civilization. Indeed, it is somewhat surprising that an as astute observer as Hart should fail to include an appreciation of this in his list of truisms which formed the basis for his 'minimum content of natural law' (McCormick 1982). As Balint (1957) has put it: sexual restrictions 'protect the structure of society against the onslaught of sexually highly excited individuals, that is, people "on heat". At the same time they protect the individual and allow him to enjoy a modicum of sexual pleasure in comparative peace and security'.

Sexual deviance, conflict, and interest groups

Generally speaking the law in this area is secondary. It follows; it does not lead. It obtains its legitimacy, or seeks to do so in a more primary reference point, the moral order. It is thus seen as reinstitutionalizing custom (Bohannan 1967) and purports to act as a reinforcement agency. As such it will, in most societies, have the support of the majority and problems of law enforcement will focus on a deviant minority. There are exceptions to this; it is thought that the puritanical sex code in much of the United States is completely out of touch with mainstream culture. The classic study by Kinsey *et al.* (1948) exposed the hypocrisy inherent in this by suggesting that nine out of ten Americans were sex criminals.

But the American situation draws attention to what, in less acute form, is a very real problem. For, if the law follows conventional morality, *whose* standards is it following? Contemporary society is pluralistic, heterogeneous; there are numerous, often overlapping cultural standards and reference groups. Outside a practically universal core, one finds not consensus but conflict. It is clear that this problem has usually been glossed over. The morality of 'middle Britain' has been taken as a norm. As Troy Duster put it (1970): 'so long as an activity is engaged in predominantly by those in the "centre" social categories the likelihood of moral condemnation for the activity is minuscule.' He traced the history of narcotics legislation in the United States and showed how, until 1914, the taking of heroin was the prerogative of the upper and middle classes; legislation to outlaw its use followed the trend for medical journals to report that the 'overwhelming' majority of users came from 'unrespectable' parts of society. And his comment can be generalized. 'Middle America's moral hostility comes faster and easier when directed toward a young, lower-class, Negro male than toward a middle-aged, middle-class, white female.' And the middle classes are assumed to have a monopoly of moral indignation (Ranulf 1938). Thus, surprisingly, eugenic considerations were by no means crucial to the passage of the law in 1908 making incest a criminal offence. Rather it can be attributed to a social-purity alliance between the National Vigilance Association and the NSPCC. Bailey and Blackburn comment (1979, p. 718) that the Act was 'a public affirmation of the moral values associated with reactionary vigilance work on behalf of social purity'. It was 'less an act of rational social policy than a manifestation of the strength and status of the social purity movement' (see also Pivar, 1973).

This perspective has often been ignored in the past, because of the tendency to characterize the social problem in individualistic terms, to assume that it can be fully explained by reference to the supposed special characteristics or stigmata of the offender. Yet one cannot have violations without norms, and violations are relatively meaningless if they do not lead to action by social control agencies or members of society. Rule-makers, 'whistle-blowers' (Becker 1963), and rule-enforcers must, however, be upholding certain sets of values and collective interests, and this must redound to the detriment of other interest groups. Within the last couple of decades, movements committed towards the 'politicization of deviance' (Horowitz and Liebowitz 1968) have grown up. Where once those considered deviants accepted the prevailing definitions of their behaviour, and 'status degradation' (Garfinkel 1956) led to identity reconstruction (Schur 1971), now the tendency is to resist, to organize collectively, and to sound the trumpet of liberation (Humphreys 1972; Altman and Weeks 1973; Millett 1973). A striking illustration of this is the movement towards gay liberation and 'gay pride'. Of course, 'if one accepts the view that dominant social and legal norms emerge out of conflicts or contests between competing interests and values, then it would seem to follow that the very meaning of the term "problem" is similarly problematic' (Schur and Bedau 1974). Lawyers working within the dominant positivistic paradigm are blind to the implications of this. Thus, legal treatises analyse sexual deviance as a 'given'. But a perspective which is sceptical of posited classifications will be used in this chapter.

The law and sexual morality

'When the mores are adequate, laws are unnecessary; when the mores are inadequate, the laws are ineffective' (Sutherland and Cressey 1970). This aphorism captures succinctly a contemporary dilemma. What ends should the law promote? Are there spheres of activity with which it would be wrong for the law to interfere? Are there areas where the law's intervention is self-defeating? What are the results of intervention and non-intervention? The debate has a long heritage, and has frequently found its inspiration in questions of legislation on matters of sexual morality. Mill (1859) argued that 'the only purpose for which power can be rightfully exercised over any member of a civilised community against his will is to prevent harm to others'. This essentially utilitarian approach was echoed in the Wolfenden report on Homosexual Offences and Prostitution (1957). The Committee stated: 'unless a deliberate attempt is to be made by society, acting through the agency of the law, to equate the sphere of crime with that of sin, there must remain a realm of private morality and immorality which is . . . not the law's business . . .' (para. 61). 'It is not the duty of the law to concern itself with immorality as such . . . It should confine itself to those activities which offend against public order and decency, or expose the ordinary citizen to what is offensive or injurious' (para. 257).

This liberal position was challenged by the English judge Lord Devlin (1965). His premise is that a society is not just a people but also a community of ideas. Shared attitudes about right and wrong and common standards of conduct are prerequisites of social life. So, he argued, a society is morally justified in punishing immorality as it is in extirpating that most heinous of offences, treason, for failure to root out either will lead to the disintegration of that society. Devlin thus rejected pluralism (Wollheim 1959; Hart 1963). He would, however, tolerate a good deal of immorality before invoking the sanction of the criminal law. His criterion for intervention was widespread intolerance, indignation, and disgust of the particular activity. His model of rational judgment was the jury man. But Devlin had elsewhere (1956) described the jury as predominantly male, middle-aged, middle-class, and middle-minded. The composition of the jury has changed since: eligibility for jury service no longer depends on a property qualification but on inclusion in the electoral register subject to exemptions and disqualifications.

Devlin's arguments have been attacked by Hart (1963, 1965, 1967), who took a modified utilitarian position. He dismissed Devlin's disintegration thesis as lacking empirical foundation. His own assumption was that depriving individuals of their autonomy requires justification. Laws designed to enforce sexual morality interfere with sexual expression, and deprive individuals of sexual outlets. Such laws, and the coercive measures that may be used to enforce them, 'may create misery of a quite special degree' (Hart 1963). They, therefore, require justification of a weighty nature. He was not convinced by Devlin's arguments. Devlin appeals to the existence of laws that enforce morality. But this is merely to invoke 'the innocuous (*sic*) conservative principle that there is a presumption that common and long-established institutions are likely to have merits not apparent to the rationalist philosopher' (Hart 1963). The present existence of such laws, and indeed their long history, says nothing about their normative value. Devlin asserted also that the function of the criminal law is only to enforce moral principles. He cited the conviction of a sadist who caned a masochist with her consent (*R.* v. *Donovan* [1934]) as proof of this. But Hart argued that there may be another reason for invoking the criminal law in these circumstances, namely, paternalism. Hart supported legal paternalism on the ground that it is not always true that the individual is the best judge of his own interests. Laws 'excluding the victim's consent as a defence to charges of murder and assault may perfectly well be explained as a piece of paternalism, designed to protect individuals against themselves' (Hart 1963). But what is paternalism other than the enforcement of a moral principle? Can one support moral individualism and physical paternalism at the same time? As Devlin (1965) wrote: 'What, alas, I did not foresee was that those who sailed under Mill's flag of liberty would mutiny and run the flag of paternalism up the mast.'

To this, two comments may be offered. First, Mill himself recognized certain exceptions to his 'harm' principle: children, the feeble-minded, and backward people. In these cases he allows paternalism. These people may be restrained for their own good. Further, Mill qualified his simple principle. He admitted 'that the mischief which a person does to himself may seriously affect, both through their sympathies and their interests, those nearly connected with him, and, in a minor degree, society at large'. Such an injury would be contingent only, an 'inconvenience' which society must accept for the sake of the greater good of human freedom *unless* the individual violates a 'specific duty to the public' or a 'distinct and assignable obligation to any other person or persons'. But this admission would seem to cut the ground from under Mill's feet. Secondly, it has been argued (Ten 1969) in defence of Hart's stand on paternalism that it can be justified in terms of the individual's inability, because of his emotional or physical state, to make a rational decision. To argue this, however, is surely to invoke a moral principle.

The debate is inconclusive. The contestants do not define their terms clearly enough. Hart did not spell out the scope of paternalism—many socially useful activities and heroic acts of selfless abnegation are not self-interested. Mill seems to have called for a 'weighing', but how can a balancing take place with such ill-defined concepts as 'harm', 'inconvenience', and the like? Each contains within itself certain unspecified moral and social assumptions (Nagel 1969; Golding 1975). Devlin may have over-identified a society with its morality. The 'community of ideas' which he treasured is not to be found in contemporary, secular, heterogeneous society, but although much separates the contestants ideologically, there are few substantive issues which divide them. Both Hart and Devlin favoured privacy—another imprecise concept which limps badly out of the debate (and see Moore 1984; Schoeman 1984). Hart supported the use of the law to preserve a 'minimum content of natural law' (1961), 'universal values' (1963), and even particular institutions which are deeply embedded within a society—such as monogamy (1967). This is not to underestimate the importance of the debate, for the issues discussed here are never far below the surface when matters concerned with social policy in connection with sexual behaviour are disputed. (See also George 1993.)

More recently Karst (1980) has put forward a different justification for non-interference: the principle of 'intimate association'. But he distinguished 'intimate associations' (where there is commitment) from 'casual associations', although he admits it is necessary also to protect the latter because they may ripen into the former. But Karst is unwilling to protect all enduring intimate associations. Thus, for example, sibling marriage (incest) can be forbidden because the 'force of conventional morality' acts as a 'political constraint' (Karst 1980, p. 673). The state can, he argues, 'legitimately seek to foster a particular morality' (p. 690) but for Karst the key question is whether it has 'offered sufficient justification for a given type of impairment of intimate associational values' (p. 691).

The law's concern with sexual deviance

> Culture, in the sense of the public, standardized values of a community, mediates the experience of individuals. It provides in advance some basic categories, a positive pattern in which ideas and values are tidily ordered. And above all, it has authority, since each is induced to assent because of the assent of others. But its public character makes its categories more rigid . . . They cannot . . . easily be subject to revision. Yet they cannot ignore the challenge of aberrant forms. Any given system of classification must give rise to anomalies and any given culture must confront events which seem to defy its assumptions . . .' (Douglas 1966)

The problem of anomaly may be solved in a number of ways; by settling for a different interpretation it may be reduced; it can be physically controlled; it can be avoided; and fourthly, anomalous events may be labelled dangerous. Sexual deviance may be construed as a anomaly and, as an event which disturbs reality, it constitutes a threat to the social order and occasions the intervention of social control.

A good example of this is our classification of sex identity. Sexual attributes are neatly categorized in contemporary society. One is either male or female and one's life is structured on the classification. The hermaphrodite, the transsexual, the homosexual threaten this pattern and ordering; so, in similar ways, do the mentally ill and prostitutes (Lofland 1969).

This theme is pursued by Garfinkel in his study of the transsexual, Agnes (Garfinkel 1967). He has constructed a list of 'properties of "natural, normally sexed persons" as cultural objects'. He argues that

> the population of normal persons is a morally dichotomised population. The question of its existence is decided as a matter of motivated compliance with this population as a legitimate order. It is not decided as a matter of biological, medical, [or] sociological fact . . . The adult member includes himself in this environment and counts himself as one of the other . . . as a condition whereby the exercise of his rights to live without excessive risks and interference from others are routinely enforceable . . . For normals, the presence in the environment of sexed objects has the feature of a 'natural matter of fact'. This naturalness carries along with it, as a constituent part of its meaning, the sense of its being right and correct; i.e. morally proper that it be that way.

This analysis of sexual typifications could be the inarticulate premise underlying Ormrod J's judgment in the April Ashley case (*Corbett* v. *Corbett* [1970] 2 All E.R. 33). It could also explain attitudes towards prostitution—she does not behave as a 'normal' woman—and homosexuality—he is a 'role-player, who attempts to refute the conception that the world is dichotomized into discrete sexes with their peculiar sets of characteristics. He poses the possibility of a midway position which is neither fully male nor fully female, and, by so doing, threatens the classification scheme with an anomalous case' (Rock 1974).

Some effects of legal intervention

Many reasons have been suggested why the law should interfere with sexual deviance. But what happens when it does? It is now generally accepted that legal intervention does not work. Thus, Packer (1968) described the operation of the criminal process in this area as 'an extraordinarily difficult and costly method of social control'. Morris and Hawkins (1970) see it as an 'unwarranted extension' of the criminal law and as 'expensive, ineffective, and criminogenic'. And Schur, describing much of this area as 'crimes without victims' (Schur 1965, 1969, 1973), has argued strongly for 'decriminalization'. A distinction has to be drawn between offences such as rape, indecent assault, and paedophilia on the one hand, where there are victims and where, on any test, the case for legal intervention is strong, and those such as homosexuality, prostitution, and some forms of incest. It is the latter category where the non-intervention school are on the strongest ground and, indeed, where on the whole they rest their case.

They argue that these are crimes without victims in the sense that the persons who are the objects of the crime do not see themselves as victims (see Quinney 1972; Schur and Bedau 1974). Schur (1965) defines a victimless crime as an offence arising in 'situations in which one person obtains from another, in a fairly direct exchange, a commodity or personal service which is socially disapproved and legally proscribed'. There are no complainants, so the police must ferret out those they intend to prosecute. How do the police decide which crimes, many of which such as obscenity and conspiracy to corrupt public morals are loosely defined, to discover and prosecute? It seems that customary morality (that is, middle-class morality) tends to define law enforcement. Thus, Lambert (1970) argues that 'the police force . . . tends to be an agency committed to establishing moral conformity; or in some instances achieving and maintaining social stability, by tolerating to a greater or lesser extent certain legal infractions—such as prostitution or some "social" violence—if such does not threaten the sense of well-being of the dominant moral community'. Offences such as these generate more work for the police (Reiss 1971). 'Lacking direct complainants, law enforcers become dependent for evidence on a variety of unsavoury techniques—use of informers and decoys, clandestine surveillance, wiretapping and other types of "bugging", surprise ("no-knock") raids and the like' (Schur and Bedau 1974). Skolnick (1993) found that half of the arrests of prostitutes resulted from decoy activity. Entrapment techniques are the norm to catch homosexuals (Gallo *et al.* 1966). Laws outlawing activities like prostitution and homosexuality cannot be enforced. The police recognize this. Arrests and prosecutions take place, but these are gestures 'to keep up the façade of public morality' (Millett 1973). Indeed, by using the informer system the police are giving indirect support to criminality. The laws can be harmful in another way. They 'can be used against those who violate inter-racial sex taboos, against political opponents and against welfare recipients and job applicants' (Sagarin 1974).

The economic effects of legislating in this area are equally great (Packer 1968; Rogers 1973). For 'regardless of what we think we are trying to do, when we make it illegal to traffic in commodities for which there is an inelastic demand, the effect is to secure a kind of monopoly profit to the entrepreneur who is willing to break the law' (Packer 1968). There is no doubt that the demand for illicit sex is inelastic. The result is the development of a black market and organized crime. A crime tariff is created and this has a number of unintended consequences.

The crimes under discussion are what is usually termed 'expressive' offences. That is to say that 'the act is committed because it is pleasurable in and of itself and not because it is a route to some other good' (Chambliss 1967). There is evidence to suggest that punishment does not deter in this situation (Chambliss 1967). Looked at from the seller's point of view, for instance, the prostitute or purveyor of pornography, every increase in risk increases his potential gain. Packer (1968) therefore has argued that the harder we strain to make sales risky 'the higher we drive the price that makes the risk worthwhile'. So 'the theory of deterrence, however useful it may be in the ordinary run of crimes, breaks down.' The inflation in the price and the absence of legitimate outlets, however, make it more difficult for the purchaser. He may be forced to commit other crimes. And there may begin a spiralling of deviant activities which sociologists of deviance have come to describe as 'secondary deviance' or amplified deviance (Lemert 1967; Wilkins 1964). A major consequence of legal intervention in this area is thus the creation of much additional crime that would not exist if the behaviour in question were not proscribed. A wide range of criminal occupations is given impetus: the opportunities for blackmail are increased; the customer, identified by the law as a criminal, takes on this imputation as his own self-identity. He becomes more and more antisocial. He is subject to constant discrediting processes, to exploitation, and to discrimination. It should not, however, be thought that 'decriminalization' necessarily stems these deleterious effects. The legalization of consenting homosexual behaviour in England has not noticeably ameliorated the status of the homosexual (Plummer 1975). Social control continues unabated: there is still stigma, harassment, and limited employment opportunities (see Humphreys 1970, 1972).

A final effect of the crime tariff, which cannot be ignored, is the impact it has on the credibility of the legal institutions. The opportunities for police corruption are wide. Police have been known to take a 'cut', to accept protection money (Cox *et al.* 1977). The deviant pays rather as one pays an insurance premium. This inevitably breeds cynicism and produces a backlash against the whole system. This is not helped when it is realized that the laws are unevenly enforced. There are socio-economic differentials as well as those grounded in race and sex. The rich not only obtain a better quality of illicit goods, but they also stand a greater chance of concealing their activity and of not being subject to formal status degradation ceremonies. (See also Freeman 1974.)

Classification of deviant sexual behaviour

There are two types of classification that might be attempted. The legal approach is to characterize sexual deviance in terms of overt behaviour problems. The psychiatrist and the psychoanalyst, on the other hand, are concerned to classify according to underlying clinical factors. It may be, therefore, that classification according to legally defined offences indicating the end behaviour will bear little relation to treatment requirements (Scott 1964). But, as James (1964) has remarked, 'the tracing of sexual perversions, which the law under various statutes or at common law proscribes, to infantile sexuality is too refined an approach to be incorporated on the statute books'. The Danish Penal Code of 1930 (ss. 16 and 17) does make an attempt in this direction, but this is not the English approach. To the psychologist, the English lawyer's approach will appear crude and lacking in scientific foundation, rather as the psychologist would take exception to legal concepts concerned with mental health.

The official English Home Office publication *Criminal statistics* is not particularly helpful. It lists sexual offences under just one category. Many offences against the person and some offences against property can, however, be regarded as sexual offences in the widest sense of this term, since sexual motivation or an element of sexual perversion is the precipitatory factor (Schmideburg 1956). This complex dimension is omitted from the discussion which follows.

We do not, and cannot, know how many deviant sexual offences are committed. *Criminal statistics* (Home Office 1991) reveal that in 1991 29 400 sexual offences were recorded as known to the police, an increase of only 1 per cent from the figure of the previous year. The clear-up rate is high (76 per cent), exceeded only by offences involving violence to the person, which is an indication of the seriousness with which the police view such crimes. Criminal statistics are socially constructed and notoriously unreliable (Box 1971; Douglas 1971). Estimates of sexual offences must be egregiously susceptible to error; perhaps only one-fifth of rape victims (or their families) notify the police, a large amount of incest goes undetected, and many other sexual offences do not come to the attention of control agencies.

The following classification is based on that of James (1964); and as James states, 'words such as "normal", "perverted", "homosexuality", etc. are here intended to indicate the overt behaviour problem, as seen by the court, and not the underlying clinical factors'. But, as James indicated, 'the law does seem to accept implicitly in its system of values that the genitally oriented adult is the normal'.

Offences against the accepted standards of family life:
- (a) bigamy
- (b) incest
- (c) adultery
- (d) fornication

Offences which display the normal sexual drive in a distorted or unacceptable manner:
- (a) rape
- (b) indecent assault on a woman
- (c) unlawful sexual intercourse
- (d) sexual murder
- (e) paedophilia
- (f) prostitution by females to males

Offences which display what is considered to be a perverted sexual drive:
- (a) homosexuality (including indecent assault by males on males and importuning)
- (b) lesbianism

(c) transvestism
(d) fetishism
(e) voyeurism
(f) exhibitionism
(g) bestiality
(h) sodomy with a woman
(i) necrophilia
(j) sado-masochism
(k) making obscence telephone calls

The historical background

In earlier times, the ecclesiastical courts exercised jurisdiction of a wide nature relating to the formalities of marriage, to problems arising from the status of marriage, and in connection with incontinence in general. Earlier still, the more primitive law punished the cruder sexual offences with great severity. Between 1558 and 1640 the Court of High Commission also dealt with sexual offences. It concerned itself with the immoral practices of the wealthy and the penalties imposed were accordingly more severe. Thus adultery, incest, excessive drinking, swearing, and blasphemy came within its purview. Hale, in his *Ecclesiastical precedents* (1736), reports cases relating to incest, bigamy, acting as a procuress, procuring abortion, and a case of assault with intent to ravish, among other offences.

The ecclesiastical jurisdiction gradually fell into decay. The ecclesiastical courts were abolished in 1640 and, although revived in 1661, were never a force again. The 19th century saw their final demise. Their jurisdiction in matrimonial causes was transferred to the secular courts in 1857, and by 1876 Lord Penzance was able to remark that 'a recurrence of the punishment of the laity for the good of their souls by ecclesiastical courts would not be in harmony with modern ideas, or the position which ecclesiastical authority now occupies' (*Phillimore* v. *Machon* 1 P.D. 481).

However, even before Cromwell, incursions had been made into ecclesiastical jurisdiction. Thus in 1603 bigamy was made a crime by statute, and unnatural offences were proscribed under a statute of Henry VIII's reign. The preamble to the latter statute states as justification for the new statutory offence that 'there is a suggestion in earlier writers (Fleta, Britton, both *circa* 1290–2) that burying alive or burning may have been the punishment, though this may be doubted' (Stephen 1883). After 1640, the common law intervened to fill in the gaps left by statute. The judges assumed wider-ranging powers to protect society against what they deemed was immorality. Typical of the attitude was Lord Mansfield's judgment in *R.* v. *Delaval* in 1763 (3 Burr. 1435). The case concerned procuration. 'It is true', said the Lord Chief Justice, 'that cases of this incontinent kind fall properly under the jurisdiction of the ecclesiastical courts and are appropriate to it, but, if you accept those appropriated cases, this court is the *custos morum* of the people and has the superintendency of offences *contra bonos mores*'.

This reasoning is no longer acceptable. But it was used again in the notorious Ladies' Directory Case in 1961 (*Shaw* v. *D.P.P.* [1962] AC220), when the House of Lords convicted Shaw of conspiring with prostitutes to corrupt public morals by publishing a pamphlet which was a guide to their activities and contained vital information about them. Viscount Simonds asserted the existence in the court of a residual power, where no statute has intervened to supersede the common law, to superintend those offences which are prejudicial to the public welfare . . . No one can foresee every way in which the wickedness of man may disrupt the order of society . . . Must we wait until Parliament finds time to deal with such conduct? . . . If the common law is powerless in such an event, then we should no longer do her reverence. But I say that her hand is still powerful and that is for Her Majesty's judges to play the part which Lord Mansfield pointed out to them.

Lord Reid powerfully dissented, but the other judges agreed. Lord Hodson, for example, saw no reason why a conspiracy to encourage fornication and adultery should be regarded as outside the ambit of a conspiracy to corrupt public morals. The ideology, seeing the courts as the upholder of public morality, was expressed strongly also in the recent *Brown* decision ([1993] 3 WLR 556). The existence of the offence of conspiracy to corrupt public morals was confirmed by the House of Lords in 1972 (*Knuller* v. *D.P.P.* [1973]) where advertisements in the *International Times* for homosexual contacts were held to come within its scope. Apparently, some 40 cases involving charges of conspiracy to corrupt public morals were brought in the decade between these two cases. One was the famous *Oz* case (*R.* v. *Anderson* [1972] 1 Q.B. 304). Two-thirds of the cases related to the showing of pornographic films in private, unlicensed premises to which members of the public were admitted on payment (Law Commission 1974).

Knuller's case is also important in that the majority of the House of Lords held that there was also a common law offence of conspiracy to outrage public decency, and, perhaps, the generalized offence of outraging decency. It is not clear from *Knuller* precisely what meaning is to be attributed to 'outrage decency'. To Lord Morris, printed matter which 'could rationally be regarded as lewd, disgusting and offensive', and which would outrage 'the sense of decency of members of the public' would be caught by the offence. Lord Simon, on the other hand, argued that 'outrage' was a 'very strong word'. So 'outraging public decency" goes considerably beyond offending the susceptibilities of, or even shocking, reasonable people'.

The offence is concerned, he said, with 'recognized minimum standards of decency, which are likely to vary from time to time'. And he opined that juries should be invited to remember that they lived in a 'plural society, with a tradition of tolerance towards minorities, and that this atmosphere of tolerance is itself part of public decency'.

The Law Commission (1974) recommended the abolition of both conspiracy offences, as well as the general offences of corrupting public morals and outraging public decency. It recommended the filling in of various lacunae this would leave with new statutory offences. These recommendations were not implemented. Indeed, the Criminal Law Act 1977 (s. 5(3)) expressly preserved both conspiracy offences referred to in this section (Smith 1977).

The history of the law in the area of sexual deviance thus presents a picture of an emergent statutory code swamping earlier ecclesiastical jurisdiction and powers cherished by the judges. But the common law lives on and ecclesiastical jurisdiction disappeared as recently as 1963, although it had long fallen into desuetude.

THE OFFENCES

Bigamy

Bigamy was in earlier times exclusively an ecclesiastical offence. Only in 1603 did it become a felony. The 1603 statute recited that men had been committing bigamy 'to the great dishonour of God, and utter undoing of divers honest men's children'. The traditional rationale of the crime is well stated by Chief Justice Cockburn in *R.* v. *Allen* ([1872] L.R. 1 C.C.R. 367): 'it involves an outrage on public decency and morals, and creates a public scandal by the prostitution of a solemn ceremony, which the law allows to be applied only to a legitimate union, to a marriage at best but colourable and fictitious, and which may be made and too often is made, the means of the most cruel and wicked deception'.

The offence is committed by anyone who being married marries some other person during the life of the first spouse. It does not matter where the second marriage takes place. The maximum sentence for this is seven years' imprisonment. Glanville Williams (1945) has described bigamy as 'the only surviving offence . . . based on word-fetishism'. He argues that 'the only anti-social consequences that are necessarily involved in the mere celebration of a bigamous marriage are (1) the falsification of the State records, and (2) the waste of time of the Minister of Religion or Registrar'. He concludes that it 'does not make sense except on the supposition that the marriage ceremony is a magic form of words that has to be protected from profanation at almost any cost in human suffering'. The situation is the more striking in that no criminal offence is committed in deserting a spouse or committing adultery. But by making the position more regular the bigamist brings into potentiality the full opprobrium of the criminal law.

However, it is probable that few bigamists are detected. It is relatively easy in a country which shuns identity cards to disappear, and it is equally simple to effect a change of name. And there is a reluctance to prosecute, particularly where the second 'spouse' has not been deceived (Wilcox 1972). But of 91 offences known to the police in 1993, 87 were cleared up.

The English law of bigamy has in recent years had to contend with the problem of immigrants whose own personal law permits polygamy. In the case of *R.* v. *Sagoo* ([1975] 2 All E.R. 926) the Court of Appeal held that, where a potentially polygamous marriage has been converted (in this case both by legislation and a change of domicile) into a monogamous marriage, it prevents a man from contracting a valid union in this country and exposes him to a charge of bigamy. Many Muslims, however, remain domiciled in their own country of origin notwithstanding lengthy sojourns in England. A marriage contracted in England by such a person would be void, but it is probable that the second marriage would not be bigamous (Pearl 1976). It seems that the assumption of a Pakistani domicile of choice, together with conversion to Islam by an Englishman would be sufficient to entitle him to marry in Pakistan a second 'wife' while still married to his first wife (*Cheni* v. *Cheni* [1965] P.85). Whether such a person commits bigamy is not settled: on principle, there seems no reason why he should.

Incest

Incest was also in earlier times exclusively (except for a short period from 1650 to 1660) an ecclesiastical offence. It was not made a criminal offence until the Punishment of Incest Act 1908 (Bailey and Blackburn 1979). Stephen (1883) explains this in terms of the existence of ecclesiastical jurisdiction. But there is no evidence that the laity were being punished for such moral offences in the second half of the 19th century. So, as James (1964) has suggested, 'this leaves open an interesting legal and sociological consideration as the incidents and legal control of incest between 1876 (the date of *Phillimore* v. *Machon*, referred to above), if not earlier, and the statute of 1908'. However, it is thought such cases were frequently prosecuted as rape or unlawful sexual intercourse. (West 1974).

In English Law, a man commits incest if he has or attempts to have sexual intercourse with a female whom he knows to be his daughter, sister, half-sister, grand-daughter or mother (Sexual Offences Act 1956 s.10). It is also an offence for a man to incite to have sexual intercourse with him a girl under 16 whom he knows to come within these categories (Criminal Law Act 1977 s.54). A woman aged 16 or over who permits a man, who stands in such a relationship to her, to have sexual intercourse with her also commits an offence (Sexual Offences Act 1956 s.11). In Scotland the law of incest was based on Leviticus xviii (Incest Act 1567) until 1986 and was punishable by death until 1887 (Sellar 1978). Blom-Cooper and Drewry (1976) report a case where a man and his daughter-in-law were prosecuted under this Act, remanded in custody for a month and then 'admonished' for 'this wretched affair'. The Incest and Related Offences (Scotland) Act 1986 limited forbidden degrees to parents and children, grandparents and grandchildren, great-grandparents and great-grandchildren, aunts and nephews, uncles and nieces. Incest by a man with a girl under 13 is punishable by up to seven years' imprisonment. Some legal systems, for example the French and Dutch, do not punish incest as such, although the conduct concerned is covered by more generalized criminal law prohibitions. There have been proposals in Scotland to replace incest with a new offence of 'sexual abuse of care'. This would cover unwelcome sexual acts other than penetration and would protect all young people in a position of trust and care within the family, including foster children (Mason 1980).

We do not know how much incest there is. Most offences are never revealed and when revealed are either ignored or not reported. A large percentage is dismissed for lack of proof and, even when proof is established, many are dropped because of the pressure and humiliation forced on the victim and family by the authorities. The incidents of incest which come to the attention of doctors or police or the courts tend to arise from situations of obvious family conflict. Where the behaviour involves adults and there is mutual consent and, hence, no victim, agencies of control are less likely to hear about it or take action. Even where cases are reported to the police, there is an almost constant ratio of nearly 2:1 between this number and the number subsequently convicted. There were 484 reported cases in 1993, and a high clear-up rate of 93 per cent. The laws of evidence require the victim's statements to be corroborated, and there is considerable discretion exercised by the police, and the Director of Public Prosecutions to whom all cases must be referred, in instituting proceedings (Manchester 1977). Some cases may also be dealt with informally by doctors, social workers, or the police. Flexibility is important for penal measures and, indeed, prosecution is sometimes inappropriate, as where, for example, brother and sister meet for the first time in adulthood and marry. There have, however, been recent examples of prosecutions in such situations. Known cases are essentially adult. We do not know the ages of the victims, although we may surmise from the fact that over two-thirds of those convicted were men aged between 30 and 50 years that teenage daughters form a high proportion of the victims. This is borne out by Manchester's research (Manchester 1977). In Hall Williams' study (1974), the victim was the offender's own child in 53 per cent of cases: 60 per cent of the victims were in the 10–16 age group.

Sentences for incest are extremely variable and they can be most severe, although it appears that no one is receiving the statutory maximum sentence. But Thomas (1970) noted that in all cases involving parents and children sentences in the region of between four and six years' imprisonment were commonly confirmed, even where there was no question of threat or force. For examples of more lenient treatment see *R.* v. *Huchison* ([1972] 56 Cr. App. R. 307) and *R.* v. *Winch* ([1974] Crim. L.R. 487). However, West (1974) believes that the Court of Appeal is more horrified by incest than the trial courts, for the sentences which it approves are much longer than those received by the majority of incest offenders.

There is strong revulsion felt against incest. Despite this, suggestions have been made that incest should not be a specially designated criminal offence when committed between mutually consenting persons over 14 (Sexual Law Reform Society Working Party Report 1975). Card (1975) argues that 'if incest is a crime because society finds it repulsive even among consenting adults this is an insufficient reason to invade their privacy' (see also Morris and Hawkins 1970; Packer 1968.) But other reasons are put forward in favour of the retention of incest as a crime. Anthropology suggests the origin of the taboo lies in the disruption and strife which incest generates in family groupings. There is evidence that this happens, although it is taken from prosecuted cases. The taboo is very widespread although not universal (Maisch 1973). The argument that inbreeding leads to a deterioration of the stock (see Lord Normand in *Phillips' Trustees* v. *Beaton* [1938] S.C. 733, 745–6) is commonly put although is difficult to prove. Allen (1969) has stated: 'studies of the offspring of incestuous unions among those of normal intelligence are probably impossible since they do not occur with any frequency' (see also Aberle 1963). But there are findings which suggest a high risk of mental retardation (Carter 1967; Adams and Neel 1967; Seemanova 1971) and it is thought that the offspring of incestuous unions have a greater mortality and morbidity than the average. Further, Lukianowicz (1972) found a 4 per cent incidence of paternal incest among an unselected group of female psychiatric patients. Weinberg (1963) suggests that most victims of father–daughter incest settle later to a normal heterosexual life, but this has now been doubted.

The disruptive effect of a prosecuted incest on the family is not in doubt. Homes and marriages are broken up. The offender's chances of parole are adversely affected (Williams 1974). His chances of being divorced are high. Even if the home is kept together the social service departments may think it necessary to remove children from the home of a convicted incest offender. The repercussions of incest are thus manifold.

Adultery

Adultery in English law connotes voluntary or consensual sexual intercourse between a married person and a person (whether married or unmarried) of the opposite sex not being the other's spouse (Cretney and Masson 1990). This definition has been criticised as 'legalistic' (Freeman 1971). Acts which do not constitute adultery in England have been held to do so in other systems. In New York sodomy has been held to constitute adultery (Ploscowe *et al.* 1972). In New Zealand an attempt by a father to have sexual intercourse with his 9-year-old daughter was held to constitute adultery. He had failed to achieve penetration but had deposited sperm around her vaginal opening (*A* v. *A* [1943]). In England sexual familiarity or masturbation is not adultery. Insemination with the semen of a third party donor (A.I.D.) is probably not adultery according to English law. It is in Canada (*Orford* v. *Orford* (1921) 58 D. L. R. 251), though it has been held not to be in Scotland (*MacLennan* v. *MacLennan* [1958] S. Cl. 105).

It seems the public is equally bemused as to what constitutes adultery. In *Barnacle* v. *Barnacle* in 1948 ([1948] P.257), it transpired that one petitioner thought adultery involved illicit connection between two unmarried persons with the consequent production of a child. Others had thought that it was not adultery 'during the day-time', or it was 'drinking with men in public houses': yet another averred that it was not adultery if the woman was 'over 50' (Megarry 1955). Lawson in 1988 found there was still uncertainty about what adultery meant (1988, ch. 1).

What is not in doubt is that adultery is quite common. Thus Kinsey *et al.* found that 26 per cent of his sample of married women had had extramarital coitus by the age of 40. He estimated that 50 per cent of married men had committed adultery by that age (Kinsey *et al.* 1948). De Wolf (1970) claims that 63 per cent of all husbands and 29 per cent of all wives have had an 'affair'. Johnson, on the other hand, reports that of those he interviewed only 24 per cent of men and 13 per cent of women had extramarital coitus (Johnson 1970). To an extent adultery is acceptable. There is a double standard involved here. As Kinsey *et al.* (1953) put it 'most societies recognise the necessity for accepting some extramarital coitus as an escape valve for the male, to relieve him from the pressures put on him by society's insistence on stable marital relationships. These same societies, however, less often permit it for the female'. Even then it may be 'covertly condoned if it is not too flagrant and if the husband is not particularly disturbed'. Gorer's studies of English life (1955, 1971) confirm this duality of standards. In his 1971 study he found that 22 per cent of his respondents disapproved of casual adultery in a man and 23 per cent disapproved of it in a woman. But men disapproved of women committing adultery more than they censured men (17 per cent and 27 per cent) and women also disapproved of female adultery more (18 per cent and 27 per cent). Confronted by serious adultery 29 per cent would 'talk it over with the spouse' and 24 per cent would 'analyse the situation'. Only 15 per cent advocated immediate separation and 7 per cent immediate divorce. Five per cent, on the other hand, believed in using physical violence on the spouse and another 2 per cent on the intervener.

Adultery is not a crime in England. It was at one time an ecclesiastical offence and was a capital crime in the period of the Commonwealth. Whether there were any convictions under the Commonwealth Act of 1650 seem doubtful (Megarry 1973). Ecclesiastical courts, however, certainly punished adulterers.

There are records of a series of indictments and in at least one case a sentence is recorded, namely, that the male adulterer should be carted (Cleveland 1913). As recently as 1959, the Archbishop of Canterbury suggested that adultery could become 'such a public menace' as to necessitate it becoming a crime. Attempts were made in the late 18th and early 19th centuries to make it impossible for the *female* adulterer to marry her 'seducer'. Bills passed the Lords (but failed in the Commons) in 1771, 1779, and 1800.

In the United States, adultery is still a crime in most states. Only in five is it not a crime. But, where once the death penalty was imposed (see *Commonwealth* v. *Call*, 38 Mass. (21 Pick) 509 (1839), today penalties range from a 10 dollar fine in Rhode Island to three years' imprisonment in Arizona. In most states adultery is rarely prosecuted. Thus, in New York between June 1959 and June 1960 there were 1700 divorce cases based on adultery (at that time the only ground), but no adultery prosecutions. But in some areas, such as Boston, prosecutions have been more frequent (Ploscowe 1962). In *Kraus* v. *Village of Barrington Hills* (571 F. Supp. 538 (1982)) the principle was upheld that the 'State may make adultery a criminal act without violating the constitutional rights of adulterers' and in *Commonwealth* v. *Stowell*. (499 N.E. 2d.357(1983)) the defendant argued unsuccessfully that the adultery statute violated the constitutional right of privacy (the police had spied on the couple in the back of a van). Other countries have also regarded adultery as a crime; Sweden did until 1937 and Yugoslavia until 1945. In France, only a wife can commit the crime of adultery, though, if convicted, her sentence, which could be two years, is remitted if her husband agrees to take her back (French Penal Code Arts 336–7). A husband who keeps a mistress at the matrimonial home also commits an offence but not one punishable by imprisonment (Art. 339).

This dual standard is common. It is found in countries influenced by Roman law. It is found also in Jewish law, under which a husband is obliged to divorce an adulterous wife, although this is not the case where he is the adulterer (Naamani 1963). It was also reflected in English law until 1923 (McGregor 1957): while a husband could divorce his wife on the ground of her adultery *simpliciter*, she had to prove aggravated adultery, for example, adultery accompanied by incest or bigamy. A double standard was found in the law of Kentucky until recently. There was an eloquent defence of the distinction by the English Lord Chancellor (Lord Thurlow) in 1779: adultery by a wife, he averred, 'not only subverts domestic tranquillity, but has a tendency, by contaminating the blood of illustrious families, to affect the welfare of the nation in its nearest interests'. Crozier (1935) argues that 'it is not immorality which is punished but theft. As the act of the wife, adultery is a revolt against the husband's property rights'. Neither argument is persuasive today.

English law then does not punish adultery as a crime. Indeed, since 1970 it has even been impossible to procure damages for adultery. It does, however, in common with most systems, permit the 'wronged' spouse to use the act of adultery as a vehicle for securing matrimonial relief. The standard of proof is high, although in most contested cases the court will have to infer adultery from circumstantial evidence. Once it was enough to prove adultery but, since the Divorce Reform Act 1969 came into operation in 1971, it has been necessary to prove additionally that one finds it intolerable to live with the respondent. However, the petitioner need not prove that cohabitation is intolerable as a result of the adultery, for the Court of Appeal, wrongly it is submitted (Freeman 1972), has held that the adultery and intolerability limbs must be construed disjunctively (*Cleary* v. *Cleary* [1974] 1 W.L.R. 73, *Carr* v. *Carr* [1974] 1 W.L.R. 449). There is only one ground of divorce in England: that the marriage has irretrievably broken down. Proof of adultery plus intolerability, however, raises a strong presumption of irretrievable breakdown. Some systems, such as in California, do not specify individual grounds or facts such as adultery but require proof generally of irreparable breakdown. English law recognized adultery as the only ground until 1937. Now there are five facts which may be relied upon; these include separation periods, but adultery is still the most popular fact relied on. Husbands still rely on their wives' adultery to a much greater extent than any of the other facts. 41.8 per cent of husbands' petitions are based on adultery, whereas only 23.2 per cent of wives' petitions are similarly based (Lord Chancellor's Office 1993). Whether this reflects less adultery by husbands, or their lower threshold of tolerance, cannot be determined.

Fornication

Fornication (or incontinence) was yet another offence that formerly fell within the jurisdiction of the ecclesiastical courts. In England today it is not in itself a criminal offence, although it may in certain circumstances amount to some specific crime such as indecent assault or procuration. Again, as with adultery and incest, it was a crime under the Commonwealth. Blackstone (1765), referring to this, states that 'when the ruling power found it for their interest to put on the semblance of a very extraordinary strictness and purity of morals', it made the commission of fornication on a second conviction a felony without benefit of clergy.

It was also a crime under a statute of Elizabeth I to have a bastard child. Both the mother and reputed father were punishable. A statute of James I provided for her committal to a House of Correction. The offence was only punishable if the child became chargeable to the parish.

In the United States fornication is still a crime in some of the states. As with adultery, the penalties vary from nominal to severe. However, the offence is rarely prosecuted.

Rape

Of all behaviour which exhibits sexual deviation, rape is the one which currently excites most interest. The interest is world-wide (Fargier 1976; Solat 1977) and the literature voluminous. Of the many collections of materials on the subject, perhaps the best, and certainly the most representative, is that by Chappell and Geis (1977). Rape has become a rallying subject for the women's movement and much of the literature is accordingly feminist in orientation (see Griffin 1971); Medea and Thomson 1974; Brownmiller 1975; Reynolds 1974; Schwendinger 1974; Weis and Borges 1973; Toner 1977; Estrich 1989). This is certainly one of the main reasons for the dramatic shift in emphasis in recent materials. Where once they were 'largely concerned with the difficulties of protecting a man accused of rape from a spurious or vindictive charge', now they 'emphasize the problems involved in protecting raped females from what is seen as particularly odious behaviour on the part of components of the criminal justice system' (Chappell *et al.* 1974). In England, attention was focused on rape by the decision in *D.P.P.* v. *Morgan* ([1975] 61 Cr. App. R. 136). This held that a man could not be convicted of rape if he in fact believed the woman consented, even if he had no reasonable grounds for so believing. This decision engendered widespread concern, although it is perfectly consistent with existing English criminal law principles (Smith 1975; Williams 1975). *D.P.P.* v. *Morgan* led to a Home Office enquiry (Heilbron Report 1975) and ultimately to legislation, but on the issue of the substantive elements of the offence, this merely confirmed what the House of Lords had said (see Sexual Offences (Amendment) Act 1976).

Rape has been understood to 'consist in intentionally having sexual intercourse with a woman who does not consent, knowing that she does not consent or being reckless whether she consents or not' (Smith 1976). Until recently it was thought that rape, by definition, could not exist within marriage, although it was accepted that the behaviour itself—forced intercourse—was functionally equivalent to a comparable behaviour committed outside the bounds of marriage and given the official label of rape. In *R.* v. *Reid* ([1972] 2 All E.R. 1350), Cairns L.J. expressed the opinion that 'the notion that a husband can, without incurring punishment, treat his wife . . . with any kind of hostile force is obsolete'. He held that the crime of kidnapping and rape are not *in pari materia*, but Cairns L.J's dictum was wide enough to cast doubts on the propriety of exempting husbands from prosecution for rapes upon their wives. The law rested on a fiction and was clearly inconsistent with civil law principles: a wife, for example, is not bound to submit to inordinate or unreasonable remands by her husband (*Holborn* v. *Holborn* [1947] 1 All E.R. 32) and she may refuse intercourse if he is suffering from a venereal disease (*Foster* v. *Foster* [1921] P. 438). The immunity was repudiated in a large number of countries. An attempt to abolish the exemption by legislation failed in England in 1976. But in 1991 The House of Lords decided that 'in modern times the supposed marital exemption in rape forms no part of the law of England' (*R.* v. *R.* [1991] 3 W.L.R. 767). The highest court described marriage as 'partnership of equals, and no longer one in which the wife must be the subservient chattel of the husband'. And of Hale's dictum that 'by their mutual matrimonial consent and contract the wife hath given up herself in this kind to her husband which she cannot retract', the House of Lords responded: 'In modern times any reasonable person must regard that conception as quite unacceptable'. This conclusion is accepted by the Law Commission (1992) and was encoded in legislation in 1994 (Criminal Justice and Public Order Act s. 142).

Rape as an offence has been hitherto limited in that it can only be committed by a male upon a female. 'In reality', as McCaghy (1976) notes, 'despite the daydreams of many men, females rarely force sexual intercourse on males'. The rape of males by males is, however, not so unusual. It is also vastly under-reported. Both Genet (1951) and T. E. Lawrence (1935) describe personal incidents, and prison rapes are known to be common (Brownmiller 1975): indeed, one former prisoner who alleged he was twice raped by a cellmate is currently suing the Home Office for negligence (*The Times* 12 July 1994). Davis's study (1973) of Philadelphia prisons found that 'virtually every slightly built young man committed by the courts is sexually approached within a day or two after his admission to prison. Many of these young men are repeatedly raped by gangs of inmates'. If we search for reasons why such acts have not been regarded by the law as rape we find three.

There is, first, the historical argument and the supposed novelty of homosexual rape. Secondly, there is, what one may call, a structural argument. Rape has been defined to require penetration of a vagina by a penis. According to Brownmiller (1975) 'one inch is the usual standard'. Oral and rectal insertions, whether they be male or female, have not, therefore, been perceived as 'rape'. And thirdly, the legal approach to rape categorizes its motivation as sexual. But much rape is not sexual at all. Eldridge Cleaver in *Soul on ice* (1968) describes his rapes of white women as 'insurrectionary'. 'It delighted me that I was defying and trampling upon the white man's law, upon his system of values, and that I was defiling his women.'

However, in 1994 English law was radically reformed to recognize for the first time male rape. The Criminal Justice and Public Order Act of 1994 will extend the law of rape to include all acts of non-consensual intercourse, whether anal or vaginal, against men and women. Male rape victims will get the same treatment in courts as female victims, with their identity and address kept secret. The maximum sentence becomes life imprisonment.

The Schwendingers (1974) argue: 'it should be kept in mind that the rapist's motives involve feelings of domination, regardless of whether the "victim" is a man or woman. Rape is a power trip—an act of aggression and an act of contempt—and in most cases is only secondarily sexual'. Much homosexual rape, then, is not overtly sexual, although some of it clearly is. Davis (1973) did not find homosexual rape in prison to be primarily motivated by the need for sexual release: 'autoerotic masturbation to orgasm being much easier and more normal'. The greatest proportion of assaults in his study involved blacks attacking whites. 'A primary goal of the sexual aggressor . . . is the conquest and degradation of his victim . . . Sexual assaults . . . are expressions of anger and aggression prompted by the same basic frustrations . . . summarised as an inability to achieve masculine identification and pride through avenues other than sex.' Feminist writers generalize this assertion. To them the act of rape is a cameo of male–female relationships, forcible penetration being at one end of the spectrum of male sexual dominance (Greenwood and Young 1975). 'It is the final expression in a series of indignities and prejudices heaped on women' (Melani and Folaski 1974), 'a form of mass terrorism' (Griffin 1971). In other words, they see rape as representing conflict, the supreme act of domination.

The other critical element of the offence of rape is the absence of woman's consent. The test is not 'was it against the woman's will?' but 'was it without her consent?' So the prosecution does not have to prove positive dissent: it is enough that she did not assent (Smith and Hogan 1973). It is not rape if she consents even if her will is weakened, unless fraud or threats are used to that end (*R. v. Lang* [1976] Crim. L. R. 65). Seduction is not rape: 'the seducer may resort to various devices in order to obtain the consent of his victim—soft lights, sweet music, flattery, and drink' (Smith 1976). An apparent consent arising from a fundamental error, induced by fraud, is no consent: thus it is rape where a man induces a woman to have sexual intercourse with him by impersonating her husband, or where he deceives her as to the nature of the transaction. Thus, the choir master of a Presbyterian church, who had intercourse with a 16-year-old pupil under the pretence that it was a surgical operation which would improve her voice, was convicted of rape (*R. v. Williams* [1923] 1 K. B. 340). 'She was persuaded to consent to what he did because she thought it was not sexual intercourse and because she thought it was a surgical operation' (*per* Lord Hewart C. J.).

The question of consent will often turn on conflicting testimony and the question then becomes one of whom to believe. Thus, a jury's concept of 'consent' is likely to be based on its interpretation of the moral character. Kalven and Zeisel (1966) note in their monumental study *The American Jury* that 'the jury . . . does not limit itself [to the law]: it goes on to weigh the woman's conduct in the prior history of the affair. It . . . scrutinizes the female complainant and is moved to be lenient with the defendant whenever there are suggestions of contributory behaviour on her part'. Leaving aside cases where there was extrinsic violence, or where the victim and defendant were total strangers, as well as group rapes, they found that, whereas judges would have convicted 22 out of 42 cases, the jury convicted in only 3. But, as Brownmiller (1975) argues, 'while most rational people might be able to agree on what constitutes rash, reckless, or precipitant behaviour leading to a homicide, in rape the parameters are indistinct and movable'. The US National Commission on the Causes and Prevention of Violence (1969) found less victim precipitation in rape than other crimes of violence (4.4 per cent, as against 22 per cent in homicide and 10.7 per cent in armed robbery). Brownmiller quotes the case of a girl on a 'date' confronted with 'if you don't let me, I'll put it in your mouth'. She gave in and then his two friends took their turn. 'I wasn't screaming or fighting any more. I just wanted to get it over with and not have anything worse happen to me', she said. Was she raped? It is certainly arguable that, according to legal definitions, she consented to sexual intercourse taking place. A study of 80 rape victims found their primary reaction to be fear (Burgess and Holmstrom 1973). They later documented what they called a 'rape trauma syndrome' (Burgess and Holmstrom 1974). 'A quid pro quo—rape in exchange for life, or rape in exchange for a good-faith guarantee against hurtful or disfiguring physical damage—dominates the female mentality in rape' (Brownmiller 1975). Nor do potential victims behave rationally under stress: 'all I could think of was my new dress' . . . I kept saying over and over "Don't rip my nylon stockings"' (quoted in Brownmiller 1975). In this light, consent is an artificial concept. The law is crude and glosses over dimensions of the female psyche.

Some of these difficulties are reflected in the statistics. Thus, of 4631 offences reported as known to the police in England and Wales in 1993 (over four times as many as in 1981) 74 per cent were cleared up. The maximum sentence is life imprisonment, although since 1986 (*R. v. Billam* (1986) 82 Cr. App. R. 347) the normal starting point has been set at five years' or, if one of certain *aggravating* features are present, at eight years imprisonment. Court of Appeal decisions on rape suggest that it will not generally be appropriate for a court—even where a mitigating factor is present—to impose a sentence of less than three years (*R. v. Roberts* (1982) 4 Cr. App. R. (S) 6) 'Wholly exceptional circumstances' are necessary to justify such a low sentence (*R. v. Bigby, The Times*, October 14, 1993). There are some *mitigating* factors. A plea of guilty is one: the young age of the offender another. In *Billam* the court accepted that the sentence might be mitigated where the victim 'has behaved in a manner which was calculated to lead the defendant to believe that she would consent to sexual intercourse'. A prior intimate relationship is also a ground of mitigation, though it is less powerful (in *R.* v. *Thornton* (1990) 12 Cr. App. R (S) 1 a mitigation of some six months was allowed). Robertshaw (1994) has found that sentences are lower than might have been expected. Both non-custodial sentences and sentences of less than three years occur, the latter not at all infrequently. The occasional sentence provokes critical comment. Thus, when a man who raped a student hitch-hiker was given a suspended sentence by Mr Justice Melford Stevenson (known as one of the severest of judges at the time), the Press was very critical. But the judge opined, for what it is worth, that it was, 'as rape goes, a pretty anaemic affair. The man had made a fool of himself but the girl was almost equally stupid'. An MP commented that perhaps he would like to have handed down a sentence for the grievous crime of hitch-hiking! (Philip Whitehead MP, H.C. vol. 905, col 822). Another recent case, which provoked angry press and backbench comment, was that of the self-confessed, double rapist who assaulted women at knife point and whom Judge Christmas Humphreys saw no reason to send to prison. Fifty-four per cent of the victims in the cases tried, on the other hand, had to go through the ordeal of seeing their names and other details printed in the Press (Soothill and Jack 1975). This latter practice has now been proscribed by the Sexual Offences (Amendment) Act 1976: anonymity will now be preserved in nearly all cases. The injustice of denying anonymity to rape defendants (Mairs 1975) was recognized by the same Act, although defendants to other charges are not protected.

The women, it is often said, are made to feel that it is they who are on trial. Brownmiller (1975) quotes one victim as saying: 'I don't understand it. It was like I was the defendant and he was the plaintiff. I wasn't on trial. I don't see where I did anything wrong. I screamed. I struggled. How could they have decided that he was innocent, that I didn't resist'. The tendency in trials is to scrutinize the victim's past sexual history. The theory is that this is suggestive of whether she is likely to have consented. It is said to reflect on her credibility, even her predisposition to tell the truth. Women are made to feel their own moral character is on trial (Berger 1977). In English law it has been long recognized that evidence may be adduced as to the victim's 'notorious bad character' (*R.* v. *Cockcroft* (1870) 11 Cox 410). As far as cross-examination as to the victim's relationship with other men is concerned, the law has been that she might be asked questions about her previous sexual activities, but if she denied their existence evidence could not be called to rebut what she said (*R.* v. *Holmes* (1871) LR 1 CCR 334). But, as Heilbron (1975) conceded, 'the difficulty in practice [was] that her denials may not be believed by the jury, and they may react adversely to her demeanour which may possibly be caused by the shock and dismay of this line of questioning'. Heilbron recommended 'that [such] questions ought not to be asked, no evidence admitted, except with the leave of the trial judge on application made to him in the absence of the jury'. A total ban was, therefore, not advocated as situations were foreseen (for example, where the victim was a prostitute) where such evidence would be relevant. This recommendation has now been implemented by the Sexual Offences (Amendment) Act 1976.

The trial, however, is only the culmination of a process that begins with the decision to report the rape. Women claim that their complaints are met by insensitive, often hostile policemen. Police manuals have tended to warn that rape is one of the most falsely reported crimes (Payton 1966). The consequences of such a warning are alarming. 'The tragedy for the rape victim is that the police officer is the person who validates her victimization' (Brownmiller 1975). But if the police believe that complainants are 'prostitutes who didn't get their money' (quoted in Brownmiller 1975). women can hardly expect a sympathetic response. A study in the *University of Pennsylvania Law Review* (1968) showed that the police declared one-fifth of complaints to be unfounded. Rapes reported promptly, and cases involving strangers, weapons, and violence stood the highest chance of being validated. Rapes in cars were considered dubious and where the man was a 'date' every instance in a car was held to be false. The police were more ready to believe a complainant who screamed than one who silently struggled. The veracity of black women and women who had been drinking was frequently doubted.

In addition to police interrogation, there will be further questioning by a police surgeon, and an intimate gynaecological examination. Apparently, the facilities for such examinations are sometimes inadequate and unsuitable (Heilbron 1975). Against this background it is not surprising that only one-fifth of rape incidents are reported to the police. In spite of Hale's 'old saw' (Le Grand 1973), women do not find it 'an accusation easily to be made'. But this myth persists. As do others: that women need to be raped (Gebhard 1965), or deserve to be raped (Kanin 1967; Amir 1971), or even want to be raped (Russell 1973). Yet the statistics suggest the number of rapes is rising, that half of the victims are raped by acquaintances, and that a larger proportion of reported rapes involve more than one offender (Geis and Chappell 1971). The 'gang-bang' rape may well be the pattern for the future.

Indecent assault on a woman

Under the Sexual Offences Act 1956 as amended by the Sexual Offences Act 1985, it is an offence punishable with 10 years imprisonment to commit an indecent assault on a woman (s. 14). 'Assault' means assault or battery. If there is touching, it is not necessary to prove that the victim was aware of the assault or the circumstances of the indecency. But if there is no touching then to constitute an indecent assault, the victim must be shown to have been aware of the assault and of the circumstances of indecency (*R.* v. *Court* [1987] 1 All E.R. 120, 122). Generally, consent is a defence, but neither persons under 16 years of age nor defectives can give any consent. Consent is not a defence where it is exacted by force, or fraud as to the nature of the transaction, nor is it where the probable consequence of the assault is the infliction of bodily harm. (*R.* v. *Donovan* [1934] 2 K. B. 498). It was formerly the law that boys under 14 could not be convicted of rape (*R.* v. *Groombridge* (1836) 7 C & P 582), although they could be convicted of indecent assault on evidence that they did in fact have intercourse (*R.* v. *Waite* [1892] 2 Q.B. 600). However, indecent assault is an aggravated assault and, accordingly, requires an attempt to apply force of some kind to another person. There must be an act done to the person of the defendant, as distinct from an accepted invitation to do something to the person of the accused. So in *Fairclough* v. *Whipp* ([1951] 2 All E.R. 834), the accused was acquitted where he invited a 9-year-old girl to touch his exposed penis. However, a new offence has been created by the Indecency with Children Act 1960: committing an act of gross indecency with or towards a child *under the age of 14 years*, or inciting a child under that age to such an act with him or another (for example, another child), is punishable by two years' imprisonment. A man who allowed a girl aged 8 to touch his penis for five minutes was recently convicted, the court holding that inactivity could amount to an invitation to the child to do the act (*R.* v. *Speck* (1977) Crim. L.R. 689). The law as stated in *Fairclough* v. *Whipp* is still applicable so far as persons over 14 are concerned.

The meaning of 'indecent' has also caused problems. It has been held that an act decent in itself but committed for the purpose of sexual gratification, does not in itself amount to an indecent assault. For example, George (*R.* v. *George* [1956] Crim. L. R. 52) had attempted to remove girls' shoes from their feet because it gave him sexual gratification. In *R.* v. *Thomas* ([1985] 81 Cr. App. Rep. 331) it was held that touching the bottom of a girl's skirt was not indecent, even though the defendant may have had an indecent purpose. Where the manner or the external circumstances of an assault are ambiguous, the assault is indecent only if the offender has an indecent purpose. In *Court*, a shop assistant put a 12-year-old girl who was in the shop across his knee and spanked her on her bottom over her shorts. When asked why he did it, he said 'buttock fetish'. This question was held to be admissible in evidence because, it was said, the act was ambiguous and it was necessary to prove an indecent intention. Had he taken her shorts down, the question whether his intention was indecent would not have been an issue. Thus, an indecent motive cannot convert an objectively decent act into an indecent assault. A decent motive, however, may justify what would otherwise be an indecent act. Medical examinations are, therefore, not indecent assaults, irrespective of consent. In the Supreme Court of Canada, there was held to be no assault where a doctor obtained a patient's consent to his friend's presence at her vaginal examination by falsely pretending he was a medical student. The court said the fraud did not go to the nature and quality of what was done (*R.* v. *Bolduc* and *Bird* [1967] 63 DLR (2d) 82). English principles suggest he would have been convicted in this country.

The number of cases reported to the police has increased sharply. In 1993 there were 17 378, up by 50 per cent in 10 years. In 1993 56 per cent of the 31 380 'known' indictable sex offences involved indecent assault on a female. The clear-up rate has risen to 69 per cent. Fewer than one-third were proceeded against and of these some 600 men only were sent to prison. Some, notably the Sexual Law Reform Society (1975), would like to see the offence abolished as a separate offence. It advocates charges relating to sexual assaults being dealt with as common assaults or assaults occasioning actual bodily harm, as appropriate. The maximum sentence for assaults occasioning actual bodily harm is five years' imprisonment. But most indecent assaults will only be common assaults, on this criterion, and attract a maximum of one year's imprisonment.

Unlawful sexual intercourse

This offence is known as 'statutory rape' in the United States. There, ages of consent range from the ludicrously low (it was 7 in Delaware until 1973), to ages well above that provided by English law (for example, it is 21 in Tennessee). According to English law, a man may not have intercourse with a girl under 16 years of age (s. 6 of Sexual Offences Act 1956). If she is under 13 years of age, the offence is punishable with life imprisonment (s. 5). The girl cannot, by law, consent. Belief that the girl is over 13 years old, no matter how reasonable it may be, is no defence to a charge (s. 5): belief that the girl is over 16 years old is a defence to a charge (s. 6) only if it is reasonable, and held by a man under 24 who has not previously been charged with a like offence (s. 6(3)). The offence dates from 1885. It was tied then, as it is now, to the minimum age of marriage. Intercourse with a girl under 16 will not be unlawful where she is validly married under her personal law (*Mohamed* v. *Knott* [1969] 1 Q.B. 1.), nor where the man reasonably believes that the girl, who is under age, is his wife (s. 6(2) of S.O.A. 1956).

Under s. 6, 1448 offences were recorded as known to the police in 1993 (a decline of more than 50 per cent in 10 years and of 7.4 per cent since 1992): 269 offences under s. 5 were also recorded (a 38 per cent increase from 1981). The clear-up rate for both offences is high (90 and 93 per cent, respectively). Statistics do not now reveal how many men went to prison for unlawful sexual intercourse with girls under 16 years of age, but the sentences are stiffer where the girl is under 13. This crime is one which is never long out of Press comment. There is a regular crop of notorious prosecutions, usually involving a man little older than the girl, and judgements tend to be humane. One case that attracted attention concerned a man of 22 years of age who had intercourse with a 15-year-old girl. The judge, Judge McKinnon QC, said of the girl: 'she has no complaints at all; it was a thoroughly satisfactory experience so far as she is concerned'. The judge was strongly critical of the law. Indeed, he went on television to say so. 'How on earth any society can delude itself into thinking that this sort of law can have any sort of success baffles me', he commented. The defendant was conditionally discharged for 12 months (*The Times* 23 June 1976). The case sparked off a debate about whether the age of consent should be lowered. Whatever age the law selects must necessarily be arbitrary for physical and mental maturation vary so much. Any change would be resisted by powerful lobbies. What is therefore to be preferred is retention of the existing age with a flexible approach to invocation of the law. The police should be encouraged to caution rather than prosecute, and sentencers should exercise their powers flexibly, taking account of the circumstances of the individual case. This has been recognized by the Court of Appeal in the case of *R.* v. *Taylor* ([1977] 3 All E.R. 527): Lawton L.J. said that the offence covered a wide spectrum of guilt and accordingly the penalties appropriate to the offence will vary in different cases. The court confirmed short prison sentences on adult men who had used the village whore aged 14. The law, said Lawton L.J., 'exists for the protection of girls', and was particularly necessary in the case of 'wanton girls'.

Many cases of 'unlawful sexual intercourse' are paradigm examples of 'crimes without victims'. In this light, the comment of Skolnick and Woodworth (1968), although generally applicable, is particularly apposite. 'It does not matter very much if criminal law forbids various erotic activities, so long as it is impossible to see through walls. When such vision becomes possible, however, the totalitarian potential is enormous because . . . the surveillance potential of those performing police functions will be extraordinary.' They found that in one town on the west coast of the United States, the greatest single source of information in statutory rape cases was the family support division of the prosecutor's office: the adolescent girl applying for maternity assistance was sent as a matter of routine to the police, who urged her in the strongest terms to present a complaint. The impact of the cybernetic revolution on an area of law like statutory rape is thus profound. Furthermore, it means that crimes like statutory rape are punished mainly among the poorer sections of the community; their actions surface to visibility on applications for welfare benefits.

Sexual murder

English law, in common with every other system of law, proscribes murder and it does not distinguish between different motivational causes. Nor, so far as is known, does any other system. Many notorious murderers have been sexual murderers. Christie was a necrophiliac and Sutcliffe ('The Yorkshire Ripper') stabbed genitals and breasts and targeted prostitutes. It seems that neither rape nor sexual assault is necessary to make a murder 'sexual'. What is important is 'the eroticization of the act of killing in and for itself' (Cameron and Frazer 1987). One must distinguish between cases where killing is done for sexual pleasure, and cases where killing takes place in the course of some other crime or otherwise lawful action which has sexual motivation. The former type of case may result in prosecutions, or convictions for manslaughter, rather than murder, on the basis that the killer is suffering from diminished responsibility. This entails the existence of 'abnormality of mind' which 'substantially impairs . . . mental responsibility for acts or . . . omissions' (Homicide Act 1957 s. 2). In effect, the law recognizes that sexual drives may irresistibly impel one to murder. Whether the accused is to be so categorized is normally a matter for psychiatrists alone. If psychiatrists for both sides agree that a defendant is abnormal, a guilty plea is normally accepted and no jury trial takes place. This happens in 80 per cent of such cases, according to recent research (Dell 1984). A jury is only likely to consider psychiatric evidence where psychiatrists disagree. The Sutcliffe case is a rare exception to this. There the judge thought it was in the public's interest to have a jury trial although both sides agreed he was abnormal. The jury concluded he was not, and he was convicted of murder, not manslaughter. In *R.* v. *Byrne* ([1960] 2 Q.B. 396), the accused strangled a girl in a YMCA hostel and then committed horrifying mutilations on her body. There was evidence that Byrne had, from an early age, been subject to perverted sexual desires, and that the urge of those desires was stronger than normal sex-impulses, so that he found it difficult, if not impossible, to resist putting the desire into practice. It was suggested that this girl was killed under such an impulse. Lord Parker C.J. held that it was wrong to say that these facts did not constitute evidence which would bring Byrne within the purview of diminished responsibility. 'Abnormality of mind' included 'the ability to exercise will-power to control physical acts in accordance with . . . rational judgment'.

Examples of the latter category are murders committed in the course of rape or assault. An example is the case of *Bedder* v. *D.P.P.* ([1954] 2 All E.R. 801). Bedder was 18 years old, and sexually impotent. He attempted unsuccessfully to have sexual intercourse with a prostitute. She jeered at him and attempted to get away. When he tried to hold her, she kicked him in his genitals. He stabbed her with a knife and killed her. The House of Lords held this was murder. When considering provocation as a defence (which would reduce the crime to manslaughter), it was the effect that the prostitute's acts would have had on an ordinary person, not one invested with the physical peculiarities of Bedder, that was relevant.

A rather different illustration is the case of *R.* v. *Sharmpal Singh* ([1962] A.C. 188). He killed his wife in the course of sexual intercourse with her. She had consented to intercourse but he used excessive force and death resulted. He pressed on his wife's neck much too hard and went 'beyond the limits of the normal accompaniments of intercourse'. The Privy Council held his actions to constitute manslaughter.

Paedophilia

Paedophilia connotes sexual attraction to children or young persons by adult males. It can take a number of varieties: it can involve rape or unlawful sexual intercourse with young girls. Where adult females are involved it is known as korephilia. This is much less common. Both these offences have been separately considered; it can also cover indecent assault on children and indecency with them, again, both of these offences in relation to young girls have already been considered. Paedophilia, however, is usually understood to mean homosexual fixation on young boys. As the Sexual Offences Act 1967 excuses homosexual behaviour in private between consenting adults (the age of consent was reduced from 21 to 18 years in 1994), the main interest of the law in relation to homosexual practices lies in paedophilia.

Paedophilia has been openly championed by various organizations in the United States and Britain. In Britain the Paedophile Information Exchange was overtly concerned to justify paedophile relationships through the liberation of 'the positive [sexual] potential that resides in everyone' (O'Carroll 1980, p. 248). It is said that paedophiles rarely 'assault' children. Children are rather the willing partners of adults who are 'gentle, fond of children and benevolent' (Virkunnen 1975, p. 179). But can children give informed consent to sexual relationships with adults? The Paedophile Information Exchange responded that instead of informed consent we should assess 'willingness'. But, as Roberts put it in a review of O'Carroll (1980), girls are 'brought up from birth to please men and to repress sexual desires until marriage [so that they] are not going to find it easy to say no to a cajoling adult . . . To vocalise no is to both admit to the possibility of forbidden sexual feelings *and* to displease a powerful adult' (O'Carroll 1980, p. 48) (see also Jackson 1984; Walkerdine 1991; Evans 1993, 1994).

According to West (1974), paedophiliacs account for about 30 per cent of all homosexuals. Two types exist: (1) those fixated upon sexually immature children, and (2) those who choose physically responsive pubertal children. Power (1976) states that 'the paedophiliac is usually shy and timid and may show a wide range of psychopathological behaviours . . . Fear has prevented the development of adult heterosexuality and they tend to seek comfort and sexual gratification with children'. Curran and Parr (1957) found paedophiliacs to be older than the other homosexuals they studied and a higher proportion were married: many are middle-aged and have experienced heterosexual intercourse over long periods. They tended to isolate themselves from other homosexuals.

The traumatic effect on the child-victim has often been noted (Ferenczi 1949). Power

(1976) suggests they suffer 'permanent psychological harm and sexual maladjustment' and he lists some of the complications: but this need not happen. Children do not automatically recognize the experience as adults classify it. The child may experience a sexual assault in a totally 'non-sexual' way 'because [he] has not yet been fully socialized into the motives and feelings that adults routinely come to associate with sexuality, they are always learnt and constructed meanings' (Plummer 1975).

A number of crimes are associated with paedophiliac tendencies. These offences are better treated under the classification of homosexuality (discussed below). It may be noted here that the offences of indecent assault and indecency with children do apply equally to male and female victims.

Prostitution by females to males

In English law prostitution is not itself an offence against the law. It is, however, in the opinion of the Wolfenden Report (1975) 'a social fact deplorable in the eyes of moralists, sociologists and . . . the great majority of ordinary people'. At least as far as sociologists are concerned, the accuracy of this statement may be doubted (Davis 1937; Lemert 1967; Gagnon and Simon 1974). Davis (1976), for example, argues that prostitution is not only inevitable but necessary. Feminists challenges views like these; they contend that prostitution is merely another example of the general exploitation of women in sexist society. Thus, they argue, elimination of sexist biases will do away with prostitution (Klein 1973; Millett 1973; Feminist Group 1973). What such a thesis ignores is the phenomenon of male prostitution. Davis's arguments seem, therefore, to have greater force.

The literature on prostitution is strangely biased. It deals almost exclusively with the prostitutes. Their clients 'are fleeting shadows not only to prostitutes, but to researchers as well' (McCaghy 1976). The Kinsey studies (1948) are an exception. He documented the male client's motivations and found that, incredibly, 69 per cent of the white male population had had some experience with prostitutes.

In some countries, including the United States, prostitution is proscribed. In England, on the other hand, it is legal but positively discouraged. Thus, it is criminal to cause or encourage a woman to become a prostitute; it is an offence to keep a brothel; it is a crime to live on the earnings of prostitutes; it is, above all, a criminal offence to loiter or solicit for the purposes of prostitution. No statute, however, defines prostitution. Winick and Kinsie (1971) say it is 'the granting of non-marital, sexual access, established by mutual agreement of the woman, her client and/or her employer, for remuneration which provides part or all of her livelihood'. The definition commonly used in English law is more value-laden, and wider; it is the offering by a woman of 'her body for purposes amounting to common lewdness for payment in return' (*per* Darling J. in *R.* v. *de Munch* [1918] 1 K.B. 635). This definition was approved in *R.* v. *Webb* ([1964] 1 Q. B. 357): there a girl was employed as a masseuse and was expected, as part of her employment, to masturbate clients who so desired. In her defence, it was argued that the role of the prostitute must be passive, and active indecency of this type could not amount to prostitution. This argument was rejected: 'it cannot matter whether she whips the man or the man whips her, it cannot matter whether he masturbates himself on her or she masturbates him'. In Utah a woman has been held to be a prostitute even if she takes no reward (*Salt Lake City* v. *Allred* 430 P. 2d 317 (1967). Some of the offences connected with prostitution will now be surveyed.

It is an offence to procure a woman to become a common prostitute (s. 22. of Sexual Offences Act 1956). Procure is widely defined by the courts (see *R.* v. *Broadfoot* [1976] 3 All E.R. 753 where it was held that a woman employed for massage in a massage parlour is procured by her employer for prostitution if she is masturbating clients). The offence is not complete until the woman becomes a common prostitute. According to Wolfenden (1957) very few cases of procuration come to the notice of the police, presumably because most woman who become prostitutes do so because they want to and need no persuading (Davis 1976). Sections 33 to 36 of the 1956 Act deal with the use of premises for prostitution. Thus, it is an offence to keep or manage a brothel ('a place resorted to by persons of both sexes for the purpose of prostitution' *per* Wills J. in *Singleton* v. *Ellison* ([1895] 1 Q.B. 607); ' a nest of prostitutes' in *Donovan* v. *Gavin* ([1965] 2 Q.B. 684): there must be at least two prostitutes in the place). It is also an offence to let premises knowing they are to be used as a brothel, or to sub-let with that knowledge.

The prostitute's employer (the pimp) commits a crime in knowingly living, wholly or in part, on her earnings (Sexual Offences Act 1956 s. 30). If he lives with her or is habitually in her company or exercises control, direction, or influence over her movements, he is presumed to be knowingly so living. These methods of proof are not exhaustive and the prosecution can adduce other evidence to show that a man is living on the earnings of a prostitute (see *R.* v. *Clark* [1976] 2 All E.R. 696). This offence can only be committed by a man. The offence has caused interpretational problems (Rook and Ward 1990). For example, does the landlord who lets premises for prostitution commit an offence? It seems that he does if he charges an exorbitant rent but not otherwise. Wolfenden (1957) considered whether this ought to be an offence. It is thought not for 'as long as society tolerates the prostitute, it must permit her to carry on her business somewhere'. However, a landlord who lets premises for prostitution cannot recover the rent however reasonable, nor can he recover possession of the premises until the lease is terminated (*Alexander* v. *Rayson* [1936] 1 K.B. 169).

The one relevant offence that is directed against the prostitute herself is found in the Street Offences Act 1959 s. 1: 'it shall be an offence for a common prostitute to loiter or solicit in a street or public place for the purpose of prostitution'.

The expression 'common prostitute' is said to be at best derogatory and at worst prejudiced. It is, however, only applied to someone who has been twice formally cautioned by the police for loitering or soliciting and who has to some extent invited the label. But she has not been convicted or any offence; as such the procedure offends against the principle of equality before the law. The cautioning system is extra-statutory, and its impact is somewhat attenuated by the ease with which new aliases can be adopted and new environments sought. In a Working Paper, the Home Office (1974) suggested a power of arrest for cautioning, a power to fingerprint, and a national cautions register, although it subsequently conceded that such innovations would be far too draconian.

The word 'solicit' has not caused many problems. It is clear that the prostitute must be physically present. The offence is, therefore, not committed where she displays a card on a notice board, inviting men to visit her for the purpose of prostitution (*Weisz* v. *Monahan* [1962] 1 All E.R. 664). The owner of the notice board may be convicted of conspiring to corrupt public morals (*Shaw* v. *D.P.P.* [1962] A. C. 220) publishing an obscene article (*idem*), and, if a man, living on the earnings of a prostitute. Further, solicitation may be by acts done and it is unnecessary to prove that the prostitute used any words. In *Horton* v. *Mead* ([1913] 1 K.B. 154), a case on importuning, it was enough that he 'smiled in the faces of gentlemen, pursed his lips and wriggled his body'. And in *Behrendt* v. *Burridge* ([1976] 3 All E.R. 285), a prostitute, who sat still on a stool in a bay window in a low-cut top and mini-skirt with a red light in the window, 'might as well have had a notice saying she was available'. It was held that she was soliciting in the sense that she was tempting and alluring prospective customers. She made no gesture or other form of communication with men in the street.

The question as to whether solicitation has taken place in a street or public place has also caused problems. In *Smith* v. *Hughes* ([1960] 2 All E.R. 859) a prostitute attracted the attention of men in the street by tapping on her window pane. She was convicted of soliciting.

Other criticisms levelled at the soliciting offence are: (1) that it is differently drafted from comparable legislation controlling male importuners and there is no offence of a man importuning a woman, so that it is in effect discriminatory; and (2) that the necessity to prove annoyance or nuisance (which existed until 1959) showed a concern for the liberty of the individual which is now missing. As far as (1) is concerned, offensive propositioning of women by men for sexual intercourse could, until 1966, be prosecuted as soliciting or importuning in a public place for immoral purposes (s. 32 of Sexual Offences Act 1956). But in *Crook* v. *Edmondson* ([1966] 2 Q.B. 81) the Divisional Court ruled that heterosexual intercourse was not an immoral purpose. The police were then forced to use s. 5 of the Public Order Act 1936 (which deals with threatening, abusive, or insulting words or behaviour in a public place and was passed to deal with Mosley's 'Blackshirts'), as well as road traffic legislation on obstruction, and binding over to keep the peace, until a new offence of kerb crawling was introduced in 1985 to deal with this problem. A Home Office Report (1976*b*) argued that any re-introduction of the 'annoyance' element in soliciting would be retrograde since it would lead to the return of prostitutes to the streets, the very mischief which the Street Offences Act tried to remove. The Sexual Offences Act 1985 provides that a man commits an offence if he solicits a woman, or different women, for the purposes of prostitution from a motor vehicle while it is in a street or public place, or in a street or public place while in the immediate vicinity of a motor vehicle that he has just got out of or off, persistently or in such a manner or in such circumstances as to be likely to cause annoyance to the woman or any of the women solicited or nuisance to other persons in the neighbourhood. It also provides (in s. 2) that a man commits an offence if in a street or public place he persistently solicits a woman or different women for the purpose of prostitution.

English legislation is directed mainly against the old-fashioned street-walker and those who sponge on her. In reality, of course, the true professional has found newer, safer, and more profitable pastures. The growth of massage parlours and escort agencies, call girls, and clip-joints has assumed major importance. The law tackles none of these directly although it intervenes when, as often happens, crimes are committed as incidents of these institutions. Thus, owners of escort agencies have been convicted of living off immoral earnings.

There are some who argue for the total repeal of all laws against prostitution. The feminist movement is to the fore in the agitation for decriminalization. It finds itself in a difficult position: on the one hand, its philosophy dictates that a woman should be able to do whatever she likes with her body; on the other hand, it sees prostitution as dehumanizing and sexist. Prostitutes themselves also support decriminalization and, in the United States and France, have formed pressure groups geared towards that end. *Coyote* (Call Off Your Old Tired Ethics) is one such American organizations (Anderson 1975). In England, the Sexual Law Reform Society (1975) is also pledged to decriminalization. The law, it argues, should be based on 'annoyance, injury or nuisance to specific citizens and no person should be convicted of such annoyance without the evidence of the person aggrieved'.

There is also a rather different movement committed to regularization of prostitution. It envisages government licensing of prostitutes, statutory medical examinations, and other controls. In this country such movement is very much in its infancy, although it recalls similar movements in the 19th century. There is no evidence that regulation is successful at controlling prostitution (Sion 1977). France abolished controls in 1946, Italy in 1958 (Honoré 1978)

Homosexuality

Homosexuality, according to Plummer (1975), 'refers to sexual experience, actual or imagined, between members of the same sex, which may be accompanied by emotional involvements'. As a clinical entity it does not exist, for its forms are as varied as heterosexuality (Hooker 1957; Sagarin 1974). Discussion of homosexuality is usually found within the rhetoric of either sin or mental health—the American Psychiatric Association dropped it from its list of mental disorders as late as 1974 (see Chapters 1, 9, and 11). Gagnon and Simon (1974), who are critical of these approaches, attack the existing literature for being 'ruled by a simplistic and homogeneous view of the psychological and social contents of the category of "homosexual" ' and at the same time for concentrating of the 'least rewarding of all questions, that on etiology'. There is too much emphasis on 'homosexuality' as a condition and too little understanding of it as process (Plummer 1975). It may well be that our very sense of boundary derives from the existence of legal sanctions (Gagnon and Simon 1974).

Kinsey *et al.*'s studies (1948) demonstrate that homosexuality and heterosexuality are not polar concepts. He showed that the behaviour of many was not an either/or proposition. He found that only 4 per cent of the male white population were exclusively homosexual throughout their lives, yet 37 per cent had had at least one homosexual experience to the point of orgasm: 50 per cent had had some homosexual experience during their adult life. The figures for females were lower, respectively 2, 13, and 28 per cent in 1953. 'Legal literature commonly thinks of homosexual activity as being performed for orgastic pleasure whereas this may be insignificant . . . The mutual dependency, which is often intense, may be far more important than sexual activity' (Slovenko 1965).

The dilemma of the homosexual has been graphically described by Plummer (1975).

> Around the subject of homosexuality has emerged a vast superstructure of beliefs and imagery which help to conceal an underlying relationship by which dominant heterosexual groups tacitly but persistently oppress and attack homosexual groups. Whether this domination takes the form of being burnt at the stake as a heretic or murdered on a common by 'queer-bashers'; whether it takes the form of penitential in medieval cloisters or exclusion from employment and country; whether it takes the form of being pilloried in the market square or mimicked and mocked on television and radio; whether it takes the form of trial and imprisonment or psychiatric examination and therapy; whether it is devalued as sin, sickness, crime or simply a sorrowful state—in each and every case the structure of the relationship is politically similar; a dominant group, probably unwittingly, coerces and controls a subordinate one.

To this may be added exposure to blackmail (Gagnon and Simon 1974, suggest as many as 15 per cent of all homosexuals have been blackmailed at some time: the Dirk Bogarde film *Victim* did much to bring this evil to public attention), police harassment (Gallo *et al.* 1966), entrapment, (Szasz (1970) suggests the episode in Sodom is the earliest account of entrapment of homosexuals, the law enforcement agents being 'God's plainclothes men'), and ostracism. Homosexuals appear to be victimized with considerable frequency (Sagarin and Macnamara 1975).

Other societies have been more tolerant of homosexuality. Ford and Beach (1952) found that in 64 per cent of the 72 similar societies they studied, homosexuality was considered acceptable for some groups. Gebhard's (1956) survey of 193 world cultures showed that only 14 per cent rejected homosexuality. Yet in England and the United States the reaction has been extremely hostile. Simmons (1965) asked American respondents: 'What is deviance?' More identified homosexuals than any other stereotypical category. Gorer's English study (1971) found that over half his male respondents, and just under half his female respondents, viewed homosexuality in strong, negative terms of disapproval. Another one-third saw homosexuals as sick. Schofield (1973) found the young to be more tolerant.

The law in England no longer punishes homosexual behaviour in private between consenting adults (Sexual Offences Act 1967). Nor does it in Illinois, New York, Connecticut, or six other US states. It has not been a crime in France, Belgium, or the Scandinavian countries for some considerable time. In England, homosexuality came within the province of the ecclesiastical courts until 1533. They handed over convicted homosexuals to the civil authorities for burning, however, apparently, this rarely happened (Pollock and Maitland 1898). The 1533 Act, part of Henry VIII's campaign to assert royal supermacy over the authority of the church (Hyde 1970), imposed the death penalty for buggery (i.e., anal connection). The death penalty was removed in 1861 (the maximum sentence then became penal servitude for life). The scope of the law was extended from buggery to all homosexual practices by the Criminal Law Amendment Act 1885. The change was the result of a peripheral amendment to a bill which aimed to protect women and girls and suppress brothels. Although a major alteration in the law it was not debated. 'It is extremely doubtful if either parliament or the government of the day were aware of the substantial change they had directed in the law against homosexuality' (Robinson 1964; see also Hyde

1948). Then in 1898, the Vagrancy Act made it an offence for a male to solicit persistently in a public place for an immoral purpose. The Act was intended to prevent men from trying to obtain clients for prostitutes but it came to be widely used to stop solicitations for homosexual purposes. The equivalent Scottish Act (The Immoral Trade (Scotland) Act 1902) has not been so used (Wolfenden 1957).

The law began to be questioned in the early 1950s, and the Wolfenden committee was appointed in 1954. Its report, issued in 1957, concluded: 'we do not think it proper for the law to concern itself with what a man does in private unless it can be shown to be so contrary to the public good that the law ought to intervene in its function as the guardian of the public good'. It was another 10 years before legislation was passed to implement the proposal that the taint of criminality should be removed from homosexual acts committed in private by consenting adults (Richards 1970). 'The one determined lobby against the Bill came from the National Maritime Board and the National Union of Seamen and this was designed to exclude the Merchant Navy from its provisions' (Richards 1970). The sponsors of the Bill yielded, otherwise the whole Act could well have been lost.

Current English law is particularly complicated. One must distinguish buggery involving anal penetration and gross indecency. Buggery (or attempted buggery) with a boy under 16 years of age (or with an animal) carries a penalty of life imprisonment. Buggery with an unwilling male under 18 carries a maximum penalty of 5 years' imprisonment. Buggery with a consenting partner carries only a two-year penalty, provided that the participants are both over 21 years of age, or both under that age (subject to the exception listed below). Where one of the partners is over and the other is under 21 years of age, the older man becomes liable to five years' imprisonment.

An act of gross indecency (which is not further defined) between two consenting males is punishable by two years' imprisonment (five years if the defendant is over 18 and his partner under 18 years of age). If a male procures or attempts to procure a male under 18 years old to commit an act of gross indecency with a third party he may also be sentenced to five years' imprisonment. If the partner is a boy under 16 the maximum sentence is 10 years' imprisonment.

The Sexual Offences 1967 introduced one important exception to all this. It provided that in England and Wales, but not in Scotland or Northern Ireland, buggery and gross indecency by male couples are not offences, provided both participants are consenting civilians over 21 years of age, and provided their conduct occurs in private with no third party present. Members of the Forces were still subject to court-martial for homosexual conduct until 1994. The crews of UK merchant ships were also still exposed to the criminal sanctions listed above until 1994.

Males are also subject to criminal penalties for persistently soliciting or importuning for immoral purposes (s. 32 of Sexual Offences Act 1956 and see *R. v. Ford* (1977) Crim. L.R. 688). The maximum penalty is two years' imprisonment. The Home Office Report on Vagrancy and Street Offences (1976b) recommended the offence be retained with lower maximum penalties. In practice it means that men who loiter in the vicinity of public lavatories or 'gay' bars are liable to prosecution. It is not necessary to prove evidence of annoyance. There is no doubt that the police use decoys to secure arrests.

The law, although an improvement on the pre-1967 situation, is unsatisfactory on several counts. The law still discriminates against homosexuals (Sexual Law Reform Society Report (1975).

(i)   The age of consent is 18 years; a girl can consent to heterosexual intercourse at 16; heterosexuals can marry at 16.

(ii)   Males can solicit women with impunity (*Crook* v. *Edmondson* above) but not other men. Indeed, women can solicit men, but not if they do so in the streets for the purpose of prostitution.

(iii)   The definition of what constitutes a homosexual act 'in private' is far more narrowly drawn than in the case of heterosexual acts. Privacy requires that only two persons take part or are present (and see *R* v. *Reakes* [1974] CLY 751). Since the 1967 Act was passed the recorded incidence of the offence of indecency between males has doubled, and the number of persons prosecuted for the offence has trebled (Walmsley 1978). Nearly 1000 cases were reported to the police in 1991 and 98 per cent of the offences were cleared up.

(iv)   The penalties are still more severe than those for equivalent heterosexual offences.

(v)   It is still an offence for a third party to procure a homosexual act, even one legalized by the 1967 Act.

(vi)   Advertisements in a magazine inviting homosexual acts may amount to a conspiracy to corrupt public morals (*Knuller* v. *D. P. P.* [1973] A. C. 435).

(vii)   Although the Criminal Justice and Public Order Act 1994 s. 146 extends the liberalization of the 1967 Act to the armed forces and merchant navy, it may lead to service personnel being dismissed from the armed forces or merchant seamen being dismissed from a ship.

The effects of all this are that blackmail, for example, is still possible. Thus, a mature 16-year-old man who chooses to participate in homosexual conduct with a man aged 21 can blackmail the older man, knowing that his victim will not complain for fear of a trial and potentially heavy prison sentence. However, it is thought that blackmail is still prevalent even where the behaviour no longer constitutes a criminal offence: the threat is no longer to expose to the police but, for example, to his employers. In a society where stigma still attaches to homosexuality, such threats are very potent.

Another effect is that social workers, psychiatrists, marriage guidance counsellors, and others cannot easily provide the guidance that they might wish to give for fear of being accused of encouraging what the law still regards as a crime (Sherwin 1965). It is true that the Director of Public Prosecutions must be consulted before proceedings are taken involving a homosexual offence and a person under the age of 18. But prosecutions nevertheless take place, even where both participants are under that age. The *Criminal statistics* do not distinguish between the different offences clearly enough to draw any conclusions. For example, we no longer know how many men are sent to prison for buggery, nor attempting to commit buggery, nor for indecency between males. Such statistics were previously published: the failure to do so now creates an unfortunate knowledge gap. Sentences for deterrent purposes can be severe. (See *R.* v. *Gillespie* (1977) Crim. L. R. 429; *R.* v. *Meadows* (1977) Crim. L. R. 429). It is to be assumed that the victims of few if any of these men were consenting adults under 21 (the age of consent until the 1994 legislation): the statistics do not classify the age, sex, or willingness of the victim.

The situation in much of the United States, however, is worse. The Supreme Court has ruled in 1986 that there is no fundamental right to engage in homosexual conduct. In *Bowers* v. *Hardwick* the majority (it was a 5–4 decision) wrote: 'We register our disagreement that the Court's prior cases (of sexual privacy) have constrained the Constitution to confer a right of privacy that extends to homosexual sodomy'. But the eloquent dissent of Justice Blackmun is likely to be remembered long after the opinion of the majority. He wrote:

> Our cases long have recognized that the Constitution embodies a promise that a certain private sphere of individual liberty will be kept largely beyond the reach of government . . . We protect those rights not because they contribute, in some direct and material way, to the general public welfare, but because they form so central a part of an individual's life . . . Only the most wilful blindness could obscure the fact that sexual intimacy is 'a sensitive, key relationship of human existence central to family life, community welfare and the development of human personality' . . . The fact that individuals define themselves in a significant way through their intimate sexual relationships with others suggests, in a nation as diverse as ours, that there may be many 'right' ways of conducting those relationships, and that much of the richness of a relationship will come from the freedom an individual has to *disclose* the form and nature of these intensely personal bonds . . . What the Court . . . has refused to recognize is the fundamental interest all individuals have in controlling the actions of their intimate associations with others . . . The issue raised by this case touches the heart of what makes individuals what they are.

He called for an early reversal of *Bowers* v. *Hardwick*. This is unlikely, given the increasingly conservative composition of the Supreme Court. It should be added that some US state courts have recognized a fundamental right to engage in private consenting homosexual behaviour, and the basis of these rulings included an interpretation of the federal constitution. These states include New York and New Jersey.

Lesbianism

Lesbianism is, of course, homosexuality. It is separated here from male homosexuality not to romanticize or minimize it (Socarides 1965), but because the attitude of the law towards female homosexuality is so very different from that towards the male counterpart. Lesbianism may be seen as less of a problem than male homosexuality. Female homosexual-paedophilia is rare. Society is probably offended less by lesbianism than male homosexuality. Less is known about it and the literature is scanty (Gagnon and Simon 1974). Today it is often a 'political act' (Hite 1977). Lesbianism has never been a crime in England, nor anywhere else, so far as is known. Socarides (1965) says he has known of no instances in which female homosexuals were trapped by the police using female detectives and unmarked police prowl cars, and one suspects that this almost never happens.

The expression of lesbianism may amount to a common assault, an indecent assault, or an offence under the Indecency with Children Act 1960. If lesbian activities are carried out in the street, or any public place to the annoyance of residents or others, they would probably be classed as one of the offences created by the many by-laws which regulate conduct offensive to the public sense of decency. Lesbians are penalized by the law in other ways. Thus, it is clear that courts are reluctant to give custody of a child to a lesbian mother. An allegation that a woman is a lesbian is actionable as slander without proof of special damage (Slander of Woman Act 1891, as interpreted in *Kerr* v. *Kennedy* [1942] 1 K.B. 409).

Transvestism

Transvestites are usually males, heterosexual, and married. But marriage relationships may not be very important for them. Transvestism tends to assert itself where there is a 'perceived difficulty in establishing successful masculine and heterosexual identity, combined with a blockage of the possibility of achieving a homosexual identity' (Taylor Buckner 1970).

There are two types of transvestite: exhibitionistic and non-exhibitionistic (Enelow 1965). In the exhibitionistic form the individual, male or female, has the need to be viewed by others in the clothes of the opposite sex, and is probably less inclined to masturbatory gratification than the non-exhibitionist. The exhibitionist transvestite may be homosexual. The non-exhibitionist is usually not and is less likely to be psychotic. Masturbatory fantasies are a feature of this type of transvestism. (See Chapter 6.)

Karpman (1954) says 'transvestism as such is not likely to be involved with the law but there is definite law against it, and there are transvestites who dress up and parade the streets and are apprehended by the police'. But, as Enelow indicates (1965), 'this group of transvestites who come into conflict with the law, that is, the exhibitionist group, are apparently in the minority. The majority of people with this disorder are usually not discovered, or if they are discovered are not brought to the courts'. Men are more likely to run foul of the law than women. This is the result of greater cultural acceptance of women dressing as men than vice versa.

In England, transvestites may be charged with a number of offences ranging from behaviour likely to cause a breach of the peace, or loitering with intent to commit a felony (Vagrancy Act 1824 s. 4), to importuning (s. 32 of Sexual Offences Act 1956). It is also possible that dressing in the clothes of the opposite sex may amount to fraud or deception for the purposes of various offences of dishonesty.

Fetishism

Fetishism is a sexual affective state held by an individual towards an object or part of a person of such intensity that the object or part of the person serves as a primary source of arousal and consummation (Storr 1964; Epstein 1965). Fetishes tend to be feminine symbols: the high-heeled shoe is probably the commonest fetish of all. Nearly all fetishists are men; minor degrees of fetishism can be detected in most men. Fetishism becomes a sexual deviation when the fetish is totally substituted for the person, and becomes the end in itself rather than a means. Fetishism is neither rare nor exotic (Becker 1963). Fetishism often involves 'theft', the 'borrowing', for example, or women's panties. If they belong to a friend, relative, or lover nothing may be said: 'it is only when [the fetishist] goes outside into the community and "steals" that the fetishist and his work becomes visible' (Plummer 1975). In the same way, if a wife willingly dresses in rubber wear for her husband, the problematic nature of her husband's deviation decreases (North 1970). (See also Chapter 4.)

In itself fetishism is not a crime. Most fetishists do not run foul of the law. But fetishistic behaviour may lead to a whole gamut of crimes. A fetishist may feel an overpowering desire to grasp the object to which he is sexually attracted. Stealing women's underwear from washing lines is common. The case of *R.* v. *George* has been considered. In his pursuit of sexual gratification via girls' shoes, he was found guilty of assault. He had also been charged with attempted larceny (now theft). Potentially the cause of any crime can be attributed to fetishistic motivation (Haines and Zeidler 1961). There is a well-documented case of a variety of murders committed by an individual who exhibited fetishistic behaviour (Kennedy *et al.* 1947).

Voyeurism

Voyeurism or scopophilia is very widespread. As with fetishism, it can properly be described as deviation only where it substitutes for normal sexual activity. According to Storr (1964), in one study 65 per cent of males admitted to have engaged in voyeuristic activity, while 83 percent would have liked to do so. Striptease shows will always be popular among men. Rosen (1965) distinguishes three types of 'looking': compulsive looking, looking and touching which may involve frotteurism, and voyeurism.

The pathology of compulsive looking and 'fully developed voyeuristic perversion' (Rosen 1965) may be distinguishable, but the law does not distinguish them. Neither is in itself a crime but both may involve a number of offences. The behaviour of 'peeping toms' is apt to occasion a breach of the peace, and voyeurs may be bound over to be of good behaviour. They may be charged with being a public nuisance, but this charge will only be sustained where a large number of people has had to complain, and this will be rare. Burglary and attempted burglary are other possible charges (Theft Act 1968 s. 9). Neither are particularly likely as the voyeur would have to enter a building as a trespasser with intent to commit a specified offence, such as theft, rape, grievous bodily harm, or criminal damage. But voyeurs who are also fetishists (for example, on a panty raid), or pyromaniacs (Rubenstein 1965; Lewis 1965), which is also often connected with voyeurism, could find themselves accused of burglary or its attempt.

Looking and touching may involve other offences. It may result in the man exposing himself and then inviting the female to touch or masturbate him. This would constitute the crimes of indecent exposure (an offence at common law and under s. 4 of the Vagrancy Act 1824) and, if the female is under 14 years of age, indecency with children (Indecency with Children Act 1960). It may lead to mutual stimulation or frottage with the man stimulating himself to the point of orgasm: in so doing, the offences of common assault and indecent assault would be committed.

Exhibitionism

Exhibitionism is probably the commonest sex offence. In addition to that which comes to attention, a vast amount is unreported (Coleman *et al.* 1964). Perhaps 20–35 per cent of all sex offenders are exhibitionists. Radzinowicz (1957) found that 80 per cent of exhibitionists were first offenders. The other 20 per cent had been convicted of previous sexual offences but 78 per cent of these offences were also for indecent exposure. Thus, there is a high rate of recidivism for exhibitionists. Most exhibitionists are non-violent. Fifty per cent of their victims are under 16 years of age: but in most cases where sexual assault also takes place, the offence is of a minor nature and no physical injury is done to the child (Allen 1969). See Chapter 8.

At common law it is a misdemeanour to commit an outraging of public decency in public and in such a way that more than one person sees, or is at least able to see, the act (*R.* v. *Sedley* [1663]). Sir Charles Sedley was indicted for exposing himself naked on a balcony in Covent Garden and urinating on the crowd beneath. The offence is in the nature of a public nuisance. The essential element is publicity. It may or may not involve a sexual motive and it is not necessary that there be any intent to insult or offend any other person. A wide view is taken of 'in public' and private premises may be so regarded, provided more than one person must at least have been able to see the act (*R.* v. *Mayling* [1963] 2 Q.B. 717).

It is an offence under s. 4 of the Vagrancy Act 1824 'wilfully, openly, lewdly and obscenely' to expose ones 'person with intent to insult any female'. 'Person' means penis (*Evans* v. *Ewels* [1972] 2 All E.R. 22). 'The exposure of the backside' is not within the section (Radzinowicz 1957). The offence may be committed in public or in private (Criminal Justice Act 1925 s. 42), and the exposure is committed 'openly' even if it occurs in the exposer's own bedroom (*Ford* v. *Falcone* [1971] 2 All E.R. 1138). A specific intent to insult must be proved.

It is also an offence under the Town Police Clauses Act 1847 s. 28 and under numerous local acts and by-laws, some of which are set out in Radzinowicz (1957). Thus, the Hyde Park Regulations 1932 provide: 'no person shall sit, lie, rest or sleep on any seat or any part of the Park in any indecent posture or behave in any manner reasonably likely to offend against public decency'.

The latest criminal statistics are deficient and fail to show how many persons are found guilty of indecent exposure, nor the number sent to prison, fined, bound over, or given hospital orders under s.60 of the Mental Health Act 1983. We do not know how many were first remanded for medical and psychiatric reports. In many cases fines and short terms of imprisonment may do little harm. But where there are 'well developed perversions'; neither fines nor imprisonment 'diminish the repetition compulsion especially in the impulsive type of exhibitionist' (Rosen 1965).

Both the Law Commission (1974) and the Home Office (1976b) have made recommendations to reform this area of the law. They are broadly in agreement that the existing law should be repealed and replaced by an offence, the ingredients of which would be that a man has exposed his genital organs knowing that it is likely that other people will see him, in circumstances where those who are likely to see him are likely to be offended. The Home Office also suggests that female nudity in public in circumstances likely to cause offence should be made a criminal offence.

Bestiality

Bestiality can be committed by both men and women Dekkis (1994). It consists in having any kind of sexual intercourse with an animal (including a domestic fowl (*R.*

v. *Brown* 1889) 24 Q.B. 357). Most cases occur in the country, where farm labourers have been known to have intercourse with a wide variety of domestic animals. There are also reported instances of women having sexual relations with dogs and other animals. In *R. v. Bourne* ([1952] 36 Cr. App. R. 125), a man compelled his wife to submit on two occasions to the insertion of the male organ of an Alsatian, which he had excited, into her vagina. He was convicted of aiding and abetting her to commit buggery. She was not charged with any offence but the Court of Criminal Appeal assumed she was entitled to be acquitted.

Under the Sexual Offences Act 1956 s. 12, bestiality carries a maximum of life imprisonment. It has been proposed that the maximum sentence be reduced to six months' imprisonment (Criminal Law Revision Committee, 1989). A two-year sentence was quashed in 1984 by a Court of Appeal which, noting that it was the perpetrator and his wife who needed help (and not the Pyrenean Mountain Bitch), established a two-year probation order (*R. v. Higson*, *The Times*, 21 January 1984). It has been argued (Brazier 1975) that the crime as such should be abolished. Its retention is justified on two grounds: (1) that it is repulsive and (2) that it is cruel to animals. The first justification is not sound and the second could be taken care of by prosecuting the offender under cruelty to animals legislation. There is also a school of thought which claims that animals have 'rights', one of which might be their sexual freedom (Clarke 1977). It must be assumed that few cases are detected: the 'victims' do not usually report the offences to the police. However, if the offence were to be abolished, which is unlikely, it is difficult to see with what Bourne could have been charged.

Sodomy with a woman

This consists in sexual intercourse *per anum* by a man with a woman. Until the passing of the Criminal Justice and Public Order Act in 1994 this was a crime (see now s. 142). It could be committed by a husband with his wife. Penetration had to be proved: emission was not necessary. Consent was no defence: indeed, the consenting party was also guilty of the offence, as a principal offender. The law was thus in the highly anomalous situation that two consenting males might do with impunity what a husband and a wife risked a sentence of life imprisonment for doing. A short prison sentence was considered appropriate (see *R. v. Dixon* [1994] Crim L.R. 579) even in the year of the reform of the law.

Although not uncommon—for reasons suggested by Storr (1964)—it is still regarded by many with horror, and the change in the law is unlikely to affect this. Apparently, sodomy and heresy were frequently associated in medieval times. It has been suggested that an act of sodomy is described in *Lady Chatterley's lover* and that, if the jury had realized this, they might have found Lawrence's novel to be obscene.

Many psychiatrists and social workers must have broken the law regularly by knowing about, or encouraging for therapeutic purposes, acts of sodomy between husband and wife. It was impossible to defend the retention of this crime where adults consented to it, particularly in the light of the 1967 reforms, and few professionals will mourn its passing.

Necrophilia

Necrophilia is assumed to be rare. Two notorious murderers, Christie (Kennedy, 1971) and Nilsen (Masters, 1986) were also necrophiles. It is not specifically proscribed by English law. There may be an offence of 'outraging decency' (*Knuller* v. *D.P.P.* [1973] A.C. 435), and necrophilia might come within its contours. If carried out in public or with intent to insult a female in private, it could fall within one of the exhibitionism offences outlined above.

Sado-masochism

Hartwich (1962) defines sadism as 'the experiencing of sexual desire up to the pitch of orgasm, when accompanied by humiliations, chastisement and all manner of cruelties inflicted upon a human being or an animal', and also as 'the impulse to evoke such feelings of desire by means of the appropriate treatment'. Sadism and masochism are bipolar manifestations of the same drive (Rothman 1968; Klein 1972) The history of flagellation is now well documented (Gibson 1978) see also Chapters 1, 2, and 12). As was indicated in the discussion of rape, not all violent sexual crimes are sadistic in motivation. Sado-masochsitic practices are found in conjugal relations and in homosexual practices, and are common activities for the prostitute and her client. Flagellations do not usually cause undue physical pain for 'the environment is one of controlled violence' (Leigh 1976). There is, of course, the possibility that 'the lines of communication between the partners will become blurred, resulting in the inflicting of greater violence than was in the customer's contemplation' (Leigh 1976). It is these cases that are more likely to come to the attention of the police.

Many crimes, and not just sexual offences, maybe expression of sadism. 'Sadism *per se* is not a mental disorder within the meaning of the Mental Health Act 1983 and does not legally excuse or mitigate murder or other serious crimes against the person. It may be an expression of psychopathic disorder, psychosis, subnormality or organic brain disease' (Power 1976). But sadism more commonly expresses itself in actions which amount to common or indecent assault, or assaults occasioning actual or (more rarely) grievous bodily harm. In England the problem has had a thorough airing and has led to a controversial decision of the House of Lords (*R.* v. *Brown* [1993] 2 WLR556). The case involved a sado-masochistic homosexual group; members engaged in a number of consensual practices involving branding, use of sandpaper and candle-wax, and making incisions in the scrotums of consenting members. The activities involved bondage, bloodletting, and torture. The participants were charged with a number of offences including assault occasioning actual bodily harm and inflicting grievous bodily harm. They were convicted. Although he dissented, Lord Mustill captured the sense of the decision when he said: 'plain humanity demands that a court . . . should recognize and respond to the profound dismay which all members of the community share about the apparent increase in cruel and senseless crimes against the defenceless' (p. 601). But, of course, the participants consented. However, as the Lord Chief Justice had said in an earlier case: 'it is not in the public interest that people should cause each other actual bodily harm for no good reason'. There is no doubt that the judges were appalled by the conduct in question. 'Pleasure derived from the infliction of pain is an evil thing', said Lord Templeman (p. 566). It is not in 'public interest that deliberate infliction of actual bodily harm during the course of homosexual sado-masochistic activities should be held to be lawful', opined Lord Jauncey. And Lord Lowry added that it was not 'conducive to the welfare of society'.

Making obscene telephone calls

This may be described as the 'symbolic equivalent' of voyeurism (Power 1976). Offenders are almost exclusively male; many are young and timid, the majority are probably harmless. Offenders are difficult to trace but, if located, may be charged with insulting behaviour, or behaviour likely to cause a breach of the peace. Making obscene telephone calls is also an offence under the Post Office Act 1969 s. 78 (and see *R.* v. *Norbury* [1978] Crim. L.R. 435). The sending of any message by telephone that is 'grossly offensive, or of an indecent, obscene or menacing character' is punishable by a £50 fine, one-month's imprisonment, or both.

A note on transsexualism

The transsexual is someone who adopts totally the identity of the other sex. The majority of transsexuals are born into the male sex but have taken on a feminine gender role. Many also undergo surgical treatment to remove what, for them, are redundant appendages. There have been a number of well-publicized cases: April Ashley and Jan Morris are two of the better known, the latter has written up her experiences in *Conundrum* (1974). (See also Chapter 7.)

As far as the law is concerned the transsexual raises major problems, in particular the question of the transsexual's status. How is the law to classify him/her? Is it to characterize him/her in the same way for all purposes?

There is no doubt as to the transsexual's status in English law. Sex is fixed at birth and cannot be changed thereafter. Thus, in the only case to reach an English court, *Corbett* v. *Corbett* ([1970] 2 All E.R. 33) Ormrod J. held that April Ashley, 'a convincing feminine pastiche', was still of the male sex in spite of 'her' undoubted adoption of a feminine gender role. The judge held that sex was tested by chromosomal, gonadal, and genital factors and possibly by hormonal (secondary sexual) characteristics. Psychological considerations were irrelevant. He recognized the phenomenon of intersex, the classic case of the hermaphrodite, where there was an absence of congruence between the first three factors. In such a case, Ormrod J. opined, he would place greatest emphasis on genital considerations. But April Ashley was 'male' because there was no doubt as to the congruence of the primary factors at 'her' birth, and that was the latest time (mistakes apart) when sexual classification could be made. Ormrod J. did, however, limit himself to pronouncing on April Ashley's sex for the purpose of marriage. He was, he said, not concerned with her status 'at large'. Her marriage was declared to be no marriage (her husband was a transvestite male). Statute now declares that a marriage is void if the marriage partners are not respectively male and female (Matrimonial Causes Act 1973 s. 11(c)). Thus, the marriage of a transsexual like April Ashley or Jan Morris to a woman would be upheld as valid by an English court. It would, however, be voidable at the option of the 'wife', certainly for incapacity and more doubtfully for wilful refusal to consummate the marriage (M.C.A. 1973 s. 12(a) (b)).

Ormrod J.'s judgment, however, leaves open the status of a transsexual for purposes other than marriage. It is thought that for most other purposes, there will be recognition of gender. Thus, she would get a woman's national insurance card, go to a women's prison, etc. She could be charged with soliciting and could be the victim of rape.

The law is most unsatisfactory. It may, with justification, be asked what interest the state has got in preserving a citizen's sexual identity. One can change one's name easily and one's nationality without too much trouble, but not one's sex. Other countries, Switzerland, for example, take account of psychological considerations and the English law should follow their example. The gravest error in Ormrod J.'s reasoning was to tie the essential role of woman in marriage to the task of procreating children. The fallacies of this line of reasoning are numerous and obvious (Kennedy 1973; Smith 1971). But challenges to the European Court on Human Rights have failed.

Sex-linked defences

Some of the defences to criminal behaviour have been considered already, in particular diminished responsibility. In this section a number of other possible sex-linked defences will be discussed.

(i) Premenstrual syndrome

This was described by Greene and Dalton in 1953. Studies have found that 62 per cent of violent crimes by women are committed premenstrually (Morton *et al.* 1953) and half of all emergency room admissions of women due to accidents occur then (Dalton 1960). Furthermore, women reportedly commit suicide at this time (Dalton 1959). Half of the women convicted of committing a crime did so during the four days before or after the onset of menses (Dalton 1980). This increases to two-thirds in the case of women who reported a history of PMS. In 1981 a barmaid, Sandie Craddock, had a charge of murder reduced to manslaughter on the basis of PMS-induced diminished responsibility and she was given probation so that she could receive hormone therapy (*R.* v. *Craddock* [1981] 1 CL 49). Courts in the United States have been far more conservative in their acceptance of the PMS defence (Greene 1992). The criminal case that came closest to testing the PMS defence involved felony child beating, but prior to trial, the woman dropped that defence and pleaded guilty in a misdemeanour (*People* v. *Santos*, New York, 1982, unreported). The US Psychiatric Association Diagnostic Manual, DSMIIIR, does not include PMS as a distinct entity, though its more severe manifestations (where there is 'marked impairment in social or occupational functioning') is included under the term 'late luteal phase dysphoric disorder' in an appendix, of diagnoses needing further study.

(ii) Post-partum psychosis

This may affect one or two women in a thousand. It is more serious than post-partum depression and includes delusions and auditory hallucinations. A common delusion is that the baby is defective or dead. Hallucinations may involve voices ordering the mother to kill her baby. About 3 per cent of mothers with post-partum psychosis do kill their babies. The *Massip* case in California focused public attention on the problem (229 Cal. 3d. 1400 (1990)). According to the trial judge: 'on the day of the killing the defendant's mental condition was disrupted and delusional from a post-partum depression and at times a post-partum psychosis'. She was convicted of manslaughter, rather than murder. But for the appellate court 'the real thrust of the People's argument is that the evidence established Massip intended to kill and malice was thus necessarily present . . . The People point to conflicts in the evidence which indicate [she] was behaving in a rational manner'. In England the crime of infanticide exists specifically to tackle this problem. This is punishable as manslaughter, not murder (Infanticide Act 1938).

(iii) Acute homosexual panic

Although 'acute homosexual panic' was first described in 1920 (Kempf 1920), its diagnosis has proved elusive. It has been said that 'it is as much an interpretation as it is a diagnosis' (Glick 1959, p. 26). It is said that 'the unassertive male's conviction of inadequacy is so strong that he concedes defeat in advance. The result is chronic pseudo-homosexual anxiety that flares up acutely in self-assertive crises as a paranoid expectation of homosexual assault, often symbolized in the form of anal rape.' (Ovesey and Woods 1980). In some cases it leads to violent acts to ward off the humiliation of masculine pride. The defence was rejected by a court in California in *People* v. *Huie* (San Francisco Superior Court, 1989, unreported). The defendant pointed to events in his childhood that bore 'directly upon his state of mind at the time of the incident', but the California Penal Code excludes evidence of mental condition except where it reveals a mental disease, defect, or disorder, so the exclusion of this defence by the trial court was upheld. The defence was also run in a protracted Illinois case (*Parisie*). The defendant opined that the deceased had put his hand on the defendant's crotch and said 'John, I'd like to blow you'. His defence was that he did not have the requisite intent or mental capacity at the time of the incident because he was undergoing a 'homosexual panic', 'a state of mind in which an individual acts instinctively'. A court-appointed psychologist found the defendant to be 'a highly latent homosexual with strong feelings of inferiority and testified that a severe stress of any type could result in an acute schizophrenic reaction with accompanying amnesia'. A court-appointed psychiatrist defined homosexual panic as a fear reaction precipitated by a psychological trauma such as a homosexual advance. In such circumstances, the person . . . loses control and acts purely instinctively, 'almost like an animal', causing the person to be unable to control the nature of his acts'. (287 N.E. 2A 310 (1972)) and 705 F. 2d 882 (1982), *cert. denied* 464 US 918 (1983)).

TREATMENT OF SEX OFFENDERS

The word 'treatment' is used to conform with contemporary terminology. Medical imagery has replaced the legal-punitive in discussions about the disposition of offenders. The therapeutic model is now all-powerful: but it should not be forgotten that looked at from the viewpoint of the offender treatment may be brutal punishment. Locking up a person's mind with drugs is at least as harsh as confining his body within prison walls. Advancing technology may eventually enable us to do away with the fabric of prisons: human warehouses may be replaced by sophisticated monitoring devices (Cohen 1974). However effective this may be, we cannot pretend that it is humane.

Treatment assumes that there is something wrong with the offender: that his behaviour is inherent to his condition. 'The very fact that a person is seen to need rehabilitation implies that he was once habilitated and now needs the process to be repeated' (Bean 1976). Furthermore, no one is quite sure what constitutes rehabilitation. Decisions are, of course, based on 'a reliance of professional judgement' (Matza 1964). It is difficult for the 'patient' to refuse treatment (Plotkin 1977). The prisoner or patient is said to be rehabilitated 'when a specifically defined goal has been reached' (Rapaport 1970). Implicit in this is a sense of values and moral ordering, and a consensus. Psychiatric diagnoses are moral evaluations (Goffman 1961). But therapists act as if there were no conflict between them and their patients. For these reasons it is wrong to suppose a qualitative difference between the penal and the therapeutic, whatever the supposed difference of approach (Pearson 1975).

The legal systems of the world, together with medical and psychiatric professions of each society, have developed numerous ways of tackling sexual deviance (Bancroft 1974). One must, of course, distinguish between those who offend against the law and those who do not, or rather, given the vast amount of hidden sexual deviance, between those labelled deviants by agents of control or who identify themselves as such and those who do not surface to the attention of 'significant others'. The latter, who constitute the greatest number of sexual deviants, are not 'official deviants' (Box 1971) and do not attract treatment, although informal social control is insidious enough to affect all of us from cradle to grave. One must also distinguish different types of sexual deviance. For a start, they provoke different reactions. Rape may call forth a need for vengeance and a sense of horror. Living off immoral earnings may evoke anger and disgust. The public, aided by the Press (Cohen 1972), conjures forth stereotypes of each. On any criterion such disparate offences merit different treatment.

The Cambridge Report on Sexual Offences (Radzinowicz 1975) found that 4 in 10 of all sexual offenders who were tried were fined; one-quarter were sent to prison; and 16 per cent were put on probation. The period since this report has been one of innovation in the penal system; it has seen the development of suspended sentences and the community service order as well as an increased emphasis on the social enquiry report, on psychiatric treatment, and on the rehabilitative ideal. We have, however, no more recent study of the disposition of sexual offenders. Disparities in sentencing are common and frequently commented upon (Hood 1962; Bottomley 1973). This is not the place to account for these, although it must be noted that severe sentences are sometimes engineered by moral panics when a particular offence is prevalent in a certain place at a particular time. Offenders may be given medical or psychiatric treatment once in prison. There is, however, little provision made for sentences with specifically medical aims. One exception is the probation order with a condition for mental treatment. Hospital and guardianship orders may be made by courts under the Mental Health Act 1983. However, they rarely do this and decisions to transfer a prisoner to a mental institution tend to be left to the prison administration. Such a transfer needs the approval of the Secretary of State.

In much of the United States, there is specific legislation to deal with sexual psychopaths (Bowman and Engle 1965; Swanson 1960; Slovenko and Phillips 1962). Sexual psychopaths are defined as persons who lack the power to control their sexual impulses or who have criminal propensities towards the commission of sex offences. Most of the states require a person to have been convicted of some offence, but some simply demand that cause be shown that he is probably a sexual psychopath. The legislation is coming under increasing attack. As Slovenko (1965) puts it:

> The vagueness of the definition of a sexual psychopath has resulted in the commitment for long periods of time—at state expense—of many nuisance-type, non-dangerous sex offenders, such as the homosexual, the exhibitionist, and the peeping tom. The legislation has resulted in a round-up of the nuisance-type offender and left untouched the dangerous, aggressive offender. The purpose of the legislation has been lost in its application.

Sentences are indeterminate, and presuppose the existence of adequate psychiatric assistance, which is not always available. Perhaps the most serious criticism of this type of legislation is that it lacks 'scientific foundation', thus 'if one uses the medical framework, sexual deviation simply refers to a symptom, but if one however uses a psychosocial framework, it refers to a type of behaviour' (Slovenko 1965). It has been held constitutional to detain a sexual psychopath for treatment for a longer time than that for which he might have been sentenced if he were so classified (*Trueblood* v. *Tinsley* 366 P. 2d 655 (1961)). Reforms have been suggested. For example, Sidley and Stolarz (1973) have argued that what is required is a 'dangerous sex-offender' law. Commitment of such an offender would depend on (1) the commission of the sexual offence in which in victim was injured (but what constitues injury?; is the willing partner in a statutory rape injured?); and (2) a convincing demonstration by the person making predictions about the offender's future behaviour, that the offender will, within a period of one year, unless he is incarcerated or treated, commit a sexual offence that will result in physical injury to his victim. But how does a psychiatrist determine this? We are told that a heterosexual aggressor 'who has no insight' satisfies the second limb. What is 'insight'? The moral overtones of evaluations like this are undeniable. The truth of the matter is that legislation of this nature is apt to be dangerously vague; indefinite commitments on such criteria offend the rule of law and should be repealed. Hospital orders in this country are subject to similar criticisms (Gostin 1977; Honoré 1978). On the recommendation of the Butler report (1975) the Mental Health Act was amended so that a psychopathic disorder consisting of a sexual deviation alone should not be a ground for a hospital order A hospital order can now only be made when a court is satisfied in the evidence of two medical practitioners that the offender is suffering from mental illness, psychopathic disorder, mental impairment, or severe mental impairment and that the disorder is of 'a nature or degree which makes it apropriate for him to be detained in a hospital for medical treatment and, in the case of psychopathic disorder or mental impairment, that such treatment is likely to alleviate or prevent a deterioration in his condition' (Mental Health Act 1983 s. 37 (2) (a) (i)).

It must also be the most suitable method of disposal (s. 37 (2) (b)). A person is not to be treated as suffering from mental disorder by reason of 'sexual deviancy'. But there remains a concern that an associated condition, reactive depression or anxiety, will be used via the all-embracing 'mental illness' to justify detention.

Sexual deviance is treated in a number of other ways. Gundlach *et al.* (1962) says that analytical psychotherapy is an appropriate treatment for sex criminals in general, but, as judged by the reduction in the reconviction rate, its practical value may be doubted (Field and Williams 1971). Aversion therapy is used mainly to 'treat' homosexuality, transvestism, and fetishism (Gibbens 1967). Storr (1964) thinks 'it is too early yet to say whether it is a permanently effective treatment, or what disadvantages may accompany it'. Many will think it totally repellent (see Chapter 16). Hormonal 'treatment' is a similarly repulsive approach (see Chapter 1. Field and Williams (1970), for example, advocate subcutaneous implants of oestradiol. This induces testicular atrophy. Field and Williams' study shows that 16 out of 25 of their implant group were not reconvicted of a sex offence over a two-year period: eight were, however, convicted of non-sexual offences. It is, however, difficult to define a non-sexual offence. These individuals may now be expressing their general frustration through other criminal outlets. Twenty out of 37 of a control group, who were given a placebo, were similarly not reconvicted of a sexual offence: eight were reconvicted of a non-sexual offence; and nine were reconvicted of sex offences. Defenders of these inhuman experiments argue that 'these individuals appreciate treatment', while conceding 'dosage should be adjusted to allow some sexual activity' (Power 1976). What makes this form of experimentation all the more unacceptable is the belief that 'objective conclusions' may be reached and that 'this procedure could help decide when a sexual offender who had killed may be safely released. The view may be taken that such men should be detained until physiological waning of the sex drive occurs in old age' (Power 1976). Power is a Senior Medical officer in H. M. Prison Service. Other drugs used include benperidol and cyproterone acetate, which Power (1976) tells us 'is *alleged* not to cause any *significant undesirable* effects' (my italics). It is used apparently in the 'treatment' of sexual exhibitionism, excessive masturbation, paedophilia, and 'to relieve depression secondary to abnormal sexual practices'.

In Scandinavia, castration of sexual recidivists has been performed fairly extensively. It is usually carried out with 'consent', often influenced by promises of earlier release from prison or security hospital. Not surprisingly, 'some castrated individuals remain embittered and resentful' (Power 1976).

A 1979 review of European research on the castration of sex offenders focused on recidivism rates and on sexual functioning (Heim and Hursch 1979). Over 1000 sex offenders, castrated by court order in Germany and released from prison between 1934 and 1944, were compared to 685 sex offenders who were released uncastrated. Of the castrated men, 2.3 per cent were recidivists and repeated their offences (before castration their recidivism rate was 84 per cent), while of the non-castrated the recidivism rate was 39 per cent. Two-thirds of those interviewed (the sample was small) reported the extinction of sex drive and potency, but 18 per cent said they were able to engage in sexual intercourse more than 20 years after castration. The younger they were castrated, the more enduring was their sexual functioning. 127 castrated Swiss offenders were compared with 50 others who had refused castration and had as a result stayed in prison longer. The recidivism rate among castrates was 7 per cent (it was 77 per cent before surgery). In the non-castrated group, 52 per cent committed sexual offences again within 10 years (their prior recidivism rate was 66 per cent). Two-thirds of sexual castrates reported an extinction of sexual interest and drive, but 10 per cent reported having sexual intercourse 8–20 years after surgery. A Norwegian study (Bremer 1959) found a recidivism rate of 7 per cent after castration (before, it had been 58 per cent). For most sexual interest dissipated but one-quarter said it persisted for at least a year. A large Danish study reported a 10 per cent relapse rate for non-castrated offenders (this was higher for those who had committed more than one previous offence) (Christiansen *et al.* 1965). But where the men were castrated the recidivism rate was only 1.1 per cent and no rapist raped again (Sturup 1972).

Success has also been reported with hormonal 'castration'. Antiandrogen treatment uses the drug medroxyprogesterone (MPA). A US study found a 15 per cent recurrence of offending behaviour while on the drug. It concluded: 'In general these men appear to do well and respond to antiandrogen medication as long as they continue taking it and as long as their problems are rather clearly confined to unconventional sexual cravings' (Berlin and Meinecke 1981). A review of MPA studies in 1986 examined 10 reports and 96 offenders (25 per cent exhibitionists, 27 per cent homosexual paedophiles, 14 per cent bisexual paedophiles, 3 per cent rapists, and 4 per cent incest perpetrators). Although it is generally accepted that MPA reduces sexual interest and functioning and has minimal side-effects, Cooper (1986) concluded 'the outcome of therapy was assessed mainly using self-report questionnaires. These were of uneven quality and unproven validity'. Another drug used for chemical castration is cyprotenoe acetate (CPA). A review of studies of this points to no recidivism in five pieces of research but a recidivism rate of 17 per cent in another (Ortman 1980).

Chemical castration has provoked controversy (Alexander *et al.* 1993). To what extent can informed, meaningful consent be given when the man is in prison or it is a condition of probation or parole? (Halleck 1981). An appeal court in Michigan (*People* v. *Gauntlett* 352 N. W. 2d. 310 (1984)) ruled that probation on condition that the offender (a man convicted of sexually abusing his two step-children) be treated with MPA was unlawful. 'The Depo-Provera treatment prescribed by the trial judge fails as a lawful condition of probation because it has not gained acceptance in the medical community as a safe and reliable medical procedure' (p. 316). In *Arizona* v. *Christopher* (652 P. 2d 1031 (1982)), a paedophile on probation who committed another offence and was reconvicted for this appealed because he had not received behaviour modification or antiandrogen therapy. A pre-sentence report had recommended behaviour modification techniques and said that chemical castration could also be used. The basis of the appeal was that 'being placed on probation constitutionally entitled him to be effectively treated and rehabilitated'. The appeal court rejected the argument that constitutional rights (cruel and unusual punishment and due process) were violated. Neither constitutional provision 'requires a state to provide incarcerated prisoners with a rehabilitation program' because 'probation itself is a matter of grace and not of right' (p. 1032). In *Bowring* v. *Godwin* (551 F. 2d. 44 (1977)), a federal court in the United States saw 'no underlying distinction between the right to medical care for physical ills and its psychological or psychiatric

444	*Sexual deviance and the law*

counterpart'. It noted that 'modern science has rejected the notion that mental or emotional disturbances are the products of afflicted souls, hence beyond the purview of counselling, medication, and therapy'. It held that a prison inmate was entitled to psychological or psychiatric treatment if the 'prisoner's symptoms evidence a serious disease', if the disease 'is curable or may be substantially alleviated', and if there is 'the substantial potential for harm to the prisoner by reason of delay or denial' (p. 47).

REFERENCES

Aberle, D. W. (1963). The incest taboo and the mating pattern of animals. *Am. Anthropol.* **65**, 253.
Adams, M. S. and Neel, J. V. (1967). Children of incest. *Pediatrics*, **40**, 255.
Alexander, M., Gunn, J., Cook, D. A. G., and Taylor, P. J. (1993). Should a sexual offender be allowed castration? *Brit. Med. J.* **307**, 790–3.
Allen, C. E. (1969). *A textbook of psychosexual disorders*. (2nd edn). Oxford University Press.
Altman, D. and Weeks, D. (1973). *Homosexual: oppression and liberation*. New York.
Amir, M. (1971). Patterns in forciable rape. Chicago.
Anderson, M. (1975) Hookers, arise! *Hum. Behav.* 40.
Bailey, V. and Blackburn, S. (1979). The Punishment of Incest Act 1908: A study in Law Creation. *Crim. Law. Rev.* 708.
Balint, M. (1957), *Problems of human pleasure and behaviour*. London.
Bancroft, J. (1974). *Deviant sexual behaviour: Modification and assessment*. Oxford.
Bean, P. (1976). *Rehabilitation and deviance*. London.
Becker, H. (1963). *Outsiders*. London.
Berger, V. (1977). Man's trial, women's tribulation: rape cases in the court-room. *Columbia Law. Rev.* **77**, 1.
Berlin, F. S. and Meinecke, C. F. (1981). Treatment of sex offenders with antiandrogenic medication: Conceptualizations, review of treatment modalities, and preliminary findings. *Am. J. Psychiat.* **138**(5), 601–7.
Bieber, I., *et al.* (1962). *Homosexuality: a psychoanalytical study of male homosexuals*. Basic Books, New York.
Blackstone, Sir W. (1765). *Commentaries on the laws of England*. London.
Blom-Cooper, L. and Drewry, G. (1976). *Law and mortality*. London
Bohannan, P. (1967). The differing realms of law. *Am. Anthropol.* **67**, 33.
Bottomley, K. A. (1973). *Decisions in the penal process*. London
Bowman, K. and Engle, B. (1965). Sexual psychopath laws. In *Sexual behaviour and the law*, (ed. R. Slovenko). Springfield, IL.
Box, S. (1971). *Deviance, reality and society*. London
Brazier, R. (1975). Reform of sexual offences. *Crim. Law. Rev.* 421.
Bremer, J. (1959). *Asexualization: a follow-up of 244 cases*. London.
Britton, J. (1865). *Laws of England*, (ed. F. M. Nichols) (Original French *c.* 1290–2). Oxford.
Brownmiller, S. (1975). *Against our will—men, women and rape*. London.
Burgess, A. W. and Holmstrom, L. L. (1973). The rape victim in the emergency ward. *Am. J. Nurs.* **1740**, 73.
Burgess, A. W. and Holmstrom, L. L. (1974). Rape trauma syndrome. *Am. J. Psychiat.* **131**(9), 981–6.

Butler report (1975). *Report of the committee on abnormal offenders*, Cmnd 6244. HMSO 50, London.

Cameron, D. and Frazer, E. (1987) *The lust to kill*. Oxford.

Card, R. (1975). Sexual relations with minors. *Crim. Law Rev.* 370.

Carter, C. O. (1967). Risk to offspring of incest. *Lancet*, 436.

Chambliss, W. (1967). Types of deviance and the effectiveness of legal sanctions. *Wisc. Law Rev.* 703.

Chappell, D. and Geis, R. (1977). *Forcible rape*. New York.

Chappell, D., Geis, G., and Fogarty, F. (1974). Forcible rape: a bibliography. *J. Crim. Law*, **65**, 248.

Christiansen, K., Elers-Nielson, M., Le Maire, L., and Sturup, G. (1965). Recidivism among sexual offenders. *Scand. Studies Criminol. Oslo*, 55.

Clark, S. L. R. (1977). *The moral status of animals*. Oxford.

Cleaver, E. (1968). *Soul on ice*. New York.

Cleveland, A. (1913). Indictments for adultery and incest before 1650. *Law Q. Rev.* **29**, 57.

Cohen, S. (1972). *Folk devils and moral panics*. London.

Cohen, S. (1974). Prison as human warehouses. *New Soc.* 14 November.

Cooper, A. J. (1986). Progestogens in the treatment of male sex offenders: A review. *Can. J. Psychiat.* **31**(1), 73–9.

Cox, B., Shirley, J., and Short, M. (1977) *The fall of Scotland Yard*. Penguin, Harmondsworth.

Cretney, S. and Masson, J. (1990). *Principles of family law*, (4th ed). London.

Crozier, B. (1935). Marital support. *Boston Univ. Law Rev*, **15**, 28.

Curran, D. and Parr, D. (1957). Homosexuality: An analysis of 100 male cases seen in private practice. *Brit. Med. J.* **i**, 797–801.

Dalton, K. (1959). Menstruation and acute psychiatric illnesses. *Brit. Med. J.* **1**, 148–9.

Dalton, K. (1960). Menstruation and accidents. *Brit. Med. J.* 2, 1425–6.

Dalton, K. (1980). Cyclical criminal acts in premenstrual syndrome. *Lancet*, **2**, 1070–1.

Davis, A. J. (1973). Sexual assaults in the Philadelphia prison system. In *The sexual scene*, (ed. J. H. Gagnon and W. Simon). Chicago.

Davis, K. (1937). The sociology of prostitution. *Am. Soc. Rev.* **45**, 215.

Davis, K. (1976). Sexual behaviour. In *Contemporary social problems*, (ed. R.K. Merton and R. Nisbet). New York.

Dekkis, M. (1994). *Dearest pet*. London.

Dell, S. (1984). *Murder into manslaughter*. Oxford.

Devlin, P. (1956). *Trial by jury*. London.

Devlin, P. (1965). *The enforcement of morals*. London.

Douglas, J. (1971). *American social order*. New York.

Douglas, M. (1966). *Purity and danger*. London.

Duster, T. (1970). *The legislation of morality: Law, drugs, and moral judgement*. New York.

Enelow, M. (1965). Public nuisance offences. In *Sexual behavior and the law*, (ed. R. Slovenko). Springfield, IL.

Epstein, A. W. (1965). Fetishism, In *Sexual behavior and the law*, (ed. R. Slovenko). Springfield, IL.

Estrich, S. (1989) *Real rape*. New York.

Evans, D. T. (1933). *Sexual citizenship*. London

Evans, D. T. (1994) Falling angels?—The material construction of children as sexual citizens. *Int. J. Child. Rights*, **2**, 1.

Fargier, M.M. (1976). *Le viol*. Paris.

Feminist Group (1973). Prostitution: A non-victim crime. *Iss. Criminol*. **8**, 137.

Ferenczi, S. (1949). Confusion of tongues between the adult and the child. *Int. J. Psychiat*. **30**, 225.

Field, L. and Williams, M. (1970). The hormonal treatment of sexual offenders. *Med. Sci. Law*, **10(1)**, 27–34.

Field, L. and Williams, M. (1971). Note on the scientific assessment and treatment of the sexual offender. *Med. Sci. Law*, **11**, 180–1.

Fleta (*c*. 1290–2). (ed. H. Richardson and G. O. Sayles 1953, 1972). (In Latin). London.

Ford, C. S. and Beach, F. (1952). *Patterns of sexual behavior*. London.

Freeman, M. D. A. (1971). The search for a rational divorce law. *Curr. Legal Probl*. **24**, 178.

Freeman, M. D. A. (1972). Adultery and intolerability. *Mod. Law Rev*. **35**, 98.

Freeman, M. D. A. (1974). *The legal structure*, London.

Freeman, M. D. A. (1977). Le vice anglais—Some responses of English and American law to wife abuse. *Fam. Law Quarterly*, **11**, 199.

Fuller, L. L. (1969). Human interaction and the law. *Am. J. Jurispr*. **14**, 1.

Gagnon, J. H. and Simon, W. (1974). *Sexual conduct*. London.

Gallo, J. J., *et al*. (1966). The consenting homosexual and the law: an empirical study of enforcement and administration in Los Angeles County. *UCLA Law Rev*. **13**, 647.

Garfinkel, H. (1956). Conditions of successful degradation ceremonies. *Am. J. Sociol*. **61**, 420.

Garfinkel, H. (1967). *Studies in ethnomethodology*. New Jersey

Gebhard, P. (1956). *Sex offenders: an analysis of types*. London.

Garfinkel, H. In *The same sex: an appraisal of homosexuality*, (ed. R. W. Weltge). Boston.

Geis, G. and Chappell, D. (1971). Forcible rapes by multiple offenders. *Abst. Criminol. Penol*. **11**, 431.

Genet, J. (1951). *The miracle of the rose*. London.

George, E. (1993) *Making men moral: Civil liberties and public morality*. Oxford.

Gibbens, T. C. N. (1967). Is aversion therapy wrong? *New Soc*. **10**, 42.

Gibson, I. (1978). *The English vice*. London.

Glick, B. (1959). Homosexual panic: Clinical and theoretical considerations. *J. Nerv. Ment. Dis*. **129**, 20–8.

Goffman, E. (1961). *Asylums*. Harmondsworth.

Golding, M. P. (1975). *Philosophy of law*. New Jersey

Gorer, G. (1955). *Exploring English the Character*. London Gorer, G. (1971). *Sex and marriage in England today*. London.

Gostin, L. (1977). *The law relating to mentally abnormal offenders*. London.

Greene, R. (1992). *Sexual science and the law*. New York.

Greene, R. and Dalton, K. (1953). The premenstrual syndrome. *Brit. Med. J*. **1**, 1007.

Greenwood, V. and Young, J. (1975). Notes on the theory of rape and its policy implications. Paper to London Group on Deviancy.

Griffin, S. (1971). Rape: the all American crime. *Ramparts*, September 28.

Haines, W. H. and Zeidler, J. C. (1961). Sexual fetishism as related to criminal acts. *J. Soc. Ther. Corr. Psychiat*. **7**, 187.

Hale, Sir M. (1736). *Ecclesiastical precedents*. London.

Halleck, S. L. (1981). Ethics of antiandrogen therapy. *Am. J. psychiat*. **138(5)**, 642–3.

Hart, H. L. A. (1961). *The concept of law*. London.

Hart, H. L. A. (1963). *Law, liberty, and morality*. London

Hart, H. L. A. (1965). *The morality of the criminal law*. Jerusalem.

Hart, H. L. A. (1967). Social solidarity and the enforcement of morality. *Univ. Chicago Law Rev.* **35**, 1.

Hartwich, A. (ed.) (1965). *Aberrations of sexual life*. (After the *Psychopathia sexualis* of R. V. Krafft-Ebing) London.

Heilbron Report (1975). *Advisory group on law of rape*, (Cmnd 6352). London, HMSO.

Heim, N. and Hursch, C. (1979). Castration for sex offenders. *Arch. Sex. Behav.* **8**, 281.

Hite, S. (1977). *The Hite Report*. London.

Home Office (1974). Working Paper.

Home Office (1992). *Civil judicial statistics*. HMSO, London.

Home Office (1976*a*). *Criminal statistics*. (Annual). HMSO, London.

Home Office (1976*b*). *Report of the working party on vagrancy and street offences*. HMSO, London.

Home Office (1978). *Sentences of imprisonment—a review of maximum penalties*. HMSO, London.

Home Office (1991). *Criminal statistics*. HMSO, London.

Honoré, T. (1978). *Sex law*. London.

Hood, R. (1962). *Sentencing in magistrates' courts*. London.

Hooker, E. (1957). The adjustment of the male overt homosexual. *J. Project. Techn.* **21**, 18.

Horowitz, I. L. and Liebowitz, M. (1968). Social deviance and political marginality: towards a redefinition of the relation between sociology and politics. *Soc. Probl.* **15**, 282.

Humphreys, L. (1970). *Tea room trade: impersonal sex in public places*. Chicago.

Humphreys, L. (1972). *Out of the closets: the sociology of homosexual liberation*. New Jersey.

Hyde, H. M. (1948). *The trials of Oscar Wilde*. London.

Hyde, H. M. (1970). *The other love*. London.

Illsey, R. and Gill, D. (1968) New fashions in illegitimacy. *New Soc.* 709.

Jackson, M. (1984). Sexology and the social construction of male sexuality. In *The sexuality papers*, (ed. B. Coveney). London.

James, T. E. (1964). Law and the sexual offender. In *The pathology and treatment of sexual deviation*. (ed. I. Rosen). Oxford University Press.

Johnson, E. (1970). Extramarital sexual intercourse: a methodological note. *J. Marr. Fam.* **32**, 279.

Kalven, H. and Zeisel, H. (1966). *The American jury*. Boston.

Kanin, E. J. (1967). Reference groups and sex conduct norm violation. *Sociol. Quarterly*, **8**, 495.

Karpman, B. (1954). *The sexual offender and his offences*. New York.

Karst, K. (1980). The freedom of intimate association. *Yale Law J.* **89**, 624.

Kempf, E. (1920). *Psychopathology*. St. Louis.

Kennedy, F., Hoffman, H. R., and Haines, W. H. (1947). A study of William Heirens *Am. J. Psychiat.* **104**, 113–21.

Kennedy, I. M. (1973). Transsexualism and the single sex marriage. *Anglo-Am. Law Rev.* **2**, 112.

Kennedy, L. (1971). *Ten Rillington Place*. London.

Kinsey, A., Pomeroy, W. B., and Martin, C. E. (1948). *Sexual behavior in the human male*. Philadelphia.

Kinsey, A., Pomeroy, W. B., Martin, C. E., and Gebhard, P. H. (1953). *Sexual behaviour in the human female*. Philadelphia.

Klein, D. (1973). The etiology of female crime. *Iss. Criminol.* **8**, 19. Klein, H. (1972). Masochism. *Med. Asp. Hum. Sex.* **6**, 32.

Lambert, J. (1970). *Crime, police, and race relations in Birmingham*. London.

Law Commission (1974). *Working paper 57—Conspiracies relating to morals and decency*. London.

Law Commission (1992). *Rape in marriage*. HMSO, London.

Lawson, A. (1988). *Adultery: an analysis of love and betrayal*. New York.

Le Grand, C. E. (1973). Rape and rape laws: sexism in society and the law. *Calif. Law Rev.* **61**, 932.

Leigh, L. (1976). Sado-masochism, consent and the reform of the criminal law. *Mod. Law Rev.* **39**, 130.

Lemert, E. (1967). *Human deviance, social problems and social control*, New York.

Lewis, N. (1965). Pathological firesetting and sexual motivation. *Sexual behaviour and the law*, (ed. R. Slovenko). Springfield, IL.

Livneh, E. (1967). On rape and the sanctity of matrimony. *Israel Law Rev.* 2, 415.

Lofland, J. (1969). *Deviance and identity*. New Jersey.

Lord Chancellor's Office (1993). *Looking to the future: mediation and divorce*. London.

Lukianowicz, N. (1972). Incest. *Brit. J. Psychiat.* **120**, 301–13.

McCaghy, C. H. (1976). *Deviant behaviour: Crime, Conflict, and interest groups*. London.

McCormick, N. (1982). *H. L. A. Hart*. London.

McGregor, O. (1957). *Divorce in England*.

McGregor, O., Blom-Cooper, L., and Gibson, C. (1970). *Separated spouses*. London

Mairs, W. (1975). Letter to *The Times*, 15 July.

Maisch, H. (1973). *Incest*. London.

Manchester, A. H. (1977). *Incest and the law*. Paper presented to 2nd World Conference of International Society on Family Law, Montreal.

Mason, J. (1980). What is wrong with incest? *SLOLAG Bull.* **47**.

Masters, B. (1986). *Killing for company: The case of Dennis Nilsen*. London.

Matza, D. (1964). *Delinquency and drift*. Chichester.

Medea, A. and Thomson, K. (1974). *Against rape*. London.

Megarry, R. (1955). *Miscellany-at-law*. London.

Megarry, R. (1973). *A second miscellany-at-law*. London.

Melani, J. and Fodaski, S. (1974). Rape: the first source book for women. In (ed. N. Connell and C. Wilson).

Mill, S. J. (1859). *On liberty*. London.

Millett, K. (1973). *The prostitution papers*. New York.

Moore, B. (1984). *Privacy*. Armonk.

Morris, J. (1974). *Conundrum*, New York.

Morris, N. and Hawkins, G. (1970). *The honest politician's guide to crime control*. Chicago.

Morton, J. H., Additon, H., Addison, R. G., Hunt, L., and Sullivan, J. J. (1953). A clinical study of premenstrual tension. *Am. J. Obstet. Gynaecol.* **65(6)**, 1182–91.

Naamani, I. T. (1969). Marriage and divorce in Jewish law. *J. Fam. Law*, 3, 177.

Nagel, E. (1969). The enforcement of morals. In *Moral problems in contemporary society*, (ed. P. Kurk).

North, M. (1970). *The outer fringe of sex: a study in sexual fetishism.* London.

O'Carroll, T. (1980). *Paedophilia: the radical case.* London

Ortman, J. (1980). Treatment of sexual offenders, castration and antihormone therapy. *Int. J. Law Psychiat.* **3**, 443.

Ovesey, L. and Woods, S. (1980). Pseudohomosexuality and homosexuality in men. In *Homosexual behaviour*, (ed. J. Harmer). New York.

Packer, H. (1968). *The limits of the criminal sanction.* Stanford University Press. London.

Payton, G. T. (1966). *Patrol procedure.* Los Angeles.

Pearl, D. (1976). Polygamy and bigamy. *Camb. Law J.* **35**, 48.

Pearson, G. (1975). *The deviant imagination.* London.

Philipson, M. (1974). *Understanding crime and delinquency.* Chicago.

Pivar, D. (1973). *Purity crusade: Sexual morality and social control, 1868–1900.*

Pollock, F. and Maitland, F. (1898). *A history of English law.* London.

Ploscowe, M. (1962). *Sex and the law.* New York.

Ploscowe, M., Foster, H., and Freed, D. (1972). *Family law*, (2nd edn). Boston.

Plotkin, R. (1977). Limiting the therapeutic orgy: mental patients' rights to refuse treatment. *Northwest. Univ. Law Rev.* **72**, 461.

Plummer, K. (1975). *Sexual stigma.* London.

Power, D. J. (1976). Sexual deviation and crime. *Med. Sci. Law*, **16**, 111.

Quinney, R. (1972). Who is the victim? *Criminology*, **10**, 315.

Radzinowicz, L. (1957). *Sexual offences.* London.

Ranulf, S. (1938). *Moral indignation and the middle class psychology.* Munksgaard, Copenhagen.

Rapaport, L. (1970). Crisis intervention as a mode of treatment. In *Theories of social casework*, (ed. R. W. Roberts and R. H. Nee). Chicago.

Reiss, A. (1971). *The police and the public.* New Haven.

Reynolds, J. (1974). Rape as social control. *Catalyst*, **8**, 62.

Richards, P. G. (1970). *Parliament and conscience.* London.

Robertshaw, P. (1994). Sentencing rapists: first tier courts in 1991–92. *Crim. Law Rev.* 343.

Robinson, K. (1964). Parliamentary and public attitudes. In *The pathology and treatment of sexual deviation*, (ed. I. Rosen), PP. 451–60. Oxford University Press.

Rock, P. (1973). *Deviant behaviour.* London.

Rogers, A. J. (1973). *The economics of crime.* Hinsdale, IL.

Rook, P. and Ward, R. (1990). *Sexual offences.* London.

Rosen, I. (1965). Exhibitionism and voyeurism. In *Sexual behaviour and the law*, (ed. R. Slovenko). Springfield, IL.

Rothman, G. (1968). *The riddle of cruelty.* New York.

Rubinstein, L. H. (1965). Sexual motivations in ordinary offences. In *Sexual behaviour and the law*, (ed. R. Slovenko). Springfield, IL.

Russell, D. (1973). *Rape and the masculine mystique.* Paper presented at American Sociological Association Meeting.

Sagarin, E. C. (1974). Sexual criminality. In *Current perspectives on criminal behaviour*, (ed. A. Blumberg). Knopf, New York.

Sagarin, E. C. and Macnamara, D. (1975). The homosexual as a crime victim. *Int. J. Crimin. Penol.* **3**, 13.

Schmideburg, M. (1956). Delinquent acts as perversions and fetishes. *Brit. J. Delinq.* **7**, 44.

Schoeman, F. D. (1984). *Philosophical dimensions of privacy: An anthology.* Cambridge.

Schofield, M. (1973). *Sexual behaviour of young adults*. London.
Schur, E. (1965). *Crimes without victims*. New Jersey.
Schur, E. (1969). *Our criminal society*. New Jersey.
Schur, E. (1971). *Labelling deviant behaviour: Gender, stigma, and social control*. New Jersey.
Schur, E. (1973). *Radical non-intervention*. New Jersey.
Schur, E. and Bedau, H. (1974). *Victimless crimes: two sides of a controversy*. New Jersey.
Schwendinger, J. and H. (1974). Rape myths. *Crime Soc. Just.* **1**, 18.
Scott, P. D. (1964). Definition, classification, prognosis, and treatment. *The pathology and treatment of sexual deviation*, (ed. I. Rosen) (2nd edn), pp. 87–119. Oxford University Press.
Seemanova. E. (1971). A study of children of incestuous matings. *Hum. Her.* **21**, 108.
Sellar, D. (1978). Leviticus XVIII, the forbidden degrees and the law of incest in Scotland. *Jewish Law Ann.* **1**, 229.
Sexual Law Reform Society (1975). Working Party Report. *Crim. Law Rev.* 323.
Sherwin, R. V. (1965). Sodomy. In *Sexual behaviour and the law*, (ed. R. Slovenko). Springfield, IL.
Sidley, N. T. and Stolarz, F. J. (1973). A proposed 'dangerous sex offender' law. *Am. J. Psychiat.* **130(7)**, 765–8.
Simmons, J. (1965). *Deviants*. Los Angeles.
Sion, A. (1977). *Prostitution and the law*. London.
Skolnick, J. (1993). *Justice without trial*. (2nd edn). Chichester.
Skolnick, J. and Woodworth, R. (1968). Morality enforcement and totalitarian potential. In *Orthopsychiatry and the law*, (ed. I. Levitt and M. Rubinstein). Detroit.
Slovenko, R. (1965). *Sexual behaviour and the law*. Springfield, IL.
Slovenko, R. and Philips, (1962). Psychosexuality and the criminal law. *V. Law Rev.* **15**, 797.
Smith, D. K. (1971). Transsexualism, sex reassignment, surgery and the law. *Cornell Law Rev.* **56**, 963.
Smith, J. C. (1975). Note on D.P.P. v. Morgan. *Crim. Law Rev.* 717.
Smith, J. C. (1976). The Heilbron Report. *Crim. Law Rev.* 97.
Smith, J. C. (1977). Conspiracy under the Criminal Law Act 1977. *Crim. Law Rev.* 598.
Smith, J. C. and Hogan, B. (1973). *Criminal law*, (3rd edn). London.
Socarides, C. (1965). Female homosexuality. In *Sexual behaviour and the law*, (ed. R. Slovenko). Springfield, IL.
Solat, M. (1977). Les feministes et le viol. *Le Monde*, 8–20 October.
Soothill, K. and Jack, A. (1975). How rape is reported. *New Soc.* **32**, 663, 702.
Stephen, J. (1883). *A history of the criminal law of England*. London.
Stephens, E. (1976). Out of the closet into the courts. *Spare Rib*, September, 6.
Storr, A. (1964). *Sexual deviation*. Penguin, Harmondsworth.
Sturup, G. K. (1972). Castration: the total treatment. In *Sexual behaviours*, (ed. H. Resnik and M. Wolfgang), p. 361. Boston.
Sutherland, E. and Cressey, D. (1970). *Principles of criminology*, (8th edn). Philadelphia.
Swanson, A. H. (1960). Sexual psychopath statutes—summary and analysis. *J. Crim. Law Criminol. Pol. Sci.* **51**, 215.
Szasz, T. (1970). *The manufacture of madness*. New York.
Taylor Buckner, H. (1970). The transvestite career path. *Psychiatry*, **30**, 381. (Also in *Deviance, reality and change* 1971, New York)

Ten, C. L. (1969). Crime and immorality. *Mod. Law Rev.* **32**, 648.

Thomas, D. A. (1970). *Principles of sentencing*. London.

Toner, B. (1977). *The facts of rape*. London.

Unger, R. M. (1976). *Law in modern society*. London.

University of Pennsylvania Law Review (1968). Police discretion and the judgment that a crime has been committed. **117**, 277.

US National Commission on the Causes and Prevention of Violence (1969).

Virkunnen, M. (1975). Victim precipitated paedophilia offences. *Brit. J. Criminol.* **15**, 175.

Walkerdine, V. (1991). *Schoolgirl fictions*. London.

Walmsley, R. (1978). Indecency between males and the Sexual Offences Act 1967. *Crim. Law Rev.* 400.

Weinberg, M. and Williams, C., (1974). *Male homosexuals: their problems and adaptation*. London.

Weinberg, S. K. (1963). *Incest behaviour*. New York.

Weis, K. and Borges, S. (1973). Victimology and rape: the case of the legitimate victim. *Iss. Criminol.* **8**, 101.

West, D. (1974). Thoughts on sex law reform. In *Crime, criminology and public policy*, (ed. Hood). London.

Wilcox, A. (1972). *The decision to prosecute*. London.

Wilkins, L. (1964). *Social deviance*. London.

Williams, G. (1945). Language and the law. *Law Quarterly Rev.* **61**, 71.

Williams, G. (1975). Letter to *The Times*, 3 October.

Williams, J. E. Hall (1974). The neglect of incest: A criminologist's view. *Med. Sci. Law*, **14**(1), 64–7.

Winick, C. and Kinsie, P. (1971). *The lively commerce—prostitution in the United States*. Chicago.

de Wolf, R. (1970). *The bonds of acrimony*. Philadelphia.

Wolfenden, J. (1957). *Report on homosexual offences and prostitution*. HMSO, London.

Wollheim, R. (1959). Crime, sin and Mr. Justice Devlin. *Encounter*, 1 November, 38.

Wynn, A. and M. (1974). *Can family planning do more to reduce child poverty?* London.

18
Biological factors in the organization and expression of sexual behaviour[1]

Richard P. Michael and Doris Zumpe

INTRODUCTION

No single physical, chemical, educational, cultural, biological, or ethical factor is responsible for the expression of sex. On the contrary, the more complex the organism, the more numerous are the factors influencing the phenomenon. In some simple forms of motile, water-dwelling plants, the addition of a chemical to the medium causes the population to divide into two groups: those which attract and those which repel each other. This simple chemistry no longer holds in more complex forms; and in the human, powerful cultural as well as subtle educational influences may be just as important in determining sex role and orientation as are the genetic and endocrine factors.

Our task here is to trace the increasing complexity in both phylogenetic and ontogenetic terms. But as it would be too ambitious to do so in any systematic fashion here, we propose to take illustrative examples of some of the factors to be dealt with, and progress from simple to more complex levels of organization as one ascends the evolutionary scale. The aim is to place human sexual activity and its variations in the setting of a more general biological background.

PHYLOGENETIC ASPECTS

In primitive forms of life—viruses, bacteria, and protozoa—reproduction is carried on by binary fission, the organism simply divides into two. There is no sexual differentiation, no morphological males and females, and offspring are exact copies of their parents. In metazoa, this asexual division can be supplemented by a stage in which two cells first fuse in order later to multiply. Neither cell is capable of reproduction without the stimulus of prior fusion, and the characteristic union of gametes to form a zygote, with some parthenogenetic exceptions, is found in all but the most simple life forms. It opens the possibility of inherited variations and permits evolutionary development in place of the endless replication of progeny that are identical with parents, that is, cloning. The physical basis of inheritance is the

[1] The original work reported in this chapter was supported by US Public Health Service Grant MH 19506 to the first author.

genes, and sexual characteristics, like all others, have a genetic basis; this is equally true for both morphological and behavioural characteristics. Sexual characteristics, as Darwin emphasized, are thus subjected to the selection pressures that mold the process of evolution.

We give two examples of how a behavioural trait can lead to the isolation of a species and to the maintenance of species isolation. The first comes from the work of Crossly, cited by Tinbergen (1959), in which an artificial selection pressure resulted in sexual isolation within the laboratory. Using the technique of micro-evolution with winged and non-winged mutants of the fruitfly (*Drosophila melanogaster*) and antihybrid selection to 40 generations, decreased hybrid matings and increased homogamic matings occurred. This was due to a mating preference which developed gradually so that females became more sensitive to and repelled strange males while males became more sensitive to the repelling movements of strange females. The development of reproductive isolation in this case was due to the selection of specific sexual behavioural characteristics. Similarly, it has been shown in the laboratory that the lack of interbreeding between sympatric species of poecilid fishes (the guppy and relatives), which are closely related and never show hybridization in nature, depends on a strong mating preference shown mainly by the females, and this accounts for the lack of interbreeding. We have no reliable data on whether or not behavioural characteristics and preferences operating over evolutionary time may have played a part in isolating the races of man. But it is not impossible because in places on the earth where environmental factors are uniform, peoples with quite distinct morphological traits exist and thrive.

In reviewing the determinants of human sexuality, the schema of Money and the Hampsons (Money *et al.* 1955) is very useful: (1) genetic sex and chromosomal sex; (2) gonadal sex; (3) hormonal sex; (4) internal accessory structures; (5) external genital appearance and somatotype; (6) assigned sex and rearing (social learning); and (7) psychological orientation and gender role; but we do not follow this schema fully here.

GENETIC AND CHROMOSOMAL FACTORS

Much experimental work on inheritance is done with *Drosophila*, and the view has developed that the action of the genes in sex determination is expressed through inter-chromosomal balances, including factors in the sex chromosomes as well as in the autosomes. Changes in chromosome numbers resulting from mutations or breeding experiments are associated with the abrupt emergence of new sexual types. In this, sex determination does not differ from that of all other physical characteristics. McClung (1902) first suggested that a single chromosome might be responsible for the differentiation of fertile eggs into males or females. In addition to the homomorphic pairs of autosomes, the number being specific for the species, a common arrangement in male mammals is a pairing of single X and single Y sex chromosomes. In female mammals, two X sex chromosomes are present: the females being homogametic for sex, whereas the males are heterozygous, and this was established for the human by Painter (1921). In certain species of fishes, amphibia, and birds, the situation is reversed, the female being XY and the male XX, usually designated ZW and ZZ to avoid confusion. Thus, the basic somatotype in each vertebrate class is homozygous for sex. The theory that sex determination results from a quantitative interaction of genes present in separate chromosomes is due to the work of Morgan *et al.* (1925) working with *Drosophila*. Every grade of sex reversal and of intersexuality can be produced by subspecies crosses resulting in different combinations of genes. In fishes and amphibia, the addition of hormones to the medium during development, as well as their injection into the eggs of birds, results in marked morphological changes and sex reversals of the gonads themselves (Kozelka and Gallagher 1934); but the phenotypic modifications are independent of the chromosomal constitution of cells, which retain their original genotypes. Among mammals, intersex states can also be induced by hormonal manipulations; of particular importance in this regard was the work of Keller and Tandler (1916) and Lillie (1916, 1917) on the freemartin condition in cattle (an intersex condition occurring in one of a pair of dizygotic twin calves, the other twin always being a normal male), and will be discussed later. Sex is now regarded as a dimorphism into male and female types rather than as an entity or force in itself. The mammalian schema for sex determination is far from universal and there are many exceptions to it in other vertebrate taxa, nor is it necessarily a once-in-a-lifetime event. The teleosts (bony fishes) have many different reproductive forms: some are testis-bearing males and ovary-bearing females in the usual way, while others are sequentially hermaphroditic and their gonads change sex according to the social context. If a male blue-headed wrasse dies or is removed from a group experimentally, the dominant female undergoes sex reversal, which includes, within the next week or so, a marked male-type colour change: the transformed female which originally produced eggs thereafter produces sperm (Zumpe 1963 and unpublished observations; Warner 1984). Thus, sex reversal from functional females to functional males (certain wrasses) and vice versa (anemone fish) has been observed in the species of some 22 fish families. True hermaphroditism in which one individual simultaneously bears both male and female gonads also occurs in fish with low population densities. Non-social environmental factors such as temperature can also be crucial. In certain reptiles, a species of gecko (Bull 1987) for example, and in the alligator (Ferguson and Joanen 1983), eggs incubating at high temperatures (above 32 °C) result in male hatchlings while at lower temperatures (below 30.5 °C) female alligators are produced. These interesting sex reversals do not involve changes in the chromosomal constitution. Several species of whiptail lizards consist entirely of genetic females which reproduce parthogenetically. Their ancestry as sexually reproducing species is still in evidence because courtship and copulatory behaviour by other females (which resembles that typical of males) facilitates ovarian development and increases the number of viable eggs produced (Crew 1987).

Among mammals, intersex states are not infrequent. The classic example, the calf freemartin, is not primarily genetically determined, but goat hermaphrodites, ranging in phenotype from near-normal males to near-normal females, are due to a recessive autosomal gene acting in the female zygote (Asdell 1936; Kondo 1955), so that homozygous embryos simultaneously develop male and female characteristics with the persistence of both male and female internal structures, a condition with particular interest for intersex states in the human. Using colchicine-induced metaphase arrest, it was demonstrated in tissue cultures of human somatic cells that there are 22 paired autosomes together with X and Y sex chromosomes (Tjio and Levan 1956). It is extraordinary that, prior to this date, 48 and not 46 had been regarded as the normal human karyotype! Sexual dimorphism occurs generally within the nuclei of human somatic cells (Barr and Bertram 1949; Moore and Barr 1955) as well as in those of monkey, cat, dog, ferret, and less reliably in lagomorphs and rodents. A granule of nuclear chromatin about one micron in diameter, the Barr body, can be identified adjacent to the inner surface of the nuclear membrane in up to 80 per cent of the somatic nuclei of females but in only 10 per cent of the cell nuclei of males. This simple test has high reliability and can be carried out on buccal smears, but in difficult cases full karyotyping must be carried out. The theory of X inactivation (Lyon 1972) is that in normal females one X chromosome is inactivated and this equalizes the expression of X-linked characteristics in males and females, and studies of aneuploid states have shown there is always one less Barr body than X chromosomes.

The current view holds that the Y chromosome, or part of it, carries the genetic information needed to develop a testis. Another view is that the information is also carried elsewhere, but that the Y chromosome is needed for its activation. The hypothesis of a single testis-determining gene or factor (TDF) in the human on the short arm of the Y chromosome, which is responsible for the development of maleness, has received strong support from the isolation of the sex-determining region of the Y chromosome (*SRY*) in humans (Sinclair *et al.* 1990). The amino acid sequence encoded by these genes indicates that the proteins function as transcription factors to activate unidentified genes nearer to the testis-determining gene in the pathway towards testis formation (Lovell-Badge 1993). These act fast and early during a brief critical period in development, rather like a switch (McLaren 1988), to cause testis differentiation; otherwise an ovary develops by default. A corresponding gene *Sry* has now been cloned from mice (Gubbay *et al.* 1990) which does indeed induce testis formation experimentally, so TDF and *SRY/Sry* appear to be closely similar if not identical. Others have postulated that the testis-determining pathway requires a number of related genes acting in sequence (Eicher and Washburn 1986). Furthermore, *SRY* is present in both sexes and is clearly not all-powerful (Tiersch *et al.* Wachtel 1991; Mittwoch 1992). These more recent developments have replaced the view that weak histocompatibility antigens (H-Y antigens) play the primary role in human male sex determination.

ILLUSTRATIVE CLINICAL SYNDROMES

There are four major clinical syndromes associated with sex chromosome aneuploidy which will be briefly described: Klinefelter's syndrome (47,XXY), the 47,XYY syndrome, trisomy X, and Turner's syndrome (45, XO). In Klinefelter's syndrome (Klinefelter *et al.* Albright 1942), which is usually diagnosed in adolescence, there are small, hard, functionless scrotal testes, and a eunuchoid habitus with male differentiation of the genital tract, gynaecomastia, sparse facial hair, and a high-pitched voice. Patients are infertile, have a somewhat low IQ, learning disabilities, and poor psychosocial adjustment. There are several types of the condition, and the incidence is about 1 in 2000 live births. In the XXXY variant, more severe dysplasia occurs, suggesting that the additional X further antagonizes the action of the Y. Patients with the 47, XYY syndrome are unusually tall and, while the incidence is about 1 in 1000 male births, it is reported that 3 per cent of men in prison and mental hospital populations have the abnormality (Jacobs *et al.* 1968). They have normal intelligence and no somatic abnormalities, but are thought to be more aggressive than normal, a view that is not endorsed by all authorities. Trisomy X (47, XXX) and the rarer tetrasomy condition (48, XXXX) occurs in females who are not phenotypically abnormal, but they are generally infertile and sometimes mentally retarded (IQ about 70). They are regarded as the female equivalent of Klinefelter's syndrome in the male. Turner's syndrome (45, XO and variants) is another genetically determined abnormal sexual state in the human female which further substantiates the feminizing effect of the X chromosome. Although the reproductive tract is female, there are streak gonads consisting only of connective tissue. There are no female puberty changes and no adult secondary sexual characteristics. There is a wide gradation of defects from the near-normal to syndromes associated with multiple congenital defects—abnormal skeletal development with short stature, neck webbing, heart defects, and mental deficiency (Bishop *et al.* 1960). The incidence of Turner's syndrome is about 1 in 5000 live female births, but there is a very high frequency of spontaneous abortion. These simple descriptions do not do justice to the many variations encountered. There are two additional syndromes in the human with normal chromosome complements which are important for our understanding of sexual differentiation. The first is an X-linked condition called the androgen insensitivity syndrome (Jacobs *et al.* 1959) (one in 20 000 live births), and the second is female pseudohermaphrodism, also called congenital adrenal hyperplasia, an autosomal recessive disorder of cortisol metabolism. In the androgen insensitivity syndrome (formerly testicular feminizing syndrome), although there is a normal male karyotype (46, XY), the androgen receptors in androgen-sensitive target tissues are not functional. The result is a normal female habitus and superficially normal female external genitalia, but the vagina is blind, there are no ovaries, no uterus, and no Fallopian tubes. Axillary and pubic hair is sparse or absent, but the testes are present either intra-abdominally, or in the inguinal canal and sometimes in the labia. The testes secrete androgens but since the receptors are unresponsive, feminization proceeds in the direction of the basic female somatotype; hence the term 'ball-bearing females' which is sometimes applied. Congenital adrenal hyperplasia comprises a group of some six autosomal recessive disorders, the locus being on the short arm of chromosome 6, which result in enzyme failures in the adrenal cortex (1 in 12 000 live births). In the most common form, there is a deficiency of C_{21}-hydroxylase and defective hydroxylation of 17-hydroxyprogesterone which blocks cortisol synthesis. This results in a loss of negative feedback to the pituitary gland and hyper-secretion of ACTH occurs with an over-production of adrenal androgens and a consequent virilization of genetic females before and after birth; the rare salt-losing form can be lethal if undiagnosed. The high androgen levels do not prevent normal development of the uterus and Fallopian tubes. Effects are relatively mild in genetic males. Both the androgen insensitivity syndrome and congenital adrenal hyperplasia throw considerable light on human psychosexual development and will be considered later.

That sexual behaviour possesses an hereditary basis is clearly evident from the experimental development of strain differences by selective breeding. Grunt and Young (1952) showed that the behavioural differences between low- and high-drive strains of male guinea pigs is in the soma and independent of the amount of androgen administered after castration. Similarly, differences in the sexual behaviour of different inbred strains of female guinea pigs persist after ovariectomy and the injection of oestradiol and progesterone (Goy and Young 1957). The inherited basis of low sexual activity in certain strains of laboratory rats was established by Craig *et al.* (1954), and similar observations have been made in different breeds of farm animals. The inherited basis of any behaviour pattern in the human is difficult to ascertain but, in agreement with Kinsey, the incidence of overt homosexuality has been confirmed at about 4 per cent in an adult, college-educated, white male population (Gebhard 1972). A family study of 50 predominantly hetersexual and 50 predominantly homosexual men has shown that hetersexual men have as many homosexual brothers as predicted from the natural prevalence data, while homosexual men have four times as many homosexual or bisexual brothers as predicted (Pillard and Weinrich 1986). There were no significant differences of any kind for females. These results certainly do not exclude a role for potent environmental influences operating within a family, but they do suggest that male and female homosexuality are different traits, and that the former has a familial and perhaps a genetic basis: this latter possibility has now received support from studies on homosexual heritability in mono- and dizygotic twins (Bailey and Pillard 1991). Recently, DNA-linkage studies in the human (Hamer *et al.* 1993) have helped uncover an association between adult sexual orientation and inheritance in some families of homosexual men. Because of increased rates of homosexuality in the maternal uncles and male cousins of probands, maternal transmission by the X chromosome has been implicated: the genetic loading was highly statistically significant in the 114 families studied. This work needs replication and confirmation, but it appears to be an important first step in locating to a region containing several hundred genes those which may contribute to homosexual orientation in this subpopulation.

EMBRYOLOGICAL DEVELOPMENT: SEX REVERSALS WITHIN THE GONADS AND GONADAL SEX

Experimental sex reversals of the gonads themselves have been possible in fishes, amphibia, and birds. Working with amphibia, Burns (1925) grafted two embryos together so that they developed a common circulation and were in parabiotic union; this resulted in the masculinization of the female embryo. The gonadal primordia (Humphrey 1928, 1942), as well as the gonads themselves, can be grafted, and the embryos bearing these orthotopic transplants may then be reared to maturity together with the donor embryos so their sex can be established with certainty. In the mid 1930s, when pure hormone preparations became available, almost complete morphological transformations were produced in birds by hormone injections into incubating eggs: the chick (Willier 1933) and duckling (Wolff and Haffen 1952) have been most investigated. The situation is complicated in birds by a lateral asymmetry, particularly of the female genital tract in which the left ovary is large while the right ovary is rudimentary. The basic somatotype in birds is male, the opposite of the mammal, and removal of the chick's left ovary causes the rudimentary right one to develop into an ovotestis spontaneously. Injection of oestrogens into incubating eggs transform the testis, particularly the left, into an ovary, while they have little effect on ovaries (Dantchakoff 1935; Willier *et al.* 1935). Androgens have less effect on the embryonic ovary than do estrogens on the embryonic testis. In birds, then, the ovary is more dominant than the testis, but gonadal primordia differentiate autonomously in tissue culture according to genotype.

Experimental sex reversals of the gonads in mammals is more difficult. The young of certain marsupials are in a specially under-developed state at birth, they are accessible to hormone injections in the pouch, and sexual differentiation continues post-natally. Almost complete reversals have been produced in the North American opossum (*Didelphis viginiana*) by hormonal injections (Burns 1956). At the stage when the primitive gonad retains its bisexual potential, future testes can be transformed into ovotestes and ovaries by oestradiol administration from birth. This treatment suppresses testicular differentiation and enhances ovarian development, but if injections are delayed for only a few days after birth, they are without effect; the sensitive period has passed. In general, the administration of sex steroids to placental mammals during embryogenesis, although exerting major behavioural and morphological effects, does not transform the gonadal primordia themselves. The concept of a blood-borne agent produced by the gonads capable of controlling the sexual characteristics rested on the transplantation studies of Berthold (1849) in the cockerel. The work of Bouin and Ancel (1903) extended this concept to sexual differentiation in the embryo. The hormonal control of sexual differentiation during embryogenesis received great impetus from the studies of Keller and Tandler (1916) and of Lillie (1916, 1917) on the freemartin condition in the calf. The external genitalia and mammary glands of the freemartin are female but there may be an enlarged penis-like clitoris. Internally, male duct structures are usually wellpreserved while female duct structures are rudimentary, and the gonads are either sterile testes or poorly developed ovotestes. The freemartin is genetically female and chromatin-positive. The essential prerequisite for this condition is an anastomotic communication between the placental circulations of the twins, and the extent of this vascular interconnection determines the extent of virilization. These studies led to the view that embryonic hormones or similar morphogenetic substances could control sexual differentiation during embryonic development. But although the gonad may be extensively transformed in the naturally occurring freemartin condition, it appears to be difficult to achieve this experimentally in placental mammals. Pregnant females have been treated with hormones at different times during gestation in order to influence the course of sexual differentiation in the embryo. In guinea pig (Dantchakoff 1936), rat (Greene 1942), rabbit (Jost 1953), and monkey (Wells and van Wagenen 1954), although treatment failed to transform the gonads themselves, marked changes are produced in the accessory structures and in the external genitalia, particularly, masculinization of genetically female fetuses.

The chromosomes and the genes carried by them determine, in a way that is still not fully understood, the sex of the primordial germ cells. These have been identified in the human embryo 3–4 weeks post-conception, and are thought to originate extra-embryonically in the endoderm of the yolk sac near the allantoic origin whence they migrate under the influence of stage-specific embryonic antigens via the wall of the hindgut through the dorsal mesentery into the genital ridges on the anterior mesial side of the mesonephros (Witschi 1963). The primitive gonads develop from mesodermal coelomic epithelium, mesenchymal elements in the genital ridge, as well as from other components, and come to contain some 1000 primordial germ cells which have migrated from their site of origin. At this stage (about 40 days of gestation), they still possess a bipotential capacity which is independent of their chromosomal constitution. In the human, testis organization begins about 6–7 weeks after fertilization (45–50 days of gestation) while ovarian organization occurs considerably later, about 12 weeks after fertilization. In future males, through the brief but critical action of the testis-determining factor (TDF) on the Y chromosome, primordial spermatogonia and primordial Sertoli cells aggregate more centrally in the sex cords (which develop *in situ*) of the gonadal ridge to form primitive testes. In genetic females, the cortical region of the genital ridge develops more conspicuously as oogonia begin to develop within it while the medullary part regresses, resulting in the formation of primitive ovaries. The future Sertoli cells may secrete factors which suppress cortical development in males and, by about 60 days post-fertilization, they secrete Müllerian inhibiting factors (MIF) which suppress development of the Müllerian ducts (Josso and Picard 1986). Shortly thereafter, primitive Leydig cells in the interstitium of the testes proliferate rapidly and begin to secrete testosterone (about 63–65 days gestation): this causes differentiation and development of the Wolffian duct system, the urogenital sinus, and external genitalia. Concentrations of testosterone reach 200–600 ng/dl in human fetal plasma at 16 weeks' gestation; remarkably, this is in the range for adult human males. In fetal male cynomolgus monkeys at about 122 days' gestation, plasma testosterone levels (mean about 570 ng/dl) are also within the range for normal adult males but, in contrast, levels in fetal females remain very low throughout (mean about 34 ng/dl) (Michael *et al.* 1992). One needs to emphsize again that the ovarian developmental pathway occurs by default in mammals in the absence of the Y chromosome and in the absence of any hormonal influences. Thus, ovarian development will normally occur in the human in the absence of any genetic programming because the basic somatotype is female, provided that germ cells are present in the genital ridge. In the absence, then, of the Y chromosome and of the testis-determining switch, the primordial germ cells enlarge into oogonia. These replicate vigorously during fetal life, and some 6–7 million are present by mid-gestation. None are formed after birth, when numbers diminish rapidly, and stocks are exhausted at menopause. Because the embryonic ovary does not differentiate until several weeks after the testes have differentiated, its bipotential capacity persists for longer. In contrast to the testis, steroidogenesis by the ovary is not evident during fetal life; some authorities relate this to the maternal production of steroids during embryogenesis. Spermatogonia, unlike oogonia, do not develop further during fetal life; their proliferation is delayed for several years until pre-puberty, and their production continues into old age. Whereas differentiation and further development of the female somatotype during fetal life occurs in the absence of any embryonic hormones, all differentiation of the male fetus depends on the secretion of testosterone by the Leydig cells of the primitive testis. This was first demonstrated conclusively for rats and rabbits by the work of Jost (1947), who showed that removal of the pituitary and of the gonads in both sexes resulted in the anhormonal development of a female somatotype and accessory sexual system. When anterior pituitary tissue from adult male rats was grafted under the cut end of the pituitary stalk of hypophysectomized females, the transplants maintained oestrous cycles and some females even became pregnant (Harris and Jacobsohn 1952). This demonstrated that male pituitary tissue under the influence of a female hypothalamus could secrete gonadotropins in the cyclic female rather than in the tonic male pattern. These and other data demonstrated that the anterior pituitary gland is not sexually differentiated in the adult and possesses a bisexual potential.

EMBRYOLOGICAL DEVELOPMENT: DIFFERENTIATION OF THE ACCESSORY SEXUAL STRUCTURES

The embryonic sex ducts are derived from the primitive nephric system while the lower part of the genital tract together with its out-growths are derived from the urogenital sinus, itself originating from the primitive hindgut. In the male embryo, the duct of the primitive kidney or mesonephros becomes the mesonephric or Wolffian duct and eventually the epididymis, the vas deferens, seminal vesicles, and male urethra. In the female embryo, the paramesonephric or Müllerian duct develops as a furrow in the thickened lateral portion of the urogenital ridge, and eventually becomes the uterus and uterine tubes. The early development of these accessory structures during about the first 6–7 weeks is independent of genetic sex and occurs while a bisexual potential still exists. The somewhat later development depends on the differentiation of the gonads themselves into embryonic testes and ovaries. In males, the primitive Sertoli cells secrete a glycoprotein (MIF) which inhibits any further development of the Müllerian system, and just a few days thereafter the Leydig cells begin to secrete testosterone which causes rapid development of the Wolffian system. If the fetal testis is removed unilaterally, the Müllerian duct develops on that side, but regression occurs on the opposite side where the testis remains *in situ*; so the effect of the fetal testis on duct formation is a local one (Jost 1971). *In vitro* experiments with organ cultures confirmed that effects are independent of the influence of hormones derived from the maternal circulation (Jost and Bozic 1951; Wolff 1953). The external genitalia and lower parts of the male and female tracts derived from the urogenital sinus are sensitive to the administration of hormones, provided this is done at the appropriate stage of development, and in the human they are completely differentiated by 16 weeks. Androgens administered experimentally to female fetuses, either directly or via the maternal circulation, result in the suppression of vaginal development, prostatic hypertrophy, and external masculinization, but only partial and incomplete suppression of Müllerian duct structures for which the specific secretions of Sertoli cells are needed. The administration of oestrogens to male fetuses produces some degree of vaginal development and external feminization. The effects of castrating male fetuses prevents the development of male duct structures while the same procedure in females has little effect. The genital tubercle, the simple primordium present in both sexes from which the penis or clitoris develops, is itself highly susceptible to modification by hormone administration.

SENSITIVE PERIODS DURING PRENATAL DEVELOPMENT

Much of what has been stated already concerning the effects of hormones during development has referred to the induction of structural or somatic modifications in the sexual apparatus. These must in themselves affect the behavioural capacities of the individual: the absence of a vagina or the induction of a phallus must profoundly alter the behavioural potential. We have seen that there are developmental stages during fetal life, for example, when bipotential capacities are lost and when tissues attain an especial sensitivity to hormonal effects. It has now become clear that hormones can exert equally profound effects on behavioural mechanisms, particularly the neural mechanisms, which underlie the expression of sexual orientation and libido; and for these mechanisms too, the concept of sensitive or critical periods has emerged. Depending on the species and gestational length, a sensitive period may be confined to fetal life or extend, usually briefly, into the neonatal period, but in either case the effects on behaviour are not usually expressed until much later on when sexual maturity is reached. W. C. Young and co-workers pioneered experiments in which pregnant guinea pigs were treated with intramuscular injections of testosterone propionate between 30 and 65 days of gestation. Female pups showed clear evidence of external masculinization and, in some cases, vaginas were absent, while Wolffian duct structures were hypertrophied. Male littermates were unaffected and the treated mothers showed no evidence of masculinization unless treatment was continued until after delivery of the young (Diamond and Young 1963). When such females reached maturity, they failed to show normal ovarian function and, of considerable interest, their capacity to show normal female sexual behaviour was much reduced. There was a decrease in the number of positive tests for oestrous behaviour, a decrease in the duration of oestrus and in the duration for which the maximum lordosis response could be elicited. These females were said to be defeminized but they were in addition masculinized, and this was indicated by a marked increase in the numbers of male-like mounting attempts they made on receptive females (Phoenix *et al.* 1959). These behavioural modifications were thought to depend on changes in brain function, since administration of the appropriate regimen of oestrogen and progesterone to ovariectomized animals when adult failed to restore behaviour to normal. It was also noteworthy that females androgenized during fetal development also showed increased responsiveness to androgens in adulthood—to a level comparable to that of normal males. Permanent effects were obtained in guinea pigs only when treatment was given before birth, the critical period probably being the middle trimester, and no permanent effects on adult sexuality resulted if treatment was delayed until the 50–65th day of the 68 day gestation, or if it was given after birth. In the rat, with its shorter 21.5-day gestation, the critical period for early hormone-induced effects extends for a week or so after birth: a single injection of testosterone propionate (0.1–1.2 mg) to female rat pups between birth and 5 days of age produced permanent infertility.

After puberty, these testosterone-treated females developed polycystic ovaries, failed to ovulate and did not show oestrous behaviour with active males (Segal and Johnson 1959; Barraclough 1961; Barraclough and Gorski 1961). Comparable findings were reported in oestrogen-treated males (Harris and Levine 1965), 50 per cent of which no longer showed any signs of male sexual behaviour in adulthood. Although the critical period in the rat extends post-natally, no irreversible behavioural changes resulted when treatment was delayed until 20 days after birth, and the overall picture is closely similar in rat and guinea pig.

Attention has been drawn to the analogy between the critical periods for hormone action on the morphogenesis of the genital tract and the critical period for hormone action on the neural tissues mediating the eventual expression of adult sexual behaviour. Harris has referred to *inductive* effects on the undifferentiated brain and to the *excitatory* effects on behaviour in adult life. Young has put this more usefully by contrasting their *organizational* and *activational* roles. The notion that embryonic hormones influence sexual differentiation of the brain, especially of the hypothalamus, stems from the observations of Everett *et al.* (1949) who were mainly concerned with the differentiation of cyclic patterns of gonadotropin secretion that characterizes the female mammal compared with the continuous or tonic pattern of secretion that characterizes the male (pulsatile LH release in the male was not then known). Although Pfeiffer (1936) had demonstrated in a series of beautiful grafting experiments in rats that males, castrated at birth and transplanted with an ovary when adult, could ovulate and develop corpora lutea, that is, they could produce a surge of LH (as in normal females), he attributed this to changes in the hypophysis rather than to changes in the hypothalamus. We now know from pituitary grafting experiments (Harris and Jacobsohn 1952) that the pituitary is not sexually differentiated and takes its secretory pattern from the sex of the hypothalamus to which it is juxtaposed.

The behavioural effects of hormones on the non-human primate fetus have been investigated systematically in a long series of studies initiated by W. C. Young. By the use of testosterone propionate and procedures similar to those of Wells and van Wagenen (1954), fetal female rhesus monkeys were made pseudohermaphroditic by the masculinizing effects of testosterone reaching them via the placental circulation. Beginning about the day 40 of gestation, testosterone propionate was injected daily for varying periods of from 25 to 50 days (Young *et al.* 1964; Goy 1968). The external genitalia were masculinized and resembled those of a male neonate except for an empty scrotum. The vagina was absent and menstruation occurred via the phallus when the somewhat delayed puberty was reached. The ontogeny of behaviour patterns after birth was observed very carefully for many years. During the first year of life, when comparisons were made between normal males and normal females on the one hand and female pseudohermaphrodites on the other, the frequencies of rough-and-tumble play, chasing play, threatening, and mounting by pseudohermaphrodites were intermediate between those of normal males and normal females. Unlike hormonal effects in fetal rodents, which appear permanent and irreversible, those in the longer-lived rhesus monkey become less obvious with increasing maturity. Between 5 and 11 years of age, gonadectomized pseudohermaphrodites tested with two normal females simultaneously showed increases in masculine sexual behaviour such as mounting when treated with testosterone propionate, as did neonatally gonadectomized, testosterone-treated normal males but not normal females: moreover, levels of behaviour were intermediate between those of the males and normal females (Pomerantz *et al.* 1988). When 15 years or older, however, the behaviour of gonadectomized pseudohermaphroditic monkeys, treated with either oestradiol benzoate or testosterone propionate and paired either with normal females (Phoenix and Chambers 1982) or with normal males (Phoenix *et al.* 1983), more closely resembled the behaviour of similarly treated normal females than that of similarly treated normal males: they rarely mounted a receptive female partner but, although lacking a vagina, were receptive to and mounted by males. It is thought that masculinization of the genital tract in fetal female rhesus monkeys exposed to testosterone may occur earlier than the masculinization of behaviour (Goy *et al.* 1988). Although some uncertainties remain concerning the persistence into adult life of the behavioural changes observed during the first year in these experimental pseudohermaphrodites, non-human primate studies have great importance because of the broader perspective they have provided by extending the findings in rodents to a species in which experiential factors and social learning play a much larger role. More recent work with the non-human primate fetus has addressed the question of the developing brain as a target for embryonic hormones (Michael and Rees 1986; Michael *et al.* 1992). Male and female macaque fetuses at around 120 days gestation (gestation length 163–168 days) were gonadectomized *in utero*, the pregnancies were stablized and maintained for about a week thereafter, when tritiated testosterone (^{3}H-T) was injected directly into the fetus. One hour later, brain and genital tract samples were examined by autoradiography and by high-performance liquid chromatography (hplc). Autoradiographic analyses clearly demonstrated the presence of receptors in neuronal nuclei of the medical preoptic area, lateral part of the hypothalamic ventromedial nucleus, arcuate nucleus, premammillary nuclei, and in the cortical and medial amygdaloid nuclei (Michael *et al.* 1989): all these brain regions have been implicated in the regulation of sexual behaviour in adult mammals. Unlike autoradiograms which can precisely locate the site and distribution of radioactivity, hplc analyses determine the chemical identity of radioactive metabolites in tissue samples. In the fetal primate brain, as in the adult, hplc analyses of fractions containing cell nuclei showed that the majority of the ^{3}H-T administered was converted to ^{3}H-oestradiol (^{3}H-E$_2$) by aromatization. In the male genital tract, on the other hand, the majority of the ^{3}H-T administered was converted to ^{3}H-dihydrotestosterone (^{3}H-DHT) by 5α-reduction. Hypothalamic nuclear concentrations of ^{3}H-E$_2$ in intact male fetuses were 62 per cent lower than those of intact female fetuses, and fetal gonadectomy completely abolished the difference in steroid uptake between males and females (Michael *et al.* 1992). This supported the view that the hypothalamus of the normal male fetus at this stage of gestation is heavily loaded with oestradiol derived by aromatization of the testosterone produced by fetal Leydig cells. These data indicate that masculinization of the fetal primate brain may be induced not by testosterone but by its oestrogenic metabolite: this paradoxical finding differs radically from the earlier view that testosterone *per se* is the masculinizing hormone. The relation of these endocrine–brain interactions to the development of sexually dimorphic behaviour patterns remains unknown.

In the congenital adrenal virilizing syndrome diagnosed in neonatal girls, both the neural and genital tissues are exposed to abnormally high concentrations of adrenal androgens before birth, and certainly a pseudohermaphrodite condition results which should be immediately corrected by surgery of the external genitalia and cortisone replacement treatment. Careful studies with matched control groups using a range of different behavioural criteria, along with follow-ups, have shown that the sexual orientation (gender-identity, gender-role) of these girls is not substantially changed in the male direction (Ehrhardt *et al.* 1968; Money and Ehrhardt 1972; Ehrhardt and Baker 1974); they do not have gender-identity disorders and become normal wives and mothers. Nevertheless, other behaviours were masculinized to some degree: in childhood, girls with this syndrome were regarded as tomboys and some showed high energy expenditure levels in rough outdoor play with a preference for boys over girls as playmates; however, in more recent studies the high energy expenditure pattern has not been fully validated (Dittman *et al.* 1990). Despite early androgen exposure, these girls clearly identified themselves, and were identified by others, as female and their behaviour was socially acceptable and not regarded as abnormal. The human differs from most other mammals in that puberty is delayed for many years, and perhaps this provides a greater opportunity for learning and psychosocial factors to modify hormonal influences occurring during intra-uterine life.

It is well established that testosterone is converted into 5α-dihydrotestosterone (DHT) in the peripheral tissues of the male genital tract. A genetic abnormality occurs in normal 46, XY males with deficiency of the enzyme 5α-reductase as a consequence of which DHT is lacking (Walsh *et al.* 1974; Imperato-McGinley *et al.* 1974). This condition is inherited as an autosomal recessive attributed to a founder effect in several somewhat isolated island populations in different parts of the world, the most well-known being villages in the south-west Dominican Republic, and in the Sambia tribe of Papua (Herdt and Davidson 1988). Affected children are brought up as girls with a small hypospadic phallus, blind vaginal pouch, a bifid scrotum, and the ejaculatory ducts open into a urogenital sinus which itself opens on the perineum. All Wolffian duct derivatives are normal, while Müllerian duct derivatives are absent. There are normal testes either in the inguinal region or in the labio-scrotal folds, but no prostatic development (which depends on DHT). Although these individuals are reared as girls, as the number of affected families has increased, the local population has come to recognize that they will change into boys at puberty, when plasma testosterone increases into the normal adult male range; nevertheless, DHT levels remain very low. After puberty, virilization occurs, the voice deepens, the muscle mass increases notably, and the penis enlarges considerably. There is no adolescent facial acne, no prostatic enlargement, the body hair is sparse, and male temporal baldness patterns do not develop. It is clear that DHT is needed for the pre-natal development of normal male genitalia; but the low levels of DHT do not preclude the massive somatic changes induced by testosterone in these individuals at puberty. The majority of males are sterile because, although penile insertion can be achieved, ejaculation via the penis is impossible without surgical correction. Although raised for the most part as girls, they change to a male gender-identity and -role after puberty without, according to the earlier reports (Imperato-McGinley *et al.* 1979), any major psychological impairment. This view has now been challenged (Ehrhardt 1985; Herdt and Davidson 1988), and some authorities feel that these young people are subjected to intense social and cultural pressures before and during puberty which distorts the natural development of their core gender-identity; this is thought to be established normally during the first 2–3 years of life (Hampson *et al.* 1956).

IATROGENIC EFFECTS OF HORMONAL SUBSTANCES *IN UTERO*

There are two iatrogenic conditions which deserve attention. In the first of these, synthetic progestins, alone or in combination with oestrogens, were administered to women either for the purpose of pregnancy testing or for the treatment of threatened abortion early in pregnancy, and varying degrees of impairment in the genitals of male offspring were reported (Courrier and Jost 1942; Aarskog 1979). Seventeen cases of pseudohermaphrodism in children of mothers receiving 17-α-ethinyltestosterone for threatened abortion during the early weeks of gestation were described by Wilkins (Wilkins *et al.* 1958). A further study of 70 cases reported external masculinization (masculinized clitoris and some degree of labial fusion) of female infants whose mothers had been given both 17-α-ethinyltestosterone and 17-α-ethinyl-19-nortestosterone orally, either alone or combined with oestrogens, during gestation (Wilkins 1960). In a study of 10 daughters of progestin-treated mothers, tomboyish traits were exhibited when young, but little abnormal sexual behaviour was found at follow-up when adult (Ehrhardt and Money 1967; Money and Ehrhardt 1972). The second iatrogenic condition concerns pseudohermaphrodism in the male children of mothers given diethylstilboestrol (DES) orally during pregnancy (Kaplan 1959). DES was introduced as the first powerful orally active oestrogen in 1938 and its obstetrical use occurred mostly in the 1940–60s. The unforseen problems associated with its use will resolve in time, but the lessons should not be forgotten. Since DES is a stilbene (not a steroid), it is less bound by sex hormone-binding globulin in maternal blood and therefore more readily enters the fetus where its low affinity for human α-fetoprotein in fetal plasma results in greater entry into the fetal brain where it is metabolically active. We know from autoradiographic and hplc studies in which ^{3}H-DES was injected directly into nonhuman primate fetuses that it localizes in the nuclei of neurones in the hypothalamus, preoptic area, and amygdala (but not in the cerebral cortex) at about 120 days of gestation (Michael and Bonsall 1990): all are limbic system sites thought to be involved in the control of sexual behaviour. A report by Herbst *et al.* (1972) describing vaginal and cervical cell dysplasia or adenosis (clear cell adenocarcinoma) in the daughters of mothers given DES raised widespread public health concerns. The now adult daughters became afraid of cancer, and several follow-up studies were conducted. One of the more comprehensive (Ehrhardt *et al.* 1985) suggested that some of these 'DES daughters' showed increased levels of bisexual and homosexual behaviour, and were regarded as 'less maternal' than controls, but about 75 per cent were more or less completely heterosexual. In another follow-up study on these women (Ehrhardt *et al.* 1989), there were no consistent differences in most domains of gender-role behaviour except for a decreased orientation towards parenting compared with controls. The authors were cautious about their results in daughters, and results in sons have been even more tenuous. Several of the early reports of semen and anatomical abnormalities including cryptorchidism, testicular hypoplasia, and hypospadias, as well as testicular cancer, have not been readily confirmed in more recent large-scale studies (Leary *et al.* 1984). Reinisch *et al.* (1991) reviewed 19 studies on the pre-natal effects in males and females of hormones administered to mothers during pregnancy. They found a potential for an *in utero* antiandrogenic effect on the fetus of both progesterone and progesterone-based synthetic progestins, resulting in some degree of later feminization or demasculinization of behaviour. But the results of different studies on different populations varied considerably, and effects were not robust. Although some of the offspring of DES-treated mothers have recently been successful in obtaining favourable judgments in court, the long-term biological consequences now seem to be milder than once was thought.

Particularly since the thalidomide crisis, we are much more alert than formerly to the sensitivity of the fetus to exposure to drugs taken by the mother during pregnancy. The fetal alcohol syndrome is now a well-recognized entity, but other abused or illicit drugs can readily cross the placenta including: nicotine, marijuana, cocaine, and the opiates. One thousand babies are born daily in the United States to addicted mothers. All these substances can reduce plasma testosterone in fetal male rats either by direct inhibition of testicular steroidogenesis or by disrupting the hypothalamic-pituitary-gonadal axis: the potential for demasculinization and incomplete defeminization of the human fetus is quite real, but hard evidence comes from laboratory studies in rodents (Ward 1992). Male rat pups that have been exposed to ethanol during gestation have lower testis weights and plasma testosterone levels than do controls (Kelce *et al.* 1989) and, in some cases, there are also effects on genital morphology: similar findings have been reported with nicotine, marijuana, and the opiates. Male rats from pregnant females fed ethanol showed double the lordosis response of controls when adult (Broida *et al.* 1988). Another aspect of the fetus' vulnerability concerns the role of maternal stress during pregnancy on the subsequent sexual behaviour of offspring. Again, the model is the pregnant rat, and the pre-natal stress syndrome (Ward 1972) is seen in the male offspring of mothers stressed during days 14–21 of gestation (23 days in this species). Female offspring are not affected. The syndrome comprises variable feminization (high levels of lordosis) and demasculinization (low levels of ejaculation) in males when they become adult without any morphological effects on the genitalia. Other components of normal female proceptive behaviour such as hopping, darting, and ear-wiggling are lacking. Different types of stress are effective, including physical restraint, bright lights, over-crowding, and conditioned emotional responses (Herrenkohl and Whitney 1976; Ward 1977; Gotz and Dorner 1980). The demasculinization of behaviour induced during gestation by maternal stress cannot easily be reversed by testosterone treatment in adulthood. The pre-natal male rat normally experiences a brief two-day tostosterone surge on days 17–18 of gestation, but in stressed males, plasma testosterone levels are significantly lower than normal on days 18–19 due, it is thought, to an enzymatic inhibition of steroidogenesis (Orth *et al.* 1983). The absence of the testosterone surge on critical days of gestation was regarded as responsible for the behavioural syndrome (Ward and Weisz 1980). Dorner (1980) has postulated in a series of papers that the syndrome produced experimentally in rats might, when combined with genetic factors, help us understand the causes of certain types of homosexual behaviour in the human male (Dorner *et al.* 1980). But this view has been strongly contested (Gooren *et al.* 1990). In addition, there is good evidence that the control system initiating the luteinizing hormone surge in rats is quite different from that in primates, including man (Karsch *et al.* 1973), which further weakens Dorner's position. Neither the data nor the arguments are clear-cut, and they depend on cross-taxa inferences which are notoriously prone to error. Interest also developed in the masculinization of fetal females by their proximity to males *in utero* in multi-gestational species (Clemens 1974; Gandelman *et al.* 1977). Female rats can be masculinized both morphologically and behaviourally by testosterone released from fetal males situated in the same uterine horn (cf., freemartin condition in cattle), but this is probably due to the cephalad direction of vascular flow in the horn (Meisel and Ward 1981): it occurs when male fetuses are positioned more caudally than the female, and is not the result of contiguity as such. The validity of some of the earlier reports in mice has been questioned, but different strains were used in the different studies (Simon and Cologer-Clifford 1991).

SENSITIVE PERIODS DURING POST-NATAL DEVELOPMENT

The concept of periods of special sensitivity to events occurring after birth is of importance in the quite separate fields of animal behaviour and psychoanalysis. While hormonal or chemical changes affecting the internal environment have, as we have seen, very great importance before birth, the effects of early experiences on the developing organism may have equally profound effects in the neonatal period. This is illustrated by the sensitive period which characterizes the imprinting phenomenon, first discovered and described by Lorenz (1935, 1937). Imprinting describes a process by which certain stimuli to which an animal is exposed during a sensitive period in early post-natal development very rapidly and irreversibly determine the orientation or form of specific behavioural responses for the rest of life. It is thought that imprinting may be a specialized type of early learning occurring during a time of special vulnerability. It may be critical for the recognition of the species to which an individual belongs, for the formation of bonds between mother and young, and for the organization of later social behaviour including courtship and mating. The phenomenon has been studied most intensively in birds. In chickens, for example, filial imprinting (of young on to mother) occurs within about 13–16 hours of hatching, and during this time hatchlings will imprint on to any individual or conspicuous feature in the environment, including inanimate objects or an individual of a different species: all filial responses are subsequently directed towards that individual, in preference even to members of its own species. A critical period for primary socialization appears to be quite general and has been identified in birds as well as in some mammals (howling monkey, Carpenter 1934; dog, Scott 1962; mouse, Williams and Scott 1953). In several species, filial imprinting onto foster species results in long-term effects on sexual behaviour in adulthood, whereby courtship is preferentially directed towards the foster species rather than towards conspecifics. For example, male mallards hatched by a chicken and raised without visual access to their own species will sexually imprint on to chickens and when adult will attempt to court and mate with them (Schutz 1965a). Male woodducks raised together in the absence of other individuals will be imprinted on to male woodducks, and will attempt to copulate with other male woodducks throughout their adult lives; although they will mate with females if denied access to males for long enough, the preference for males remains (Schutz 1965*b*). They show male courtship and copulatory patterns but the object is another male, so this is a model for one type of homosexual behaviour. It was initially thought that filial and sexual imprinting were two expressions of one underlying process, but they are now regarded as two separate, partially overlapping processes, and sexual imprinting occurs somewhat later than filial imprinting (Bateson 1979, 1981; ten Cate 1989). The role of imprinting in modulating behaviour in mammals is less understood, but there are many examples of the acquisition of specific pieces of information during brief periods early in development. Patterns of colour, movement, and sound are important in birds, while olfactory cues are also important in mother–offspring recognition in mammals. In shrews (Zippelius 1972) and the precocial spiny mouse (Janus 1988), for example, filial imprinting during the first few days of life depends on maternal odour. In wolves and some breeds of dog (chow-chow), puppies will bond to the human caretaker up to about 6 weeks of age but not thereafter (Lorenz 1950), and if semi-feral farm cats do not bring their kittens into the house to meet people within a few weeks of birth, they remain forever wild and fearful of humans. Maternal imprinting (of mother on to newborn) differs from filial and sexual imprinting because it occurs in the mature adult and reappears with each parturition. For 1–2 hours after parturition in goats, an alien kid will be accepted (Klopfer and Klopfer 1968; Gubernick 1980). Women are also able to recognize their newborn babies by olfaction after 10–60 minutes exposure to them (Kaitz *et al.* 1987). We know little about these mechanisms in the human, but studies on rhesus monkeys (Harlow and Harlow 1962) have special importance because they were concerned with the maturation of social and sexual behaviour in a primate. Harlow and colleagues were concerned with what they called the 'affectional system' in the monkey, and gave particular emphasis to the infant's relationship with its mother. During the first year there is crude sexual play with peers and inappropriate sexual posturing, but infant males show earlier and more aggressive sexual behaviour than females and very rarely assume the female posture. Females, on the other hand, display both male and female patterns. Although these early expressions of sexual behaviour are fragmentary, they are very important for the subsequent development of adult sexuality, and this was demonstrated by Harlow's observations on infant primates reared in states of semi-isolation. Infants were separated from their mothers shortly after birth and were reared by hand without physical contact with other monkeys (Harlow and Zimmermann 1959). When mature, animals reared in this way showed a wide variety of grossly disturbed behaviours, including such autistic patterns as withdrawal, self-sucking, stereotyped movements, persistent masturbation, uncontrolled episodes of frenzy and self-mutilation, and an almost total loss of the capacity to socialize with other monkeys: they also lost the ability to engage in any form of sexual activity other than masturbation. Females had menstrual cycles and appeared to ovulate normally, but were quite unreceptive to male courtship approaches. Thus, they were rendered incapable of behaviour which involved relating to another member of the species. The importance for adequate adult sexual behaviour of early exposure to social experiences and to opportunities for cognitive rehearsals and learning could not be more convincingly demonstrated. The nature of the infant's relationship to its mother and siblings has, of course, engaged the interest of psychiatrists and psychoanalysts for many years, and it now seems self-evident that healthy infant- and child-rearing practices are essential for the development of normal heterosexuality; but one sometimes wonders.

STRUCTURAL DIFFERENCES IN THE BRAINS OF MALES AND FEMALES

Hypotheses about structural differences in the brains of male and female rats stemmed from the finding that the hypothalamus and related structures are programmed during development to initiate in the female a preovulatory surge of luteinizing hormone (LH) which is lacking in the male (Harris and Campbell 1966; Barraclough 1967). In a pioneering effort at the ultrastructural level, Raisman and Field (1971) examined synapses in the preoptic area and elsewhere which receive efferent projections from the stria terminalis using orthograde degeneration and electron microscopy: these projections are thought to be essential for ovarian cyclicity in rats (Halász 1969), but not in monkeys. Non-amygdaloid axodendritic synapses occur more frequently on dendritic spines in females, whereas they occur more frequently on dendritic shafts in males. Raisman and Field concluded that the preoptic neuropil was sexually dimorphic, and sought to relate this to the sex difference in the control of pituitary gonadotropin secretion. A group of densely-staining neurones within the medial preoptic area of the rat, identified in Nissl-stained sections, is 3–8 times larger in males than in females (Gorski *et al.* 1978): other species (but not all), including gerbil (Yahr and Commins 1982), guinea pig (Hines *et al.* 1985), and ferret (Tobet *et al.* 1986) show similar dimorphisms. The pattern of dendritic branching is also sexually dimorphic in the preoptic area of the macaque (Ayoub *et al.* 1983) and, using the freeze-fracture technique, Naftolin and colleagues (Naftolin *et al.* 1990) have demonstrated sexual dimorphism in neuronal membranes from the infundibular hypothalamus of African green monkeys. With all this, investigations have moved on to the human brain and, since the original report (de Lacoste-Utamsing and Holloway 1982) that the splenium of the corpus callosum in women is larger and more bulbous than in men when measured in the midsagittal plane, there have been many studies on callosal sex differences, but interpretations differ sharply. Although men in general have larger brains than women, this difference diminishes when corrected for body size. Even so, males have about 8 per cent greater brain weight from the second year onward when corrected for differences in height (Swaab and Hofman 1984). Some studies report that cognitive abilities, visual-spatial function, and language are more lateralized in the male's than in the female's brain (Geschwind and Levitsky 1968), but other studies have not confirmed this. In addition to the corpus callosum, the anterior commissure, which is also involved in inter-hemispheric transfer (and the massa intermedia), are reported to be larger in post-mortem brains from women than from men (Allen and Gorski 1986). Structural differences involving cortical mechanisms remain very difficult to assess, but there is much better agreement on sexual dimorphism in the human diencephalon. Morphometric analyses have revealed a sexually dimorphic nucleus in the preoptic area which is twice the size and contains twice as many neurones in men than in women (Swaab and Fliers 1985; Allen and Gorski 1990). These nuclei are of approximately equal size in boys and girls up to about four years of age, but there after a sex difference develops due to a decrease in cell numbers in females during development (Hofman and Swaab 1991). The suprachiasmatic nucleus is important for the regulation of circadian rhythms as well as for the control of longer-term environmental influences such as the photoperiod, and it is more elongated in human females and more spherical in males. An enlarged suprachiasmatic nucleus has now been reported in homosexual men compared with a reference group of heterosexual males (Swaab and Hofman 1990). Four small cell groups (interstitial nuclei of the anterior hypothalamus) have been described in the preoptic-anterior hypothalamic region of the human brain, and two of these appear to be sexually dimorphic, being larger in males than in females (Allen *et al.* 1989). These nuclei have been investigated further in heterosexual and homosexual men (LeVay 1991), and one of the four nuclei was found to be more than twice the size in heterosexual than in homosexual men, which, the author proposes, indicates a dimorphism in respect of sexual orientation; much of the material came from homosexual individuals who died from the complications of AIDS, and a replication of these provocative results is needed.

SEXUAL BEHAVIOUR IN LABORATORY MAMMALS

In 1923 Allen and Doisy extracted a hormone from four tons of sow ovaries which they crystallized and found to be responsible for mating behaviour in ovariectomized mice and rats (Allen and Doisy 1923): this discovery inaugurated the biochemistry of sexual behaviour. The early work of Calvin Stone emphasized the importance of two systems underlying sexual behaviour, namely, the endocrine system and the central nervous system. Marshall, in 1922, wrote 'little or nothing is known concerning the chain of causation leading to that disturbed state of the nervous mechanism the existence of which during oestrus is so plainly manifest in the display of sex feeling'. But this situation has now changed dramatically. Oestrus (Greek: gadfly) or heat describes a behavioural state, namely, periods of intense sexual arousal which many female mammals exhibit when receptive to the male. In oestrus, they adopt specialized postures permitting intromission, and these are associated with specialized movements, calls, and odours that signal receptivity to the male. These behavioural patterns are controlled by hormones liberated by follicles and corpora lutea in the ovaries, which are themselves under the control of the pituitary gonadotropins regulating the oestrous cycle. Many male mammals, on the other hand, have months of sexual quiescence, but the testes become active seasonally, at which time males are said to rut. There are internal biological clocks regulating some of these phenomena, but the long-term physiological and behavioural rhythms are entrained by exteroceptive factors (Marshall 1922), including the photoperiod. Data are now available which suggest that mood and activity generally are also influenced by exteroceptive factors in the human.

A great deal is known about the behavioural changes induced by androgens and oestrogens when given, over a wide dose-range, to intact and gonadectomized animals of both sexes at different stages of development. This work has been brilliantly reviewed by Frank A. Beach (1948) and by William C. Young (1961), and at intervals thereafter by several less distinguished successors. There are noteworthy species differences, exemplified by the role of progesterone on behaviour in the female. Oestradiol alone induces oestrous behaviour in spayed female guinea pigs, but if its administration is followed a few hours later by an injection of progesterone, much lower priming doses of oestradiol are effective, more females come into oestrus, and the latency to oestrus is reduced by several hours; thus, oestradiol and progesterone act synergistically in mouse, rat and, guinea pig to facilitate receptivity, but the reverse occurs in rabbit and ferret, in which progesterone antagonizes the action of oestrogen on receptivity. In ewes, progesterone and oestrogen again act synergistically, but to do so progesterone administration must precede the administration of oestrogen, so timing is the opposite of that in rat and guinea pig. In domestic cats, progesterone has little effect either way on behaviour, and in primates it again tends to antagonize the effects of oestrogen. It is difficult to understand the basis for these differences without some knowledge of the reproductive strategies (solitary or social) and reproductive cycles (reflex or spontaneous ovulation) of the species concerned (which is outside our present scope). But it becomes clear why it is unwise to extrapolate across species, particularly from lower mammals to the human.

Evidence has gradually accumulated indicating that certain parts of the brain have special importance for organizing the total pattern of sexual behaviour. The presence of the genital tract itself is not necessary for the manifestation of sexual excitation in the female, and surgical removal of the uterus and vagina in rats does not prevent oestrous behaviour, nor does total deafferentation of the pelvis by combined sacral cord section and abdominal sympathectomy. Heat behaviour can occur in animals that are both deaf and blind and in the absence of olfactory bulbs and neocortex. It seems, therefore, that neither the distance receptors nor any one sensory modality is in itself essential for the expression of sexual excitement in lower mammals, although all may contribute to it. Data have been collected from patients following penectomy, vulvectomy, and from both paraplegics and quadruplegics, and they are in line with the animal observations, namely, that sensory input from the genitalia is not essential for sexual activity, sexual fantasy, and sexual climax.

Spinal and low midbrain transections prevent the expression of integrated oestrous behaviour in female guinea pigs and cats, but complete removal of the neocortex, part of the rhinencephalon, striatum, and rostrolateral thalamus does not prevent the manifestation of oestrous behaviour in rat, rabbit, and cat. Males depend more on neocortical mechanisms than females to mate efficiently because they need to orient actively to the female, whereas the latter generally maintains a somewhat more static posture during mating. The view developed that it was essential for the hypothalamus and related parts of the diencephalon to be in contiguity with the midbrain and lower neuroaxis for integrated oestrous postures and reflexes to be expressed. Using modern stereotaxic methods, localized lesions have been placed within the hypothalamus in an effort to block the behavioural effects associated with the administration of gonadal hormones. But the hypothalamus is a relatively small structure and is concerned with many behavioural, autonomic, endocrine, and regulatory mechanisms (feeding, drinking, temperature regulation, fluid balance, etc.), and interference with these other functions makes for difficulties in interpreting behavioural deficits: obviously, if an animal is sick and not eating, its mating behaviour may also be impaired.

A more fruitful approach has been to implant minute fragments of solid hormone directly into the brain, and to search for neural sites from which a positive behavioural reaction could be evoked. Michael and colleagues (Harris *et al.* 1958; Michael 1961; Harris and Michael 1964) were the first to do this with implants of stilboestrol esters into the brains of ovariectomized cats. The use of solid implants was preferred to the injection of solutions since the former provide both a higher degree of localization and a more prolonged period of action. By this technique an oestrogen-sensitive neurological system was identified in the brain from which the complete pattern of oestrous behaviour and mating could be evoked while the genital tract of the female remained in an atrophic, anoestrous condition; this indicated that oestrogen was not being released from the brain implant in sufficient quantities to oestrogenize the vagina. Identical, control implants in other brain sites generally failed to promote any behavioural changes. This technique was subsequently refined and utilized in elegant studies in fish, amphibia (Wada and Gorbman 1977), reptiles (Friedman and Crews 1985), birds (Hutchison 1967; Barfield 1969), and mammals (Davidson and Sawyer 1961; Lisk 1962; Davis and Barfield 1979) of both sexes and different stages of development.

The advent of ^{3}H-labelled hormones with very high specific activity in the early 1960s marked the next step in the resolution of problems concerning the interactions between hormones and the brain (Michael and Glascock 1961). It became possible to identify in both male and female brains individual neurones possessing receptors for the major steroids produced by ovaries and testes. Work with ^{3}H-steroids in several laboratories largely confirmed the implantation studies, but with the much higher localization and finer microscopical resolution provided by autoradiography (Michael 1962, 1965; Pfaff 1968), and also the metabolic resolution provided by high-performance liquid chromatography. Steroid receptor-containing neurones are distributed in systems which are similar in male and female brains, involving the medial group of amygdaloid nuclei and preoptic-anterior hypothalamic area in the male, with extensions into the hypothalamic ventromedial nucleus and midbrain particularly in the female. Neurones with steroid receptors are present in the primate fetus in mid-gestation, although it is not possible to determine their function (pituitary regulation or behaviour) at this stage (Michael *et al.* 1989). Now that antibodies to the androgen, oestrogen, and progestin receptors are available, immunocytochemical methods have identified steroid receptor-immunoreactive neurons in the brains of several species (Blaustein and Turcotte 1989; Balthazart *et al.* 1991; Clancy *et al.* 1992): in general, results have confirmed and supplemented the autoradiographic findings. Expression of the immediate-early proto-oncogene c-*fos* can be visualized in neurones by immunocytochemistry about an hour after exposing an animal to any of several sensory stimuli. This index of increased neuronal activity has been used in both males and females after mating to localize regions in the brain which are directly and immediately involved in sexual excitation and consummation (Baum and Everitt 1992). Within a few years, application of modern molecular biological techniques will establish the neurological concomitants of orgasm in males and females and resolve the age-old question of sex differences in this regard.

STUDIES IN ANTHROPOID NON-HUMAN PRIMATES

These include the Old World (catarrhine) monkeys and apes. There has been a significant increase in the number of high-quality field and laboratory studies on primate sexual behaviour during the last 20 years, and there is a widely held view that, as one ascends the phylogenetic scale, the role of hormones in controlling behaviour is reduced, while the role of brain mechanisms and learning increases. These are, of course, broad generalizations, and we now know that a significant component of the sexual behaviour of non-human primates is heavily influenced by gonadal hormones. It should also be mentioned that only the anthropoid monkeys and apes share, in common with the human, the reproductive characteristic of a menstrual cycle which is absent in the majority of mammals, although oestrous cycles are a constant feature of mammalian reproductive life. Several species of monkey show periods of heightened sexual activity near mid-cycle around the time of ovulation. These may be fairly well circumscribed, particularly in species showing marked mid-cycle swellings of the specialized perineal sexual skin (mangabeys, some macaques, baboons, chimpanzees, etc.). However, in related species (some other macaques), sexual interactions between males and females may continue throughout the whole course of the female's cycle, although intensity and frequency fluctuate, increasing near ovulation. In macaques, this cyclicity occurs under natural conditions (Carpenter 1942), in social groups housed in large outdoor enclosures (Gordon 1981), and when one male and one female are paired together in an observation cage in the absence of conspecifics (Michael *et al.* 1967; Zumpe and Michael 1983). Ovariectomy abolishes the behavioural rhythms of the pair (but not all the sexual interactions), and small amounts of oestradiol benzoate (1–3 μg/kg/day s.c.) restore female sexual motivation (proceptivity and receptivity) as well as her attractiveness as a partner for the male. Although results are variable, it appears that large amounts of progesterone (2–5 mg/kg/day s.c.) partly antagonize oestradiol's effects (Michael *et al.* and Zumpe 1968). These observations have a bearing on the human situation, when women are consuming oral contraceptive preparations containing oestrogens and progestins. Because of some earlier clinical impressions which, nevertheless, were uncontrolled of the effects of testosterone on the libido of women suffering from menorrhagia (Greenblatt *et al.* 1942), the view developed that testosterone, and not oestradiol, was the important libidinal hormone in the female (Money and Ehrhardt 1972; Money 1987). We believe this view has been over-stated, and that the positive association between plasma testosterone levels and sexuality in young women is less than compelling (Bancroft *et al.* 1991). In macaques, as in the human, testosterone increases clitoral size and sensitivity, without necessarily increasing either female attractiveness (Michael and Zumpe 1977) or the sexual interactions of the pair. The effect of androgen on libido in the human female remains an open question.

Our understanding of the role of the female's cycle in integrating the behavioural interactions of the pair has been increased by the development of what are called 'artificial menstrual cycles' (Michael *et al.* 1982). These are induced by injecting *ovariectomized* females once daily for 28-day periods with mixtures of oestradiol, progesterone, and testosterone whose concentrations are changed daily so as to produce in blood 8 hours later the changing levels of hormones occurring in intact females during natural cycles. These ovariectomized females 'menstruate' every 28 days and show the characteristic physiological and behavioural changes of intact females. The virtue of the artificial cycle is that it is timed precisely and can be used in social groups to assess the influence of one female's cycle stage on the behaviour of the male with a female in a different cycle stage. Modern sociobiological theory predicts that, to maximize their reproductive success, males will mate with as many females as possible while females conserve their time and energy by mating only periodically at the time of maximal fertility with the 'best' males. This hypothesis has been confirmed experimentally, in groups consisting of one male and four ovariectomized females, by offsetting the artificial cycles of two of the females by 7-day intervals. It was seen that males were indeed successful in maintaining high constant levels of sexual activity by moving from one female to another as each came into full receptivity whereas when a female's receptivity declined with her cycle phase, she was able to move away from the male so as no longer to be the focus of his attentions (Michael and Zumpe 1988). Several studies have examined the effect of ovarian hormones on libido and sexual behaviour during the human menstrucal cycle in stable cohabiting pairs. Again, results have not been clear-cut, but there is some evidence for a mid-cycle peak in sexual fantasy and in some types of sexual activity (see Matteo and Rissman 1984; Stanislaw and Rice 1988). Results obtained in non-human primates imply that the behavioural changes associated with the human cycle might be more readily identified in polygynous mating systems.

Many social primates live in semi-closed groups containing several adult males and females together with their young. In macaques, shortly after adolescence and about every four years thereafter, males emigrate voluntarily into another social group whereas females remain in their natal group for life. The immigrant male's social integration into a new group depends on his acceptance by resident females, which show greater interest in new males than in familiar, resident ones (Bernstein *et al.* 1977; Wilson and Gordon 1979). There appears to be incest avoidance (different from an incest taboo, which is a socially imposed prohibition) between an adult male and his sisters and mother (Sade 1972; Missakian 1973), and there is a similar avoidance of homosexual mounting between female kin (Chapais and Mignault 1991). The degree of familiarity between potential mates appears to be a common factor in these and other observations. Westermarck (1891) was the first to point out for the human that familiarity between kin, rather than consanguinity *per se*, might be responsible for inhibiting sexual desire between siblings after adolescence, as well as between parents and their adolescent offspring. Studies on adult and childhood Chinese marriages (Wolf 1970) and on Israeli kibbutzim (Shepher 1971; Parker 1976) have provided evidence supporting this view: in 2769 marriages of second-generation kibbutz adults, none was between those raised in the same kibbutz peer group. If this effect operates between adult humans, as it appears to do in adult macaques (Michael and Zumpe

1978; Zumpe and Michael 1984), it could add to our understanding of human mating systems which, despite impressions to the contrary, are not primarily monogamous. Polygynous marriage practices have been reported for 708 of 849 societies (83 per cent) (Murdock 1967), and analysis of divorce in 58 peoples and populations between 1947 and 1981 revealed a marked tendency towards serial pair-bonding, with a modal length of four years for marriages ending in divorce, and most divorces occurred at the height of the reproductive years in both men and women (Fisher 1989).

The sexual activity of males depends on the secretory activity of the testes, as does the manifestation of male aggression. Thus, the castration of farm animals has been employed since antiquity to make them more tractable, but effects depend on whether castration is performed before or after puberty. Castration of a boy before puberty results in the classical eunuch: a high soprano voice, lack of facial hair, lack of libido, and a tendency towards the female distribution of subcutaneous fat. Castration of adults, for medical or other reasons, may not have such obvious effects, and changes develop slowly: however, there are enormous individual differences. Studies in macaques have been helpful. Castration of adult males causes a decline in mounting and ejaculation in a few weeks, as it does in male rats; however, ejaculations may occur intermittently for up to two years after surgery (Michael *et al.* 1973). Injections of testosterone can restore sexual behaviour in some 12 weeks, but the role of testosterone (T) is complicated because it is metabolized both to dihydrotestosterone (DHT) by 5α-reduction and to oestradiol by aromatization. As we have already seen in men with a genetic defect, DHT is critically important for the masculinization of peripheral genital structures, including those derived from the urogenital sinus, but its role in regulating behaviour via brain mechanisms remains open to question. In castrated macaques, for example, injections of DHT in the physiological dose-range do not increase ejaculatory activity, but injections of T in its physiological dose-range do so quite markedly (Michael *et al.* 1986). Concerning the role of testosterone's aromatized product, oestradiol, there is no doubt it acts synergistically with both T and DHT in several lower mammals to enhance male sexual behaviour (Larsson *et al.* 1973; Baum *et al.* 1982; Whalen *et al.* 1985), and the use of aromatase inhibitors has recently shown that E_2 contributes to the expression of sexual motivation in male primates also (Zumpe *et al.* 1993). Although hormones appear to have a 'necessary and sufficient' function in the male primate, this is not the whole story. For example, plasma T levels do not correlate well with male potency, and it is difficult to increase the potency of a low-potency macaque or human male by T administration. The best way to enhance male potency is to find the right female partner. If the sexual activity of a male macaque with one female is low, levels of sexual arousal and activity increase dramatically when the partner is exchanged for a 'favourite' (Michael *et al.* 1972) or for a novel one (Michael and Zumpe 1978). Individual differences and partner preferences play a much greater part in the sexual interactions of primates than in those of lower mammals. It is the view of the authors, in summary, that unmetabolized T together with E_2 activates brain mechanisms responsible for libido in the male primate, while DHT is primarily responsible for peripheral mechanisms necessary for male potency. Adrenal steroids are essential for feelings of well-being and strength, but are not importantly involved in the behavioural changes associated either with the menstrual cycle or with season.

COMMUNICATION BETWEEN THE SEXES

In many invertebrates and vertebrates including mammals, elaborate courtship displays serve to attract individuals of the opposite sex and help to synchronize their reproductive physiology. These displays have evolved from conflicts between sexual (approach) and aggressive (agonistic) tendencies aroused by a prospective mate. Different sensory cues are involved: changes in colour (e. g., fishes), specialized movements (invertebrates to the human), elaborate sounds (e. g., bird song), and tactile and odour stimuli (e. g., mammals). Many courtship displays co-evolved with specialized morphological features (e. g., tails of peacocks, antlers of deer) which exaggerate the display's communicatory impact. Human mammary glands, in contrast to those of other mammals, are conspicuously positioned and serve a signalling function: breasts have evolved functions in courtship and love-making that are independent of nutrition and feeding Both men and women enhance their physical characteristics by costume, dress (or the lack of it), and other adornments (make-up, jewellry) utilized in both heterosexual and homosexual contexts. Although distance communication by posture, movement, and sound is found in all the vertebrate taxa, olfactory communication is particularly important in mammals. The pheromone concept, originally used in insect communication, has been applied more recently to mammals and involves signalling by chemicals which are often airborne. It is now known that the vomeronasal organ, which is connected by its own nervous pathway to the accessory olfactory bulb, influences many reproductive activities in rodents (Bronson 1971). For example, dimethyl disulphide, which has been identified in hamster vaginal secretions, probably acts on nasal chemoreceptors connected to the main olfactory bulb and promotes sexual approaches by males (Singer *et al.* 1976). On the other hand, a protein (aphrodisin), which has also been isolated from hamster vaginal discharge, elicits actual copulation by males, and this response is mediated by the vomeronasal organ and the accessory olfactory bulb (Singer *et al.* 1986). Homologous proteins, which are also thought to serve a signalling function, are present in the urine and scent glands of mice, rats, and voles (Singer 1991). In primates, a collection of short-chained, fatty acids (copulin) have been isolated from oestrogen-stimulated vaginal secretions of several species including macaques, chimpanzees, and women (Michael *et al.* 1976). They certainly serve a signalling function in the macaque, and males will consort preferentially with a female in a group if that female is treated with them (Michael and Zumpe 1982). In the vaginal secretions of women, they show a well-marked mid-cycle maximum (Michael *et al.* 1974), but there is no evidence that they have any communicatory significance in the human and, in high concentrations, they are not pleasant. The size of the perfume industry attests to the importance of olfactorily active substances detected by their odour, but we can now give credence to the possibility that, in the human, non-olfactorily active substances detected by the vomeronasal organ influence behaviour. Although controversial for many years, the existence of a vomeronasal organ in men and women has been established beyond doubt in a study of over 1000 human subjects (Garcia-Velasco and Mondragon 1991), its ultrastructure has been largely established, but its nervous connections to the brain have not. Some putative pheromones extracted from human skin can elicit specific, electrical responses from the vomeronasal organs of conscious human subjects of both sexes (Monti-Bloch and

Grosser 1991). Although these are intriguing findings, the functional significance of this system and its role, if any, in communication between men and women has yet to be determined.

REFERENCES

Aarskog, D. (1979). Maternal progestins as a possible cause of hypospadias. *N. Engl. J. Med.* **300**, 75–8.

Allen, E. and Doisy, E. A. (1923). An ovarian hormone: preliminary report on its localization, extraction and partial purification, and action in test animals. *J. Am. Med. Assoc.* **81**, 819–21.

Allen, L. S. and Gorski, R. A. (1986). Sexual dimorphism of the human anterior commissure. *Anatom. Rec.* **214**, 3A.

Allen, L. S. and Gorski, R. A. (1990). Sex difference in the bed nucleus of the stria terminalis of the human brain. *J. Comp. Neurol.* **302**, 697–706.

Allen, L. S., Hines, M., Shryne, J. E., and Gorski, R. A. (1989). Two sexually dimorphic cell groups in the human brain. *J. Neurosci.* **9**, 497–506.

Asdell, S. A. (1936). Hermaphroditism in goats. *Dairy Goat J.* **14**, 3–4.

Ayoub, D. M., Greenough, W. T., and Juraska, J. M. (1983). Sex differences in dendritic structure in the preoptic area of the juvenile macaque monkey brain. *Science*, **219**, 197–8.

Bailey, J. M. and Pillard, R. C. (1991). A genetic study of male sexual orientation. *Arch. Gen. Psychiat.* **48**, 1089–97.

Balthazart, J., Foidart, A., Surlemont, C., and Harada, J. (1991). Neuroanatomical specificity in the co-localization of aromatase and estrogen receptors. *J. Neurobiol.*, **22**, 143–57.

Bancroft, J., Sherwin, B. B., Alexander, G. M., Davidson, D. W., and Walker, A. (1991). Oral contraceptives, androgens, and the sexuality of young women: II. The role of androgens. *Arch. Sex. Behav.* **20**, 121–35.

Barfield, R. J. (1969). Activation of copulatory behaviour by androgen implanted into the preoptic area of the male fowl. *Horm. Behav.* **1**, 37–52.

Barr, M. L. and Bertram, E. G. (1949). A morphological distinction between neurones of the male and female, and the behaviour of the nucleolar satellite during accelerated nucleoprotein synthesis. *Nature (London)*, **163**, 676–7.

Barraclough, C. A. (1961). Production of anovulatory, sterile rats by single injections of testosterone propionate. *Endocrinology*, **68**, 62–7.

Barraclough, C. A. (1967). Modifications in reproductive function after exposure to hormones during the prenatal and early postnatal period. In *Neuroendocrinology*, Vol. II, (ed. L. Martini and W. F. Ganong), pp. 61–99. Academic Press, New York.

Barraclough, C. A. and Gorski, R. A. (1961). Evidence that the hypothalamus is responsible for androgen-induced sterility in the female rat. *Endocrinology* **68**, 68–79.

Bateson, P. (1979). How do sensitive periods arise and what are they for? *Anim. Behav.* **27**, 470–86.

Bateson, P. (1981). Control of sensitivity to the environment during development. In *Behavioral development*, (ed. K. Immelman, G. W. Barlow, L. Petrinovich, and M. Main), pp. 432–53. Cambridge University Press.

Baum, M. J. and Everitt, B. J. (1992). Increased expression of *c-fos* in the medial preoptic area after mating in male rats: role of afferent inputs from the medial amygdala and midbrain central tegmental field. *Neuroscience* **50**, 627–46.

Baum, M. J., Tobet, S. A., Starr, M. S., and Bradshaw, W. G. (1982). Implantation of dihydrotestosterone propionate into the lateral septum or medial amygdala facilitates copulation in castrated male rates given estradiol systemically. *Horm. Behav.* **16**, 208–23.

Beach, F. A. (1948). *Hormones and behavior*. Paul B. Hoeber, New York.

Bernstein, I. S., Rose, R. M., and Gordon, T. P. (1977). Behavioural and hormonal responses of male rhesus monkeys introduced to females in the breeding and non-breeding seasons. *Anim. Behav.* **25**, 609–14.

Berthold, A. A. (1849). Transplantation der Hoden. *Arch. Anat. Physiol. Wissensch. Med. Leipzig*, **16**, 42–6.

Bishop, P. M. F., Lessof, M. H., and Polani, P. E. (1960). Turner's syndrome and allied conditions. In *Memoirs of the Society for Endocrinology*, No. 7: *Sex differentiation and development*, (ed. C. R. Austin), pp. 162–72. Cambridge University Press.

Blaustein, J. D. and Turcotte, J. C. (1989). Estradiol-induced progestin receptor immunoreactivity is found only in estrogen receptor-immunoreactive cells in guinea pig brains. *Neuroendocrinology*, **49**, 454–61.

Bouin, P. and Ancel, P. (1903). Sur la signification de la glande interstitielle du testicule embryonnaire. *C. R. Hebdomad. Séanc. Mém. Soc. Biol. (Paris)*, **55**, 1682–4.

Broida, J. P., Churchill, J, and McGinnis, M. (1988). Prenatal exposure to alcohol facilitates lordosis in male rats. Poster presented at the *Annual Conference on Reproductive Behaviour*. Omaha, Nebraska.

Bronson, F. H. (1971). Rodent pheromones. *Biol. Repro.* **4**, 344–58.

Bull, J. J. (1987). Temperature-sensitive periods of sex determination in a lizard: similarities with turtles and crocodilians. *J. Exp. Zool.* **241**, 143–148.

Burns, R. K. (1925). The sex of parabiotic twins in Amphibia. *J. Exp. Zool.* **42**, 31–89.

Burns, R. K. (1956). Hormones versus constitutional factors in the growth of embryonic sex primordia in the opossum. *Am. J. Anat.* **98**, 35–67.

Carpenter, C. R. (1934). A field study of the behavior and social relations of howling monkeys (*Alouatta palliata.*). *Comp. Psychol. Mon.* **10**, 1–168.

Carpenter, C. R. (1942). Sexual behavior of free ranging rhesus monkeys (*Macaca mulatta*). I. Specimens, procedures and behavioral characteristics of estrus. *J. Com. Psychol.* **33**, 113–42.

Chapais, B. and Mignault, C. (1991). Homosexual incest avoidance among females in captive Japanese macaques. *Am. J. Primatol.* **23**, 171–83.

Clancy, A. N., Bonsall, R. W., and Michael, R. P. (1992). Immunohistochemical labeling of androgen receptors in the brain of rat and monkey. *Life Sci.* **50**, 409–17.

Clemens, L. G. (1974). Neurohormonal control of male sexual behavior. In *Reproductive behavior*, (ed. W. Montagna and W. A. Sadler), pp. 23–53. Plenum, New York.

Courrier, R. and Jost, A. (1942). Intersexualité foetale provoquée par la prégnéninolone au cours de la grossesse. *C. R. Séanc. Mém. Soc. Biol. Fil. (Paris)*, **136**, 395–6.

Craig, J. V., Casida, L. E., and Chapman, A. B. (1954). Male infertility associated with lack of libido in the rat. *Am. Natural.* **88**, 365–72.

Crews, D. (1987). Diversity and evolution of behavioral controlling mechanisms. In *Psychobiology of reproductive behavior. An evolutionary perspective*, (ed. D. Crews), pp. 88–119. Prentice Hall, Englewood Cliffs, NJ.

Dantchakoff, V. (1935). Sur les différences de sensibilité des récepteurs tissulaires envers la folliculine, divers stades embryonnaires. *C. R. Acad. Sci.* **201**, 161–3.

Dantchakoff, V. (1936). Réalisation du sexe à volonté par inductions hormonales. I. Inversion du sexe dans un embryon génétiquement mâle. *Bull. Biol. Fr. Belg.* **70**, 241–307.

Davidson, J. M. and Sawyer, C. H. (1961). Effects of localized intracerebral implantation of estrogen on reproductive function in the female rabbit. *Acta Endocrinol.*, **37**, 385–393.

Davis, P. G. and Barfield, R. J. (1979). Activation of masculine sexual behavior by intracranial estradiol benzoate implants in male rats. *Neuroendocrinology*, **28**, 217–27.

de Lacoste-Utamsing, C. and Holloway, R. L. (1982). Sexual dimorphism in the human corpus callosum. *Science*, **216**, 1431–2.

Diamond, M. C. and Young, W. C. (1963). Differential responsiveness of pregnant and nonpregnant guinea pigs to the masculinizing action of testosterone propionate. *Endocrinology*, **72**, 429–38.

Dittman, R. W., *et al.* (1990). Congenital adrenal hyperplasia. I: gender-related behavior and attitudes in female patients and sisters. *Psychoneuroendocrinology*, **15**, 401–20.

Dörner, G. (1980). Sexual differentiation of the brain. *Vit. Horm.* **38**, 325–81.

Dörner, G., *et al.* (1980). Prenatal stress as possible aetiogenetic factor of homosexuality of human males. *Endokrinologie*, **75**, 365–8.

Ehrhardt, A. A. (1985). The psychobiology of gender. In *Gender and the life course*, (ed. A. Rossi), pp. 81–96. Aldine, New York.

Ehrhardt, A. A. and Baker, S. W. (1974). Fetal androgens, human central nervous system differentiation, and behavior sex differences. In *Sex differences in behavior*, (ed. R. C. Friedman, R. M. Richart, and R. L. Vande Wiele), pp. 33–51. Wiley, New York.

Ehrhardt, A. A. and Money, J. (1967). Progestin-induced hermaphroditism: IQ and psychosexual identity in a study of ten girls. *J. Sex. Res.* **3**, 83–100.

Ehrhardt, A. A., Epstein, R., and Money, J. (1968). Fetal androgens and female gender identity in the early-treated adrenogenital syndrome. *Johns Hopkins Med. J.* **122**, 160–7.

Ehrhardt, A. A., *et al.* (1985). Sexual orientation after prenatal exposure to exogenous estrogen. *Arch. Sex. Behav.* **14**, 57–75.

Ehrhardt, A. A., *et al.* (1989). The development of gender-related behavior in females following prenatal exposure to diethylstilbestrol (DES). *Horm. Behav.* **23**, 526–41.

Eicher, E. M. and Washburn, L. L. (1986). Genetic control of sex determination in mice. *Ann. Rev. Genet.* **20**, 327–60.

Everett, J. W., Sawyer, C. H., and Markee, J. E. (1949). A neurogenic timing factor in control of the ovulatory discharge of luteinizing hormone in the cyclic rat. *Endocrinology*, **44**, 234–50.

Ferguson, M. W. J. and Joanen, T. (1983). Temperature-dependent sex determination in *Alligator mississipiensis*. *J. Zool. (London)*, **200**, 143–77.

Fisher, H. E. (1989). Evolution of human serial pairbonding. *Am. J. Phys. Anthropol.*, **78**, 331–54.

Friedman, D. and Crews, D. (1985). Role of the anterior hypothalamus-preoptic area in the regulation of courtship behavior in the male Canadian red-sided garter snake (*Thamnophis sirtalis parietalis*): intracranial implantation experiments. *Horm. Behav.* **19**, 122–36.

Gandelman, R., vom Saal, F. S., and Reinisch, J. M. (1977). Contiguity to male foetuses affects morphology and behaviour of female mice. *Nature (London)*, **266**, 722–4.

Garcia-Velasco, J. and Mondragon, M. (1991). The incidence of the vomeronasal organ in 1000 human subjects and its possible clinical significance. *J. Ster. Biochem. Mole. Biol.* **39(4B)**, 561–3.

Gebhard, P. H. (1972). Incidence of overt homosexuality in the United States and western Europe. In *National Institute of Mental Health Task Force on Homosexuality: Final report and background papers*, (ed. J. M. Livingood), publication 72–9116, pp. 22–9.

Department of Health, Education and Welfare, Washington, DC.

Geschwind N. and Levitsky, W. (1968). Human brain left-right symmetries in temporal speech region. *Science*, **161**, 186–7.

Gordon, T. P. (1981). Reproductive behavior in the rhesus monkey: social and endocrine variables. *Am. Zool.* **21**, 185–95.

Gooren, L., Fliers, E., and Courtney, K. (1990). Biological determinants of sexual orientation. *Ann. Rev. Sex Res.* **1**, 175–96.

Gorski, R. A., Gordon, J. H., Shryne, J. E., and Southam, A. M. (1978). Evidence for a morphological sex difference within the medical preoptic area of the rat brain. *Brain Res.* **148**, 333–46.

Götz, F. and Dörner, G. (1980). Homosexual behaviour in prenatally stressed male rats after castration and oestrogen treatment in adulthood. *Endokrinologie*, **76**, 115–17.

Goy, R. W. (1968). Organizing effects of androgen on the behaviour of rhesus monkeys. In *Endocrinology and human behaviour*, (ed. R. P. Michael), pp. 12–31. Oxford University Press.

Goy, R. and Young, W. C. (1957). Strain differences in the behavioral responses of female guinea pigs to alpha-estradiol benzoate and progesterone. *Behaviour*, **10**, 340–54.

Goy, R. W., Bercovitch, F. B., and McBrair, M. C. (1988). Behavioural masculinization is independent of genital masculinization in prenatally androgenized female rhesus macaques.*Horm. Behav.* **22**, 552–71.

Greenblatt, R. B., Mortara, F., and Torpin, R. (1942). Sexual libido in the female. *Am. J. Obstet. Gynecol.* **44**, 658–63.

Greene, R. R. (1942). Hormonal factors in sex inversion: the effects of sex hormones on embryonic sexual structures of the rat. *Biol. Symp.* **9**, 105–23.

Grunt, J. A. and Young, W. C. (1952). Differential reactivity of individuals and the response of the male guinea pig to testosterone propionate. *Endocrinology*, **51**, 237–48.

Gubbay, J., *et al.* (1990). A gene mapping to the sex-determining region of the mouse Y chromosome is a member of a novel family of embryonically expressed genes. *Nature (London)*, **346**, 245–50.

Gubernick, D. J. (1980). Maternal "imprinting" or maternal "labeling" in goats? *Animal. Behav.* **28**, 124–9.

Halász, B. (1969). The endocrine effects of isolation of the hypothalamus from the rest of the brain. In *Frontiers in neuroendocrinology*, (ed. W. F. Ganong and L. Martini), pp. 307–42. Oxford University Press, New York.

Hamer, D. H., Hu, S., Magnuson, V. L., Hu, N., and Pattatucci, A. M. L. (1993). A linkage between DNA markers on the X chromosome and male sexual orientation. *Science*, **261**, 321–7.

Hampson, J. G., Money, J., and Hampson, J. L. (1956). Hermaphrodism: recommendations concerning case management. *J. Clin. Endocrinol.* **16**, 547–56.

Harlow, H. F. and Harlow, M. K. (1962). Social deprivation in monkeys. *Sci. Am.* **207**, 136–46.

Harlow, H. F. and Zimmermann, R. R. (1959). Affectional responses in the infant monkey. *Science*, **130**, 421–32.

Harris, G. W. and Campbell, H. J. (1966). The regulation of the secretion of luteinizing hormone and ovulation. In *The pituitary gland*, (ed. G. W. Harris and B. T. Donovan), pp. 99–165. Butterworths, London.

Harris, G. W. and Jacobsohn, D. (1952). Functional grafts of the anterior pituitary gland. *Proc. Roy. Soc. B*, **139**, 263–76.

Harris, G. W. and Levine, S. (1965). Sexual differentiation of the brain and its experimental control. *J. Physiol.* **181**, 379–400.

Harris, G. W. and Michael, R. P. (1964). The activation of sexual behaviour by hypothalamic implants of oestrogen. *J. Physiol.* **171**, 275–301.

Harris, G. W. Michael, R. P., and Scott, P. P. (1958). Neurological site of action of stilboestrol in eliciting sexual behaviour. *The neurological basis of behaviour*, (ed. G. E. Wolstenholme and C. M. O' Connor), pp. 236–51. J. & A. Churchill, London.

Herbst, A. L., Kurman, R. J., Scully, R. E., and Poskanzer, D. C. (1972). Clear cell adenocarcinoma of the genital tract in young females. Registry report. *New Engl. J. Med.* **287**, 1259–64.

Herdt, G. H. and Davidson, J. (1988). The Sambia "Turnim-Man": sociocultural and clinical aspects of gender formation in male pseudohermaphrodites with 5-alpha-reductase deficiency in Papua New Guinea. *Arch. Sex. Behav.* **17**, 33–56.

Herrenkohl, L. R. and Whitney, J. B. (1976). Effects of prepartal stress on postpartal nursing behavior, litter development and adult sexual behavior. *Physiol. Behav.* **17**, 1019–21.

Hines, M., Davis, F. C., Coquelin, A., Goy, R. W., and Gorski, R. A. (1985). Sexually dimorphic regions in the medial preoptic area and the bed nucleus of the stria terminalis of the guinea pig brain: a description and an investigation of their relationship to gonadal steroids in adulthood. *J. Neurosci.* **5**, 40–7.

Hofman, M. A. and Swaab, D. F. (1991). Sexual dimorphism of the human brain: myth and reality. *Exp. Clin. Endocrinol.* **98**, 161–70.

Humphrey, R. R. (1928). Sex differentiation in gonads developed from transplants of the intermediate mesoderm of Amblystoma. *Biol. Bull.* **55**, 317–39.

Humphrey, R. R. (1942). Sex inversion in the Amphibia. *Biol. Symp.* **9**, 81–104.

Hutchison, J. B. (1967). Initiation of courtship by hypothalamic implants of testosterone propionate in castrated doves (*Streptopelia risoria*). *Nature (London)*, **216**, 591–2.

Imperato-McGinley, J. L., Petersen, R. E., Gautier, T., and Sturla, E. (1974). Steroid 5α reductase deficiency in man: an inherited form of male pseudohermaphroditism. *Science*, **186**, 1213–43.

Imperato-McGinley, J. L., Guerrero, L., Gautier, T., and Petersen, R. E. (1979). Androgens and the evolution of male-gender identity among male pseudohermaphrodites with 5α-reductase deficiency. *New Engl. J. Med.* **300**, 1233–7.

Jacobs, P. A., *et al.* (1959). Chromosomal sex in the syndrome of testicular feminisation. *Lancet*, **ii**, 591–2.

Jacobs, P. A., Price, W. H., Court-Brown, W. M., Brittain, R. P., and Whatmore, P. B. (1968). Chromosome studies on men in a maximum security hospital. *Ann. Hum. Genet.* **31**, 339–58.

Janus, C. (1988). The development of responses to naturally occurring odors in spiny mice, *Acomys cahirinus*. *Animal Behav.* **36**, 1400–6.

Josso, N. and Picard, J-Y. (1986). Anti-Müllerian hormone. *Physiol. Rev.* **66**, 1038–90.

Jost, A. (1947). Recherches sur la différenciation de 1' embryon de lapin. II. Action des androgènes synthèse sur l'histogénèse génitale. *Arch. Anat. Microscop. Morphol. Exp.* **36**, 242–70.

Jost, A. (1953). Problems of fetal endocrinology: the gonadal and hypophysical hormones. *Rec. Prog. Horm. Res.* **8**, 379–418.

Jost, A. (1971). Embryonic sexual differentiation (morphology, physiology, abnormalities). In *Hermaphroditism, genital anomalies and related endocrine disorders*, (ed. H. W. Jones and W. W. Scott), pp. 16–64. Williams & Wilkins, Baltimore.

Jost, A. and Bozic, B. (1951). Données sur la différenciation des conduits génitaux du foetus de rat etudiée *in vitro*. *C. R. Soc. Biol.* **145**, 647–50.

Kaitz, M., Good, A., Rokem, A. M., and Eidelman, A. I. (1987). Mothers' recognition of their newborns by olfactory cues. *Dev. Psychobiol.* **20**, 587–91.

Kaplan, N. M. (1959). Male pseudohermaphrodism: report of a case, with observations of pathogenesis. *New Engl. J. Med.* **261**, 641–4.

Karsch, F. J., Dierschke, D. J., and Knobil, E. (1973). Sexual differentiation of pituitary function: apparent difference between primates and rodents. *Science*, **179**, 484–6.

Kelce, W. R., Rudeen, P. K., and Ganjam, V. K. (1989). Prenatal ethanol exposure alters steroidogenic enzyme activity in newborn rat testes. *Alcoholism, Clin. Exp. Res.* **1**, 617–21.

Keller, K. and Tandler, J. (1916). Über das Verhalten der Eihäute bei der Zwillingsträchtigkeit des Rindes. *Wiener tierärzt. Wochenschr.* **3**, 513–26.

Klein, M. (1948). *Contributions to psychoanalysis 1921–1945.* Hogarth Press, London.

Klinefelter, H. F., Reifenstein, E. C., and Albright, F. (1942). Syndrome characterized by gynecomastia, aspermatogenesis without A-Leydigism, and increased excretion of follicle-stimulating hormone. *J. Clin. Endocrinol.* **2**, 615–27.

Klopfer, P. H. and Klopfer, M. S. (1968). Maternal "imprinting" in goats: fostering of alien young. *Zeitschr. Tierpsychol.* **25**, 862–6.

Kondo, K. (1955). The frequency of occurrence of intersexes in milk goats. *Jap. J. Genet.* **30**, 139–46.

Kozelka, A. W. and Gallagher, T. F. (1934). Effect of male hormone extracts, theelin and theelol, on the chick embryo. *Proc. Soc. Exp. Biol. Med.* **31**, 1143–4.

Larsson, K., Södersten, P., and Beyer, C. (1973). Sexual behavior in male rats treated with estrogen in combination with dihydrotestosterone. *Horm. Behav.* **4**, 289–99.

Leary, F. J., Resseguie, L. J., Kurland, L. T., O'Brien, P. C., Emslander, R. F., and Noller, K. L. (1984). Males exposed *in utero* to diethylstilbestrol. *J. Am. Med. Assoc.* **252**, 2984–9.

LeVay, S. (1991). A difference in hypothalamic structure between heterosexual and homosexual men. *Science*, **253**, 1034–7.

Lillie, F. R. (1916). The theory of the freemartin. *Science.* **43**, 611–13.

Lillie, F. R. (1917). The freemartin: a study of the action of sex hormones in the foetal life of cattle. *J. Exp. Zool.* **23**, 371–452.

Lisk, R. D. (1962). Diencephalic placement of estradiol and sexual receptivity in the female rat. *Am. J. Physiol.* **203**, 493–6.

Lorenz, K. (1935). Der Kumpan in der Umwelt des Vogels. *J. Ornithol.* **83**, 137–213, 289–413.

Lorenz, K. (1937). The companion in the bird's world. *Auk*, **54**, 245–73.

Lorenz, K. (1950). *So kam der Mensch auf den Hund.* Borotha–Schoeler, Vienna.

Lovell-Badge, R. (1993). Sex determining gene expression during embryogenesis. *Phil. Trans. Roy. Soc. London B.* **339**, 159–64.

Lyon, M. F. (1972). X chromosome inactivation and development patterns in mammals. *Biol. Rev. Camb. Phil. Soc.* **47**, 1–35.

Marshall, F. H. A. (1922). *The physiology of reproduction.* Longman, London.

Matteo, S. and Rissman, E. F. (1984). Increased sexual activity during the midcycle portion of the human menstrual cycle. *Horm. Behav.* **18**, 249–55.

McClung, C. E. (1902). The accessory chromosome—sex determinant? *Biol. Bull.* **3**, 43–84.

McLaren, A. (1988). Sex determination in mammals. *Trends Genet.* **4**, 153–7.

Meisel, R. L. and Ward, I. L. (1981). Fetal female rats are masculinized by male littermates located caudally in the uterus. *Science*, **213**, 239–42.

Michael, R. P. (1961). An investigation of the sensitivity of circumscribed neurological areas to hormonal stimulation by means of the application of oestrogens directly to the brain of the cat. In *Regional neurochemistry*, (ed. S. S. Kety and J. Elkes), pp. 465–80. Pergamon, Oxford.

Michael, R. P. (1962). Estrogen-sensitive neurons and sexual behaviour in female cats. *Science*, **136**, 322–3.

Michael, R. P. (1965). Oestrogens in the central nervous system. *Brit. Med. Bull.* **21**, 87–90.

Michael, R. P. and Bonsall, R. W. (1990). The uptake of tritiated diethylstilbestrol by the brain, pituitary gland, and genital tract of the fetal macaque: a combined chromatographic and autoradiographic study. *J. Clin. Endocrinol. Metabol.* **71**, 868–74.

Michael, R. P. and Glascock, R. F. (1961). The distribution of ^{14}C- and ^{3}H-labelled oestrogens in brain. *Proc. Int. Cong. Biochem.* **5**, 11.37.

Michael, R. P. and Rees, H. D. (1986). Neurons in the brain of fetal rhesus monkeys accumulate ^{3}H-testosterone or its metabolites. *Life. Sci.* **38**, 1673–7.

Michael, R. P. and Zumpe, D. (1977). Effects of androgen administration on sexual invitations by female rhesus monkeys. (*Macaca mulatta*). *Animal Behav.* **25**, 936–44.

Michael, R. P. and Zumpe, D. (1978). Potency of male rhesus monkeys: effects of continuously receptive females. *Science*, **200**, 451–3.

Michael, R. P. and Zumpe, D. (1982). Influence of olfactory signals on the reproductive behaviour of social groups of rhesus monkeys (*Macaca mulatta*). *J. Endocrinol.* **95**, 189–205.

Michael, R. P. and Zumpe, D. (1988). Determinants of behavioral rhythmicity during artificial menstrual cycles in rhesus monkeys (*Macaca mulatta*). *Am. J. Primatol.* **15**, 157–70.

Michael, R. P., Herbert, J., and Welegalla, J. (1967). Ovarian hormones and the sexual behaviour of the male rhesus monkey (*Macaca mulatta*) under laboratory conditions. *J. Endocrinol.* **39**, 81–98.

Michael, R. P., Saayman, G., and Zumpe, D. (1968). The suppression of mounting behaviour and ejaculation in male rhesus monkeys (*Macaca mulatta*) by administering progesterone to their female partners. *J. Endocrinol.* **41**, 421–31.

Michael, R. P., Zumpe, D., Keverne, E. B., and Bonsall, R. W. (1972). Neuroendocrine factors in the control of primate behavior. *Rec. Prog. Horm. Res.* **28**, 665–706.

Michael, R. P., Wilson, M., and Plant, T. M. (1973). Sexual behaviour of male primates and the role of testosterone. In *Comparative ecology and behaviour of male primates*, (ed. R. P. Michael and J. H. Crook), pp. 235–313. Academic Press, New York.

Michael, R. P., Bonsall, R. W., and Warner, P. (1974). Human vaginal secretions: volatile fatty acid content. *Science*, **186**, 1217–19.

Michael, R. P., Bonsall, R. W., and Zumpe, D. (1976). Evidence for chemical communication in primates. *Vit. Horm.* **34**, 137–86.

Michael, R. P., Zumpe, D., and Bonsall, R. W. (1982). The behavior of rhesus monkeys during artificial menstrual cycles. *J. Comp. Physiol. Psychol.* **96**, 875–85.

Michael, R. P., Zumpe, D., and Bonsall, R. W. (1986). Comparison of the effects of testosterone and dihydrotestosterone on the behavior of male cynomolgus monkeys (*Macaca fascicularis*). *Physiol. Behav.* **36**, 349–55.

Michael, R. P., Bonsall, R. W. and Rees, H. D. (1989). The uptake of ^{3}H-testosterone and its metabolites by the brain and pituitary gland of the fetal macaque. *Endocrinology*, **124**, 1319–26.

Michael, R. P., Zumpe, D., and Bonsall, R. W. (1992). The interaction of testosterone with the brain of the orchidectomized primate fetus. *Brain Res.* **570**, 68–74.

Missakian, E. A. (1973). Genealogical mating activity in free-ranging groups of rhesus monkeys on Cayo Santiago. *Behaviour*, **45**, 225–41.

Mittwoch, U. (1992). Sex determination and sex reversal: genotype, phenotype, dogma and semantics. *Hum. Genet.* **89**, 467–79.

Money, J. (1987). Human sexology and psychoneuroendocrinology. In *Psychobiology of reproductive behavior. An evolutionary perspective*, (ed. D. Crews), pp. 324–44. Prentice Hall, Englewood Cliffs, NJ.

Money, J. and Ehrhardt, A. A. (1972). *Man and woman, boy and girl*. The Johns Hopkins University Press, Baltimore, MD.

Money, J., Hampson, J. G., and Hampson, J. L. (1955). An examination of some basic sexual concepts: the evidence of human hermaphroditism. *Bull. Johns Hopkins Hosp.* **97**, 301–19.

Monti-Bloch, L. and Grosser, B. I. (1991). Effect of putative pheromones on the electrical activity of the human vomeronasal organ and olfactory epithelium. *J. Ster. Biochem. Molec. Biol.* **39(4B)**, 573–82.

Moore, K. L. and Barr, M. L. (1955). Smears from the oral mucosa in the determination of chromosomal sex. *Lancet*, **ii**, 57–8.

Morgan, T. H., Bridges, C. B., and Sturtevant, A. H. (1925). Genetics of Drosophila. *Biblio. Genetica*, **2**, 1–262.

Murdock, G. P. (1967). *Ethnographic atlas*. University of Pittsburgh Press.

Naftolin, F., Perez, J., Leranth, C. S., Redmond, D. E., and Garcia-Segura, L. M. (1990). African green monkeys have sexually dimorphic and estrogen-sensitive hypothalamic neuronal membranes. *Brain Res. Bull.* **25**, 575–9.

Orth, J. M., Weisz, J., Ward, O. B., and Ward, I. L. (1983). Environmental stress alters the developmental pattern of Δ^5-3β-hydroxysteroid dehydrogenase activity in Leydig cells of fetal rats: a quantitative cytochemical study. *Biol. Reproduct.* **28**, 625–31.

Painter, T. S. (1921). The Y chromosome in mammals. *Science*, **53**, 503–4.

Parker, S. (1976). The precultural basis of the incest taboo: toward a biosocial theory. *Am. Anthropol.* **78**, 285–305.

Pfaff, D. W. (1968). Autoradiographic localization of radioactivity in the rat brain after injection of tritiated sex hormones. *Science*, **161**, 1355–6.

Pfeiffer, C. A. (1936). Sexual differences of the hypophyses and their determination by the gonads. *Am. J. Anat.* **58**, 195–225.

Phoenix, C. H. and Chambers, K. C. (1982). Sexual behavior in adult gonadectomized female pseudohermaphrodite, female, and male rhesus monkeys (*Macaca mulatta*) treated with estradiol benzoate and testosterone propionate. *J. Comp. Physiol. Psychol.* **96**, 823–33.

Phoenix, C. H., Goy, R. W., Gerall, A. A., and Young, W. C. (1959). Organizing action of prenatally administered testosterone propionate on the tissues mediating mating behavior in the female guinea pig. *Endocrinology*, **65**, 369–82.

Phoenix, C. H., Jensen, J. N., and Chambers, K. C. (1983). Female sexual behavior displayed by androgenized female rhesus macaques. *Horm. Behav.* **17**, 146–51.

Pillard, R. C. and Weinrich, J. D. (1986). Evidence of familial nature of male homosexuality. *Arch. Gen. Psychiat.* **43**, 808–12.

Pomerantz, S. M., Roy, M. M., and Goy, R. W. (1988). Social and hormonal influences on behavior of adult male, female, and pseudohermaphroditic rhesus monkeys. *Horm. Behav.* **22**, 219–30.

Raisman, G. and Field, P. M. (1971). Sexual dimorphism in the preoptic area of the rat. *Science*, **173**, 731–3.

Reinisch, J. M., Ziemba-Davis, M., and Sanders, S. A. (1991). Hormonal contributions to sexually dimorphic behavioral development in humans. *Psychoneuroendocrinology*, **16**, 213–78.

Sade, D. S. (1972). A longitudinal study of social behavior of rhesus monkeys. In *The functional and evolutionary biology of primates*, (ed. R. Tuttle), pp. 378–98. Aldine-Atherton, Chicago.

Schutz, F. (1965*a*). Sexuelle Prägung bei Anatiden. *Zeitschr. Tierpsychol.* **22**, 50–103.

Schutz, F. (1965*b*). Homosexualität bei Enten. *Psychol. Forsch.* **28**, 439–63.

Scott, J. P. (1962). Critical periods in behavioral development. *Science.* **138**, 949–58.

Segal, S. J. and Johnson, D. (1959). Inductive influence of steroid hormones on the neural system. Ovulation controlling mechanisms. *Arch. Anat. Microscop. Morphol. Exp.* **48**, 261–74.

Shepher, J. (1971). Mate selection among second generation kibbutz adolescents and adults: incest avoidance and negative imprinting. *Arch. Sex. Behav.* **1**, 293–307.

Simon, N. G. and Cologer-Clifford, A. (1991). *In utero* contiguity to males does not influence morphology, behavioral sensitivity to testosterone, or hypothalamic androgen binding in CF-1 female mice. *Horm. Behav.* **25**, 518–30.

Sinclair, A. H., *et al.* (1990). A gene from the human sex-determining region encodes a protein with homology to a conserved DNA-binding motif. *Nature (London)*, **346**, 240–4.

Singer, A. G. (1991). A chemistry of mammalian pheromones. *J. Ster. Biochem. Molec. Biol.* **39(4B)**, 627–32.

Singer, A. G., Agosta, W. C., O'Connell, R. J. Pfaffmann, C., Bowden, D. V., and Field, F. H. (1976). Dimethyl disulphide: an attractant pheromone in hamster vaginal secretion. *Science*, **191**, 948–50.

Singer, A. G., Macrides, F., Clancy, A. N., and Agosta, W. C. (1986). Purification and analysis of a proteinaceous aphrodisiac pheromone from hamster vaginal discharge. *J. Biol. Chem.* **261**, 13323–6.

Stainislaw, H. and Rice, F. J. (1988). Correlation between sexual desire and menstrual cycle characteristics. *Arch. Sex. Behav.* **17**, 499–508.

Swaab, D. F. and Fliers, E. (1985). A sexually dimorphic nucleus in the human brain. *Science*, **228**, 1112–1115.

Swaab, D. F. and Hofman, M. A. (1984). Sexual differentiation of the human brain. A historical perspective. In *Progress in brain research*, Vol. 61, (ed. G. J. de Vries, J. P. C. de Bruin, H. B. M. Uylings, and M. A. Corner), pp. 361–74. Elsevier, Amsterdam.

Swaab, D. F. and Hofman, M. A. (1990). An enlarged suprachiasmatic nucleus in homosexual men. *Brain Res.* **537**, 141–8.

ten Cate, C. (1989). Behavioral development: toward understanding processes. In *Perspectives in ethology*. Vol. 8: *Whither ethology?* (ed. P. P. G. Bateson and P. H. Klopfer), pp. 243–69. Plenum, New York.

Tiersch, T. R., Mitchell, M. J., and Wachtel, S. S. (1991). Studies on the phylogenetic conservation of the SRY gene. *Hum. Genet.* **87**, 571–3.

Tinbergen, N. (1959). Comparative study of the behaviour of gulls (*Laridae*): a progress report. *Behaviour*, **15**, 1–70.

Tjio, J. H. and Levan, A. (1956). The chromosome number in man. *Hereditas*, **42**, 1–6.

Tobet, S. A., Zahniser, D. J., and Baum, M. J. (1986). Sexual dimorphism in the preoptic/anterior hypothalamic area of ferrets: effects of adult exposure to sex steroids. *Brain Res.* **364**, 249–57.

Wada, M. and Gorbman, A. (1977). Relation of mode of administration of testosterone to evocation of male sex behavior in frogs. *Horm. Behav.* **8**, 310–19.

Walsh, P. C., Madden, J. D., Harrod, M. J., Goldstein, J. L., MacDonald, P. C., and Wilson, J. D. (1974). Familial incomplete male pseudohermaphroditism, type 2: decreased dihydrotestosterone formation in pseudovaginal perineoscrotal hypospadias. *N. Engl. J. Med.* **291**, 944–9.

Ward, I. L. (1972). Prenatal stress feminizes and demasculinizes the behavior of males. *Science*, **175**, 82–4.

Ward, I. L. (1977). Exogenous androgen activates female sexual behavior in noncopulating prenatally stressed males. *J. Comp. Physiol. Psychol.* **91**, 465–71.

Ward, I. L. and Weisz, J. (1980). Maternal stress alters plasma testosterone in fetal males. *Science*, **207**, 328–9.

Ward, O. B. (1992). Fetal drug exposure and sexual differentiation of males. In *Handbook of behavioral neurobiology,* Vol. 11: *Sexual differentiation*, (ed. A. A. Gerall, H. Moltz, and I. L. Ward), pp. 181–219. Plenum, New York.

Warner, R. R. (1984). Mating behavior and hermaphroditism in coral reef fishes. *Am. Sci.* **72**, 128–36.

Wells, L. J. and van Wagenen, G. (1954). Androgen-induced female pseudohermaphroditism in the monkey (*Macaca mulatta*); anatomy of the reproductive organs. *Contrib. Embryol., Carnegie Inst. Wash.* **35**, 93–106.

Westermarck, E. (1891). *The history of human marriage.* Macmillan, New York.

Whalen, R. E., Yahr, P. and Luttge, W. G. (1985). The role of metabolism in hormonal control of sexual behavior. In *Handbook of behavioral neurobiology*, Vol.7, (ed. N. Adler, D. Pfaff, and R. W. Goy), pp. 609–63. Plenum, New York.

Wilkins, L. (1960). Masculinization of the female fetus due to the use of orally given progestins. *J. Am. Med. Assoc.* **172**, 1028–32.

Wilkins, L., Jones, H. W., Holman, G. H., and Stempfel, R. S. (1958). Masculinization of the female fetus associated with administration of oral and intramuscular progestins during gestation: nonadrenal female pseudohermaphrodism. *J. Clin. Endocrinol. Metab.* **18**, 559–85.

Williams, E. and Scott, J. P. (1953). The development of social behavior patterns in the mouse, in relation to natural periods. *Behaviour*, **6**, 35–65.

Willier, B. H. (1933). Potencies of the gonad-forming area in the chick as tested in chorio-allantoic grafts. *Wilhelm Roux' Arch. Entwick. mech. Org.* **130**, 616–49.

Willier, B. H., Gallagher, T. F., and Koch, F. C. (1935). Sex-modification in the chick embryo resulting from injections of male and female hormones. *Proc. Nat. Acad. Sci. USA* **21**, 625–31.

Wilson, M. E. and Gordon, T. P. (1979). Sexual activity of male rhesus monkeys introduced into a heterosexual group. *Am. J. Phys. Anthropol.* **50**, 515–24.

Witschi, E. (1963). Embryology of the ovary. In *The ovary*, (ed. h. G. Grady and E. D. Smith), pp. 1–10. Williams & Wilkins, Baltimore.

Wolf, A. P. (1970). Childhood association and sexual attraction: a further test of the Westermarck hypothesis. *Am. Anthropol.* **72**, 503–15.

Wolff, E. (1953). La croissance et différenciation des organes embryonnaires des vertébrés amniotes en cultur *in vitro. J. Suisse Med.* **83**, 171–5.

Wolff, E. and Haffen, K. (1952). Sur le dévelopment et la différenciation sexuelle des gonades embryonnaires d' oiseau en culture *in vitro. J. Exp. Zool.* **119**, 381–404.

Yahr, P. and Commins, D. (1982). The neuroendocrinology of scent marking. In *Chemical signals in vertebrates*, Vol. 2, (ed. R. M. Silverstein and D. Müller-Schwarze), pp. 119–33. Plenum, New York.

Young, W. C. (1961). The hormones and mating behavior. In *Sex and internal secretions*, (ed. W. C. Young), pp. 1173–239. Williams & Wilkins, Baltimore.

Young, W. C., Goy, R. W., and Phoenix, C. H. (1964). Hormones and behavior. *Science*, **143**, 212–18.

Zippelius, H. (1972). Die Karawanenbildung bei Feld- und Hausspitzmaus. *Zeitschr. Tierpsychol.* **30**, 305–20.

Zumpe, D. (1963). Über das Ablaichen von *Thalassoma bifasciatum*. *Aqua. Terra. Zeitschr.* **16**, 86–8.

Zumpe, D. and Michael, R. P. (1983). A comparison of the behavior of *Macaca fascicularis* and *Macaca mulatta* in relation to the menstrual cycle. *Am. J. Primatol.* **4**, 55–72.

Zumpe, D. and Michael, R. P. (1984). Low potency of intact male rhesus monkeys after long-term visual contact with their female partners. *Am. J. Primatol.* **6**, 241–52.

Zumpe, D., Bonsall, R. W., and Michael, R. P. (1993). Effects of the nonsteroidal aromatase inhibitor, Fadrozole, on the sexual behavior of male cynomolgus monkeys (*Macaca fascicularis*). *Horm. Behav.* **27**, 200–15.

Index